Exercise and Sport Sciences Reviews

Volume 21, 1993

EXERCISE AND SPORT SCIENCES REVIEWS

Volume 21, 1993

Editor

JOHN O. HOLLOSZY, M.D.

Professor of Medicine
Department of Internal Medicine
Washington University School of Medicine
St. Louis, Missouri

American College of Sports Medicine Series

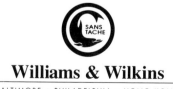

Williams & Wilkins
BALTIMORE • PHILADELPHIA • HONG KONG
LONDON • MUNICH • SYDNEY • TOKYO
A WAVERLY COMPANY

Editor: Deanna F. Gemmill
Associate Editor: Carole E. Pippin
Copy Editor: Shelley Potler
Designer: Norman W. Och
Illustration Planner: Lorraine Wrzosek
Production Coordinator: Charles E. Zeller

Copyright © 1993
American College of Sports Medicine

Printed in the United States of America

Library of Congress Catalog Card Number (ISBN 0-683-00035-7)

93 94 95 96 97
1 2 3 4 5 6 7 8 9 10

Preface

Exercise and Sport Sciences Reviews, an annual publication sponsored by the American College of Sports Medicine, reviews current research concerning behavioral, biochemical, biomechanical, clinical, physiological, and rehabilitational topics involving exercise science. The Editorial Board for this series currently consists of 15 recognized authorities who have assumed responsibility for one of the following general topics: athletic medicine, biochemistry, biomechanics, environmental physiology, epidemiology, exercise physiology, gerontology, growth and development, metabolism, molecular biology, motor control, physical fitness, psychology, rehabilitation, and sociology. The organization of the Editorial Board should help foster the commitment of the American College of Sports Medicine to publish timely reviews in areas of broad interest to clinicians, educators, exercise scientists, and students. The goal for this Editorial Board is to provide reviews in each of these 15 areas whenever sufficient new information becomes available on topics that are likely to be of interest to the readership of *Exercise and Sport Sciences Reviews.* Further, the Editor selects additional topics to be developed into chapters based on current interest, timeliness, and importance to the above audience. The contributors for each volume are selected by the Editorial Board members and the Editor.

John O. Holloszy, M.D.
Editor

Contributors

Jay Coakley, Ph.D.
Center for the Study of Sport and Leisure
University of Colorado at Colorado Springs
Colorado Springs, Colorado

Steven T. Devor, M.S.
Department of Physical Education
University of California at Berkeley
Berkeley, California

Trevor Drew , Ph.D.
Faculty of Medicine
Centre Recherche Science Neurologiques
University of Montreal
Montreal, Canada

William J. Evans, Ph.D.
Human Physiology Laboratory, USDA
Human Nutrition Research Center on Aging
Tufts University
Boston, Massachusetts

Cyril B. Frank, M.D.
Department of Surgery
University of Calgary
Calgary, Alberta, Canada

Susan George
Metabolism Unit
Shriner's Burns Institute
University of Texas Medical Branch
Galveston, Texas

G. Geelen, Ph.D.
Laboratoire de Physiologie
Universite Claude Bernard
Lyon, France

John E. Greenleaf, Ph.D.
National Aeronautics and Space Administration
Moffett Field, California

Tessa Gordon, Ph.D.
Department of Pharmacology
Division of Neuroscience
University of Alberta
Edmonton, Alberta, Canada

Robert Hickson, Ph.D.
Department of Physical Education
University of Illinois
Chicago, Illinois

Michael J. Joyner, M.D.
Department of Anesthesia Research
Mayo Clinic
Rochester, Minnesota

John F. Kalaska, Ph.D.
Faculty of Medicine
Centre Recherche Science Neurologiques
University of Montreal
Montreal, Canada

Margaret A. Kolka, Ph.D.
Thermal Physiology and Medicine Division
Department of the Army
U.S. Army Research Institute of Environmental Medicine
Natick, Massachusetts

Barbara J. Loitz, Ph.D.
Department of Surgery
University of Calgary
Calgary, Alberta, Canada

Jane R. Marone, M.D.
Department of Physical Education
University of Illinois
Chicago, Illinois

Timothy David Noakes, M.B., Ch.B., M.D., F.A.C.S.M.
Bioenergetics of Exercise Research Unit
Department of Physiology
University of Cape Town Medical School
Cape Town, South Africa

Mary C. Pattullo, Ph.D.
Department of Pharmacology
Division of Neuroscience
University of Alberta
Edmonton, Alberta, Canada

Marc A. Rogers, Ph.D.
Exercise Physiology Laboratory
Department of Kinesiology
University of Maryland
College Park, Maryland

Marcia L. Stefanick, Ph.D.
Stanford Center for Research in Disease Prevention
Palo Alto, California

Lou A. Stephenson, Ph.D.
Thermal Physiology and Medicine Division
Environmental Physiology and Medicine Directorate
Department of the Army
U.S. Army Research Institute of Environmental Medicine
Natick, Massachusetts

Timothy P. White, Ph.D.
Department of Physical Education
University of California at Berkeley
Berkeley, California

Robert R. Wolfe, Ph.D.
Department of Surgery
University of Texas Medical Branch
Shriners Burn Institute
Galveston, Texas

Contents

1
Stable Isotopic Tracers as Metabolic Probes in Exercise

ROBERT R. WOLFE, Ph.D.
SUSAN GEORGE

INTRODUCTION

Atoms are generally composed of a dense core of positively charged protons and uncharged neutrons. In lighter elements, there are approximately equal numbers of neutrons and protons. Certain elements are composed of atoms that are chemically identical but differ slightly in weight, due to different numbers of nuclear neutrons. Elemental atoms with differing number of neutrons, and thus weight, are called isotopes. The number of neutrons in the atom does not affect the chemical properties of the atom, which are determined by the electronic configuration. Thus, a commonly used radioactive isotope of carbon (^{14}C) is the same mass as the most abundant isotope of nitrogen (^{14}N), yet those two atoms are as chemically distinct as carbon and nitrogen. Isotopes are either radioactive or stable. A radioactive nuclide spontaneously disintegrates to form an atom of another element, with the occurrence of the emission of radiation. The radioactive tracers most commonly used in metabolic studies are ^{14}C and ^{3}H (tritium). Stable isotopes do not spontaneously disintegrate, but in some cases may be present in sufficiently low natural abundance to be useful in tracer studies. The stable isotopes, which, with their naturally occurring abundances, are most commonly used in metabolic studies are: ^{2}H (deuterium), 0.015%; ^{13}C, 1.11%; ^{15}N, 0.37%; and ^{18}O, 0.204%.

The most obvious advantage of stable isotopes is that they are naturally occurring, nonradioactive, and present little or no risk to human subjects. Furthermore, since there are no radioactive isotopes of nitrogen or oxygen that could be used as tracers, the use of stable isotope technology is the only way in which these elements can be studied. On the other hand, there are some difficulties in using stable isotopes, mostly stemming from the need to use mass spectrometry to quantify their abundance. Because precision of analysis is lacking, it is often necessary to use rather large doses of tracer, thereby raising into question the assumption that the metabolism of the endogenous substrate is not affected by the tracer. Furthermore, the natural occurrence of stable isotopes requires that account must be taken of the "natural enrichment." On the other hand, the nature of analysis by gas-chromatography mass spectrometry enables several tracers with the same label to be infused simultaneously, and to be distinguished analytically. These issues are discussed in detail in another source [59].

STABLE ISOTOPES IN EXERCISE

Despite the use of stable isotopes as tracers for metabolic studies as early as the 1930s [46], only a minimal number of investigators have capitalized on these useful tools to investigate the human metabolic response to exercise. Such studies fall into the general categories of total energy expenditure; glucose kinetics and oxidation (and, related to this topic, $^{13}CO_2$ kinetics); fatty acid metabolism; and amino acid/protein metabolism. Each of these general topics will be discussed from the methodological perspective, and then the physiological information obtained will be described.

TOTAL ENERGY EXPENDITURE

The metabolic cost of exercise can be estimated by means of the measurement of oxygen consumption ($\dot{V}O_2$) by indirect calorimetry. Whereas this approach has been widely used, several important aspects of energy metabolism and exercise remain unresolved with only the measurement of $\dot{V}O_2$. Indirect calorimetry cannot be performed in the free-living situation. Thus, whereas the measurement of $\dot{V}O_2$ allows the calculation of the metabolic cost of exercise in a laboratory setting, it cannot reveal the total caloric requirement of exercise training or competition. For extension of energy expenditure measurements to actual caloric requirements, the rate of total energy expenditure (TEE) in the free-living state is needed. Attempts have been made to determine TEE by compiling an accurate record of food intake over a period of several days and measuring any changes in body composition that occur over time. Whereas this has been a useful approach to establish general guidelines of energy requirements, it suffers from obvious limitations. Accurate dietary records are difficult to obtain in free-living subjects, and the act of keeping a diary might well affect food intake. Also, over relatively short periods of time, potentially important changes in body composition cannot be accurately measured.

The so-called doubly-labeled water (DLW) method for measuring TEE in the free-living situation was first described over 20 years ago [31], but it did not become widely used in humans until the early 1980s [43]. The fundamental observation underlying the DLW technique is that oxygen atoms in exhaled CO_2 and in body water are in isotopic equilibrium [30], because of the action of the enzyme carbonic anhydrase. Thus, a dose of $H_2{}^{18}O$ will be eliminated from the body as both CO_2 and H_2O, whereas water labeled in the hydrogen position will be eliminated solely as a function of water turnover. Thus, the difference between the elimination rates is a measure of CO_2 flux. This concept can be represented graphically as the difference in the rates of decline in isotopic enrichment following a simultaneous bolus of ^2H_2O.

The basic principle underlying the calculation of the $\dot{V}CO_2$ from data such as those illustrated in Figure 1.1 is that the tracers are distributed in a single pool (total body water, TBW), and in this case, the loss from the pool is equal to the rate constant k times the pool size. Thus, the rate of loss of water (rH_2O) is the fractional turnover rate of ^2H_2O (k_h) times the TBW. The abbreviation N is conventionally used for TBW. Thus,

$$rH_2O = k_h \cdot N$$

The rate of loss of water $+ CO_2$ ($\dot{V}CO_2$) is the product of the fractional turnover rate of oxygen of body water (k_o) $\cdot$ N:

$$rH_2O + 2\dot{V}CO_2 = k_o \cdot N$$

The factor 2 is required since each mole of CO_2 contains oxygen equal to 2 mol of water. The difference between the two products (divided by 2) is thus equal to $\dot{V}CO_2$:

FIGURE 1.1
The basic principle of the doubly-labeled water (DLW) technique is that the enrichment in ^2H_2O declines as a function of water turnover, whereas $H_2{}^{18}O$ enrichment declines as a function of both water and CO_2 turnover.

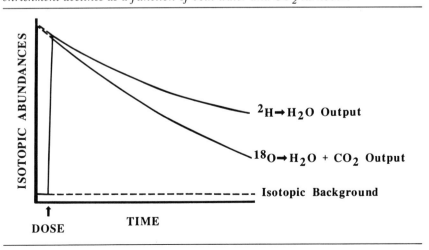

$$\dot{V}CO_2 = \frac{k_o \cdot N \cdot (k_h \cdot N)}{2}$$

$$\dot{V}CO_2 = \frac{N}{2}(k_o \cdot k_h)$$

The $\dot{V}CO_2$ enables calculation of TEE. For this purpose, an average respiratory quotient (RQ) must be assumed. Then, the equation of DeWeir [15] can be used:

$$\text{TEE (k/cal/day)} = 3.941\ \dot{V}CO_2/RQ + 1.106\ \dot{V}CO_2 - 2.17\ \text{UN}$$

where $\dot{V}CO_2$ is expressed in liters/day, and UN is urinary nitrogen excretion (in g/day). An assumed value for UN will not significantly affect the calculated TEE.

Whereas the general principles of the method, as outlined previously, are simple, there are a number of necessary assumptions and potential pitfalls of which one must be aware.

1. It is necessary that the subject background enrichment of water remain constant throughout, because cost and availability of $H_2^{18}O$ restricts the amount of tracer given, and thus, the enrichment above baseline is small. Changes in the source of drinking water during the course of the experiment should, therefore, be prevented.
2. As presented previously, it is assumed that there is a single compartment in which the isotopes are distributed and from which the isotopes are lost. However, it is well known that the isotope distribution volume of ^2H_2O is about 4% greater than TBW, and the $H_2^{18}O$ distribution volume is 1% greater than TBW. Whereas these general observations are agreed upon, the optimal manner in which to account for volume distributions is controversial. Briefly, a fixed relationship between ^2H_2O and $H_2^{18}O$ dilution spaces can be assumed, or accounted for by direct measurement in each individual experiment. Whereas the latter approach may seem intuitively more rational, measurement errors can make implementation of this approach impractical.
3. Account must be taken of fractionation in the process of evaporation. Thus, water containing heavier isotopes of H or O will evaporate more slowly than their unenriched counterparts. Here again, there are different approaches proposed to account for fractionation, and whereas under normal circumstances they all yield similar values [59], in exercising subjects who are sweating a great deal, this could be more of a problem.
4. The calculations assume a constant TBW (N). Whereas account can

be taken for changes in N [14], errors in the final calculated TEE will be greater if there are changes in body water.

Beyond problems related to uncertain assumptions, additional sources of errors must be recognized. Most importantly, if the water turnover rate is high, relative to $\dot{V}CO_2$, it will be difficult to calculate the difference between the k_o and k_h accurately (Fig. 1.2). In the case of exercising subjects, this is not likely to be a problem, because of the high $\dot{V}CO_2$. Other sources of error, including miscalculation of the tracer dosage, incorrect estimation of the extent of fractionation, and errors in the

FIGURE 1.2
The differences between k_h and k_o are small when the water turnover is high, relative to the rate of CO_2 production, as illustrated in the **bottom panel.** *This makes the calculation of TEE imprecise.*

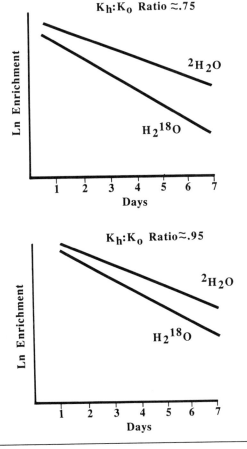

measurement must all be carefully considered [48]. Despite all of these potential problems, the measurement of TEE by the DLW method has been validated by comparison to measurement of TEE by indirect calorimetry performed in subjects who lived several days in a chamber [45]. Given that regular exercise will generally make the difference between k_o and k_h greater and, therefore, improve the precision of the method, it seems likely that this method should be useful for assuming many aspects of the effects of exercise on TEE.

The apparent potential of the DLW method to investigate the effect of exercise on energy expenditure is substantiated by the few studies that have addressed this topic. Thus, it was found that, during heavy exercise, the DLW method could be performed accurately over extremely short periods. Stein et al. [51] compared the calculation of TEE by indirect calorimetry with the DLW method over 8 hr of continuous exercise at 55% $\dot{V}o_2$. TEE was found to be 735 ± 118 kcal/hr by the DLW method, which compared favorably with the value of 735 ± 82 kcal/hr determined by indirect calorimetry. They also showed that careful sample collection enabled distinction of daytime and nighttime energy expenditure with the DLW method. Favorable comparison of the results from the DLW method and indirect calorimetry in exercising subjects by Westerterp et al. [54] adds further support for the application of the DLW method in free-living exercising subjects. Finally, the DLW method produced results comparable to those obtained by careful dietary intake/balance recording in exercising soldiers [23]. Thus, both theoretically and empirically, the DLW method appears to be well suited to the determination of TEE in exercising subjects over periods of time ranging from 1–14 days.

Despite the numerous questions that might be addressed regarding the effect of exercise on TEE using the DLW technique, little actual experimentation has been performed. Westerterp et al. [54] used the DLW method to determine energy expenditure in cyclists racing in the Tour de France. The TEE during this gruelling effort was found to be, on average, four to five times the basal value, which was considered to be the energetic ceiling of performance in humans. This is about the same energetic ceiling, relative to basal, as in birds, with their energy-consuming flight behavior [16].

In a more recent study [47], the DLW technique was used to help determine if female endurance athletes (runners) have unusually low energy requirements, as suggested by many food intake studies [5]. Energy expenditure and body weight changes (and thus, intake estimated from the DLW technique) were significantly in excess of those calculated from food records. They found that, contrary to popular belief, these female runners had no metabolic adaptations that lowered energy requirements, and that the metabolic cost of physical activity (1087 ± 244 kcal/day) was even greater than that calculated on the basis of the net caloric expenditure required to run their training distance (an average of 10 miles/day.

The DLW technique has two important advantages: it can be used in free-living subjects; and it enables calculation of TEE over several days, thereby allowing an accurate estimate of caloric requirements. On the other hand, $H_2^{18}O$ is both expensive and in short supply. Furthermore, energy expenditure during exercise cannot be quantified, because the time interval is too short to distinguish adequately between k_o and k_h. However, it is possible that use of $NaH^{13}CO_3$ as a tracer of bicarbonate kinetics may be of use in this regard. Administration of $NaH^{13}CO_3$, either as an infusion [28] or as a bolus [3] enables the calculation of $\dot{V}CO_2$ by classical isotope-dilution methodology with only the measurement of the enrichment of expired CO_2. This method has the advantage that the tracer is cheap and readily available, and the collection of breath for the measurement of CO_2 enrichment is simple [59]. The disadvantage of the methodology is that all labeled CO_2 is not immediately recovered in the breath. The reason(s) for this includes incorporation of labeled carbon into metabolic products such as glucose and urea, and also, delayed equilibration with slowly turning over pools. Thus, if $NaH^{13}CO_2$ is infused for 24 hr, the recovery of labeled $^{13}CO_2$ in the breath is almost 100% [56]. In this case, the rate of production of CO_2 can be accurately calculated. However, after only a few hours of infusion, or in the 2 hr after a bolus injection, recovery of label is only about 75–80% (e.g., [3]). Correction for this incomplete recovery will improve the accuracy of the calculated value of $\dot{V}CO_2$ (e.g., [28]. However, this is a moot point, since $\dot{V}CO_2$ is needed to calculate recovery. It so happens, however, that this problem is minimized in exercise. The kinetics of the bicarbonate pool are more rapid in exercise, and therefore, recovery of tracer in breath is greater [3, 66]. Consequently, during exercise, the labeled bicarbonate technique can be used simply and cheaply to determine $\dot{V}CO_2$ approximately [11]. The calculated value may underestimate the true values however, by as much as 15%, because of uncertainties regarding tracer recovery. This level of precision nonetheless may be sufficient for field studies, where indirect calorimetry equipment is not available. Collection of breath samples is made particularly easy by the fact that the volume of expired air per unit time need not be determined.

SPECIFIC SUBSTRATE OXIDATION

Knowledge of the rates of oxidation of specific substrates is important in understanding the mechanisms of metabolic regulation that enable sustained utilization of energy at high rates during exercise. To this end, studies have used ^{13}C-labeled compounds to quantify substrate oxidation for almost 20 years (e.g., [36, 37], particularly involving the measurement of the oxidation of exogenously administered glucose. These studies are hindered, in general, by many theoretical limitations, which will be discussed later.

The general principle underlying the use of a ^{13}C-labeled compound to quantify oxidation is that the rate of excretion of $^{13}CO_2$ is divided by the isotopic enrichment of the precursor. Implicit in this approach are several assumptions: (*a*) there must be no influence of the bicarbonate kinetics on the observed CO_2 enrichment (i.e., whatever $^{13}CO_2$ is produced at the cellular level is immediately and quantitatively reflected in the breath); (*b*) that the true precursor enrichment is identified; (*c*) that isotopic exchange does not occur in the pathways of oxidation; and (*d*) the background enrichment of (naturally occurring) $^{13}CO_2$ remains constant over the experimental collection period. Finally, in most applications, it is necessary that $\dot{V}CO_2$ is measured accurately to compute total $^{13}CO_2$ excretion, which is the product of $^{13}CO_2$ enrichment and $\dot{V}CO_2$.

Any $^{13}CO_2$ produced at the cellular level must transit through the bicarbonate pool before exiting in the breath. Two aspects of bicarbonate kinetics complicate the quantification of substrate oxidation rates. First, the bicarbonate kinetics are complex, requiring a compartmental model of at least three pools to describe the disappearance of a labeled bolus of $NaH^{13}CO_3$ adequately [3, 24]. Thus, whereas it is feasible to account for the delay in transit of $^{13}CO_2$ through the bicarbonate pool in a nonsteady state during exercise, the necessary modeling is complex (e.g., the 10-pool model described by Cobelli et al. to quantify the kinetics and oxidation of ^{13}C-leucine [10]). Even if a physiological steady state can be produced during exercise, an isotopic steady state may not apply if the tracer has been given orally, along with exogenous substrate (e.g., [20]). Efforts to account for the problem in exercise have been limited to a two-pool model [34], which is probably not of sufficient complexity to allow accurate quantification.

Recognizing the limitation in quantifying the oxidation of a ^{13}C-labeled substrate given orally does not eliminate the use of such compounds to make qualitative or comparative observations. For example, oral administration of ^{13}C-labeled glucose [36, 37] showed that it was readily available as an energy substrate during exercise in normal subjects, and also in well-insulinized diabetic subjects [29]. Furthermore, comparable labeling of oral fructose and glucose indicated that each were equally well metabolized during exercise [50]. ^{13}C-labeled sucrose given orally can also be used as an energy substrate during exercise, and its use is significantly inhibited by Acarbose, a potent α-glucosidase inhibitor used to slow sugar absorption in diabetics [20].

These sorts of qualitative observations are useful, but a good understanding of metabolic regulation requires accurate quantitative values of substrate oxidation rates. For several reasons, including the problem with the bicarbonate kinetics cited earlier, these oral ^{13}C-sugar studies have likely provided approximations of the true rates of substrate oxidation. Many problems not accounted for in these studies must be considered for the determination of accurate quantitative data.

Identification of the enrichment of the true precursor for the production of $^{13}CO_2$ is a problem because one generally does not have access to the intracellular pool from which oxidation occurs. With certain amino acids, such as leucine, the problem can be overcome to a considerable extent by using a metabolite (e.g., α-ketoisocaproate, KIC) derived entirely from the intracellular pool of the precursor, which presumably is the same pool from which the substrate is oxidized. This approach is necessary to account for the fact that there may be an intracellular pool of the substrate not in equilibration with the plasma pool, and also that not all tracer entering an organ or tissue will be taken up by the tissues. Thus, when ^{13}C-pyruvate or ^{13}C-lactate is given and the arteriovenous balance across the leg is determined, only about 50% of the tracer is taken up by muscle tissue [9]. The rest is functionally shunted from the artery to the vein. These two sources of dilution of the intracellular enrichment of the tracer may be quite large. In the case of ^{13}C-pyruvate, the enrichment in the intracellular compartment (muscle—obtained by biopsy) is only 20% of that in arterial blood [57]. During exercise, the intracellular ^{13}C-glucose enrichment will be diluted by muscle glycogen breakdown, before oxidation, yielding spuriously low rates of glucose oxidation. Thus, at a given rate of total glucose oxidation (plasma plus muscle glycogen), more $^{13}CO_2$ will be produced the higher the proportion of (labeled) plasma glucose that is oxidized, as opposed to the (unlabeled) muscle glycogen that does not enter the plasma pool. The same complication is true for the measurement of fatty acid oxidation using ^{13}C-labeled fatty acids [22]. On the other hand, if total carbohydrate and total fat oxidation can be quantified by indirect calorimetry (see below), the additional use of a ^{13}C-labeled plasma substrate may allow the distinction of intracellular (i.e., muscle) vs. plasma glucose and fat oxidation (see later in this chapter).

Another problem that can arise when using stable isotope tracer methodology is that the background $^{13}CO_2$ enrichment can change during exercise. Approximately 1.1% of all naturally occurring carbon is ^{13}C. Furthermore, the natural enrichment of carbon from various sources, such as different plants, atmospheric CO_2, and so forth, differs significantly in relation to the magnitude of change in enrichment by an isotope infused in a tracer dose. This problem is normally accounted for by taking background samples prior to the start of isotope infusion and then subtracting the enrichment of the background sample from all of the samples obtained after the isotope infusion. Whereas this approach is satisfactory for experiments in which no aspects of the metabolic state changes from the time at which the background sample is drawn until the enriched samples are collected, serious errors may arise if a treatment intervenes between the collection of the background and enriched samples. This is because the treatment may affect the background enrichment, independent of the tracer administration. The naturally occurring enrichments of various carbohydrates and fats are different [25], and if there is a shift in the relative rates of metabolism of these substances in the body, a corresponding change in the background enrichment would be expected. Such a shift will confound the interpretation of the $^{13}CO_2$ data obtained during an isotope infusion.

One must be concerned about the possibility that exercise may cause a shift in the background enrichment of CO_2. This has been demonstrated to occur during exercise in the fasting state, due to an increase in the proportion of carbohydrate oxidation [65]. The problem may be amplified when exogenous carbohydrate is given during exercise [35], since the natural ^{13}C abundance in the carbohydrate is likely to be high [44]. Some studies have failed to account for possible changes in background enrichment properly (e.g., see [35] for discussion), and the quantitative aspects of such studies could be in question [35]. Thus, two factors must be considered in the correction of expired $^{13}CO_2$ data: possible changes in background enrichment over the course of the experiment and the percentage of recovery in breath of $^{13}CO_2$ produced at the cellular level. To determine if changes in background enrichment occur as a consequence of the experimental perturbation, studies in which nonenriched tracers are infused must be performed. The need for this correction is particularly important when the enrichment of CO_2 resulting from the infusion of isotope is in the same range as the change in background enrichment resulting from the experimental perturbation. This was the problem in the exercise study cited earlier in that natural abundance of ^{13}C in ingested carbohydrate was being used as a "tracer." Changes in background enrichment resulting from the oxidation of a substrate infused in greater than tracer quantities can be accounted for in the calculations of the oxidation rate if the isotopic tracer is chemically identical to the infused substrate (see [49]).

The major limitation in using either ^{13}C-labeled glucose or ^{13}C-labeled fatty acids to quantify substrate oxidation is the likelihood that isotopic exchange will result in the spurious underestimation of the true oxidation rates. This is particularly true when the label enters the tricarboxylic acid (TCA) cycle, for reasons shown in Figure 1.3. There are two CO_2 molecules produced for every molecule of acetyl CoA that enters the cycle. Thus, for a tracer to yield a correct value for oxidation of a labeled substrate, it is necessary that a labeled CO_2 molecule be produced for every labeled carbon that enters the cycle via acetyl CoA. However, there are two prominent pathways whereby label that enters the cycle via acetyl CoA can leave the cycle by a route other than CO_2 (Fig. 1.3). The incorporation of label from acetate (via acetyl CoA) into glucose is well established [12]. This occurs in the liver via the

FIGURE 1.3

Schematic diagram of potential pathways whereby label entering the TCA cycle in acetyl CoA might not be excreted as labeled CO_2.

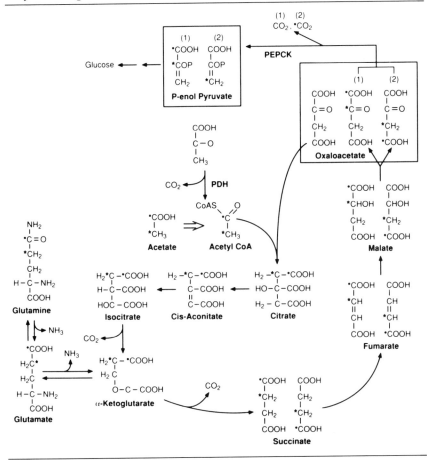

oxaloacetate pool of the TCA cycle, which is the same as the oxaloacetate pool for gluconeogenesis. The other route by which loss of label from the TCA cycle can occur is via exchange between α-ketoglutarate, glutamate, and glutamine. This pathway can occur throughout the body.

Because of the various pathways of possible isotopic exchange, the extent of underestimation of oxidation caused by the loss of label from the TCA cycle by the exchange reactions described earlier depends on the position of the label within the acetyl CoA entering the TCA cycle. When the rate of oxidation of acetate labeled in the 1 position was compared with the rate of oxidation as calculated with the tracer labeled in the 2 position, a 50% difference was observed [61]. Acetate is directly converted to acetyl CoA and then enters the TCA cycle, so the difference in labeled CO_2 production rates is a direct reflection of the isotopic exchange in the TCA cycle. The reason the 2 carbon is subject to greater exchange reactions than the 1-position carbon is that many more spins of the cycle are necessary to lose the 2 carbon completely to CO_2. The 1 carbon is entirely lost to CO_2 in the second spin. On the first spin of the cycle there is an equal chance that the 1 carbon and the 2 carbon will be lost to glutamate/glutamine or to the gluconeogenic pathway. On the second spin of the cycle, however, half of the remaining 1 carbon is lost to CO_2 before the production of α-ketoglutarate (and, thus, possible exchange with glutamate and glutamine), and the other half is lost before the formation of oxaloacetate (and, thus, possible loss of label to the gluconeogenic pathway). Meanwhile, none of the 2 carbon is lost to CO_2 on the second spin. It is only on the third spin of the cycle that label originally in the 2 position begins to be lost to CO_2, and many more spins are needed until the label is completely lost. The result is that the 2 position of acetyl CoA has many more chances to participate in exchange reactions than the 1 position.

The effect of the isotopic exchange reactions in the TCA cycle is evident not only for calculation of acetate oxidation but also more generally for carbohydrate or fat oxidation. Carbohydrate oxidation determined by indirect calorimetry should equal the rate of pyruvate oxidation calculated from the tracer technique, corrected appropriately for the fact that there are 6 carbons in glucose and 3 in pyruvate. However, whereas 1-^{13}C-pyruvate yields values roughly equal to those from indirect calorimetry both in the fasting state and during the infusion of glucose, the 3-^{13}C-pyruvate (which produces 2-^{13}C-acetyl CoA before entry into the TCA cycle for complete oxidation) underestimates the rate of pyruvate oxidation, determined by indirect calorimetry, by 50% in the fasting state and by 70% during glucose infusion.

The magnitude of differences in oxidation rates between tracers with labels in different positions may seem surprisingly large, but in fact, such differences are expected. A large difference in excreted CO_2 can be accounted for by consideration solely of the rate of loss of label via exchange from the oxaloacetic acid pool. The rate of formation of phosphoenolpyruvate from oxaloacetic acid is in the range of 6 μmol/kg^{-1}/min^{-1} in postabsorptive human subjects and might be as high as 15 μmol/kg^{-1}/min^{-1} in fasting subjects. Because the rate of entry of acetyl CoA into the TCA cycle would be $\sim$45 μmol/kg^{-1}/min^{-1}, based on an average value of 90 μmol/kg^{-1}/min^{-1} value for $\dot{V}CO_2$, then anywhere from 13% to 33% of the carbons reaching oxaloacetic acid in each spin of the cycle would be likely to be directed to phosphoenolpyruvate. Keeping in mind that the 2-carbon position of acetyl CoA can reach oxaloacetic acid on each of several spins of the TCA cycle, the basis for a substantial amount of tracer being lost to the gluconeogenic pathway is obvious. Furthermore, from the simple example provided earlier, it would be predicted that the relationship between the rate of the phosphenolpyruvate creatine kinase reaction and the TCA cycle activity in the liver would have an effect on the ratio of labeled carbon dioxide excreted when the 1 carbon, as opposed to the 2 carbon, of acetyl CoA is labeled. Thus, errors in the calculation of the rate of oxidation would not be expected to be consistent in different physiological states, and certain oxidation measurements would not be expected to be useful even in a comparative sense. For all of the reasons cited previously, precise quantitation of substrate oxidation rates using traditional tracer techniques are probably not accurate. The traditional method of calculation of substrate oxidation based on measurement of total $\dot{V}O_2$ and $\dot{V}CO_2$ is possible [19], but the validity of results obtained during exercise has long been questioned because of the possibility of excessive CO_2 excretion to balance pH, thereby leading to an overestimate of the true RQ, and therefore, an overestimate of carbohydrate oxidation. To circumvent the use of $\dot{V}CO_2$ and the multiple problems of traditional isotopic tracer methods, we developed an alternative approach to the determination of substrate oxidation at rest and during exercise [41]. The basic principle is that the naturally occurring enrichment of $^{13}C/^{12}C$ in carbohydrate (R_c), fat (R_f), and protein (R_p) all differ, and that the $^{13}C/^{12}C$ ratio in the breath (R_b) is ultimately the result of the relative contributions of $^{13}C/^{12}C$ ratios derived from combustion of the various substrates [41]:

$$R_b = R_c + Y R_f + z R_p \qquad (1)$$

The sum of the relative contributions of the $^{13}C/^{12}C$ ratios of glucose, fat, and protein to the breath $^{13}C/^{12}C$ ratio equals 1:

$$x + y + z = 1 \qquad (2)$$

The relative contribution of glucose, fat, and protein to CO_2 production can be calculated from the following stoichiometric equation [14]:

$$\dot{V}CO_2 = 0.746\,c + 1.43\,f + 0.744\,n\ 6.25 \qquad (3)$$

In equation 3, $\dot{V}CO_2$ represents carbon dioxide production (liters/min), c and f represent carbohydrate and fat oxidation (g/min) in respiration, and n represents urinary nitrogen excretion (g/min). From these relationships, the following equation can be derived to quantify carbohydrate and fat oxidation [41]:

$$\text{Carbohydrate oxidation (g/min)} =$$
$$\frac{0.944 \ VO_2 \ (R_f - R_b) + n \ [6.555 \ (R_p - R_b) - 5.703 \ (R_f - R_b)]}{R_b - R_c + 0.704 \ (R_f - R_b)} \quad (4)$$

$$\text{Fat oxidation (g/min)} = .493 \ \dot{V}O_2 - .367 \ c - 2.975 \ n \quad (5)$$

Thus, with these equations, it is possible to calculate the rates of carbohydrate and fat oxidation independently of the $\dot{V}CO_2$, which is the parameter of questionable validity in the calculation of substrate oxidation rates by indirect calorimetry during strenuous exercise. The relative contribution of carbohydrates and fat to energy production can even be calculated completely independently of both $\dot{V}O_2$ and $\dot{V}CO_2$, and thus of indirect calorimetry, using the $^{13}C/^{12}C$ ratios in the breath, endogenous fat, and glucose (equation 6). The contribution of protein oxidation to energy expenditure during strenuous exercise is relatively small and therefore has not been taken into account [7].

$$\text{Carbohydrate oxidation (\%)} = \frac{(R_b - R_f)}{(R_c - R_f)} \times 100 \quad (6)$$

The use of this approach requires knowledge of the values of R_c, R_f, R_p, and R_b. R_b can easily be determined on small samples (1–2 liters) of expired air [59]. R_p and R_f are determined on plasma protein and plasma triglyceride, respectively, and will be representative of their total body stores [41]. R_c can be determined from plasma glucose [41]; however, this value may not necessarily be representative of the ratio in the glycogen stored in the muscle. The plasma glucose is derived from the liver, and therefore will predominantly reflect the enrichment of hepatic glycogen, as well as any gluconeogenic precursors. Since hepatic glycogen is largely depleted after an overnight fast, the plasma glucose $^{13}C/^{12}C$ ratio will be a direct reflection of the $^{13}C/^{12}C$ ratio of the last meal. In contrast, muscle glycogen is rather stable and becomes depleted only by strenuous exercise, meaning that the $^{13}C/^{12}C$ ratio of muscle glycogen may be different than that of plasma glucose. This potential problem can be overcome by having the subjects perform a glycogen-depleting exercise the day before the study, and then repleting the glycogen stores with a carbohydrate of known $^{13}C/^{12}C$ ratio. Because of the small total pool of carbohydrate in the body, one depletion/repletion protocol can result in relatively complete replacement, so that all carbohydrates in the body will have almost the same $^{13}C/^{12}C$ ratio as the ingested carbohydrate. This protocol also has the advantage that if carbohydrate is given that has been enriched in ^{13}C, a greater difference between R_c and R_f will be achieved, thereby increasing the precision and accuracy of the method.

The assumptions of this method, along with assumptions that are not required, have been discussed in detail [41]. Furthermore, the results with the ratio method have been validated against indirect calorimetry at rest [41], and the latter technique is known to be valid at rest [19]. Thus, this new ratio method enables the determination of substrate oxidation at any intensity of exercise without the necessity of determining $\dot{V}CO_2$. Surprisingly, in well-trained athletes, the same values for carbohydrate and fat oxidation were obtained with the ratio method and indirect calorimetry, indicating the validity of indirect calorimetry in the athletes exercising at a high intensity [40].

Quantification of Plasma and Intracellular Kinetics and Oxidation of Glucose
Once it is possible to quantify substrate oxidation in exercise, it becomes possible to obtain estimates of the sources of carbohydrate and fat when the oxidation measurements are coupled with measurements of plasma kinetics.

The rate of appearance of glucose into the plasma, and rate of tissue uptake, can be quantified by traditional tracer techniques using 6, 6-d_2-glucose [59]. Although widely used in a variety of circumstances, this methodology has been infrequently used in exercise. One major problem has been the complications arising from the nonsteady state kinetics induced by exercise. The limitations in calculating glucose kinetics in the nonsteady state have been well documented (e.g., [1]). The problems caused by rapid changes in plasma enrichment can be overcome to a great extent, however, by appropriate changes in tracer infusion rate. We first applied this general principle to the quantification of glucose kinetics in exercise using 1-^{13}C-glucose as a tracer [62]. By first running a pilot study to determine the magnitude of change in enrichment caused by exercise, it was possible to adjust the tracer infusion rate appropriately to maintain a relatively steady state in isotopic enrichment during exercise, even when large changes in plasma glucose concentration were occurring [62]. This approach enables accurate calculation of glucose appearance and uptake, even in strenuous exercise.

The regulation of glucose production and uptake in humans has been rather well documented in exercise with stable isotope methodology, despite the absence of a large number of studies. The rate of production is only modestly increased at low intensity exercise, but is increased by as much as 10-fold or more in high intensity work [13]. Despite the marked increase in plasma glucose production with increasing intensity, the relative importance of plasma glucose as a substrate fails to increase. During high-intensity exercise, glucose uptake does not increase as much as production, as reflected by the increase in plasma concentration [13]. Muscle glycogen breakdown becomes increasingly important in high-intensity exercise [4], perhaps indirectly contributing to the increase in plasma glucose concentration by impeding glucose uptake. An increase in the concentrations of plasma glucagon or a small decrease in plasma insulin concentration is responsible for the stimulation of glucose production in exercise. When changes in these hormones are prevented in exercise, glucose production fails to increase despite the development of hypoglycemia and total catecholamine concentrations in excess of 2000 pg/ml [62]. Acute exposure to altitude caused an increase in glucose production and uptake, both at rest and during exercise at the same work level as at sea level [6]. Upon adaptation to altitude for 3 weeks, resting glucose production was further increased and, during exercise, glucose production and uptake were also elevated even more than after acute exposure, reaching values almost double those attained at sea level during the same work load [6].

Stable isotopic tracers can also be used to measure hepatic glucose substrate cycling, which involves the simultaneous conversion of glucose to glucose 6 P to glucose in the liver. The rate of this cycle can be quantified by simultaneously infusing 2-^2H_1-glucose and $6,6\text{-}^2H$-glucose and calculating the difference between the rates of glucose flux (Ra glucose) calculated with each tracer [42]. This is because the ^2H in the 2 position is lost in the hexoseisomerase reaction (glucose-6P $\leftrightarrow$ fructose-6P). In contrast, ^2H-in the 6 position of glucose is not lost in the process of glycolysis, but can be lost at two possible sites in the process of gluconeogenesis. Thus, if a molecule labeled with ^2H in the 2 position enters the liver and is metabolized as far as fructose-6P, and is then recycled back out into the blood as glucose, the label will be lost. In contrast, a glucose tracer labeled with ^2H in the 6 position will not lose its label in the glucose cycle. Thus, Ra glucose calculated with $6,6\text{-}^2H_2$-glucose will not include the glucose cycle, whereas glucose flux calculated with 2-^2H_1-glucose will induce the glucose cycle [42].

The potential role of substrate cycling in amplifying metabolic control has been discussed extensively on a theoretical basis [33]. Conceptually, a high rate of cycling means that net flux can change both as a consequence of a change in the rate of flux in the forward direction (i.e., glucose production) or by a change in the reverse direction (i.e., glucose phosphorylation). If simultaneous changes occur, then the magnitude of change in net flux is amplified. Numerous studies have established that about 30% of glucose production in resting man recycles directly back into glucose-6P [32]. Thus, if a decrease in glucose phosphorylation accompanies the increase in glucose production, the amount of net glucose output into blood would be amplified. However, we found that during exercise at 70% $\dot{V}O_2$max, the rate of glucose cycling increased directly in proportion to the increase in the rate of glucose production [53]. Consequently, whereas a significant rate of glucose cycling occurs at rest, this does not serve to amplify the magnitude of the glucose output to exercise, since the reverse direction (glucose → glucose-6P) is apparent-ly a direct function of glucose production.

FATTY ACID KINETICS

Fatty acids are the predominant energy substrate in almost all circum-stances in the fasting state, except during extremely strenuous exercise. Understanding the factors controlling the release of fatty acids as a result of the breakdown of stored triglyceride to release fatty acids (lipolysis) and the oxidation of fatty acids thus is central to understanding the metabolic response in exercise. Recent advances in stable isotope methodology now allow the quantitative aspects of many components of fatty acid kinetics and oxidation to be determined.

Lipolysis can be quantified by means of the determination of the rate of appearance of glycerol, as determined by a stable isotope tracer of glycerol such as $^2H_5$ or 2-^{13}C-glycerol. This is because glycerol can only be metabolized in the liver, because the enzyme glycerol kinase is necessary for the first step in the metabolism of glycerol, and this enzyme is only in the liver [17]. Furthermore, since glycerol dissolves freely in water, there is no limitation to the amount of glycerol that can diffuse from the intracellular site of lipolysis into the plasma. Only an insignificant portion of glycerol is released in the gut and is directly cleared in the liver [52], thereby causing the tracer technique using only peripheral blood to miss that amount of R_a glycerol. Also, there is no endogenous metabolic production of glycerol [63]. Finally, there is virtually no partial hydrolysis of triglyceride [2] meaning that for every glycerol that is released, three fatty acids were also released.

The fatty acids released into the intracellular space of the adipocyte have two potential fates—release into the plasma, or reesterification into triglycerides within the adipocyte. The process of reesterification involves the attachment of three fatty acids to α-glycerol phosphate derived from the metabolism of plasma glucose. This may occur because of an abundance of α-glycerol phosphate, as occurs during hyperglyce-mia [63], or because of a deficient rate of blood flow through the fat. A decrease in blood flow is important because free fatty acids are not soluble in water. They are carried in plasma bound to albumin, and availability of binding sites on albumin can be rate limiting for transport when blood flow is low.

Once released into the plasma, the fatty acids can be cleared by tissues such as muscle for oxidation, or they can be cleared by the liver and reesterified into triglyceride and transported back to the periphery as very low density lipoprotein. Thus, in the general sense, we can consider triglyceride/fatty acid cycling to involve the reesterification of fatty acids that have been initially released as a consequence of lipolysis. There are two routes of recycling in vivo (Fig. 1.4):

1. Intracellular, wherein fatty acids are reesterified within the adipocyte in which the lipolysis occurred; and
2. "Extracellular," where the fatty acid is released into plasma and transported to another tissue (predominantly liver) for clearance and reesterification.

The difference between the total release of fatty acids and the rate of appearance of fatty acids into the plasma (RaFFA) is equal to the rate of reesterification of fatty acids within the adipocyte. The RaFFA can be determined by means of a labeled tracer of any individual free fatty acid (FFA) (e.g., $[1-^{13}C]$-palmitate); and then converted to total FFA turnover by dividing Ra palmitate by the fraction of the total FFA concentration represented by palmitate (determined by gas chromatography). This calculation presumes that all fatty acids released by lipolysis either enter the plasma or are reesterfied. It is also possible that fatty acids might be "directly" oxidized without entering the plasma. This would cause an overestimation of the intracellular recycling of FFA. However, it seems unlikely that this pathway of oxidation occurs to a great extent at rest. Over a large number of experiments, the ratio of RaFFA/Ra glycerol is about 3/1 [32, 64]. Biopsy data indicate that virtually all fat is in the form of triglyceride (TG) [2], meaning that no partial hydrolysis of TG occurs. Since "direct" oxidation of FFA would therefore also involve the release of glycerol into the plasma, the ratio of RaFFA/Ra glycerol would be significantly less than 3 if there was much of this type of oxidation. This is precisely the observation, however, in strenuous exercise (see later in this chapter).

The TG/FA (fatty acid) cycle can result in the availability of FAs in excess of requirement at rest, so that uptake by active muscle can increase immediately at the start of exercise, before any change occurs in the rate of lipolysis. At rest, about 70% of fatty acids released in the process of lipolysis are reesterified rather than oxidized, meaning that all those FAs are potentially available for oxidation in case of a sudden increase in demand. Thus, the TG/FA cycle theoretically should amplify the response of FA oxidation to a sudden change in the requirement for oxidative energy substrates, as compared with the situation if only enough FAs were released at rest to correspond exactly to the rate of FA oxidation. If the TG/FA cycle plays any role in matching FA availability and energy requirements, one would anticipate that the response to exercise would be one such circumstance. Therefore, we have investigated the response of normal volunteers to 4 hr of moderate exercise (40% $\dot{V}O_2$ max) [64]. Total TG/FA cycling was quantified as (3 × Ra glycerol)

FIGURE 1.4
Potential pathways of triglyceride/fatty acid (TG/FA) cycling.

Intracellular (━) And Extracellular (┈) TG/FA Cycling

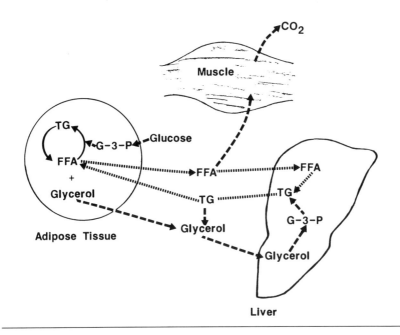

— fat oxidation (μmol/kg · min). Exercise intensity of 40% $\dot{V}O_2$max was chosen to maximize the reliance on fat as an energy substrate. If TG/FA cycling amplifies responsiveness, one would expect the percentage of reesterification to fall during exercise in conjunction with the stimulation of lipolysis (to amplify the availability of FAs for oxidation). In recovery, the percentage of reesterification should rise as the rate of lipolysis falls (to reduce the elevated plasma FFA level more rapidly than could be accomplished by only a reduction in lipolysis).

The results indicated that lipolysis was stimulated significantly at the start of exercise, but did not reach its maximal level until 4 hr of exercise, despite the constant energy requirement throughout. In recovery, lipolysis gradually declined, but 2 hr after exercise had stopped the value was still significantly greater than the resting value (Fig. 1.5). Changes in RaFFA corresponded to the stimulation of lipolysis (Fig. 1.5). Accompanying these responses of lipolysis, there were reciprocal changes in the percentage of reesterification. The value dropped from the resting value of 70% to 25–35% throughout exercise (Fig. 1.6). In recovery, almost 90% of fatty acids released by lipolysis were reesterified

FIGURE 1.5

*Response of lipolysis (**Ra glycerol**) and free fatty acid appearance (**RaFFA**) in exercise (40% V̇O₂max) and in recovery.*

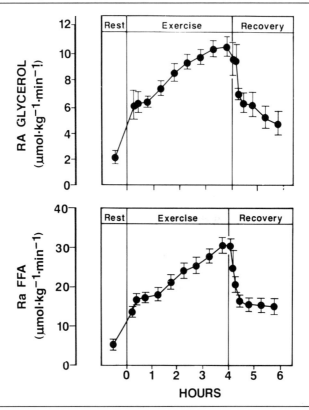

FIGURE 1.6

Effects of exercise on the percentage of free fatty acids released that are reesterified (recycled) as opposed to oxidized.

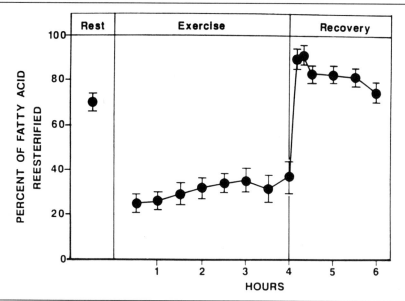

(Fig. 1.6). In exercise, approximately 55% of total FA oxidation was attributable to the decrease in the percentage of reesterification (Fig. 1.7). In other words, FA oxidation increased by twice as much as it would have, had the same stimulation of lipolysis occurred in a system in which total flux = net flux (i.e., oxidation) in the resting state. In recovery, the increased reesterification was important in enabling the FAs to return toward the basal level, despite the sudden decrease in demand for energy substrates and the sluggish responsiveness of the rate of lipolysis. The amplification of control was achieved almost entirely via changes in the percentage of reesterification via the extracellular route.

At 40% $\dot{V}O_2$max in untrained subjects, RaFFA still exceeded the rate of fat oxidation, meaning that at least theoretically all FA oxidation could be derived from plasma. At higher intensity exercise in trained subjects, however, oxidation becomes markedly greater than 3 × RaFFA [40], meaning that there must be some intramuscular hydrolysis of TG and direct oxidation of the fatty acids. In a manner analogous to the calculation of the rate of intramuscular glycogen utilization, the minimal amount of intramuscular fat oxidation can be calculated as the difference between total fat oxidation (determined by either indirect calorimetry or the ratio method described earlier) and RaFFA. The rate of intramuscular lipolysis is thus equal to the rate of intramuscular fat

FIGURE 1.7

The total rate of fat oxidation in exercise (●—●) and the rate of fat oxidation that would have occurred had there been no change in the percent of recycling (○—○). The shaded area represents the amount of fat oxidation that could be attributed to the change in the rate of TG/FA cycling.

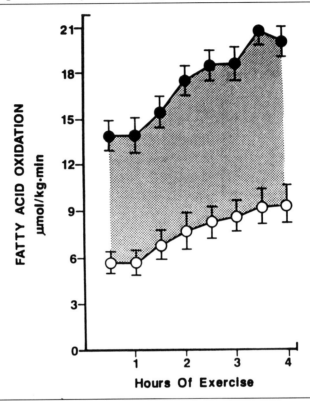

oxidation divided by 3, and thus peripheral lipolysis is equal to total Ra glycerol-intramuscular Ra glycerol. Using this approach in well-trained cyclists, it was possible to document that peripheral lipolysis is maximally stimulated at an exercise rate as low as 25% $\dot{V}O_2$max. However, only at higher intensity efforts does intramuscular lipolysis become stimulated [40]. At 85% $\dot{V}O_2$max, despite a stimulation of lipolysis similar to that at 65% $\dot{V}O_2$max, fat oxidation falls, suggesting an impairment in the ability to oxidize FAs in high-intensity exercise [40].

ASSESSMENT OF AMINO ACID/PROTEIN METABOLISM

Exercise was considered to have an unimportant effect on protein metabolism until the late 1970s. This perception was primarily based on the minimal changes that occur in urinary urea excretion (e.g., [67]). However, this perception was challenged by some studies that coupled the measurement of urea excretion in sweat with urinary excretion, and came to the conclusion that although urinary excretion, and came to the conclusion that although urinary urea excretion may be unaffected or reduced in exercise, total urea excretion may be increased, thereby indicating an increase in net protein breakdown [38]. Subsequently, a number of stable isotope experiments have been performed to address the general issue of protein metabolism in exercise. Stable isotopes are particularly important in this regard, because ^{15}N is a useful stable isotope of nitrogen, and there is no radioactive counterpart.

The first use of stable isotopes to assess protein metabolism in exercise was by Rennie et al. [39], who used ^{15}N-glycine to trace whole body protein synthesis and breakdown. They concluded that prolonged exercise led to net proteolysis [39]. This methodology, however, depends on the measurement of the enrichment of either urea or ammonia acid products and also on the actual rate of urea excretion. Theoretically, the same values should be obtained for either ammonia or urea enrichment, but in practice considerable discrepancies are obtained [18]. Urea excretion is difficult to quantify in exercise, given the uncertainties in measuring sweat losses, and changes in kidney blood flow during exercise make urinary excretion difficult to interpret. Furthermore, there is no assurance that total N, or urea excretion, is a direct reflection of protein breakdown over a short period of time. Thus, we have recently shown that not only is the rate of delivery of amino acids (i.e., glutamine and alanine) to the liver important in the regulation of urea production, but also factors such as hormones can acutely regulate urea production, independent of amino acid delivery [27]. Consequently, over the past several years, we have performed a series of experiments in exercising human volunteers using stable isotopic tracers with the goal of extending the study of the effect of exercise on protein metabolism as assessed by the measurement of urea production alone to the study of other aspects of protein metabolism. In all experiments, the subjects were normal, healthy males, who were not involved in any sort of organized physical training. The exercise in all of the studies summarized was moderate, ranging from 30–40% of the $\dot{V}O_2$max. The data from our own studies will be stressed, since other studies using stable isotopic tracers of amino acids and/or protein in exercise have been minimal.

Our original isotopic studies focused on the assessment of the rate of urea production using an isotopic technique that does not require collection of urea excretion [60]. Simultaneously, 1-^{13}C-leucine was used to estimate whole-body protein synthesis and breakdown, and the net balance between these two processes. The results indicated that exercise has no effect on urea production, and minimal effect an leucine flux, but a marked increase in leucine oxidation occurred [60]. Thus, the rate of net protein breakdown was not altered by exercise if it was calculated from the urea data, but net protein breakdown appeared to be markedly increased if calculated from the leucine data. We performed several experiments in an attempt to reconcile these apparently discordant data.

Any tracer model relies on assumptions that may not hold under certain conditions, such as exercise. Therefore, we performed a series of experiments to assess the validity of the ^{15}N-technique further to quantitate urea production [26]. Briefly, these experiments demonstrated that the isotopic data responded quickly and appropriately to known changes in urea production. Thus, when urea production was stimulated by alanine infusion, the isotopic enrichment of urea immediately fell, and when urea production was inhibited by glucose infusion, urea enrichment promptly increased [26]. When no perturbation was performed, urea enrichment remained constant for the 8 hr of infusion [26]. Therefore, we are confident in the validity of the ^{15}N-urea method, and thus we can conclude that during prolonged, moderate exercise, there is no increase in total urea production.

Several aspects of the ^{13}C-leucine data involve assumptions that may be invalid during exercise. Potential problems with changes in bicarbonate retention have been discussed previously. These were accounted for in revised calculations of leucine oxidation [58], with only minimal changes in the absolute values and no change in the conclusion that leucine oxidation was increased in exercise. The use of $1-^{13}C$-leucine eliminates worry about isotopic exchange diluting the expired CO_2 enrichment, since the carbon is lost directly to CO_2 without entering the TCA cycle. Account must be taken of altered ^{13}C-bicarbonate kinetics (i.e., recovery) during exercise, but this was done in the original study [66]. Finally, the true precursor enrichment was determined by measuring the enrichment of KIC. KIC is derived entirely from the intracellular leucine pool, and thus serves as a direct reflection of the precursor enrichment for leucine oxidation, since the next step in the metabolism of leucine is the irreversible loss to CO_2 of the 1 carbon of KIC. Thus, despite all of the potential pitfalls of measuring oxidation by collecting $^{13}CO_2$ and measuring the precursor enrichment, this approach seems to be generally valid in the case of $1-^{13}C$-leucine when ^{13}C-KIC enrichment is measured as an indicator of precursor enrichment.

There is one aspect of the model of leucine oxidation that could be a problem in exercise. Leucine oxidation at rest occurs to a great extent in the liver [21]. During exercise, one would expect that if there is an increase in leucine oxidation, it would occur in muscle. The oxidation rate is calculated by dividing the rate of $^{13}CO_2$ excretion by the isotopic enrichment of the precursor, which is taken to be the plasma KIC enrichment [60]. However, plasma KIC enrichment is not representative of any specific tissue, but is a pooled value. After only a few hours of infusion of labeled amino acid, enrichments within different tissues differ [Wolfe, unpublished data]. This could potentially result in an overestimation of leucine oxidation in exercise if the intracellular enrichment of free leucine in muscle was higher than the intracellular free pool of the liver. When the predominant site of oxidation shifts from the liver to the muscle, the true precursor for oxidation would increase, but this would not be reflected in the pooled central enrichment of KIC. Consequently, the true rate of leucine oxidation would be overestimated. To assess the likelihood of this potential problem, we recently performed a study in anesthetized dogs. Animals were given a primed-constant infusion of $1\text{-}^{13}C$-leucine in a manner analogous to the procedure we have used in the exercise study. After 4 hr, several tissues, including liver and skeletal muscle, were freeze-clamped for subsequent determination of the free leucine enrichment in the intracellular compartment. Results indicated that the liver free-leucine enrichment was about 70% of the mixed venous enrichment, and the muscle free-leucine was about 60% of the plasma value (unpublished observations). Thus, even if the pooled venous enrichment does not precisely reflect the intracellular precursor pool, the differences are not large and therefore of little reason for concern regarding the qualitative nature of the conclusions.

It seems, therefore, that there is little doubt that there is an increase in the oxidation of leucine during exercise. Furthermore, when we simultaneously infused ^{15}N-leucine and ^{13}C-alanine during exercise, only about 15% of the nitrogen contained in the increased alanine flux could be accounted for by the oxidation of leucine [66]. The oxidation of amino acids other than leucine, therefore, must also be accelerated during exercise. In the absence of exogenous input of amino acids, an increased oxidation of essential amino acids would be expected to result in an increase in net protein breakdown, which, in turn, would be expected to be reflected in an increased rate of urea production. One possible explanation for those apparently discordant results is that there is an inhibition of urea production during exercise that is counteracted by the increased delivery of amino-N to the liver. Therefore, we performed an experiment designed to test this hypothesis.

The rationale we used in an attempt to uncover an underlying inhibition of urea production during exercise was to infuse amino acids at a rate sufficient to obscure any change in endogenous amino acid flux that might occur during exercise. If changes in endogenous flux were normally counteracting an inhibition of urea production, this counteracting influence would be eliminated and urea production would fall. Four volunteers were given a primed-constant infusion of $^{15}N_2$-urea. On one occasion, they performed 4 hr of treadmill exercise without any other infusion. In another protocol, they received an infusion of mixed amino acids at the rate of 1.25 g protein/kg·day, starting 8 hr before exercise and continuing throughout exercise and 4 hr of recovery. In addition, each subject was also studied under resting conditions throughout, with and without the amino acid infusion, to control for time effects of the 16-hr protocol. Even in this circumstance, urea production during exercise was not different from either the resting value or from the values before and after exercise [Wolfe, unpublished data]. These results do not support the notion of an inhibition of urea production during exercise.

Another possible explanation that could at least partially reconcile the increased flux of N to the liver during exercise and the absence of a change in urea production is that amino acids within the liver are directed toward plasma protein synthesis rather than toward urea synthesis. Therefore, we performed a study to explore this hypothesis. In addition, we evaluated the effect of a high-protein diet (2.5 vs. 1.1 g protein/kg·day) on the response of protein metabolism to exercise [7]. Dietary control was maintained for 5 days before the experimental day. The primed-constant infusion of ^{15}N-glycine was used to quantify the synthetic rate of fibronectin and fibrinogen, two plasma proteins produced in the liver that have high rates of turnover. The urinary hippurate enrichment was used to represent the precursor enrichment for isotope incorporation into protein. Hippurate is a useful probe of intracellular liver enrichment of glycine, since it is synthesized entirely from glycine and benzoic acid in the liver. The rate of albumin synthesis was also measured in this experiment, and whole-body protein turnover was estimated from the enrichment of urinary ammonia. Urinary ammonia was chosen as an end-product because it is largely produced in muscle during exercise. Neither exercise nor recovery had an effect on whole-body protein turnover or on albumin fractional synthetic rate (FSR), but the FSR of fibronectin was significantly elevated at the end of exercise, and fibrinogen synthesis was significantly elevated in recovery (Fig. 1.8). Dietary protein intake had no effect on the response to exercise [8]. Thus, there appears to be a stimulation of the synthesis of some acute phase proteins during exercise, which may serve to explain, to some extent, the disposition of an increased delivery of N to the liver. However, since the increased flux of N is not in a balanced mixture of amino acids, with the increase in alanine flux predominating, it is unlikely that the stimulation of synthesis of plasma proteins can entirely explain the absence of an increase in urea production.

The increased oxidation of amino acids during exercise, presumably in muscle, might be expected to result in a decreased rate of muscle protein synthesis during exercise. On the other hand, repetitive exercise training does not cause muscle wasting. One possibility is that accelerated muscle protein breakdown in exercise is balanced by a subsequent

FIGURE 1.8

Fractional synthetic rates of fibrinogen and fibronectin in normal volunteers in exercise k (4 hr at 40% $\dot{V}O_2$max) and recovery (4 hr).

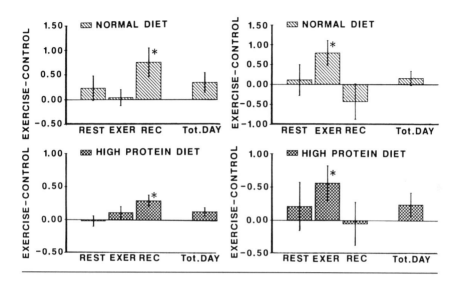

PROTEIN KINETICS IN EXERCISE

stimulation of muscle protein synthesis in recovery. This notion is supported by one human study in which amino acid uptake by the muscle assessed using ^{13}C-leucine was increased in the recovery period following exercise [8]. However, no direct determination of the response of muscle protein synthesis to exercise or recovery from exercise has been previously made in either intact animals or in humans. Therefore, we recently determined the rate of ^{13}C-leucine incorporation into muscle protein during 4 hr of aerobic exercise and throughout the following 4 hr of recovery [8]. The muscle FSR was slightly, but not significantly, decreased during exercise, as compared with the control value, but there was a significant increase in FSR in the exercise group during the recovery period (Fig. 1.8) [8]. These results indicate that whereas aerobic exercise may stimulate muscle protein breakdown and amino acid oxidation, this does not result in a significant depletion of muscle mass because muscle protein synthesis is stimulated in recovery.

Thus, it seems that during aerobic exercise there is a modest increase in both muscle protein breakdown and the oxidation of amino acids, including leucine. Nitrogen is transported to the liver at an increased rate, predominantly in the form of alanine, were acute phase plasma protein synthesis (rather than urea production) is stimulated. Muscle protein synthesis is essentially maintained during exercise, and is stimulated during recovery.

REFERENCES

1. Allsop, J. R., R. R. Wolfe, and J. F. Burke. The reliability of rates of glucose appearance in vivo calculated from constant tracer infusions. *Biochem. J.* 172:407–416, 1978.
2. Arner, P., and J. Ostman. Mono and di-acyl glycerols in human adipose tissue. *Biochim. Biophys. Acta* 369:209–221, 1974.
3. Barstow, T. J., D. M. Cooper, E. M. Sobel, E. M. Landaw, and S. Epstein. Influence of increased metabolic rate on ^{13}C bicarbonate washout kinetics. *Am. J. Physiol.* 259:R163–R171, 1990.
4. Bergstrom, J., and E. Hultman. A study of glycogen metabolism during exercise in man. *Scand. J. Clin. Lab. Invest.* 19:218–223, 1967.
5. Blair, S. N., N. M. Ellsworth, W. L. Haskell, M. P. Stern, J. W. Farquhar, and P. D. Wood. Comparison of nutrient intake in middle-aged men and women runners and controls. *Med. Sci. Sports Exerc.* 13:310–315, 1981.
6. Brooks, G. A., G. E. Butterfield, R. R. Wolfe, B. M. Groves, R. S. Mazzeo, J. R. Sutton, R. R. Wolf, and J. T. Reeves. Increased dependence on blood glucose after acclimatization to 4,300 m. *J. Appl. Physiol.* 70:919–927, 1991.
7. Carraro, F., W. Hartl, C. A. Stuart, D. K. Layman, F. Jahoor, and R. R. Wolfe. Whole-body and plasma protein synthesis in exercise and recovery in human subjects. *Am. J. Physiol.* 258:E821–E831, 1990.
8. Carraro, F., C. A. Stuart, W. H. Hartl, J. Rosenblatt, and R. R. Wolfe. Effect of exercise and recovery on muscle protein synthesis in human subjects. *Am. J. Physiol.* 259:E470–E476, 1990.
9. Chinkes, D. L., X. J. Zhang, J. A. Romijn, and R. R. Wolfe. In vivo determination of pyruvate/lactate production, interconversion and transmembrane transport in muscle. *Diabetes* 41(s):10A, 1992. (Abstract).
10. Cobelli, C., M. P. Saccomani, P. Tessari, G. Biolo, L. Luzi, and D. E. Matthews. Compartmental model of leucine kinetics in humans. *Am. J. Physiol* 261:E539–E550, 1991.
11. Coggan, A. R., D. L. Habash, L. A. Mendenhall, S. C. Swanson and C. L. Kien. Isotopic estimation of CO_2 production during exercise before and after endurance training. *Med. Sci. Sports* 24:S141, 1992.
12. Consoli, A., F. Kennedy, J. Miles, and J. Gerich. Determination of Krebs cycle metabolic carbon exchange in vivo and its use to estimate the individual contributions of gluconeogenesis and glycogenolysis to overall glucose output in man. *J. Clin. Invest.* 80:1303–1310, 1987.
13. Cooper, D. M., T. J. Barstow, A. Bergner, and W. N. P. Lee. Blood glucose turnover during high- and low-intensity exercise. *Am. J. Physiol.* 257:E405–E412, 1989.
14. Coward, W. A., T. J. Cole, H. Gerber, S. B. Roberts, and I. Flect. Water turnover and the measurement of milk intake. *Pflugers Arch.* 393:344–347, 1982.
15. DeWeir, J. B. New methods for calculating metabolic rate with special reference to protein metabolism. *J. Physiol.* 109:1–9, 1949.
16. Drent, R. H. and S. Daan. The prudent parent: energetic adjustments in avian breeding. *Ardea* 68:225–252, 1980.
17. Dixon M., and E. L. Webb. *Enzymes.* New York: Academic Press, 1979.
18. Fern, E. B., P. J. Garlick, M. A. McNurlen, and J. C. Waterlow. The excretion of isotope in urea and ammonia for estimating protein turnover in man with ^{15}N glycine. *Clin. Sci.* 61:217–228, 1981.

19. Frayn, K. N. Calculation of substrate oxidation rates in vivo from gaseous exchange. *J. Appl. Physiol.* 55:628–634, 1993.
20. Gerard, J., B. Jandrain, F. Pirnay, N. Pallikarakis, G. Krzentowski, M. Lacroix, F. Mosora, A. S. Luyckx, and P. J. LeFebvre. Utilization of oral sucrose load during exercise in humans. Effect of the α-glucosidase inhibitor acarbose. *Diabetes* 35:1294–1301, 1986.
21. Harper, A. E., and C. Zapalowski. Metabolism of branched chain amino acids. In J. C. Waterlow, and J. M. L. Stephen (eds.). *Nitrogen Metabolism In Man*. London: Applied Science Publishers, 1981, pp. 97–115.
22. Heiling, V. J. and J. M. Miles. How valid are isotopic measurements of fatty acid oxidation? *Am. J. Physiol.* 1992. (in press)
23. Hoyt, R. W., T. E. Jones, T. P. Stein, G. W. McAninch, H. R. Lieberman, E. W. Askew, and A. Cymerman. Doubly labeled water measurement of human energy expenditure during strenuous exercise. *J. Appl. Physiol.* 71:16–22, 1991.
24. Irving, C. S., W. W. Wong, R. J. Schulman, E. O. Smith, and P. D. Klein. [^{13}C] bicarbonate kinetics in humans: intra- vs. inter-individual variations. *Am. J. Physiol.* 14:R190–R202, 1983.
25. Jacobson, B. S., B. N. Smith, S. Epstein, and G. G. Laties. The prevalence of carbon-13 in respiratory carbon dioxide as an indicator of the type of endogenous substrate. *J. Gen. Physiol.* 55:1–17, 1970.
26. Jahoor, F. and R. R. Wolfe. Re-assessment of primed-constant infusion tracer method to measure urea kinetics. *Am. J. Physiol.* 252:E557–E564, 1987.
27. Jahoor, F, and R. R. Wolfe. Regulation of urea production by glucose infusion in vivo. *Am. J. Physiol.* 253:E543–E550, 1987.
28. Kien, C. L. Isotopic dilution of CO_2 as an estimate of CO_2 production during substrate oxidation studies. *Am. J. Physiol.* 257:E296–E298, 1989.
29. Krzentowski, G., F. Pirnay, N. Pallikarakis, A. S. Luyckx, M. Lacroix, F. Mosora, and P. J. LeFebvre. Glucose utilization during exercise in normal and diabetic subjects: the role of insulin. *Diabetes* 30:983–989, 1981.
30. Lifson, N., G. B. Gordon, M. B. Visscher, and A. O. Nier. The fate of utilized molecular oxygen and the source of heavy oxygen of respiratory carbon dioxide, studied with the aid of heavy oxygen. *J. Biol. Chem.* 180:803–811, 1949.
31. Lifson, N. and R. McClintock. Theory of use of turnover rates of body water for measuring energy and material balance. *J. Theor. Biol.* 12:46–74, 1966.
32. Miyoshi, H., G. I. Schulman, E. J. Peters, M. H. Wolfe, D. Elahi, and R. R. Wolfe. Hormonal control of substrate cycling in humans. *J. Clin. Invest.* 81:1545–1555, 1988.
33. Newsholme, E. A., and B. Crabtree. Substrate cycles in metabolic regulation and in heat generation. *Biochem. Soc. Symp.* 41:61–109, 1992.
34. Pallikarakis, N., N. Sphiriks, and P. LeFebvre. Influence of the bicarbonate pool on the occurrence of $^{13}CO_2$ in exhaled air. *Eur. J. Appl. Physiol.* 63:179–183, 1991.
35. Peronnet, F., D. Massicotte, G. Brisson, and C. Hillaire-Marcel. Use of ^{13}C substrates for metabolic studies in exercise: methodological considerations. *J. Appl. Physiol.* 69:1047–1052, 1990.
36. Pirnay, F., M. Lacroix, and F. Mosora. Glucose oxidation during prolonged exercise evaluated with naturally labeled ^{13}C glucose. *J. Appl. Physiol.* 43:258–261, 1977.
37. Pirnay, R., M. Lacroix, and F. Mosora. Effect of glucose ingestion on energy substrate utilization during prolonged muscular exercise. *Eur. J. Appl. Physiol.* 36:247–254, 1977.
38. Refsum, H. E., R. Gjessing, and S. B. Stromme. Changes in plasma amino acid distribution and urine amino acid excretion during prolonged heavy exercise. *Scand. J. Clin. Lab. Invest.* 39:407–413, 1979.
39. Rennie, M. J., R. H. T. Edwards, S. Krywawych, C. T. M. Davies, D. Halliday, J. C. Waterlow, and D. J. Millward. Effect of exercise on protein tumors in man. *Clin. Sci.* 61:627–639, 1981.

40. Romijn, H. A., E. F. Coyle, L. Sidossis, J. F. Horowitz, and R. R. Wolfe. Effects of exercise intensity on fat metabolism. *Med. Sci. Sports* 24:S72, 1992. (Abstract)

41. Romijn, J. A., E. F. Coyle, J. Hibbert, and R. R. Wolfe. Comparison of indirect calorimetry and a new breath $^{13}C/^{12}C$ ratio method during strenuous exercise. *Am. J. Physiol.* 1992. (in press)

42. Royle, G. T., R. R. Wolfe, and J. F. Burke. Glucose and fatty acid kinetics in fasted rats: effects of previous protein intake. *Metabolism* 31:279–283, 1982.

43. Schoeller, D. A. Energy expenditure from doubly-labeled water: some fundamental considerations in humans. *Am. J. Clin. Nutr.* 38:999–1005, 1983.

44. Schoeller, D. A., P. D. Klein, J. B. Watkins, T. Heim, and J. Maclean. ^{13}C abundances of nutrients and the effect of variations in ^{13}C isotopic abundances of test meals formulated for $^{13}CO_2$ breath tests. *Am. J. Clin. Nutr.* 33:2375–2385, 1980.

45. Schoeller, D. A., E. Ravussin, Y. Schutz, K. J. Acheson, P. Baertschi, and E. Jequier. Energy expenditure by doubly-labeled water: Validation in humans and proposed calculation. *Am. J. Physiol.* 250:R823–R830, 1986.

46. Schoenheimer, R. and D. Rittenberg. Deuterium as indicator in study of intermediary metabolism. *Science* 82:156, 1935.

47. Schulz, L. O., S. Alger, I. Harper, J. H. Wilmore, and E. Ravussin. Energy expenditure of elite female runners measured by respiratory chamber and doubly-labeled water. *J. Appl. Physiol.* 72:23–28, 1992.

48. Seale, J., C. Miles, and C. E. Bodwell. Sensitivity of methods for calculating energy expenditure by use of doubly-labeled water. *J. Appl. Physiol.* 66:644–653, 1989.

49. Shangraw, R. E., C. A. Stuart, M. J. Prince, E. J. Peters, and R. R. Wolfe. Insulin responsiveness of protein metabolism in vivo following bedrest in humans. *Am. J. Physiol.* 255:E548–E558, 1988.

50. Slama, G., J. Boillot, I. Hellal, D. Darmoun, S. W. Rizkalla, E. Orvoen-Frija, M. F. Dore, G. Guille, J. Fretault, and J. Coursaget. Fructose is as good a fuel as glucose for exercise in normal subjects. *Diabete Metab.* 15:105–106, 1989.

51. Stein, T. P., R. W. Hoyt, R. G. Settle, M. O'Toole, and W. D. Hiller. Determination of energy expenditure during heavy exercise, normal daily activity, and sleep using the doubly-labeled water ($^2H_2^{18}O$) method. *Am. J. Clin. Nutr.* 45:534–539, 1987.

52. Wasserman, D. H., D. B. Lacy, R. E. Goldstein, P. E. Williams, and A. P. Cherrington. Exercise-induced fall in insulin and increase in fat metabolism during prolonged muscular work. *Diabetes* 38:484–491, 1989.

53. Weber, J. M., S. Klein, and R. R. Wolfe. Role of the glucose cycle in control of net glucose flux in exercising humans. *J. Appl. Physiol.* 68:1815–1819, 1990.

54. Westerterp, K. R., F. Brouns, W. H. Saris, and F. Ten-Hoor. Comparison of doubly labeled water with respirometry at low- and high-activity levels. *J. Appl. Physiol.* 65:53–56, 1988.

55. Westerterp, K. R., W. H. Saris, M. Van-Es, and F. Ten-Hoor. Use of the doubly labeled water technique in humans during heavy sustained exercise. *J. Appl. Physiol.* 61:2162–2167, 1986.

56. Whitelaw, F. G., J. M. Brockway, and R. S. Reid. Measurement of carbon dioxide production in sheep by isotope dilution. *Q. J. Exp. Physiol.* 57:37–55, 1972.

57. Williams, B., I. Plag, J. Troup, and R. R. Wolfe. Lactate kinetics in humans during exercise: measurement of muscle intracellular lactate enrichment. *The Physiologist* 1992. (in press)

58. Wolfe, R. R. Does exercise stimulate protein breakdown in humans? Isotopic approaches to the problem. *Med. Sci. Sports Exerc.* 19:S172–S178, 1987.

59. Wolfe, R. R. *Radioactive and Stable Isotope Tracers in Biomedicine: Principles and Practice of Kinetic Analysis.* New York: Wiley-Liss, 1992.

60. Wolfe, R. R., R. D. Goodenough, M. H. Wolfe, G. T. Royle, and E. R. Nadel. Isotopic analysis of leucine and urea metabolism in exercising humans. *J. Appl. Physiol.* 52:458–466, 1982.

61. Wolfe, R. R. and F. Jahoor. Recovery of labeled CO_2 during the infusion of C-1 versus C-2-labeled acetate. Implications for tracer studies of substrate oxidation. *Am. J. Clin. Nutr.* 51:248–252, 1990.

62. Wolfe, R. R., E. R. Nadel, J. H. F. Shaw, L. A. Stephenson, and M. H. Wolfe. Role of changes in insulin and glucagon in glucose homeostasis in exercise. *J. Clin. Invest.* 77:900–907, 1986.

63. Wolfe, R. R., and E. J. Peters. Lipolytic response to glucose infusion in human subjects. *Am J. Physiol.* 252:E218–E223, 1987.

64. Wolfe, R. R., E. J. Peters, S. Klein, O. B. Holland, J. Rosenblatt, and H. Gary, Jr. Effect of short-term fasting on the lipolytic responsiveness in normal and obese human subjects. *Am. J. Physiol.* 252:E189–E196, 1987.

65. Wolfe, R. R., J. H. F. Shaw, E. R. Nadel, and M. H. Wolfe. Effect of substrate intake and physiological state on background $^{13}CO_2$-enrichment. *J. Appl. Physiol.* 56:230–234, 1984.

66. Wolfe, R.R., M.H. Wolfe, E.R. Nadel, and J.H.F. Shaw. Isotopic determination of amino acid-urea interactions in exercise in humans. *J. Appl. Physiol.* 56:221–229, 1984.

67. Zuntz, N. Uber die Bedentung der verschiedener Nahr-Stoffe als Erzeuger der Muskeldraft. *Pflugers Arch.* 83:557–582, 1900.

2
Biology and Mechanics of Ligament and Ligament Healing

BARBARA J. LOITZ, Ph.D.
CYRIL B. FRANK, M.D.

Ligament biology is relevant not only to exercise and sports medicine specialists, but because of various congenital anomalies, rheumatological disorders, and neurological conditions that involve ligaments and their support of joints, an understanding of normal ligament biology is critical to a broader range of specialists than is recognized customarily. The contribution of ligaments to normal joint kinetics and kinematics and how the same joint qualities may, in turn, influence ligament healing have been the focus of a wealth of research investigations. Many questions remain unanswered, however, particularly concerning the mechanisms that link mechanical stimuli and cellular processes. This review concatenates previous works [4, 14, 27] and highlights the most recent information on ligament biology, mechanics, and healing.

By far the most common ligaments used in connective tissue research are those of the knee joint because of the relative accessibility to the structures, the joint's suitability for mechanical testing, and its reputation for injury, disabling instability, and arthritis [14, 26, 49, 56]. However, differences between the biomechanical and healing behaviors of the individual knee ligaments suggest that caution be observed when generalizing findings to all ligaments. The paucity of data describing ligaments other than those of the knee certainly presents a challenge to clinicians and exercise specialists interested in the normal and healing behaviors of ligaments of other joints.

The contemporary researcher is interested primarily in the type of cells present in the ligament tissue, what the cells produce, and whether or not that which is produced fulfills the functional need of the ligament under different circumstances. Is the ligament providing adequate support to its corresponding joint and doing so without undue risk of damaging itself? The following discussion, therefore, includes descriptions of ligament morphology (cells and fibrils), biochemistry (the matrix components), and mechanical behavior.

NORMAL LIGAMENT

Morphology

GROSS STRUCTURE AND APPEARANCE. Skeletal ligaments (L. *ligare:* to bind) are dense connective tissue bands that attach bone to bone and function in concert with muscles and bony geometry to direct and to limit joint motions [17, 23, 78]. Ligaments are critical in optimizing joint function, a role perhaps best illustrated by the disability and degenerative changes that may result from ligament injury. A ligament is often described by its shape (deltoid ligament), bony attachments (glenohumeral ligament), or location relative to a joint (collateral) or joint capsule (intrinisic or extrinsic). The latter classification is particularly interesting because of the implications that the intra- vs. extra-capsular environment may have on the ligament nutrient supply and other factors that may influence a ligament's healing potential (e.g., exposure to synovial fluid).

Grossly, ligaments appear as white, parallel-fibered bands. Distinct borders allow some ligaments to be identified easily, while others are defined less clearly and often blend with surrounding tissues, particularly the joint capsule, along bony attachments. Despite their appearance as single structures, most ligaments do not function as single units to resist a discrete range of joint motion. Rather, at a particular joint position, one portion of a ligament may be taut while another portion is slack [2, 20, 26, 30, 97]. This "functional heterogeneity" is pertinent to our understanding of how particular joint motions may contribute to ligament injury and also implies that certain positions or motions may need to be avoided to optimize ligament healing. Joint position influences anterior cruciate and medial collateral ligament behavior during mechanical testing [93, 97], suggesting that one also must consider the relationship between joint position and ligament orientation when interpreting biomechanical data collected from in vitro ligament tests.

Ignoring specific anatomical differences among ligaments, it is important to recognize that each ligament is actually part of an anatomical and functional complex that includes not only the ligament itself and the bones to which it attaches, but the osteoligamentous insertions that are the transitions between the ligament ends and the bones. Interactions between these regions are critical in determining how the complex reacts to various mechanical stimuli and, clinically, how the complex responds when injured. Descriptions of ligament healing are perhaps more appropriately described as healing of the bone-ligament-bone complex because even grossly uninjured structures may be influenced when the ligament alone is damaged.

HISTOLOGY. With light microscopy, the ligament midsubstance is a fibrous network, with relatively few cells, and an intercellular/interfibrillar matrix. A loose connective tissue layer recently called the epiligament [32], formerly called a paratenon [34], can be seen enveloping the ligament and extending septa into the ligament substance thereby enclosing the collagen bundles into discrete fascicles [32, 99]. The epiligament supports a neurovascular network that occasionally sends small nerve or vascular branches along the septa deep into the ligament [32]. Collagen fascicles and cells orient roughly parallel to the ligament long axis to provide resistance to tensile loads. However, specific collagen and cell orientation, cell number, and cell shape differ within and among ligaments. The following discussion refers specifically to the rabbit anterior cruciate (ACL) and medial collateral ligaments (MCL) unless otherwise stated.

Ligament sections stained with hematoxylin and eosin reveal primarily spindle-shaped fibroblasts lying among the collagen fibrils in the MCL whereas the ACL contains both the spindle-shaped cells and ovoid, fibrocartilage-like cells [10, 55]. The ACL fibroblasts are more numerous [10, 89] and tend to cluster in the loose connective tissue layers between the collagen bundles rather than among the fibrils as in the MCL [47]. Superficial areas of the MCL tend to be more cellular than deep layers [23], suggesting that care must be taken when comparing histological sections to ensure that samples were taken from similar areas of the ligament. It is unclear how this cellular heterogeneity within regions of the same ligament and between different ligaments influences each ligament's mechanical behavior or healing potential.

Transmission electron microscopy (TEM) is often used to examine cell and matrix ultrastructure in greater detail than is possible with the light microscope. With TEM, the MCL and ACL fibroblasts appear metabolically active, with abundant organelles and microvilli that extend into the surrounding areas. ACL fibroblasts send short cellular processes only into areas of small diameter reticular fibers, distant from collagen fibrils. In contrast, the MCL fibrolast processes are more extensive and lie packed among the collagen fibrils, in much closer proximity to the collagen that is being produced [8]. These differences in cell shape and proximity to collagen fibrils may alter the interactions between cells and the surrounding matrix elements, which may, in turn, contribute to the differing mechanical and healing behaviors of these two ligaments.

The collagen fibrils range in diameter from 10–1500 nm, a range that appears to be age-, tissue-, and species-specific [41, 70, 71, 99]. In the human ACL, 85% of the fibrils in a specific cross-sectional area were less than 100 nm in diameter, while in a similar cross-sectional area of the human patellar tendon, 45% of the fibrils had diameters greater than 100 nm [47]. The larger fibrils in the patellar tendon are likely reflected in the greater maximum stress in the tendon compared with the ACL [29].

Frank et al. [41] reported a bimodal distribution of collagen fibril diameters in the rabbit MCL, similar to distributions reported previously in the rat [19] and horse [71]. This distribution shifted during maturation, with a greater percentage of both small- and large-diameter fibrils and fewer intermediate fibrils in older rabbits (Fig. 2.1). This was attributed to the aggregation of intermediate fibrils into larger ones, possibly mediated by increased mechanical stress, and a concomitant degradation of intermediate fibrils into smaller ones. Alternatively, the shift may reflect production of a different collagen type or changes in interactions between the individual collagen molecules leading to the formation of smaller or larger fibrils [41]. These shifts in fibril diameter are thought to be important functionally because of the contribution of collagen size to mechanical strength and elasticity [71], in which the large-diameter fibrils reportedly increase tissue strength and the small fibrils, because of increased surface area and interaction with the surrounding matrix elements, offer the tissue greater elasticity.

In addition to the TEM measurement of fibril diameter, collagen morphology can be examined with polarized light microscopy. In normal ligament, the collagen fibrils assume a characteristic wavy or crimp pattern that can be described by its amplitude and period. MCL and ACL crimp period is similar (45–60 μm, but MCL crimp amplitude (10 μm) is twice that of the ACL (5 μm) [8], giving MCL collagen a wavier appearance. Although its functional significance continues to be investigated, crimp is believed to influence the low load, toe portion of the load-elongation curve and may play an important protective role during rapid loading. Interestingly, restoration of normal crimp has not been reported in healing ligaments. The implications of this in terms of the mechanical behavior of scarred ligament, particularly at low loads, are unclear.

Ligament insertions examined with light microscopy can be divided into two distinct types: direct and indirect. The tibial insertion of the rabbit MCL is a good example of a direct insertion in which, in a skeletally mature animal, most of the collagen fibrils of the ligament course directly into the insertional bone [57]. The remaining fibers that do not attach to bone blend with the periosteal layer of connective tissue found on the bone surface. In contrast, indirect insertions include a zone of fibrocartilage and mineralized fibrocartilage between the ligament and the bone. In this type of insertion, as the ligament approaches the bone, the fibroblasts gradually change from a spindle-shape to more ovoid and the matrix stains more intensely, suggesting that the matrix is becoming cartilaginous. In skeletally mature animals, a line called the tidemark separates clearly the zones of nonmineralized and mineralized fibrocartilage, yet the cell morphology is similar between these areas. The calcified fibrocartilage then blends directly into the lamellar bone itself. The femoral insertion of the rabbit MCL is an indirect insertion.

The morphology of the direct and indirect insertions changes during skeletal maturation [94]. Matyas and colleagues [57] characterized

FIGURE 2.1

Histograms of MCL fibril diameter distributions for 3-month-old (**A**) *and 10-month-old* (**B**) *rabbits. Note the shift in the distribution of fibrils in the older ligaments to greater numbers of small and large diameter fibrils. From Frank et al. Electron microscopic quantification of collagen fibril diameters in the rabbit medial collateral ligament: a baseline for comparison.* Connect. Tissue Res. *19:11–25, 1989, with permission.*

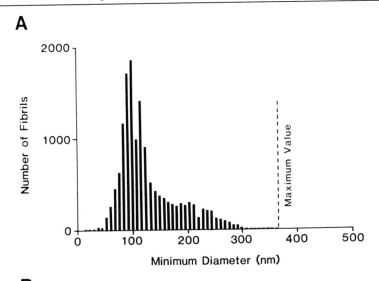

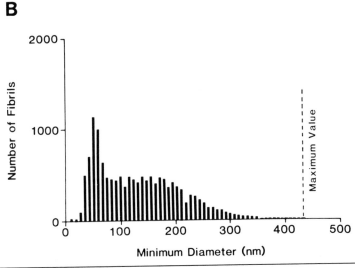

changes in the MCL tibial insertion in rabbits between 1 and 27 months of age. Of particular relevance in terms of the mechanical properties of the ligament complex is their definition of a "functional insertion length," which was the length of the insertion where the ligament collagen fibrils inserted directly into the tibial cortex rather than into the tibial periosteum. The ratio of the functional insertion length to the total histological insertion length increased from 45% in 1-month-old animals to 87% by age 9 months. These histological data support the findings from mechanical tests that describe the changes in ligament strength and the relative frequency of insertional failures during maturation [96].

NEUROVASCULARITY. Historically, ligaments have been described as passive stabilizers to joints [14, 23], yet there is growing evidence that ligaments influence muscle activation patterns through reflex loops originating as sensory endings within the ligament and synapsing on motoneurons within the spinal cord. Symptoms of joint instability following ligament injury than may be attributed not only to the obvious loss of mechanical support but also to the absence of sensory input from the ligament to the muscles [17].

Early research [76] identified primarily the role of periarticular tissues (particularly the articular capsule) in joint proprioception but it was not until the 1950s to 1960s that the contribution of ligament afferents was investigated systematically [36, 69]. From observations of reflex firing of various thigh muscles elicited by MCL stretch in cats, Palmer postulated a "ligamentomuscular reflex" [69] that, to date, has not been refuted. More recently, sensory afferents have been identified in the cat posterior cruciate [77] and anterior cruciate [52] ligaments. Sojka and colleagues [77] noted that fusimotor neurons were reflexively activated by posterior cruciate ligament receptors, suggesting that a spinal cord link exists that may allow ligament afferents to influence muscle activity during normal movements. However, in most of these studies, ligament afferent activity was elicited during passive movements in anesthetized animals and, given the diverse input to the interneuronal and motoneuronal pools within the spinal cord, the contribution that the relatively few ligament afferents may make to the muscle activation patterns remains unknown.

In humans, Abbott and associates [1] described articular receptors as part of a kinetic chain that functions to initiate a defensive strategy to prevent joint injury, but these conclusions were reached without evidence that sensory endings actually existed within the ligament. Schultz et al. [74] and Zimney et al. [101] provided the first such histological evidence of receptors in autopsied human cruciate ligaments. The receptors were found on the ligament surface deep to the synovial membrane and measured 75 μm in diameter and 200 μm in length.

Solomonow and co-workers [78] recorded electrical activity of the hamstrings and quadriceps in human subjects during quasi-isometric knee flexion and extension. By comparing data from subjects free of knee pathology with subjects that had documented ACL deficiency, the researchers concluded that, in the normal subjects, a rapid reflex arc between the ACL and the hamstrings limited anterior tibial translation during maximal quadriceps contraction. This primary reflex arc was disrupted in the ACL-injured subjects and excessive tibial motion was checked only by a secondary, slower reflex that likely originated from the knee joint capsule. One question that remained unanswered by this study was whether the primary reflex arc could respond fast enough during rapid, high load activities to prevent ACL injury. The implications of these studies are especially critical in terms of rehabilitation because, to date, therapeutic modalities aimed at restoring "ligamentomuscular" connections after injury do not exist.

The vascular anatomy of the patellar tendon, ACL, and MCL have been well characterized because of the frequency of ACL and MCL injuries and the widespread use of patellar tendon autografts in ACL reconstructions. While changes in vascular anatomy during healing have been described, quantification of actual blood flow and how the delivery of blood to the tissues may be altered by clinical interventions have not been investigated thoroughly.

The MCL derives its blood flow from the inferior geniculate artery and from the periosteum around the ligament insertions, but no vessels have been observed crossing the actual osteoligamentous junction [23]. As noted previously, the vessels form an extensive network on the ligament surface and a few vascular channels course within interfascicular septa into the ligament midsubstance [23, 32].

Alm and Stromberg [6] and Arnoczky et al. [16] studied the vascularity of the canine anterior and posterior cruciates. Both described a rich vascular network that coursed within the synovial membrane surrounding the ligaments and sent frequent vascular branches into the ligament substance. The central core of both cruciates, however, was poorly supplied, especially the core of the midsubstance compared to the insertional areas. The ligaments' bony attachments contributed little to the overall vascular supply. In general, the PCL was found to be more vascular than the ACL, although recent evidence suggests that the ACL may derive nutrients from synovial fluid [7]. This finding may be particularly important in the healing of ACL injuries in which blood supply has been disrupted.

Biochemistry

The functional behavior of normal ligament cannot be understood fully until examining its biochemical composition. This includes a characterization of collagen type, the nature and quantity of bonds between the collagen fibrils, and the various substances within the ground substance [8]. How these constitutive biochemical elements influence the biomechanical behavior of ligaments is understood incompletely but is certainly the focus of much contemporary research. Collagen biochemistry, in particular, receives tremendous attention and is an area in which understanding is changing rapidly.

Collagen provides an extracellular framework for all multicellular organisms and thus is the most abundant protein in animal tissues [37]. Fourteen collagen types have been identified, forming a broad variety of structures that ranges from the fibrils found in most connective tissues to the sheets constituting basement membranes and the organic exoskeleton of sponges [84]. In tendon, ligament, cartilage, and skin, collagen comprises 65–80% of the tissue mass by dry weight [8]. Type I collagen comprises 88% of the rabbit ACL and 91% of the rabbit MCL, with type III collagen comprising most of the remaining portion [10]. Bray and colleagues [22] recently identified type VI collagen in rabbit MCL, but its relative concentration has not been quantified.

The collagen molecule is an extracellular aggregate of protein subunits (tropocollagen), with each subunit comprised of a triple helix of polypeptide (α) chains [59]. Each polypeptide chain, with its characteristic amino acid sequence, forms a left-handed helix that aligns each third amino acid residue. When three α-chains coil to form a right-handed tropocollagen molecule, the aligned residues are brought to the center of the superhelix. Steric limitations of this configuration require that these aligned, central elements be glycyl residues, thus giving rise to collagen's well-recognized amino acid sequence of Gyl-Xaa-Yaa, where Xaa and Yaa represent the second and third amino acids in the sequence. The triple helical configuration is stabilized by the presence of imino acids in the Xaa and Yaa positions, with 30% of these positions occupied by prolyl and hydroxyprolyl residues [84]. This arrangement also provides for lateral interactions between the outwardly pointed side chains of amino acids in the remaining two-thirds of the Xaa and Yaa positions and other proteins, particularly other triple helices. The glycyl residues, therefore, are important for the close-packed configuration of collagen, and the hydroxyprolyl and prolyl residues give collagen its stiffness and strength by cross-linking with adjacent proteins [8].

α-Chains within each tropocollagen subunit are connected by intramolecular cross-links, while adjacent tropocollagen units are bound by intermolecular cross-links. These connections are critical in determining collagen tensile strength and its resistance to chemical or enzymatic breakdown [8]. After the exocytosis of tropocollagen molecules, lysyl oxidase acts on the terminal amine of lysine and hydroxylysine to form an aldehyde. The aldehyde residues then either condense to form the intramolecular (aldol) bonds, or react with lysine or hydroxylysine to form intermolecular (Schiff-base) bonds. The Schiff-base cross-links have historically been believed to have the greatest significance in soft tissue [47], particularly lysinonorleucine, hydroxylysinonorleucine

(HLNL), and dihydroxylysinonorleucine (DHLNL). A more complex, tetramolecular cross-link, histidinohydroxymerodesmosine (HHMD), may also be important in ligament. With maturation, the reducible Schiff-base cross-links decrease in number and a more stable trivalent cross-link (3-hydroxypyridinium) forms. The functional significance of this change is unknown and the role that such cross-link maturation may play in improving ligament strength during healing needs to be described more thoroughly.

Cross-link profiles differ dramatically between ligament and tendon and are believed to reflect the differing functional loading environments that these tissues experience [10]. When expressed as ratios, ligaments have 12–17 times the DHLNL/HLNL ratio of tendons, and 3–4 times greater (DHLNL + HLNL)/HHMD ratio then tendon [8].

The final major component of the extracellular matrix is the ground substance found between the collagen fibers and around the cells. The ground substance contains glycoproteins (proteoglycans, structural glycoproteins, and glycoslylated collagens) and water (60–80%). Interaction between these components, particularly between proteoglycans and water, plays a critical role in a tissue's viscoelastic mechanical behavior [8, 23]. To date, this area of ligament biochemistry has been examined minimally, but recent important work, particularly that of Bray and colleagues [21, 22], suggests that the constituents of the ground substance may play a much larger part in the overall biology of ligament than has been recognized.

Proteoglycans account for the greatest percentage of the matrix glycoproteins. Each proteoglycan consists of a core protein to which specialized carbohydrate side chains are bonded. The side chains are simply repeating disaccharide units of one amino sugar (galactosamine or glucosamine) and uronic acid [8] that, when bonded together, form glycosaminoglycans called hyaluronate, chondroitin sulfate, or keratan sulfate. The core protein of each proteoglycan has specialized keratan sulfate- or chondroitin sulfate-binding regions, but does not bind directly to hyaluronate. Instead, another protein, the "link protein," serves as an intermediate structure to bind the core protein and hyaluronate. These interactions create a large protein-carbohydrate aggregate that is highly negatively charged and, because the hydroxyl groups of the glycosaminoglycans (GAGs) are highly hydrophilic, is an important site for the binding of water.

Glycosaminoglycan content is greater in the ACL than MCL, and tends to be greater in ligament than tendons [10]. Similar to other constituents, collagen concentration and GAG and water content differ along the length of the rabbit MCL and change during growth and maturation [44]. Water content is generally greatest at the ligament's femoral insertion, and decreases up to 10% toward the tibial end. GAG content, measured by hexosamine concentration, is greatest in both insertions, least in the ligament midsubstance, and tends to decrease with maturation. Conversely, collagen concentration increases with age and is greater in the midsubstance than in the insertions. These findings are consistent with the cellular heterogeneity described previously and may help explain some of the variability reported in the material and structural behaviors of a variety of connective tissues during maturation [80, 85, 95–97].

Fibronectin is another glycoprotein found within the ligament extracellular matrix. It plays an important role in the interaction between cells and the extracellular matrix, particularly in cell to cell adhesion, fibroblast attachment to matrix collagen, and cell migration [8]. In addition, fibronectin facilitates wound healing and is important in mesenchymal cell differentiation and proliferation [88].

Interactions between the various components and the ultrastructure of the extracellular matrix received little attention until a recent study by Bray and colleagues [22]. The researchers examined the "ground substance" of the rabbit MCL, paying particular attention to proteoglycan location and interaction with other matrix components. Through a combination of cationic stains and enzymatic digestion, a network of electron-dense "seams" was found interconnecting cells and subdividing the matrix into irregularly sized compartments. The seams contained varying amounts of microfilaments, microfibrils, and granular material. With high power magnification, the granules appeared to be suspended on the microfilaments and were believed to be large chondroitin sulfate-containing proteoglycans. The beaded microfilaments spiraled through the seams and formed the primary structural framework. The authors believe that these microfilaments are type VI collagen based on this morphology and on a more recent immunogold labeling experiment [21].

These findings by Bray and co-workers are important because of the implications that a fine filamentous network may have on ligament mechanical behavior, particularly the viscoelastic properties. Proteoglycans attached to the microfilament network may provide functional divisions within the matrix and, because of the hydrophilic nature of proteoglycans, water bound within the seams may act as a "lubricant" to facilitate sliding between adjacent collagen fascicles, thereby making the seams an integral part of ligament's viscous element. Proteoglycan-bound water may also act as a diffusion barrier to the flow of certain substances through the tissue, or a diffusion pathway for wastes, nutrients, and chemicals. Yet to be quantified are the relative concentrations of each of these substances within the whole ligament and how these quantities may change during maturation or following alterations in the ligament's mechanical stress state, such as following immobilization.

Mechanical Properties

Ligament function can be assessed with both in vivo and in vitro techniques. A commonly used in vivo technique is to compare joint kinetics and kinematics between normal subjects and subjects with known ligament pathology. The technique is limited, however, by the inability to control extraneous variables, such as damage to surrounding joint structures that may have occurred with the initial ligament injury. Certainly, manipulation of factors that may influence ligament healing cannot be done effectively with this approach.

In vitro testing of cadaveric bone-ligament-bone complexes is perhaps the most common tool used to test ligament mechanical behavior. By applying loads with a calibrated and tightly controlled system, the effects of extraneous variables, such as joint position, can be minimized while the specific variables of interest are accurately and reproducibly quantified. Recent reviews of mechanical testing principles have been written by Butler et al. [27] and Akeson et al. [4] and the reader is referred to these previous works for more in-depth presentations of this topic. The following review will familiarize the reader with the basic terminology and concepts of in vitro mechanical testing that are necessary to understand the subsequent discussions of changes in ligament mechanical properties following exercise and during healing.

A load-elongation curve generated during tensile tests to failure can be divided into three areas: the toe region; the linear region; and a prefailure, nonlinear region. As described previously, the toe region is characterized by relatively large tissue elongation with small magnitude loads and reflects straightening of the collagen crimp and reorientation of the collagen fibrils into line with the applied load. Because only low loads are sustained by the tissue, the toe region may be considered a "buffer" for the ligament to prevent damage to collagen fibrils during rapid loading. When the crimp is completely removed and the fibrils are aligned, the collagen fibrils themselves begin to take up load. Subsequently, load and elongation increase linearly. The slope of this linear region represents the tissue stiffness. As load continues to increase, microfailure of individual collagen bundles begins, resulting once again in greater elongation with only small increases in load. Complete tissue rupture eventually occurs and is accompanied by a precipitous decrease in load. Maximum load refers to the peak load sustained by the tissue. If the ligament fails abruptly at the peak load, maximum and failure loads are the same. If load decreases slightly after maximum and before gross tissue disruption, maximum and failure loads represent unique points on the load-elongation curve. The area under the load-elongation curve is a measure of the energy absorbed by the tissue during loading. Maximum and failure loads, stiffness, and energy absorbed describe a tissue's structural properties and are strongly influenced by tissue geometry.

Normalizing load with respect to tissue cross-sectional area (stress) and elongation relative to initial tissue length (strain) eliminates some influences of tissue geometry and expresses mechanical behavior in terms of the tissue material itself. Stress, strain, and chord or tangent modulus (slope of the stress-strain curve) are referred to as material properties.

Accurate measurement of ligament strain continues to present a challenge to researchers. Because of testing complete bone-ligament-bone complexes and the potential for deforming the bone and testing fixtures, the expression of strain in terms of fixture-to-fixture displacement is invalid. This demands that strain be measured directly on the soft tissue itself. The most common method of strain measurement during in vitro mechanical tests is to track the displacement of dye lines placed on the tissue surface. Tracking can be done with either high-speed cinematography [28, 100] or with an automated video dimension analyzing system [91]. The advantage of this type of strain measurement is the relative ease with which it is implemented. Unfortunately, at low strains typically measured in the toe portion of a load-elongation curve, especially during cyclic testing, this method may introduce very large errors [53]. In addition, because the dye lines are placed only on the tissue surface, the strains cannot reflect deformation occurring deeper in the tissue. Given the heterogeneity documented for ligament morphology [99] and biochemistry [44], surface strains likely do not represent the strain behavior of the entire structure. Unfortunately, at present, a better technique to measure strain during mechanical testing does not exist.

Measurement limitations aside, strain topography has been characterized along the length of various human tissues (isolated semitendinosus and gracilis tendons, bone-patellar tendon-bone, fascia latae) and found to range (at failure) from 6.9–12.9% along the length of the same tissue and from 30.7–52.4% among different tissues [28]. These data have several important implications. First, caution should be observed when interpreting strains collected during isolated ligament or tendon tests because variability in technique will influence the strain measured. Second, attempts to characterize in vivo strains with tools such as Hall effect transducers [18, 73] are likely to be influenced by site-specific variability. Furthermore, because strain is expressed as a change in tissue length relative to an arbitrary initial length, initial length strongly influences the final strain value computed. For example, if the ligament is slack when a transducer is inserted, the transducer may deform before the ligament begins to take up load and elongate, producing an erroneously high strain reading. Conversely, if the ligament is under load prior to transducer placement, strain already present in the tissue is not recorded. Thus, initial ligament condition is critical in the accuracy of strain measurement.

In addition to the ultimate or failure properties, changes in a ligament's behavior over time and with repeated load applications are important. This behavior is the ligament viscoelasticity. If a tissue is viscous, sustained load results in tissue "flow," known as creep (deformation that changes with time). An elastic tissue returns to its original shape or length after load removal and its stress-strain behavior is unchanged with repeated, nondestructive loading cycles. Time-dependent viscoelasticity can be assessed with a creep test in which load is applied to the tissue and maintained while the tissue deforms, or a static load-relaxation test in which a specific deformation is maintained while the change in load sustained by the tissue is measured for a given time interval. The influence of load history on mechanical behavior is measured with a cyclic load-relaxation test. The tissue is repeatedly loaded and unloaded to the same elongation and the load-relaxation is then expressed as the load of the final cycle relative to the initial cycle.

Ligament viscoelastic behavior is also evident in the tissue's strain rate dependency. When loads are applied slowly, the complex usually fails by a bony fracture or disruption of the insertion. During rapid loading, although ligament stiffness and strength increase, bone is much stronger and stiffer, and the ligament actually becomes the weak link. This property is highly age dependent, with younger animals demonstrating significantly greater strain-rate sensitivity than older animals [96].

Failure and cyclic testing of ligaments are equally important in characterizing fully the ligament's mechanical behavior. However, because there is a strong interaction between tissue structure and function, mechanical tests do not stand alone. Rather, the three basic components—morphology, biochemistry, and mechanical behavior—must be considered together to understand ligament biology fully.

Influences of Mechanical Stress on Ligament
One area of ligament biology that remains poorly understood is the mechanism linking a ligament's mechanical loading environment and its cellular processes. How do ligament fibroblasts know to alter collagen production when the ligament sustains an altered load or load history? Historically, one approach taken to investigate this relationship has been to manipulate the ligament's load through exercise or joint immobilization and then evaluate changes in ligament morphology or mechanical behavior. Use of this approach assumes that the ligament load is actually influenced by the specific exercise or immobilization imposed. It is unclear, for example, whether treadmill running with dogs increases the load on the medial collateral ligament. Equivocal conclusions, particularly from studies examining exercise and ligament adaptation, suggest that more work must be done to link joint kinematics with the actual load sustained by the particular ligament and in the specific animal model of interest.

Exercise-related changes in the MCL have been reported in dogs [79] and rats [81]. Daily bouts of moderately intense treadmill running increased MCL failure load by 7% in rats after 10 weeks of training and by 12% in the dogs after 6 weeks of training. In these dogs, lateral collateral ligament hydroxyproline levels increased by 15% in the exercised animals compared with sedentary controls. These findings suggest that the MCL can respond to exercise, although it is unclear whether exercise-related changes in load, blood flow, or systemic factors provide the actual adaptive stimulus.

Tipton and co-workers [79, 81] also quantified immobilization-related changes in the rat and canine MCL. MCL strength decreased 18% in the rats and 40% in the dogs after 6 weeks of immobilization. Immobilization did not change lateral collateral ligament hydroxyproline content in the dogs. A comprehensive examination of immobilization-induced changes in primate ligament strength was undertaken by Noyes [64]. Rhesus monkeys were maintained in full-body casts for 8 weeks then immediately euthanized or allowed 5 or 12 months of free cage activity. Mechanical tests of the femur-ACL-tibia were completed as well as analysis of whole bone volume and ash weight, and histological examination of the ACL insertions and surrounding bone. Eight weeks of immobilization resulted in a 39% decrease in complex load to failure. If the immobilization was followed with 5 months of reconditioning, ACL failure load improved but remained 21% less than controls. Twelve months of reconditioning improved failure load to within 9% of normal. Energy absorbed to failure changed similarly. Complex stiffness significantly decreased during immobilization, but regained a normal value after 5 or 12 months of reconditioning. The site of failure also appeared to be influenced by immobilization. In normal controls, most failures occurred through the ligament midsubstance. After 8 weeks of immobilization, one-third of the complexes failed by femoral avulsion. Five months of remobilization resulted in 27% tibial avulsions, whereas 12 months of reconditioning returned the failure mode to normal.

Histological examination of the ACL insertions and surrounding bone revealed changes that paralleled the failure mode data. Immobilization resulted in marked resorption of the tibial and femoral cortical bone but the ACL insertions themselves appeared to change only minimally. The cortical loss was reversed in the remobilized groups, with normal histological appearance after 12 months of recovery. Ash weights of the femur, tibia, and fibula did not differ significantly between normal and immobilized specimens.

In the same study, Noyes examined the effects of cage confinement alone on the femur-ACL-tibia complex mechanical behavior. The complex load and energy at failure were evaluated in animals confined from 10–218 weeks; small but statistically significant negative correlations existed between the mechanical measures and duration of captivity.

These data emphasize the exquisite sensitivity of the bone-ligament-bone unit to disuse. Furthermore, the findings suggest that this sensitivity must be considered when describing caged controls as representative of a normal population of unconfined animals.

Similar immobilization-induced changes in the rabbit MCL have been reported [92]. Failure loads 29–31% of normal control values resulted after 9 or 12 weeks of immobilization. Stiffness decreased in a time-dependent manner, with a greater decrease in ligaments immobilized 12 weeks compared with those immobilized 9 weeks. Material properties of the bone-MCL-bone complex were also affected detrimentally by immobilization, with stress at failure only 48% of normal after 9 weeks of immobilization and 38% of normal after 12 weeks. Remobilization for 9 weeks returned material properties to normal, but structural measures remained significantly lower than normal controls.

The work of Noyes [64], Woo et al. [92], and earlier work by Laros et al. [54] that noted resorption of insertional bone of the canine MCL and LCL, lead to several important conclusions regarding immobilization-related changes in ligament mechanical behavior. First, the bone-ligament-bone complex changes rapidly during immobilization, with bone resorption accounting for a substantial change in the complex mechanical behavior and histological appearance. Second, normal ligament properties are regained after remobilization at a much slower rate than they are lost during immobilization. For primates, 12 months of reconditioning were needed to regain strength lost during 8 weeks of immobilization. Third, the rates at which bone and ligament respond appear to differ, suggesting that the mechanism responsible for triggering cellular response may have a tissue-specific sensitivity. These implications are far reaching in terms of how ligament injuries are managed to minimize loss of surrounding tissue without compromising healing of the injured structures.

Vailas and colleagues [82] investigated the effects of immobilization or exercise on the aerobic metabolism of rat tendon and ligament. Oxygen consumption of the patellar tendon and MCL were assessed by quantifying cytochrome oxidase activity, an enzyme related to aerobic metabolism in the tissues. After 6 or 8 weeks of immobilization, cytochrome oxidase activity decreased 36%, whereas exercising for 12 or 16 weeks increased the same enzyme level less than 10% relative to sedentary controls. These data suggest that ligament and tendon may have dramatically different thresholds to specific changes in activity, with an apparently greater sensitivity to decreased loading, consistent with the findings of Noyes [64] and Woo et al. [92] discussed previously. To date, no hypothesis has been developed to explain these differing sensitivities.

Changes in ligament mechanical behavior after immobilization imply that ligament structure or biochemistry also changes. Amiel and colleagues [13] reported that 9 weeks of immobilization increased rabbit MCL collagen synthesis and degradation 11% and 14%, respectively, resulting in only a slight decrease in MCL collagen mass. If immobilization continued for an additional 3 weeks (12 weeks total), MCL collagen degradation exceeded synthesis and a 29% decrease in total collagen mass resulted. The ACL was more sensitive to the same immobilization protocol, with a significant 15% loss in total collagen mass after 9 weeks of immobilization that increased to 25% after 12 weeks [12]. In contrast to the ligaments' mechanical properties, total collagen mass returned to normal with a remobilization period that was similar to the duration of immobilization.

An immobilization-related increase in the concentration of immature collagen cross-links in periarticular tissues [3] is consistent with the increased turnover rate and abundance of new collagen in the MCL. That is, changes in total collagen mass do not account for the entire immobilization-induced loss of ligament strength but the abundance of immature collagen suggested by the cross-link profile may be partly responsible for the decreased strength of immobilized ligaments.

TEM suggests that ACL ultrastructure is affected more dramatically by immobilization than is the ultrastructure of the MCL [62]. Immobilization induced a shift in ACL fibroblast morphology from an ovoid shape with short processes, to a spindle-shaped cell with extensive cytoplasmic processes, similar to the typical fibroblast morphology of the MCL. ACL fibroblasts became closely apposed with pericellular collagen after immobilization. Increased lysosomal vacuoles suggestive of enhanced degradation and increased rough endoplasmic reticulum suggestive of increased production of extracellular proteins were noted in both the ACL and MCL, consistent with the increased collagen turnover noted previously by Amiel and associates [13].

From these comprehensive investigations, immobilization-related changes in ligament can be characterized. Diminished mechanical stress increases collagen turnover in the ligament, resulting in an abundance of immature collagen fibrils and collagen cross-links. Osteopenia occurs as well, with increased resorption of the insertional bone. These changes decrease ligament complex structural and material properties in a time-dependent fashion, with increased immobilization duration increasing the detrimental changes. Total collagen mass returns to normal at the same rate it decreased, but return of the complex mechanical behavior requires a much longer recovery period. The insertions and insertional bone appear to recover at a much slower rate than the ligament midsubstance.

HEALING

Ligament sprains are the most common joint injury and account for 25–40% of all knee injuries [35]. Twenty percent of knee ligament injuries ultimately require operative treatment [63]. Despite this substantial morbidity, clinical management of ligament injuries has been based historically on a few basic studies [14]. It is only recently that well-controlled experiments have provided more meaningful data to clinicians and sports medicine specialists. Nonetheless, a lack of data persists, especially in the area of therapeutic interventions to enhance ligament healing.

A major problem that plagued early animal studies of ligament healing was how to create a ligament injury that was both reproducible and injured only the ligament of interest. Early on, most ligament injuries were caused by manual joint manipulation [51, 60, 61]. The compounding influences of such diffuse injuries were recognized and subsequent experiments studied injuries created simply by transecting the ligament with a scalpel [33, 65, 67]. Unfortunately, a clean scalpel cut does not mimic accurately the clinical ligament rupture that leaves the ligament ends frayed or "mopped." This led to the development of another method in which a braided metal suture or blunt metal probe was passed under the ligament and pulled abruptly through the tissue.

Using the rabbit MCL model, Walsh and Frank [86] quantified the extent of the injury created by a clean scalpel cut vs. braided suture rupture with polarized light and scanning electron microscopy. They concluded that while both methods were reproducible in terms of the damage pattern, depth in the ligament, and location, the wire suture technique produced more extensive damage that mirrored more closely the clinical condition. More recently, Weiss and associates [87] demonstrated histologically that ligament rupture caused by pulling a rigid metal bar through the MCL midsubstance induced insertional injuries as well as the midsubstance rupture. Although this type of injury may be more relevant clinically than the methods examined by Walsh and Frank, it is perhaps a less well-controlled technique that may produce a range of injuries to the ligament complex. These data are pertinent particularly when comparing findings between studies that use different techniques to induce ligament injury.

Ligament healing is similar to wound healing in that the process is basically one of initial inflammation followed by proliferation and scar remodeling or maturation. Age-, species-, and ligament-specificity influence the healing process, as do systemic factors such as nutritional status and diabetes mellitus, and local factors, including mechanical stress and blood flow [14]. The description that follows deals specifically with healing of the rabbit MCL.

Histology of Ligament Healing
Immediately following a midsubstance ligament rupture, blood clots in the space between the retracted ligament ends. Within hours, inflammatory fluid begins to collect in the area [14]. Within 3 days, the ligament

ends are bridged by a fragile fibrinous scar [45] and the overlying fascia is adhered to the ligament, helping to contain the accumulating fluid around the injury site. Polymorphonuclear leukocytes and lymphocytes increase in number, and monocytes and macrophages predominate within 3 days [39]. These early events can be attributed to the release of histamine from platelets which, in turn, causes vasodilation, increased capillary permeability, and the influx of fluid and inflammatory cells [14]. By 10 days after injury, edema and hypervascularity encompass the entire medial knee and the scar contains significantly more water than normal [40].

Reconstitution of the extracellular matrix begins within 1 week of injury. Large, active-appearing fibroblasts with abundant rough endo-plasmic reticulum are visible with electron microscopy and are likely responsible for the matrix synthesis [14]. New fibrils within the matrix apparently provide structural strength by 10 days because the scar can be handled without disruption [40].

Decreased edema and increased scar density occur during the proliferative healing phase. Hypercellularity persists, with fibroblasts beginning to predominate [14]. With polarized light microscopy, the matrix appears disorganized early in the proliferative phase but organization improves as healing continues. Elastin is also present in the extracellular matrix during this phase [14].

Between 6 and 24 weeks, cellularity and vascularity decrease, although both remain greater in the scar than in normal ligament [23]. Fibroblasts are large and arranged randomly throughout the scar, with no observed tendency toward a more mature spindle shape and longitudinal orientation [40]. Cellular changes indicative of scar maturation are present by 12 months and continue to approach normality for up to 30 months, but to date, no study has documented an end to scar remodeling and a return of the ligament to "normal" [40]. Tibial and femoral insertions return to normal histologically between 24 and 52 weeks after injury.

Examination with TEM reveals that collagen fibril diameters differ between normal ligament and ligament scars (Fig. 2.2). Improvement in ligament strength and stiffness with longer healing duration might suggest that collagen fibril diameter increases during healing. However, Frank and associates [43] have found recently that small-diameter collagen fibrils are seen from 3–40 weeks after injury in MCL midsub-stance scars. The mean fibril minimum diameter was significantly less in scars than in the contralateral, unoperated ligaments and did not change over the healing interval. Ligament mechanical properties were also tested in the same study and found to correlate poorly with mean fibril minimum diameter ($r^2 < 0.61$ for strength and stiffness measures). These findings differ from previous work of Parry et al. [70] and Flint et al. [38] that suggest a close relationship between collagen fibril diameter and

FIGURE 2.2

Transverse TEM micrographs of a control MCL and a 40-week MCL scar demonstrating differences in collagen fibril diameters. From Frank et al. Collagen fibril diameters in the healing adult rabbit medial collateral ligament. Connect. Tissue Res. *27:251–263, 1992, with permission.*

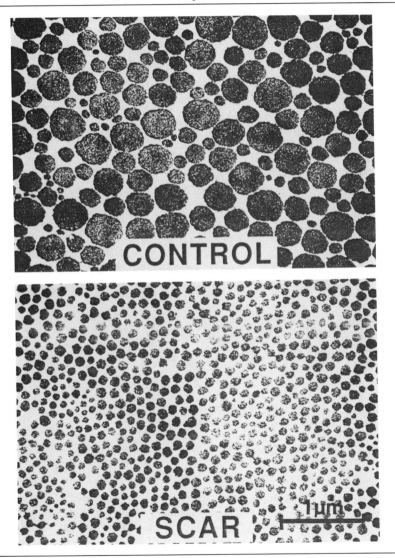

mechanical behavior of normal skin, ligament, and tendon, although the difference may represent a unique contribution of collagen in normal vs. healing ligaments.

Alignment of the new collagen fibrils changes during healing. Frank and colleagues [42] used scanning electron microscopy and an automated image analysis system to quantify the matrix fibril alignment in healing rabbit MCLs. Fibrils in the scar were found to align more randomly than fibrils of the unoperated, contralateral MCL after 3 or 6 weeks of healing (Fig. 2.3). By 14 weeks of healing, significant remodeling improved fibril alignment such that injured and contralateral ligaments were oriented similarly. The improved collagen alignment

FIGURE 2.3
*Scanning electron micrographs of a **normal MCL** and a 3-week MCL scar showing the differences in fibril alignment. Below each micrograph is the corresponding rose diagram that illustrates fibril orientation. Each petal of the rose diagram represents the relative number of fibrils in each of the 15° bands from 0–180°. The ligament longitudinal axis corresponds to 90°. From Frank et al. A quantitative analysis of matrix alignment in ligament scars: a comparison of movement versus immobilization in an immature rabbit model.* J. Orthop. Res. 9:219–227, 1991, with permission.

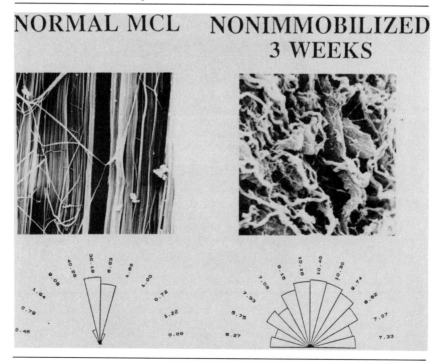

may influence ligament mechanical behavior, particularly at low loads, although this relationship has not been well established.

Biochemistry of Ligament Healing

In addition to the aforementioned morphological changes in collagen that occur during healing, the type of collagen being produced, its concentration, and rate of synthesis and degradation are important biochemical variables during healing. Amiel and associates [9] studied these changes during 40 weeks of healing in an unrepaired rabbit MCL injury model. Total collagen mass was 16% greater in the scar after 3 weeks, and continued to increase for 40 weeks, at which time it was 44% greater than normal. Collagen concentration (mass per unit dry weight), however, was 12–17% less in scars between 3 and 14 weeks of healing and returned to normal by 40 weeks. These changes in the relative amounts of collagen were reflected in the synthesis and degradation rates. Immediately after ligament transection collagen synthesis increased and, after 3 weeks of healing, was 10% greater than normal. Over the same healing interval, degradation was 5% greater in scars. The relatively greater increase in synthesis resulted in a net increased collagen mass after 3 weeks. From 3–6 weeks of healing, synthesis and degradation were essentially equal, and 8% greater than normal. Synthesis again exceeded degradation from 6–14 weeks, but both returned essentially to normal levels by 40 weeks. These data indicate that, in the rabbit MCL, collagen turnover (synthesis and degradation) is greatest during the early healing intervals and slowly approaches normal as healing progresses.

The expression of total collagen mass does not reflect differences in the relative amounts of type I and type III collagen. When examined, ligament scar was found to contain more type III collagen (40% after 14 weeks of healing) than normal ligament (less than 10%) [9]. The production of type III collagen increased steadily from the time of injury, peaked at 14 weeks, then decreased until 40 weeks. The increase in total collagen mass from 14–40 weeks suggested that the decreased type III production was concomitant with an increased production of type I collagen. Even after 40 weeks of healing, the type III: type I ratio remained elevated relative to normal ligaments [9] despite the return of collagen mass to normal.

Immature cross-links accompany the changes in collagen type. DHLNL cross-links increase significantly during early healing, increasing the ratio of (DHLNL/HLNL) for 6 weeks following injury. The ratio decreases to normal control values by 40 weeks [46].

Mechanical Properties of Healing Ligaments

Geometrically, MCLs that have healed for 3 weeks have a cross-sectional area almost four times greater than normal. After 3 weeks, cross-sectional area decreases but remains almost twice as large after 14 weeks and no further decrease is seen up to 40 weeks after injury [46].

Load-deformation curves of healing MCLs are significantly different than normal, with decreased stiffness and failure loads in the healing ligaments. Failure load improves between 3- and 14-week healing intervals, but remains only 60% of normal after 14 weeks. No further improvement occurs between 14 and 40 weeks, although at the later interval, most of the failures are femoral fractures, suggesting that the MCL midsubstance is stronger than the failure loads indicate. Recovery of the material properties is similar to structural behavior, with improvement until 14 weeks, then a plateau with little change in maximum stress or strain up to 40 weeks of healing [46].

The ACL does not recover its mechanical properties after injury as well as the MCL, with mechanical behavior of ACL scars inferior after more than 1 yr of healing. The first systematic study of canine ACL healing was reported by O'Donoghue in 1966 [66], in which the ACL tibial attachment was partially or completely transected, and nonrepaired or repaired. Inflammation and necrosis of the injured sites marked the early healing phase, with the ends of the unrepaired, completely transected ligaments retracting and never regaining continuity. Collagen was laid down in the scars of the repaired ligaments, but the scar was minimal, in contrast to the hypertrophic response typically seen in MCL healing. In the repaired ligaments, tension placed on the repair by the sutures appeared to influence healing. Ligaments repaired with increased tension healed poorly, while healing improved if tension across the repair approximated more closely the tension in an uninjured ACL.

Despite the significant findings of O'Donoghue and colleagues, their studies are not without controversy, however, because the injuries investigated were insertional, rather than midsubstance. Subsequent work demonstrated that insertional injuries account for less than 5% of ACL injuries and heal better than midsubstance injuries [75]. The practical relevance of the previous findings, therefore, is questionable.

Factors Influencing Healing

Several factors may influence the rate and extent of healing following ligament rupture, including age, general health (e.g., diabetes, cardio-vascular disease), nutritional status, and related injuries, such as a fracture, which may have occurred at the time of the ligamentous injury. While these variables may be difficult to control in clinical practice, most can be monitored in the research laboratory allowing other factors to be manipulated. Specifically, three factors are most commonly investigated: repair vs. nonrepair, joint immobilization vs. free use of the involved extremity, and degree of joint stability or instability related to simultane-ous injury to other ligaments.

The question of repair or nonrepair is not new. Clayton and Weir [33] transected MCLs and lateral collateral ligaments in dogs, then compared histologically and mechanically the effects of suturing the cut ends with leaving the ligament ends free. All animals were immobilized postoperatively for intervals from 4 days to 9 weeks. The authors reported that sutured ligaments regained "normal" strength after 6 weeks of healing, whereas nonrepaired ligaments continued to be the weak link in the bone-ligament-bone complex. Many confounding influences made data interpretation difficult, however. Because of significant interanimal differences, Clayton and Weir compared repaired and unrepaired ligaments only within the same animal. Their definition of "normal" strength, therefore, did not reflect a numerical normality but was evaluated by when failure mode was similar to the insertional failures of nonoperative controls. The repaired bone-MCL-bone complexes failed by insertional disruption after 6 weeks thus were judged to have "normal" strength when, in fact, the failure load did not reflect the ultimate strength of the ligament scar. Recent evidence suggests that ligament transection unloads the ligament insertions in a manner similar to the decreased loads caused by immobilization [58]. This decreased mechanical stress may stimulate resorption of the insertional bone, suggesting that the complex failure loads reported by Clayton and Weir may actually have been a measure of when the scar became stronger than the bone. The effect of immobilization was thus an important covariate, especially if bony or insertional failure was deemed "normal."

Apposition of torn ligament ends has been investigated more recently in a rabbit MCL model [31]. MCLs were transected with either a noncontact injury, in which a 4-mm gap was removed from the ligament midsubstance, or a 4-mm Z-plasty, in which the injury was created by a 4-mm long sagittal Z cut and the ligament ends resutured. The model incorporates not only repair of the injury, but also looks at the effect created by the scar actually having to fill in a hole or defect created by removal of actual ligament midsubstance. Morphological and biomechanical evidence of healing was described after 3, 6, 14, and 40 weeks of healing.

Histologically, both gap models were similar to previous work, which suggested that ligaments heal with scar rather than with ligament [45]. After 3 weeks of healing, the developing scar was hypercellular and incorporated the old ligament ends into the scar mass (Fig. 2.4). Even after 40 weeks of healing, the scars remained hypercellular and disorganized, with the noncontact gap having more disorganized, hypercellular areas than the contact gaps. The healing contact gaps were larger at the early intervals, suggesting that the scar mass was laid down on top of and around the cut ligament ends. In the gap injury, cross-sectional area did not exceed that of the contact scar until 6 weeks after injury, indicating that more time was needed to fill in the large defect created by removing the piece of ligament.

FIGURE 2.4

Histological sections stained with hematoxylin and eosin from **gap** *and* **contact** *scar after 3, 6, or 14 weeks of healing.* **Arrowheads** *indicate swirls of cells that form imperfections within the scar. Note that the fibers and cells are more oriented in the 3-week-old contact scars and that orientation improves in both injury models with increased healing duration. The* **arrow** *is parallel to the ligament longitudinal axis, (56 × magnification).*

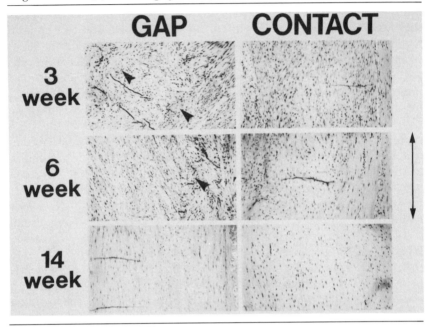

Biomechanical data paralleled the histological findings, with failure loads of the gaps improved over time, but only the contact gaps regained failure loads similar to the unoperated contralateral MCLs after 40 weeks. Maximum stress of both gaps remained significantly less than the contralaterals at all intervals, suggesting that although the structural mechanical properties improved faster in the contact gaps, the improvement in material properties did not differ between the injury types. The differences between structural and material behaviors paralleled the changes in ligament geometry. The contact gaps were stronger because they were bigger but, when load was normalized to size, the material itself was no different than in the noncontact injuries.

Findings of this study suggest that apposition of the damaged ligament ends contributes to a more rapid recovery of ligament structural behavior. The presence of old ligament apparently enhances return of these structural properties, with gap injuries that are filled with true "scar" being mechanically inferior to contacts. Interesting as well was the finding that MCL viscoelastic behavior in both injury models returned to contralateral values within 14 weeks. Thus, ligament low-load behavior returns to normal relatively soon, whereas the ultimate properties continue to be abnormal for longer durations.

The role of joint motion in ligament healing has been investigated extensively [42, 68, 72, 79, 83, 90]. Early studies of ligament healing suggested that limbs with damaged ligaments should be immobilized to optimize healing. However, the detrimental effects of immobilization on surrounding tissues [5, 13] led to investigations of whether joint motion, which may prevent atrophy of associated joint structures, compromises ligament healing.

O'Donoghue et al. [65–67] studied the effects of repair vs. nonrepair and immobilization vs. free activity on healing of the lateral collateral ligaments (LCLs) and ACLs in dogs. Their findings illustrate important differences between LCL and ACL healing. LCLs healed by a sequence of events similar to that described previously for the MCL: inflammation, proliferation, and remodeling. Histologically, repaired LCLs healed faster with more organized scar than did nonrepaired ligaments. Tensile strength improved in both repaired and nonrepaired ligaments but after 10 weeks of healing, all scars continued to be weaker than contralateral control ligaments.

The ACL data were quite different in that no transected ligament reunited unless the ligament was repaired regardless of whether the limb was immobilized postoperatively. The femoral stump of one nonrepaired ligament reattached to the synovial covering of the femur but without crossing the joint. Marked retraction in the unrepaired ligaments was noted within 10 days of transection preventing the apposition of the cut ends from ever occurring. Repair did not guarantee healing, however, as 39% of the repaired ACLs resorbed completely within 24 months. The authors attributed this to improper tensioning of the sutures at the time of repair, with increased or decreased tension increasing the likelihood of resorption. Tensile strength of repaired ACLs improved with time, although all healing ligaments remained weaker than normal after 4 yr of healing. Unfortunately, no data were collected from a repaired-nonimmobilized group, therefore the question of whether free activity compromised ACL repair was not answered with this study.

Other factors appear to influence the ACL's healing potential. The ligament is contained within the knee joint capsule but is not normally in contact with the synovial fluid of the joint because of the overlying synovial membrane. When the ligament is injured, however, the synovial membrane often tears, allowing synovial fluid to surround the damaged ligament ends. Given that synovial fluid decreases fibroblast proliferation in culture [15] the synovial fluid that bathes the ligament ends may inhibit healing. Alternatively, Amiel and co-workers [11] demonstrated increased collagenase in ACL and meniscal injuries, suggesting that the ACL itself may be responsible for its own degradation by releasing active collagenase to break down the surrounding collagen matrix.

The integrity of other supporting structures about a joint may influence a ligament's ability to heal by limiting the mechanical stress placed on the damaged structure. For example, Inoue and associates [50] compared valgus and varus laxity between intact canine knees and knees in which the MCL or ACL alone were cut or the MCL and ACL were both cut. Valgus laxity increased 21% in the isolated MCL cuts, 186% in isolated ACL transections, and nearly 300% in the combined lesions. These data illustrate the effect that combined ligament lesions have on the range of extraneous motions that the MCL and ACL may experience during healing. MCL healing in rats has been found to benefit from active motion only when the secondary supporting structures of the joint are intact [25, 48]. If the joint is unstable, such as when the MCL and ACL are both cut, MCL healing is affected detrimentally. The loss of stability following an isolated MCL injury is not dramatic and may explain why MCL injuries can heal without joint immobilization, whereas an isolated ACL injury produces a greater joint instability that may limit healing.

MCLs from an experiment similar to that of Inoue et al. [50] were mechanically tested to evaluate the effects of ACL transection on MCL healing [98]. Dogs were divided into three groups: MCL transection only, MCL transection with partial ACL transection, and complete MCL and ACL transections. After 12 weeks of healing, failure loads were 79–98% of control values for the three groups. However, because cross-sectional areas of healing ligaments were also significantly greater than controls, failure stress of isolated MCL injuries was 52% of controls, complete MCL with partial ACL transections regained only 45% of the control strength, and complete MCL and ACL lesions resulted in MCL strength returning to only 14% of controls. Varus-valgus knee laxity returned to control values in the isolated MCL and MCL-partial ACL injuries, but the complete MCL/ACL-injured knees remained three times more lax than controls after 14 weeks of healing. In addition to the mechanical data, the authors noted marked deterioration of the joint surfaces and periarticular osteophyte formation in the knees in which both ligaments were transected.

In a similar study using rabbits [24], MCL healing was examined when ACL transection was combined with joint immobilization. Following 3, 6, or 14 weeks of healing, joint immobilization appeared to limit the joint destruction that is often associated with ACL deficiency, but immobilization inhibited improvement of the MCL structural strength and stiffness. Conversely, although the MCLs of the unstable, nonimmobilized knees recovered significantly greater failure loads than the unstable, immobilized MCLs, the cartilage surfaces demonstrated marked degeneration, particularly 14 weeks after injury. In terms of material properties, both groups recovered less than 10% of the failure stress of the sham controls.

Several conclusions can be drawn from these studies. First, in the canine, the ACL appears to provide substantial support to the knee even in the absence of the MCL. Second, in the dog, an unrepaired, transected MCL will regain 50% of the failure stress of controls if the ACL remains intact, but maximum stress will return to only 14% of control if the ACL is transected. In the rabbit, maximum stress of the MCL returned to less than 10% of sham controls in the ACL-deficient knee. Third, the findings illustrate the importance of ligamentous support in limiting degeneration of articular surfaces. In the rabbit, immobilization was useful in limiting joint surface destruction but inhibited return of the MCL mechanical strength.

The numerous and varied studies that have examined ligament healing can be summarized with a few general points. First, no ligament has been found to heal with normal ligament tissue but rather, each heals with scar that remains different than noninjured tissue even after extended healing intervals. Second, the unique qualities of the ACL and MCL preclude generalizing about the advantages and disadvantages of repair and restriction of joint motion on ligament healing. Isolated MCL injuries tend to heal without repair or restriction of joint motion, whereas even repaired ACLs in immobilized joints do not tend to heal as well. Just as the morphological and biochemical characteristics of normal ligaments differ, the healing behaviors of the MCL and ACL are quite unique.

These differences provide a challenge to the investigators studying the link between mechanical stimuli and cellular responses. Whatever the transduction mechanism, it must be general enough to provide for the wide anatomical and functional ranges among ligaments. By the same token, the mechanism must also be sensitive enough to account for the unique responses of each ligament.

ACKNOWLEDGMENTS

We gratefully acknowledge The Alberta Children's Hospital Foundation, Zimmer Berlett, The Arthritis Society, The Alberta Heritage Foundation for Medical Research, and The Medical Research Council of Canada for their ongoing support of this work.

REFERENCES

1. Abbott, L. C., J. B. Sanders, F. C. Bost, and C. E. Anderson. Injuries to the ligaments of the knee joint. *J. Bone Joint Surg.* 26:503–521, 1944.
2. Ahmed, A. M., A. Hyder, D. L. Burke, and K. H. Chan. In vitro ligament tension pattern in the flexed knee in passive loading. *J. Orthop Res.* 5:217–230, 1987.
3. Akeson, W. H., D. Amiel, G. L. Mechanic, S. L.-Y. Woo, F. L. Harwood, and M. L.

Hamer. Collagen cross-linking alterations in joint contractures: changes in the reducible cross-links in periarticular connective tissue collagen after nine weeks of immobilization. *Connect. Tissue Res.* 5:15–19, 1977.

4. Akeson, W. H., C. B. Frank, D. Amiel, and S. L.-Y. Woo. Ligament biology and biomechanics. G. Finerman (ed). *Symposium on Sports Medicine. The Knee.* St. Louis: CV Mosby Co, 1985, pp. 111–151.

5. Akeson, W. H., S.L.-Y. Woo, D. Amiel, and J. V. Matthews. Biomechanical and biochemical changes in the periarticular connective tissue during contracture development in the immobilized rabbit knee. *Connect. Tissue Res.* 2:315–323, 1974.

6. Alm, A., and B. Stromberg. Vascular anatomy of the patellar and cruciate ligaments. A microangiographic and histologic investigation in the dog. *Acta Chir. Scand. (Suppl.)* 445:25–35, 1974.

7. Amiel, D., M. F. Abel, J. B. Kleiner, and W. H. Akeson. Synovial fluid nutrient delivery in the diarthrial joint: an analysis of rabbit knee ligaments. *J. Orthop. Res.* 4:90–95, 1986.

8. Amiel, D., E. Billings, and W. H. Akeson. Ligament structure, chemistry, and physiology. D. D. Daniel, W. H. Akeson, and J. J. O'Conner (ed). *Knee Ligaments: Structure, Function, Injury, and Repair.* New York: Raven Press, 1990, pp. 77–91.

9. Amiel, D., C. B. Frank, F. L. Harwood, W. H. Akeson, and J. B. Kleiner. Collagen alteration in medial collateral ligament healing in a rabbit model. *Connect. Tissue Res.* 16:357–366, 1987.

10. Amiel, D., C. Frank, F. Harwood, J. Fronek, and W. Akeson. Tendons and ligaments: a morphological and biochemical comparison. *J. Orthop. Res.* 1:257–265, 1984.

11. Amiel, D., K. K. Ishizue, F. L. Harwood, L. Kitabayashi, and W. H. Akeson. Injury of the ACL: the role of collagenase in ligament degeneration. *J. Orthop. Res.* 7:486–493, 1989.

12. Amiel, D., H. von Schroeder, and W. H. Akeson. The response of ligaments to stress deprivation and stress enhancement. Biochemical studies. D. D. Daniel, W. H. Akeson, and J. J. O'Conner (eds). *Knee Ligaments: Structure, Function, Injury, and Repair.* New York: Raven Press, 1990, pp. 329–336.

13. Amiel, D., S. L.-Y. Woo, F. L. Harwood, and W. H. Akeson. The effect of immobilization on collagen turnover in connective tissue: a biochemical-biomechanical correlation. *Acta Orthop. Scand.* 53:325–332, 1982.

14. Andriacchi, T., P. Sabiston, K. DeHaven, L. Dahners, S. Woo, C. Frank, B. Oakes, R. Brand, and J. Lewis. Ligament: injury and repair. S.L.-Y. Woo and J. A. Buckwalter (eds). *Injury and Repair of the Musculoskeletal Soft Tissues.* Park Ridge, IL: American Academy of Orthopaedic Surgeons, 1988, pp. 103–128.

15. Andrish, J., and R. Holmes. Effects of synovial fluid on fibroblasts in tissue culture. *Clin. Orthop. Relat. Res.* 138:279–283, 1979.

16. Arnoczky, S. P., R. M. Rubin, and J. L. Marshall. Microvasculature of the cruciate ligaments and its response to injury. *J. Bone Joint Surg.* 61A:1221–1229, 1979.

17. Barrack, R. L., and H. B. Skinner. The sensory function of knee ligaments. D. D. Daniel, W. H. Akeson, and J. J. O'Conner (eds). *Knee Ligaments: Structure, Function, Injury, and Repair.* New York: Raven Press, 1990, pp. 95–113.

18. Beynnon, B. D., J. G. Howe, M. H. Pope, R. J. Johnson, and B. C. Fleming. The measurement of anterior cruciate ligament strain in vivo. *Int. Orthop.* 16:1–12, 1992.

19. Binkley, J. M., and M. Peat. The effects of immobilization on the ultrastructure and mechanical properties of the medial collateral ligament of rats. *Clin. Orthop. Relat. Res.* 203:301–308, 1986.

20. Blankevoort, L., R. Huiskes, and A. deLange. Recruitment of knee joint ligaments. *Trans. A.S.M.E.* 113:94–103, 1991.

21. Bray, D. F., R. C. Bray, and C. B. Frank. Ultrastructural immunolocalization of type VI collagen and chondroitin sulphate in ligament. *J. Orthop. Res.* (in press).

22. Bray, D. F., C. B. Frank, and R. C. Bray. Cytochemical evidence for a proteoglycan-

associated filamentous network in ligament extracellular matrix. *J. Orthop. Res.* 8:1–12, 1990.

23. Bray, R., C. Frank, and A. Miniaci. Structure and function of diarthrodial joints. J. B. McGinty (ed). *Operative Arthroscopy.* New York: Raven Press, 1991, pp. 79–123.

24. Bray, R. C., N. G. Shrive, C. B. Frank, and D. D. Chimich. The early effects of joint immobilization on medial collateral ligament healing in an ACL-deficient knee: a gross anatomic and biomechanical investigation in the adult rabbit model. *J. Orthop. Res.* 10:157–166, 1992.

25. Burroughs, P., and L. E. Dahners. The effect of enforced exercise on the healing of ligament injuries. *Am. J. Sports Med.* 18:376–378, 1990.

26. Butler, D. L. Anterior cruciate ligament: its normal response and replacement. *J. Orthop. Res.* 7:910–921, 1989.

27. Butler, D. L., E. S. Grood, F. R. Noyes, and R. F. Zernicke. Biomechanics of ligaments and tendons. R. S. Hutton (ed). *Exercise and Sport Sciences Reviews.* Washington, DC: Franklin Institute Press, 1978, pp. 125–181.

28. Butler, D. L., E. S. Grood, F. R. Noyes, R. F. Zernicke, and K. Brackett. Effects of structure and strain measurement technique on the material properties of young human tendons and fascia. *J. Biomech.* 17:579–596, 1984.

29. Butler, D. L., M. D. Kay, and D. C. Stouffer. Comparison of material properties in fascicle-bone units from human patellar tendon and knee ligaments. *J. Biomech.* 18:425–432, 1986.

30. Butler, D. L., E. T. Martin, A. D. Kaiser, E. S. Grood, K. J. Chun, and A. N. Sodd. The effects of flexion and tibial rotation on the 3-D orientations and lengths of human anterior cruciate ligament bundles. *Trans. Orthop. Res. Soc.* 13:59, 1988.

31. Chimich, D., C. Frank, N. Shrive, H. Dougall, and R. Bray. The effects of initial end contact on medial collateral healing: a morphological and biomechanical study in a rabbit model. *J. Orthop. Res.* 9:37–47, 1991.

32. Chowdhury, P., J. R. Matyas, and C. B. Frank. The "epiligament" of the rabbit medial collateral ligament: a quantitative morphological study. *Connect. Tissue Res.* 27:33–50, 1991.

33. Clayton, M. L., and G. J. Weir. Experimental investigations of ligamentous healing. *Am. J. Surg.* 98:373–378, 1959.

34. Danylchuk, K. D., J. B. Finlay, and J. P. Krcek. Microstructural organization of human and bovine cruciate ligaments. *Clin. Orthop. Relat. Res.* 131:294–298, 1978.

35. DeHaven, K. E., and D. M. Lintner. Athletic injuries: comparison by age, sport, and gender. *Am. J. Sports Med.* 14:218–224, 1986.

36. Ekholm, J., G. Eklund, and S. Skoglund. On the reflex effects from the knee joint of the cat. *Acta Physiol. Scand.* 50:167–174, 1960.

37. Eyre, D. R. Collagen: molecular diversity in the body's protein scaffold. *Science* 207:1315–1322, 1980.

38. Flint, M. H., A. S. Craig, H. C. Reilly, G. C. Gillard, and D. A. Parry. Collagen fibril diameters and glycosaminoglycan content of skins—Indices of tissue maturity and function. *Connect. Tissue Res.* 13:69–81, 1984.

39. Flynn, J. E., and J. H. Graham. Healing following tendon suture and tendon transplants. *Surg. Gynecol. Obstet.* 115:467–472, 1962.

40. Frank, C., D. Amiel, and W. H. Akeson. Healing of the medial collateral ligament of the knee: a morphological and biochemical assessment in rabbits. *Acta Orthop. Scand.* 54:917–923, 1983.

41. Frank, C., D. Bray, A. Rademaker, C. Chrusch, P. Sabiston, D. Bodie, and R. Rangayyan. Electron microscopic quantification of collagen fibril diameters in the rabbit medial collateral ligament: a baseline for comparison. *Connect. Tissue Res.* 19:11–25, 1989.

42. Frank, C., B. MacFarlane, P. Edwards, R. Rangayyan, Z.-Q. Liu, S. Walsh, and R. Bray. A quantitative analysis of matrix alignment in ligament scars: a comparison of

movement versus immobilization in an immature rabbit model. *J. Orthop. Res.* 9:219–227, 1991.

43. Frank, C., D. McDonald, D. Bray, R. Bray, R. Rangayyan, D. Chimich, and N. Shrive. Collagen fibril diameters in the healing adult rabbit medial collateral ligament. *Connect. Tissue Res.* 27:251–263, 1992.

44. Frank, C., D. McDonald, R. Lieber, and P. Sabiston. Biochemical heterogeneity along the length of the rabbit medial collateral ligament. *Clin. Orthop. Relat. Res.* 236:279–288, 1988.

45. Frank, C., N. Schachar, and D. Dittrich. Natural history of healing in the repaired medial collateral ligament. *J. Orthop. Res.* 1:179–188, 1983.

46. Frank, C., S.L.-Y. Woo, D. Amiel, F. Harwood, M. Gomez, and W. Akeson. Medial collateral ligament healing. A multidisciplinary assessment in rabbits. *Am. J. Sports Med.* 11:379–389, 1983.

47. Frank, C., S. Woo, T. Andriacchi, R. Brand, B. Oakes, L. Dahners, K. DeHaven, J. Lewis, and P. Sabiston. Normal ligament: structure, function, and composition. S.L.-Y. Woo and J. A. Buckwalter (eds). *Injury and Repair of the Musculoskeletal Soft Tissues.* Park Ridge, IL: American Academy of Orthopaedic Surgeons, 1988, pp. 103–128.

48. Hart, D. P., and L. E. Dahners. Healing of the medial collateral ligament in rats. The effects of repair, motion, and secondary stabilizing ligaments. *J. Bone Joint Surg.* 69A:1194–1199, 1987.

49. Hulth, A., L. Lindberg, and H. Telhag. Experimental osteoarthritis in rabbits. *Acta Orthop. Scand.* 41:522–530, 1970.

50. Inoue, M., E. McGurk-Burleson, J. M. Hollis, and S.L.-Y. Woo. Treatment of the medial collateral ligament injury. I: The importance of anterior cruciate ligament on the varus-valgus knee laxity. *Am. J. Sports Med.* 15:15–21, 1987.

51. Jack, E. A. Experimental rupture of the medial collateral ligament of the knee. *J. Bone Joint Surg.* 32B:396–402, 1950.

52. Krauspe, R., M. Schmidt, and H.-G. Schiable. Sensory innervation of the anterior cruciate ligament. *J. Bone Joint Surg.* 74A:390–397, 1992.

53. Lam, T. C., C. B. Frank, and N. G. Shrive. Calibration characteristics of a video dimension analyser (VDA) system. *J. Biomech.* 25:1227–1231, 1992.

54. Laros, G. S., C. M. Tipton, and R. R. Cooper. Influence of physical activity on ligament insertions in the knees of dogs. *J. Bone Joint Surg.* 53A:275–286, 1971.

55. Lyon, R. M., E. Billings, S.L.-Y. Woo, K. K. Ishizue, L. Kitabayashi, D. Amiel, and W. H. Akeson. The ACL: a fibrocartilaginous structure. *Trans. Orthop. Res. Soc.* 14:189, 1989.

56. Marshall, J. L., and S.-E. Olsson. Instability of the knee. A long-term experimental study in dogs. *J. Bone Joint Surg.* 53A:1561–1570, 1971.

57. Matyas, J. R., D. Bodie, M. Andersen, and C. B. Frank. The developmental morphology of a "periosteal" ligament insertion: growth and maturation of the tibial insertion of the rabbit medial collateral ligament. *J. Orthop. Res.* 8:412–424, 1990.

58. Matyas, J. R., and C. Frank. Midsubstance injury of the rabbit MCL affects the tissue architecture of the femoral insertion. *Trans. Orthop. Res. Soc.* 15:34, 1990.

59. Miller, E. J. The structure of fibril-forming collagens. *Ann. N.Y. Acad. Sci.* 460:1–13, 1985.

60. Miltner, L. J., and C. H. Hu. Experimental reproduction of joint sprains. *Proc. Soc. Exp. Biol. Med.* 30:883–884, 1933.

61. Miltner, L. J., C. H. Hu, and H. C. Fang. Experimental joint sprain: pathologic study. *Arch. Surg.* 35:234–240, 1937.

62. Newton, P. O., S.L.-Y. Woo, L. R. Kitabayashi, R. M. Lyon, D. R. Anderson, and W. H. Akeson. Ultrastructural changes in knee ligaments following immobilization. *Matrix* 10:314–319, 1990.

63. Nielsen, A. B., and J. Yde. Epidemiology of acute knee injuries: a prospective hospital investigation. *J. Trauma* 31:1644–1648, 1991.

64. Noyes, F. R. Functional properties of knee ligaments and alterations induced by immobilization. *Clin. Orthop. Relat. Res.* 123:210–242, 1977.
65. O'Donoghue, D. H., G. R. Frank, G. L. Jeter, W. Johnson, J. W. Zeiders, and R. Kenyon. Repair and reconstruction of the anterior cruciate ligament in dogs. *J. Bone Joint Surg.* 53A:710–718, 1971.
66. O'Donoghue, D. H., C. A. Rockwood, G. R. Frank, S. C. Jack, and R. Kenyon. Repair of the ACL in dogs. *J. Bone Joint Surg.* 48A:503–519, 1966.
67. O'Donoghue, D. H., C. A. Rockwood, B. Zaricznyj, and R. Kenyon. Repair of knee ligaments in dogs. I. The lateral collateral ligament. *J. Bone Joint Surg.* 43A:1167–1178, 1961.
68. Ogata, K., L. A. Whiteside, and D. A. Andersen. The intra-articular effect of various postoperative managements following knee ligament repair: an experimental study in dogs. *Clin. Orthop. Relat. Res.* 150:271–276, 1980.
69. Palmer, I. Pathophysiology of the medial ligament of the knee joint. *Acta Chir. Scand.* 115:312–318, 1958.
70. Parry, D. A., G. R. Barnes, and A. S. Craig. A comparison of the size distribution of collagen fibrils in connective tissues as a function of age and a possible relation between fibril size distribution and mechanical properties. *Proc. R. Soc. Lond. B.* 203:305–321, 1978.
71. Parry, D. A., A. S. Craig, and G. R. Barnes. Tendon and ligament from the horse: an ultrastructural study of collagen fibrils and elastic fibres as a function of age. *Proc. R. Soc. Lond. B.* 203:293–303, 1978.
72. Piper, T. L., and L. A. Whiteside. Early mobilization after knee ligament repair in dogs: an experimental study. *Clin. Orthop. Relat. Res.* 150:277–282, 1980.
73. Renstrom, P., S. W. Arms, T. S. Stanwyck, R. J. Johnson, and M. H. Pope. Strain within the anterior cruciate ligament during hamstring and quadriceps activity. *Am. J. Sports Med.* 14:83–87, 1986.
74. Schultz, R. A., D. C. Miller, C. S. Kerr, and L. Micheli. Mechanoreceptors in human cruciate ligaments. *J. Bone Joint Surg.* 66A:1072–1076, 1984.
75. Sherman, M. F., and J. R. Bonamo. Primary repair of the anterior cruciate ligament. *Clin. Sports Med.* 7:739–750, 1988.
76. Sherrington, C. S. *The Integrative Action of the Nervous System.* New Haven: Yale University Press, 1911.
77. Sojka, P., H. Johansson, P. Sjolander, R. Lorentzon, and M. Djupsjobacka. Fusimotor neurones can be reflexly influenced by activity in receptors from the posterior cruciate ligament. *Brain Res.* 483:177–183, 1989.
78. Solomonow, M., R. Baratta, B. H. Zhou, H. Shoji, W. Bose, C. Beck, and R. D'Ambrosia. The synergistic action of the anterior cruciate ligament and thigh muscles in maintaining joint stability. *Am. J. Sports Med.* 15:207–213, 1987.
79. Tipton, C. M., S. L. James, W. Mergner, and T.-T. Tcheng. Influence of exercise on strength of medial collateral knee ligaments of dogs. *Am. J. Physiol.* 218:894–902, 1970.
80. Tipton, C. M., R. D. Matthes, and R. K. Martin. Influence of age and sex on the strength of bone-ligament junctions in the knee joints of rats. *J. Bone Joint Surg.* 60A:230–234, 1978.
81. Tipton, C. M., T.-T. Tcheng, and W. Mergner. Ligamentous strength measurements from hypophysectomized rats. *Am. J. Physiol.* 221:1144–1150, 1971.
82. Vailas, A. C., C. M. Tipton, H. L. Laughlin, T. K. Tcheng, and R. D. Matthes. Physical activity and hypophysectomy on the aerobic capacity of ligaments and tendons. *J. Appl. Physiol.* 44:R542–R546, 1978.
83. Vailas, A. C., C. M. Tipton, R. D. Matthes, and M. Gart. Physical activity and its influence on the repair process of medial collateral ligaments. *Connect. Tissue Res.* 9:25–31, 1981.
84. van der Rest, M., and R. Garrone. Collagen family of proteins. *F.A.S.E.B. J.* 5:2814–2823, 1991.

85. Vogel, H. G. Influence of maturation and age on mechanical and biochemical parameters of connective tissue of various organs in the rat. *Connect. Tissue Res.* 6:161–166, 1978.

86. Walsh, S., and C. Frank. Two methods of ligament injury: a morphological comparison in a rabbit model. *J. Surg. Res.* 45:159–166, 1988.

87. Weiss, J. A., S. L.-Y. Woo, K. J. Ohland, S. Horibe, and P. O. Newton. Evaluation of a new injury model to study medial collateral ligament healing: primary repair versus nonoperative treatment. *J. Orthop. Res.* 9:516–528, 1991.

88. Weiss, R. E., and A. H. Reddi. Role of fibronectin in collagenous matrix-induced mesenchymal cell proliferation and differentiation in vivo. *Exp. Cell Res.* 133:247–254, 1981.

89. Wiig, M. E., D. Amiel, M. Ivarsson, C. N. Nagineni, C. D. Wallace, and K. E. Arfors. Type I procollagen gene expression in normal and early healing of the medial collateral and anterior cruciate ligaments in rabbits: an in situ hybridization study. *J. Orthop. Res.* 9:374–382. 1991.

90. Woo, S. L.-Y., M. A. Gomez, M. Inoue, and W. H. Akeson. New experimental procedures to evalute the biomechanical properties of healing canine medial collateral ligaments. *J. Orthop. Res.* 5:425–432, 1987.

91. Woo, S. L.-Y., M. A. Gomez, Y. Seguchi, C. M. Endo, and W. H. Akeson. Measurement of mechanical properties of ligament substance from a bone-ligament-bone preparation. *J. Orthop. Res.* 1:22–29, 1983.

92. Woo, S. L.-Y, M. A. Gomez, T. J. Sites, P. O. Newton, C. A. Orlando, and W. H. Akeson. The biomechanical and morphological changes in the medial collateral ligament of the rabbit after immobilization and remobilization. *J. Bone Joint Surg.* 69A:1200–1211, 1987.

93. Woo, S. L.-Y., J. M. Hollis, R. D. Roux, M. A. Gomez, M. Inoue, J. B. Kleiner, and W. H. Akeson. Effects of knee flexion of the structural properties of the rabbit femur-anterior cruciate ligament-tibia complex (FATC). *J. Biomech.* 20:557–564, 1987.

94. Woo, S. L.-Y., J. Maynard, D. Butler, R. Lyon, P. Torzilli, W. Akeson, R. Cooper, and B. Oakes. Ligament, tendon, and joint capsule insertions to bone. S. L.-Y. Woo and J. A. Buckwalter (eds). *Injury and Repair of the Musculoskeletal Soft Tissues.* Park Ridge, IL: American Academy of Orthopaedic Surgeons, 1988, pp. 133–166.

95. Woo, S. L.-Y., C. A. Orlando, M. A. Gomez, C. B. Frank, and W. H. Akeson. Tensile properties of the medial collateral ligament as a function of age. *J. Orthop. Res.* 4:133–141, 1986.

96. Woo, S. L.-Y., R. H. Peterson, K. J. Ohland, T. J. Sites, and M. I. Danto. The effects of strain rate on the properties of the medial collateral ligament in skeletally immature and mature rabbits: a biomechanical and histological study. *J. Orthop. Res.* 8:712–721, 1990.

97. Woo, S. L.-Y., J. A. Weiss, M. A. Gomez, and D. A. Hawkins. Measurement of changes in ligament tension with knee motion and skeletal maturation. *Trans. A.S.M.E.* 112:46–51, 1990.

98. Woo, S. L.-Y., E. P. Young, K. J. Ohland, J. P. Marcin, S. Horibe, and H.-C. Lin. The effects of transection of the anterior cruciate ligament on healing of the medial collateral ligament. *J. Bone Joint Surg.* 72A:382–392, 1990.

99. Yahia, L.-H, and G. Drouin. Microscopical investigation of canine anterior cruciate ligament and patellar tendon: collagen fascicle morphology and architecture. *J. Orthop. Res.* 7:243–251, 1989.

100. Zernicke, R. F., D. L. Butler, E. S. Grood, and M. S. Hefzy. Strain topography of human tendon and fascia. *J. Biomech. Eng.* 106:177–180, 1984.

101. Zimney, M., M. Schutte, and E. Dabezies. Mechanoreceptors in the human anterior cruciate ligament. *Anat. Rec.* 214:204–209, 1986.

3
Changes in Skeletal Muscle with Aging: Effects of Exercise Training

MARC A. ROGERS. Ph.D.
WILLIAM J. EVANS, Ph.D.

INTRODUCTION

The decline in the physiological capacity of humans is an inevitable consequence of the biological aging process. Reductions in functional capacity can generally be attributed to loss of cardiovascular, respiratory, neuromuscular, and metabolic functions that typically occur with aging. In addition, alterations in body composition may have an impact on the physiological capacity of individuals as they age. The age-related deterioration in the capacities of the various physiological systems not only has an adverse effect on exercise performance but also results in a decreased ability to perform common activities of daily living in older individuals.

In this chapter our intent is to: *(a)* review the changes in skeletal muscle morphology and metabolic potential that occur with aging in both sedentary and active individuals; *(b)* outline the capacity of older individuals to adapt to both aerobic (endurance) and resistive (strength) exercise training; and *(c)* determine the effects of exercise training, maintained for a prolonged period of time, on the functional and metabolic capacities of skeletal muscle in older humans.

BODY COMPOSITION CHANGES WITH AGING

Aging is associated with alterations in body composition such that there is an increase in percentage of body fat and a concomitant decline in lean body mass (LBM) [104, 109]. About 60% of the body's potassium is found in skeletal muscle, and the ratio of nitrogen is higher in muscle than in nonmuscle lean tissue. Using total body potassium and nitrogen, Cohn and co-workers [29] determined that skeletal muscle protein is reduced and nonmuscle protein is maintained with advancing age. They also demonstrated that the age-related loss in total body nitrogen is closely related to the losses in total body calcium, suggesting that the loss of skeletal muscle may be related to the reduced bone density seen in the elderly. Furthermore, computed tomography of individual muscles shows that after age 30 yr, there is a decrease in cross-sectional area of

65

the thigh along with decreased muscle density associated with increased intramuscular fat [17].

In an 18-yr longitudinal study, Flynn et al. [44] found that the most rapid rate of total body potassium loss occurred between the ages of 41 and 60 yr for men while the rapid loss in the women did not take place until after the age of 60 yr. These findings suggest that there may be a gender difference in the rate of change in body composition over time. Additional support for the reduction in LBM with aging comes from the fact that total body water decreases from maturity to senescence, urinary creatinine levels decline, and resting metabolic rate is also lower in older individuals [38, 43, 112, 136, 137]. Fleg and Lakatta, using creatinine excretion, determined that muscle mass between the ages of 30 and 70 yr was reduced by 23% and 22%, respectively, in men and women [43]. Tzankoff and Norris [136, 137] measured resting metabolic rate and urinary creatinine levels in individuals aged 20–95 yr enrolled in the Baltimore Longitudinal Study of Aging (BLSA); they found that resting metabolic rate evidenced no decline up to approximately age 45 yr, but with each succeeding decade the resting metabolic rate decreased significantly. A reduction in 24-hr urinary creatinine excretion was positively correlated with the reduced resting metabolic rate and indicated that there was an approximate 30% loss in total muscle mass over the span of about 50 yr [136]. Resting metabolic rate, when corrected for the age-associated change in skeletal muscle mass, was similar in the various age groups leading the authors to conclude that the loss of muscle mass with aging accounts for most of the age-related decrease in resting metabolic rate. Aging, therefore, results in a substantial alteration in body composition, with a marked reduction in skeletal muscle mass, which we will refer to as sarcopenia. Loss of muscle mass and strength may be an important cause of the age-related loss in bone mineral density resulting in osteoporosis [117]. Muscle atrophy and weakness are more prevalent among elderly individuals who develop hip fractures than among those of a similar age who do not [10]. Sarcopenia results in profound muscle weakness and extreme difficulty in carrying out activities of daily living [66], falls [120], and institutional care among the elderly. The importance of muscle mass in maintaining basal metabolic rate, physical activity levels, and optimal body fat implicates sarcopenia in such age-associated diseases as Type II diabetes, coronary artery disease, hypertension, and their resultant array of complications.

CHANGES IN MUSCLE FUNCTION WITH AGING

Decline in Muscle Strength
It has been well established that significant losses in maximal force production (muscle strength) take place with aging [8, 30, 31, 57, 75, 78,

126] although there appear to be substantial variations in the rate of loss among muscle groups. Larsson et al. [75] studied 114 male subjects between the ages of 11 and 70 yr and found that maximal isometric and dynamic strength of the quadriceps increased up to the age of 30 yr, stayed relatively constant up to the age of 50 yr, and then decreased thereafter with increasing age (Fig. 3.1). In this study, the age-related changes in maximal isometric and dynamic muscle strength and speed of movement were quite similar, with reductions between the ages of 50 and 70 yr, ranging from 24–36%. The muscle strength and mechanical performance decrement that occurred after age 50 yr was not accompanied by significant change in thigh circumference, thus no generalized muscle atrophy had occurred, however selective muscle fiber atrophy took place as the 60-yr-old subjects had a 36% smaller Type II fiber area than the 40-yr-olds did.

Cross-sectional studies in women have also known significant losses in strength with aging [60, 73, 103, 143]. Young and co-workers [143]

FIGURE 3.1
Maximal isometric and dynamic strength **(Nm)** *and maximal knee extension velocity* **(MEV)** *for subjects in various age groups. Maximal strength was measured at 0 rad · sec^{-1} (isometric, —), $\pi/3$ (60° · sec^{-1}, — — —) and π rad · sec^{-1} (180° · sec^{-1}, — · — ·). (Reprinted with permission from Larsson, L., G. Grimby and J. Karlsson. Muscle strength and speed of movement in relation to age and muscle morphology. J. Appl. Physiol. 46:451–456, 1979.)*

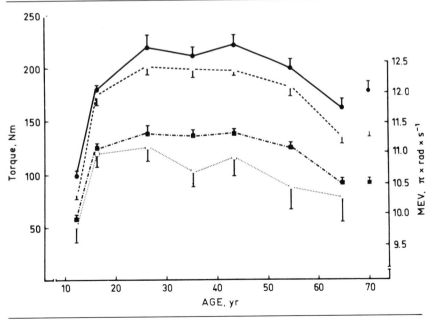

compared the voluntary isometric strength of the quadriceps of 20- and 70-yr-old healthy women and, in addition, measured midthigh cross-sectional areas (CSA) via ultrasonography. The older women had maximal isometric strength levels that were 35% lower than the young women, while mean quadriceps CSAs were 33% less. Similar differences in isokinetic [60, 73] and isometric strength [103] have been noted in women between the ages of 20 and 70 yr.

Relatively little information exists with regard to muscle strength in men and women past the age of 70 yr. Quadriceps strength in a group of healthy 80-yr-olds in the Copenhagen City Heart Study was 30% lower [31] compared with a previous population study of 70-yr-olds [3], a rather large deficit over the span of only a decade. While muscle strength levels appear to be relatively well maintained up through the 5th decade of life, the decline amounts to about 15% per decade in the 6th and 7th decade after which time the loss in muscle strength approximates 30% per decade [31, 60, 75, 103, 138].

Very few longitudinal studies have assessed the loss of muscle strength with age. Aniansson et al. [8] found that while body weight and total body cell mass were reduced by only 2% and 6%, respectively, in 23 men aged 73–83 yr over a 7-yr time span, vastus lateralis muscle strength was decreased by 10 to 22% at five different contraction velocities. During these 7 yr, Type IIa and IIb fiber areas in the vastus lateralis decreased by 14% and 25%, respectively, while Type I fiber area was unchanged. Although this longitudinal study confirmed the reductions in muscle strength and area of Type II muscle found in earlier cross-sectional investigations [57, 75], on a per-decade basis, the loss of muscle strength in these 73 to 83-yr-old subjects was approximately 23% whereas the reduction in Type II muscle fiber area was almost 56%. This implies that there may be a greater reduction in Type II fiber size than loss of muscle strength, at least in very old individuals. Furthermore, it appears that older individuals experience a generalized loss of muscle strength with aging, which is accelerated even further after the age of 70 yr.

Relationship Between Size and Strength Losses
The decline in muscle strength with aging can potentially be attributed either to the loss of muscle mass [6, 17, 45, 143, 144] or to some alteration of the muscle's capacity to generate force (because of a reduced activation of motor units and/or a loss of contractile or mechanical properties of the muscle) or to a combination of these two mechanisms thus making older muscle intrinsically weaker [22, 139]. In this context, there is some evidence to support the contention that the decline in strength with aging may be greater than the absolute loss of muscle mass [22, 92, 137]. It has been shown that the ratio of maximal voluntary force to muscle CSA [MVC/CSA] of the adductor pollicis of older subjects is about 70% that of young controls [22]. Furthermore, Vandervoort and

McComas determined that the reduction in ankle plantar and dorsiflex-or muscle strength with aging was greater than the reduction in CSA [139]. Thus, the capacity to generate force per unit of CSA was lower in the older subjects. This means that when comparing muscle strength levels between young and old subjects, some index of muscle mass should be measured [45]. Young and colleagues [143] found that maximal voluntary isometric strength of older women (74 yr) was 35% lower than that of young women (24 yr) and the older women had quadriceps CSA that were 33% smaller than that of the young women. In addition, there was no difference in MVC/CSA between the young (7.1) and old women (6.9). This evidence suggests that there was no difference in the intrinsic strength of the older women's skeletal muscle, even though they were weaker than the young women. A follow-up study in men determined that the older men had a 39% reduction in maximal voluntary isometric strength compared with their younger counterparts, while the midthigh CSA was 25% smaller [144]. The mean MVC/CSA for young men was 8.7 compared with 7.1 for the old men. The difference between the MVC/CSA ratios indicates that the old men's quadriceps muscle was approximately 19% weaker than the young men's muscle. Furthermore, the MVC/CSA ratio of the old men in this study was similar to values obtained in young and old women [143]. It is conceivable that the greater MVC/CSA ratio in young men compared with old men and young and old women may be due to differences in physical activity. Along the same lines, Frontera and co-workers [45] measured the isokinetic strength of elbow and knee extensor and flexor muscles in 200 healthy women and men (ages 45 to 78 yr) to determine the relationship between changes in muscle strength and muscle mass that occur with aging. As expected, the strength of all four muscle groups was significantly lower in the older compared with the younger subjects. However, when muscle strength was corrected for muscle mass, the significant differences between age groups were either greatly reduced or eliminated altogether. Frontera et al. concluded that the loss of muscle mass is the major factor in the age-related decline in muscle strength rather than a deterioration in the contractile capacity of the muscle [45].

In keeping with the previously mentioned whole muscle ultrasonographic studies of Young et al. [143, 144] similar reductions in the CSA of thigh muscles with age in two groups of men (30–70 yr) have been reported in a cadaver study [84]. Expanding on this earlier work, Lexell et al. performed a large cross-sectional study where frozen, whole vastus lateralis muscle cross-sections were used to determine whole muscle CSA histologically [87]. They demonstrated that the reduction in muscle size commences before the age of 30 yr and that by the age of 50 yr muscle area is reduced by about 10% (Fig. 3.2A). Furthermore, they determined that the rate of decline in muscle area becomes more rapid after the age of 50 yr and that between the ages of 20 and 80 yr, 40% of the muscle

FIGURE 3.2

A. *Relationship between age and muscle area of whole vastus lateralis muscle cross-sections (in mm²/48). Muscle area is mean taken from 48, 1 × 1 mm grid squares throughout the whole muscle.* **B.** *Relationship between total number of fibers and age in whole vastus lateralis muscle. (Reprinted with permission from Lexell, J., C. C. Taylor and M. Sjöström. What is the cause of the ageing atrophy? Total number size and proportion of different fiber types studied in whole vastus lateralis muscle from 15- to 83-year-old men.* J. Neurol. Sci. 72:211–222, 1988.

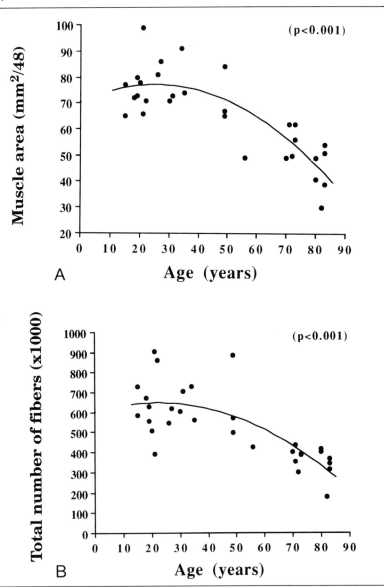

area is lost. The decrease in muscle size with aging can account for much of the reduction in muscle strength, thus, supporting this interpretation rather than the notion that skeletal muscle becomes intrinsically weaker with age [14, 138, 143, 144].

Muscle Endurance Capacity

Studies on the effects of aging on skeletal muscle have generally focused on losses in muscular strength rather than endurance or motor performance [138]. Fitts et al. showed no difference in the fatigability of the soleus muscle of 28- vs. 9-month-old rats. even though the aged muscles had higher lactate and lower glycogen levels, thus suggesting a difference in the metabolic response to prolonged contactile activity [42]. The old rats had a prolonged isometric twitch duration of both slow-twitch and fast-twitch muscle that was due to an increased one-half relaxation time. In addition, these authors found that twitch and tetanic tension, peak rate of tension development, and the maximal velocity of shortening were all maintained between 9 and 28 months of age. Furthermore, voluntary wheel running had a minimal effect on the contractile properties of the rat's muscles. In contrast, Klitgaard et al. [69] have shown that twitch and tetanic tension decreased significantly in the soleus and plantaris muscle with aging.

In the few human studies that have been performed to date, the capacity for 70-yr-old subjects to maintain voluntary isometric [6, 77, 125] and dynamic [77] muscle contractions for up to 60 seconds is similar to that of young individuals when the contractions are performed at the same percentage of MVC. In contrast, Lennmarken et al. [80] more recently found that older men (65 yr) evidenced a significantly greater force loss over 30 seconds of electrical stimulation of the adductor pollicis muscle than did young men (32 yr) (8.5 and 5.0%, respectively) and older women (3.5%), thus indicating an age and gender effect on muscle endurance. Davies and co-workers found that the ankle plantar flexors and elbow flexors of older subjects showed a greater relative force loss compared with young controls suggesting that aged muscle has a reduced capacity to resist fatigue [32, 33, 97]. In addition, the extended time course of recovery of contractile properties from contractions that induce fatigue has been studied following 10 minutes of electrical stimulation in the triceps surae muscle of men [68]. The decline in muscle force during the fatigue test was not significantly different between 25- and 65-yr-old active men (approximately 18% and approximately 22%), a finding supported by previous studies [4, 77]. However, the older individual's twitch force relaxation rate was decreased and half-relaxation time was significantly increased at 15 min and 1 hour after fatigue. These results are indicative of a slower return to resting contractile function in the skeletal muscle of older men when compared with that of young men.

MUSCLE MORPHOLOGY AND AGING

Muscle Fiber Types
Human skeletal muscle fibers can be divided into different types based on their physiological, ultrastructural, and metabolic characteristics [18, 36, 50]. Type I muscle fibers in humans have slow contractile velocities, low actomyosin adenosine triphosphatase (ATPase) activity, and a high mitochondrial density that parallels the high activity of marker enzymes for the Krebs cycle, the electron transport chain, and β-oxidation. Fast-contracting Type IIb fibers, on the other hand, have a high actomyosin ATPase activity, fewer mitochondria, and a lower mitochondrial respiratory capacity. The intermediate Type IIa fibers have a relatively fast-contraction velocity but also display metabolic characteristics similar to the Type I fiber with an enhanced capacity for aerobic metabolism. In young individuals, Type I and Type II muscle fibers also differ with respect to size and capillarization with Type II muscle fibers being approximately 20% larger than Type I muscle cells and Type I fibers having a 15–20% greater capillary/fiber ratio [53].

Distribution of Fiber Types with Aging
The distribution of fiber types in aging human muscles may potentially be altered as a result of an interconversion between Type I and Type II muscle fibers or secondary to the preferential loss of a specific muscle fiber type [52]. Initial studies on the effect of aging on fiber types determined that there is a shift toward a distribution with a higher percentage of Type I fibers and a corresponding decrease in Type II fibers. Gollnick et al. found that 24- to 30-yr-old trained and untrained men had a distribution consisting of 36% Type I fibers while 31 to 52-yr-old men had 44% Type I fibers [49]. This finding was later substantiated in a more extensive cross-sectional study by Larsson et al. in a group of sedentary males between the ages of 22 and 65 yr where there was also a higher percentage of Type I fibers in the older group [78]. Subjects in the 20 to 29-yr-old age group had 39% Type I muscle fibers while the 60 to 65-yr-old subjects had 66% Type I fibers.

More recent studies seem to contradict these early findings [55, 57, 84, 118]. Sato determined the fiber distribution in the pectoralis minor muscle after surgical resectioning in 200 women between the ages of 26 and 80 yr and found that the percentage of Type I fibers did not change with age [118]. Furthermore, Grimby et al. studied the vastus lateralis of very old (66–100 yr) patients admitted for hip surgery and found that Type I muscle fibers ranged between 52% and 58% in women of three age groups and a comparison group of men, aged 70–89 yr, thus indicating no significant alteration with age [57].

Most studies that have evaluated the effects of aging on muscle fiber type distributions have used the muscle biopsy technique. This technique allows for fresh human muscle to be studied but only a small portion of a specific muscle can be sampled, which is an obvious limitation [85, 86]. Lexell et al. have overcome this problem by excising whole vastus lateralis muscles at autopsy, cutting thin cross-sections (Fig. 3.3) and measuring the fiber type distribution [83, 84]. Using this technique, they have found that young men (24 yr) had 49% Type I fibers, middle-aged

FIGURE 3.3

Representative thin cross-section of autopsied whole vastus lateralis muscle. (Reprinted with permission from Lexell, J., C. C. Taylor, and M. Sjöström. What is the cause of ageing atrophy? Total number, size and proportion of different fiber types studied in whole vastus lateralis muscle from 15- to 83-year-old men. J. Neurol. Sci. *84:275–294, 1988.*

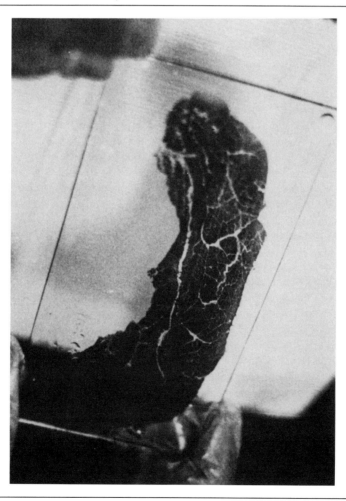

men (52 yr) had 52% Type I fibers, and the oldest men (77 yr) had 51% Type I fibers [83]. Taken together, these most recent findings [55, 57, 83, 84, 118] provide a reasonable consensus opinion that during aging when loss of skeletal muscle mass occurs, it is not because of the preferential loss of a specific fiber type but that both Type I and Type II skeletal muscle are equally affected.

Aging and Fiber Number
The utilization of the whole muscle cross-section technique by Lexell and co-workers has provided definitive information on the loss of muscle fibers that takes place with aging [83, 84, 87]. In their initial study, the authors measured muscle size and painstakingly counted fiber number in vastus lateralis muscles from six healthy men, aged 30 to 72 yr. The muscles of the older individuals contained 25% fewer muscle fibers than those of the younger subjects, thereby accounting for the 18% difference in muscle size between the two groups. These findings have since been corroborated in studies with larger sample sizes [83, 87]. By assessing the quadratic relationship between age and the total number of muscle fibers (Fig. 3.2B), Lexell et al. [87] have concluded that the loss of fibers commences at about 25 yr of age, and that between the ages of 20 and 80, total fiber number is reduced by 39%. Similar findings have been noted by Sato et al. [118] in their study of aging females who had their pectoralis minor muscle surgically resected. Total fiber number and the number of Type I and II fibers were similar in the 26- to 39-, 40- to 49- and 50- to 59-yr age groups. However, after 60 yr of age, total fiber number and the numbers of both fiber types declined significantly such that by the seventh decade there was an approximate reduction in total fiber number of 25%.

The age-related decline in total muscle fiber number could signify a preferential loss of either Type I or Type II muscle cells. As described in the previous section, results of studies using small muscle samples from biopsies have been somewhat equivocal [8, 55, 74, 106]; however, the answer to this question as provided by the whole muscle cross-section technique of Lexell et al. is more definitive [87], i.e. that there is no significant alteration in mean fiber type percentage or preferential loss of either Type I or Type II muscle fibers with age.

Denervation and Muscle Fiber Loss
What then is the cause of the generalized loss of muscle fibers with increasing age? Two potential mechanisms may account for the significant decline in the number of muscle fibers with age. Fibers could be lost as a result of: (*a*) damage to the muscle cells without regeneration; or (*b*) an interruption in the connection between the motoneuron and the fibers that it innervates [138]. Little evidence exists to suggest that

normal, aging muscle is typified by significant myopathies that could account for the decreased fiber number [3, 8, 56, 84]. It is much more likely that neuropathic changes are responsible since they are quite common in the muscle of older subjects [132, 133]. Studies utilizing electromyography (EMG) have shown that the number of active motor units decreases with age [21, 23, 96] and that the low threshold motor units that remain in older individuals become progressively larger [125]. In addition, older individuals maintain a lower number of functioning spinal cord motor neurons than do young people [134]. Stålberg et al., using EMG amplitude and fiber density as indices of the electrical size of the motor unit and the number of muscle fibers per motor unit, found an increase in both EMG amplitude and fiber density with increasing age [127]. The increase in fiber density is suggestive of a reorganization of the motor unit, which more than likely results from reinnervation, secondary to sprouting from collateral nerve fibers. The fact that older muscle displays increases in fiber-type grouping compared with young muscle [83, 88] is also consistent with a denervation-reinnervation model [87, 127]. Lexell and Downham [82] quantitatively assessed fiber-type grouping in whole vastus lateralis muscle cross-sections in men between the ages of 15 and 83 yr and found that segregated fibers were common in young muscles, a random mosaic-like pattern predominated in men between the ages of 30 and 50 yr, and over 60 yr an excess of enclosed fibers were evident. This fiber-type grouping implies that the fiber population is continually in a state of transition throughout life and that denervation and reinnervation occur in normal muscle during aging.

When a comparison was made between the Macro EMG amplitude of the young and old subjects in Stålberg's study, it was estimated that the 27–36% increase in amplitude translated into a functional dropout of approximately 25% of the motor neurons. Taken together, these findings suggest that the decline in muscle fiber number that typically occurs with aging is probably due to a neurological deficit at the level of the motor neuron. Unfortunately, the molecular mechanisms of the neuronal loss with aging have yet to be established.

Aging and Muscle Fiber Size
Human Type I muscle fibers seem to be relatively resistant to age-associated atrophy at least until the age of 60–70 yr [5, 8, 26, 56, 78, 87, 118]. Once again, Lexell's 1988 cross-sectional study with whole muscle cross-sections taken at autopsy provides definitive support for the earlier studies that relied on small muscle biopsy samples [87]. Lexell et al. determined that there was no significant change in Type I muscle fiber size with age and that Type I muscle fiber size in the 80-year-olds was almost exactly the same as that in the 20-yr-olds. Consistent with previous reports was Lexell's finding that there was a significant

reduction in Type II fiber size with advancing yrs [8, 26, 56, 78, 81, 118]. The reduction in Type II fiber size between the ages of 20 and 80 yr amounted to 26% [87]. Aniansson et al. determined that there was no change in Type I fiber area over 7 yr in 70- to 80-yr-old men but that the Type IIa and IIb fiber areas were decreased by 14% and 25%, respectively [8]. Several other studies have shown a preferential atrophy in Type IIb muscle fibers compared with IIa fibers in older individuals thus signifying that these fibers may be more susceptible to the effects of aging [26, 56]. When Coggan et al. compared IIa and IIb fiber areas between young and old men, they determined the reductions to be 13% and 22%, respectively, while the women in that study experienced a 24% decrease in IIa and a 30% decrease in IIb fiber area [26]. Thus, the reduction in Type II fiber area with age accounts for the significant decrease in muscle size and strength that occurs with aging [81].

Up until the mid-1980s, most studies dealing with aging skeletal muscle had been carried out in men with much less information available about the characteristics of aging muscle in women. Essén-Gustavsson and Borges [37] found that 20- to 70-yr-old men had a significantly greater percentage of Type I fibers (58%) as compared with women of the same age (51%) while the women evidenced a significantly higher percentage of IIa fibers (32%) vs. the men (27%). In contrast, Coggan et al. did not detect any effect of gender on fiber-type distribution in 65-year-old women and men [26]. The percentage of the different fiber types did not change in relation to age in either men or women, which is consistent with previous reports [5, 56, 66]. In Essén-Gustavsson's study, the smallest fiber areas were detected in the oldest age groups in both women and men, with 70-year-old women having smaller total fiber areas, Type I, and IIa fiber areas than 60-year-old females. The area occupied by each fiber type and the mean area were larger in men compared with women in each age group. Therefore, while men show significantly larger fiber areas than women, the aging process seems to result in similar decreases in muscle fiber size in both genders [37].

While the advance of the whole muscle cross-section methodology has provided a great deal of insight into morphological changes in aging skeletal muscle, its utility in exercise and aging muscle studies is somewhat limited. Studies in this area will continue to rely on the muscle biopsy technique and, in the future, magnetic resonance spectroscopy may provide noninvasive answers to incisive muscle morphology questions in gerontology.

Aging and Muscle Capillarization
In 1971, Parízkova et al. [110] demonstrated that muscle from young (age 20) and old (age 70) subjects had a similar number of capillaries/ mm^2 but that a concomitant reduction in fiber size and a 60% greater number of muscle fibers in the muscle sample from the older men

resulted in a significantly lower capillary/fiber ratio in the older subjects. The range in capillarization for young individuals has been reported to be between 260 and 380 capillaries/mm^2 with a capillary/fiber ratio of between 1.3 and 1.8 for both women and men [2, 5, 105]. When Grimby et al. [56] measured the capillary supply of the vastus lateralis in 78 to 81-yr-old women and men, they showed similar capillary densities (350/mm^2) and capillary/fiber ratios (1.5) as compared with young individuals [2, 5, 105]. Furthermore, 60- to 70-yr-old men have similar capillary densities to women of the same age [6, 26].

In contrast to some early reports, Coggan and co-workers have recently shown a 25% reduction in capillary density in the gastrocnemius muscle of 65-yr-old men and women as compared with 25-yr-olds [26]. Capillary/fiber ratio and the number of capillaries in contact with each fiber were also significantly lower (19–40%) in the muscles of the old men and women, thus reflecting an actual loss of capillaries in the muscle. Subjects in this study were carefully screened to be truly sedentary, a fact that was supported by the relatively low $\dot{V}O_2$max values and precise records of past physical activity. Second, the authors intentionally studied a muscle that is frequently recruited during common daily activities like walking. These measures helped to control for the confounding effects of physical activity. Even so, it is likely that the reduction in muscle capillarization in the older subjects was the result of lower levels of activity, compared with young individuals, that put less of a demand on their gastrocnemius muscle. Our current understanding of the effects of aging on muscle capillarization is somewhat incomplete since relatively few systematic studies have been conducted. Although most of the available evidence suggests that capillary supply to skeletal muscle is fairly well maintained in senescent muscle compared with muscle from young individuals, recent information indicates that there is a significant decrease in capillarization in sedentary older men and women. It remains to be determined whether this apparent decline in capillarization is because of inactivity or the effects of aging per se.

METABOLIC CAPACITY OF AGING SKELETAL MUSCLE

The enzymatic activity of various marker enzymes has been measured in skeletal muscle from individuals of different ages to quantify the effect of aging on the metabolic capacity of muscle. The following enzymes and metabolic pathways have been of most interest: citrate synthase (CS) and succinate dehydrogenase (SDH) (Krebs cycle); cytochrome oxidase (CO) and cytochrome C (electron transport chain); 3-hydroxy Co-A dehydrogenase (β-HAD) (β-oxidation); phosphorylase (PHOS), hexokinase (HK), lactate dehydrogenase (LDH), and phosphofructokinase (PFK) (glycolysis); and myokinase (MK) (ATP synthesis).

Aging and the Glycolytic Capacity of Muscle

Early studies in the area of aging and the metabolic capacity of muscle were carried out by Örlander et al. [107, 108] and Larsson et al. [78, 79] with sedentary male subjects between the ages of 25 and 65 yr. The authors collectively determined that the maximal activities of PFK, MK, and Mg^{2+} myofibrillar ATPase did not show a decrease as a function of age while total LDH activity in skeletal muscle was significantly greater in the young subjects and the muscle-specific LDH isoenzymes (LDH_4 and LDH_5) decreased with advancing age [52]. These early studies have been extended to include individuals older than 65 yr. Aniansson et al. [3] showed that there were no differences in skeletal muscle enzyme activities (Mg^{2+} ATPase, MK, and LDH) in men (ages 66–76 yr) and women (ages 61–71 yr), while Grimby came to the same conclusion with regard to HK and LDH activity in the muscle of men and women between the ages of 78 and 81 yr [56] who were compared with young subjects [108, 123]. Coggan et al. determined that PHOS, LDH, and PFK activities in the gastrocnemius muscle of 25- and 65-yr-old untrained subjects were essentially the same [26]. It also appears that aging has a minimal effect on the concentration of high-energy phosphate compounds in muscle since resting ATP, adenosine monophosphate (AMP), and the energy charge of the cell are equivalent in young and old individuals [100]. In a 7-yr longitudinal study, Aniansson et al. [8] showed that MK and LDH activity was maintained in men between the ages of 73 and 83 yr. Probably the most systematic study of the effects of aging on muscle metabolism was performed by Essén-Gustavsson and Borges in a large group of healthy men and women, stratified in 10-yr age groups from 20 to 70 yrs [37]. The enzymatic assays were performed on whole muscle homogenates and the results indicated that, in general, only minor changes in glycolytic enzyme activity occurred with aging. There were no significant differences in HK or LDH activity in the different age groups of men and women, except that the glycolytic enzyme activity was significantly lower in the 70-yr-old women. The lower glycolytic enzyme activity was probably a function of the mixed muscle homogenate technique and the fact that the 70-yr-old women experienced a significant reduction in Type II muscle fibers, known to have a high concentration of glycolytic enzymes. A second study was carried out, using the same subjects as in the previous investigation, to evaluate glycolytic enzyme activities in Type I and II skeletal muscle fibers of young and old individuals [16]. Rather than rely on enzymatic determinations in mixed muscle homogenates, 300–400 freeze-dried single muscle fibers were pooled as Type I or Type II fibers and assayed for LDH, creatine kinase (CK), and MK activities. The glycolytic enzymes were lower in Type I vs. Type II muscle in both young and old subjects. For example, the MK activity in the Type II fibers of both old and young subjects was about twice the activity in Type I muscle. As before [3], the glycolytic marker enzymes did not show any major change with age (variations on the order of 3–15% with age) except that MK activity declined markedly (approximately 45%) with age in both Type I and Type II fibers. The authors surmised that the physical activity patterns of the older subjects probably accounted for the sharp decline in MK activity since older individuals typically do not participate in activities that recruit fast-contracting Type II muscle cells with a concomitant induction of MK activity. This rationale however, does not explain the reduced MK activity in Type I muscle fibers. There was a significant correlation between MK activity in Type II fibers and the maximal capacity for torque development, thus leading the authors to suggest that perhaps a portion of the decline in force-generating capacity of the muscle could be because of the loss of MK activity in Type II skeletal muscle [14]. This hypothesis may warrant further testing in a larger group of aging individuals with varying levels of physical activity. In summary, considerable evidence exists to support the tenet that glycolytic enzyme activities and high energy phosphagens are not adversely affected by aging in sedentary humans [8, 16, 26, 37, 78, 79, 100, 108].

Aging and the Respiratory Capacity of Muscle
Örlander et al. and Larsson et al. made the initial observations that the mitochondrial respiratory capacity of human skeletal muscle is not adversely affected by age [78, 79, 108]. Grimby [56] came to a similar conclusion since he found that β-HAD and CS activity in the vastus lateralis muscle of men and women between the ages of 78 and 81 yr was no different than that in young subjects. Three other cross-sectional studies have reported data that are consistent with the notion that aging does not result in a reduction in the respiratory capacity of skeletal muscle [9, 16, 37]. However, Essén-Gustavsson and Borges [37] found that CS activity was about 20% higher in 20- to 30-yr-olds vs. 60- to 70-yr-old men and women. Most recently, Coggan et al. [26] have compared the enzymatic activities of SDH, CS, and β-HAD in the gastrocnemius muscles of 25- and 65-year-old men and women who were truly sedentary. The young men and women had $\dot{V}O_2$max values of 45 and 35 ml/kg/min, while the older subjects had values of 28 and 23 ml/kg/min, respectively. These subjects had only participated in low-intensity recreational games and had never been involved in endurance sports or activities. The oxidative muscle enzyme activities were approximately 25% lower in the older subjects when compared with the younger group (26–30% lower in men; 14–29% lower in women). These findings agree with the results of Meredith et al. [99] who determined that the O_2 uptake capacity of muscle measured in vitro was approximately 40% less in older men and women as compared with young control subjects.

Why then do the Scandinavian studies show no reduction in skeletal muscle oxidative capacity with aging [8, 16, 37, 56, 78, 79] which is in contrast to the findings of Coggan et al. [26] and Meredith et al. [99]? Since it is well known that physical activity can have a powerful effect on the oxidative capacity of skeletal muscle [62], it may be that the early studies in older Scandinavians were confounded by the physical activity habits of the subjects, whereas the studies by Coggan and Meredith controlled for the influence of physical activity by studying truly sedentary individuals. While it is difficult to attribute the decline in the respiratory capacity of skeletal muscle seen in some studies solely to either the aging process or to physical inactivity, it is likely that the decrease contributes to the reduced capacity for muscular endurance in older, sedentary individuals [26].

SKELETAL MUSCLE ADAPTATIONS TO ENDURANCE EXERCISE TRAINING IN OLDER WOMEN AND MEN

Aging, Training, and $\dot{V}O_2max$
The functional capacity of the cardiovascular system declines with age such that in healthy yet sedentary individuals, $\dot{V}O_2max$ is reduced about 10% per decade [61]. A portion of this decline in cardiovascular capacity is undoubtedly due to the effects of aging per se while some of the loss is secondary to the effects of physical inactivity. In fact, in older individuals who maintain a constant level of vigorous endurance exercise training, the reduction in $\dot{V}O_2max$ is only approximately 5% [61, 115].

Cartee and Farrar [24] have shown that the relative increase in $\dot{V}O_2max$ and muscle respiratory capacity is equivalent in young and old rats subjected to the identical training stimulus, even though the older rats had a $\dot{V}O_2max$ value that was 17% lower. Early studies in elderly humans showed that endurance exercise training did not result in significant improvements in $\dot{V}O_2max$ [70] probably because the studies employed an insufficient training stimulus, i.e., inadequate intensity and duration. More recently, Seals and colleagues [122] found that 6 months of low-intensity and 6 months of high-intensity endurance training resulted in a 30% mean increase in $\dot{V}O_2max$ in 11 healthy 60- to 70-yr-old subjects. Other studies have shown that vigorous endurance exercise training can increase $\dot{V}O_2max$ approximately 20%. In this context, Kohrt et al. trained 53 men and 57 women between the ages of 60 and 71 yr for 9–12 months [70]. The subjects participated in a progressively increasing walk/run program 4 days/week, 45 min/day at about 80% of maximal heart rate. The mean increase in $\dot{V}O_2max$ was 24% (range 0–58%), thus indicating that older individuals adapt to an endurance exercise training program in a similar fashion to young individuals. Furthermore, it was determined that the relative improvement in $\dot{V}O_2max$ in these subjects was independent of their age, gender, and initial level of cardiovascular fitness. Hagberg and co-workers [59] determined that even 70- to

79-yr-old men and women adapt to endurance training with increases in $\dot{V}O_2$max of approximately 22%.

The increase in $\dot{V}O_2$max of young individuals in response to endurance exercise training is partly due to peripheral adaptations in skeletal muscle [62]. These adaptations include a significant increase in the mitochondrial respiratory capacity [48, 49], an increase in muscle capillarization [1], and a transformation of Type IIb skeletal muscle fibers to Type IIa [2]. Studies in older men and women have presented conflicting results with regard to the adaptability of skeletal muscle to endurance exercise training. The following sections outline the adaptations to regular, vigorous endurance exercise training in older humans (summary Table 3.1). Part of the inconsistency may be due to an insufficient training stimulus that was applied by some investigators resulting in an inability to elicit skeletal muscle adaptations similar to those seen in young individuals.

Oxidative Capacity of Aging Skeletal Muscle
One of the first studies to assess whether older individuals showed adaptations in skeletal muscle after endurance exercise training was reported by Suominen et al. in 1977 [130]. They found that 8 weeks of low-intensity endurance training resulted in only a 10–15% increase in the respiratory capacity of skeletal muscle of 69-yr-old men and women. Subsequent to this study, Suominen et al. [129] found that 8 weeks of exercise training, which included about 20 minutes of jogging three to five times per week, increased the respiratory capacity of vastus lateralis muscle by approximately 45% in 56- to 70-yr-old sedentary men (Table 3.1). This training regimen also elicited a 12% increase in $\dot{V}O_2$max. In contrast, Örlander and Aniansson [107] found no increases in the volume of mitochondria, or increases in β-HAD or CS activity in the skeletal muscle of 70- to 75-yr-old men who participated in a 12-week walking/jogging program at about 70% of $\dot{V}O_2$max. More recently, Meredith et al. [99] compared the peripheral effects of vigorous endurance exercise training in young (24 yr) and older (65 yr), healthy men and women. The training program consisted of 12 weeks of stationary cycling for 45 min/day, 3 days/week at 70% of heart rate reserve. The muscle oxidative capacity of the older subjects increased 128% after endurance training, while the young subjects showed only a 27% increase. The marked increase in muscle oxidative capacity of these 65-yr-old subjects was accompanied by a 20% increase in $\dot{V}O_2$max. The authors concluded that peripheral changes do occur in the skeletal muscle of older individuals and are important in the adaptations to endurance exercise training. The intensity and duration of the training stimulus were the components of the study by Meredith et al. [99] that distinguished it from previous efforts that failed to detect enzymatic adaptations in muscle.

TABLE 3.1
Summary of Endurance Exercise Training Studies and Effects on Skeletal Muscle

Study	N	Gender	Age	Mode	Training Freq	Intensity	Duration	Length	Muscle Oxidative Capacity	V̇o₂max	Capillarization
Suominen et al. (130)	27	M	62	20 min running	3–5×		45–60 min	8W	↑ 45%	↑ 12%	
Örlander and Aniansson (107)	5	M	71 ± 1	Walk/run/static exercise	3×	70% V̇o₂max	45 min	12W	No Δ β-HAD No Δ CS ↑ 30% Cytoxidase		
Meredith et al. (99)	10	5M 5W	65 ± 3	Cycling	3×	70% HRR	45 min	12W	↑ 128%	↑ 20%	
Makrides et al. (93)	12	M	65 ± 3	Cycling	3×	5-min intervals 65–85%	60 min	12W		↑ 38%	
Coggan et al. (27)	23	12M 11W	65 ± 3	Walk/run	4×	80% MHR	45 min	40W	↑ 29–65% ↑ 17–38%	↑ 29% ↑ 26%	↑ 21%

HRR = heart rate reserve; MHR = maximal heart rate; V̇o₂max = maximal heart rate.

Probably the most comprehensive endurance exercise training study was carried out by Coggan et al. [27] in 23 healthy 65-yr-old men and women, who trained for an average of 10 months. In this investigation, where the exercise stimulus was progressively increased throughout the training program, the participants walked/jogged four times per week for 45 min/session at 80% of maximal heart rate. After endurance training, the activities of SDH, CS, and β-HAD in gastrocnemius muscle were significantly increased in both men and women, indicating a substantial improvement in mitochondrial respiratory capacity (Fig. 3.4A). A comparison of the men with the women in this study showed

FIGURE 3.4

A. *Changes in gastrocnemius muscle enzymatic activities (% △) after 10 months of endurance exercise training in older men and women (N =23). Phosphorylase* **(PHOS):** *phosphofructokinase* **(PFK):** *lactate dehydrogenase (LDH); succinate dehydrogenase* **(SDH);** *citrate synthase* **(CS);** *and β-hydroxyacyl-CoA dehydrogenase (β-HAD). Drawn from Coggan, A. R., R. J. Spina, D. S. King, M. A. Rogers, M. Brown, P. M. Nemeth, and J. O. Holloszy. Skeletal muscle adaptations to endurance training in 60- to 70-yr-old men and women.* J. Appl. Physiol. *72:1780–1786. 1992. * (p<0.05) † (p<0.001).*

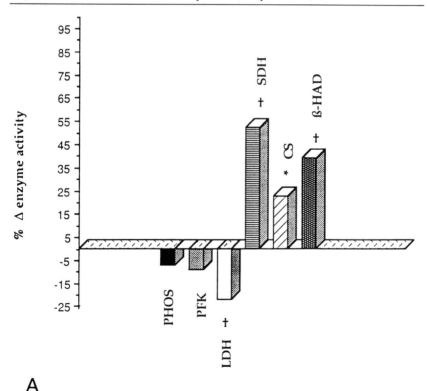

A

that the activities of SDH, CS, and β-HAD increased by 65%, 29%, and 42% for the men, and 38%, 17%, and 36% for the women. The exercise training program utilized in the study by Coggan et al. resulted in similar changes in respiratory enzyme activities for men and women [48] along with an increase in $\dot{V}O_2$max after training, which was essentially the same as the increase typically seen in young individuals who train vigorously.

Glycolytic Capacity of Aging Skeletal Muscle
Relatively few studies have examined the effects of endurance exercise training on the glycolytic capacity of skeletal muscle in older individuals. Suominen found no difference in hexokinase activity in the skeletal muscle of endurance-trained and untrained men between the ages of 33 and 70 yr [129]. Later, Suominen and co-workers determined that there was no change in HK activity as a result of 8 weeks of physical training in 56- to 70-yr-old men [130]. Total LDH activity decreased after endurance training in this study, a finding that is consistent with the results of Coggan et al. [27] but in conflict with Örlander et al. [107]. The decrease in total LDH activity in muscle after training in older people is similar to the response seen in young individuals [11]. Coggan et al. also found that 10

FIGURE 3.4
B. *Capillary density (caps/mm²) and number of capillaries in contact with each fiber for men (♂) and women (♀) pretraining and after 10 months of endurance training. Values are means ± SD for 12 men and 11 women. Drawn from Coggan, A. R., R. J. Spina, D. S. King, M. A. Rogers, M. Brown, P. M. Nemeth, and J. O. Holloszy. Skeletal muscle adaptations to endurance training in 60- to 70-yr-old men and women.* J. Appl. Physiol. *72:1780–1786, 1992. † vs. pre (p<0.001) †† vs. ♀ (p <0.001).*

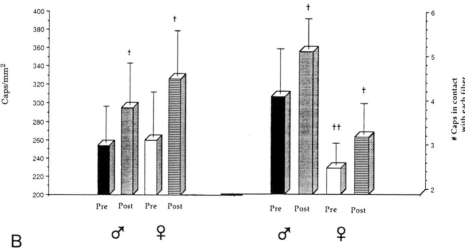

months of vigorous endurance exercise training elicited no change in PHOS or PFK activity (Fig. 3.4A) in the gastrocnemius muscle of older subjects [27], which is in conflict with the results of Örlander et al. [107]. The consensus from a limited number of studies is that, just as in young individuals, prolonged endurance exercise training has a minimal impact on glycolytic enzyme activity in the skeletal muscle of older individuals.

Endurance Training and Muscle Capillarization
Several studies in older individuals have shown no increases in capillary supply after endurance exercise training. Aniansson and Gustafsson [7] used a relatively short-term, low-intensity training program and found no change, while Denis and co-workers [34] measured capillary density in young and old subjects and also concluded that there was no increase in muscle capillarization after endurance training. A potential shortcoming of the Denis study was that many of the subjects had previously been training and, therefore, the capacity for further skeletal muscle adaptations may have been limited. Recently, Coggan et al. have shown that vigorous endurance exercise training in 60- to 70-yr-olds elicits an increase in capillary supply [27]. As shown in Figure 3.14B, capillary density per mm^2 increases in men and women by about 20% after 10 months of training. The fact that the capillary to fiber ratio and the number of capillaries in contact with each fiber increased by 25% indicates that the adaptation to endurance training in these older subjects is the generation of new capillaries, much the same response as in young individuals [1].

There is some evidence to suggest that resistive training in older men may induce capillary proliferation. Frontera et al. [46] strength trained 12 men (60–72 yr) for 12 weeks with three sets of eight repetitions at 80% of 1 repetition maximum (RM). The mean fiber area increased 28%, while there was a 15% increase in the number of capillaries per fiber.

Fiber Type Alterations with Endurance Training
Gollnick et al. [48] have shown that 5 months of endurance exercise training results in a 23% increase in the size of Type I muscle fibers, no change in Type II fiber area, and no change in the percentage of Type I muscle fibers in 30-yr-old men. There is, however, a transformation of Type IIb muscle fibers to IIa as a consequence of endurance training in young individuals [2].

None of the early studies in older people [107, 129, 130] dealing with the effect of endurance exercise training on skeletal muscle morphology evaluated changes in fiber type distribution or size. Recently, Denis and colleagues determined that moderate-intensity endurance training elicited no change in fiber type distribution in 60-yr-old subjects [34]. Along this line, Coggan et al. [27] found that the percentage of Type I muscle did not change with 10 months of intense endurance exercise training in

60- to 70-yr-old men and women (Fig. 3.5). Therefore, it is apparent that neither young nor old individuals show a change in percentage of Type I muscle with endurance training [27, 34, 48]. However, just like young individuals subjected to endurance exercise training, the 60- to 70-yr-old men and women subjects in Coggan's study experienced an approximately 8% increase in Type IIa fibers while the percentage of Type IIb fibers declined significantly. Along with this conversion of Type IIb fibers to IIa, there was a significant increase in the cross-sectional area of Type I skeletal muscle fibers that averaged approximately 12% for both men and women. Similarly, the size of Type IIa fibers was significantly increased for both men and women after training, 6% and 18%, respectively, while the Type IIb fiber area increased about 11% (Fig. 3.5). These moderate increases in muscle fiber area after endurance exercise training are similar to the changes seen in muscle from young individuals [1, 2, 48].

Considerable evidence indicates that older men and women adapt to endurance exercise training with similar relative increases in $\dot{V}O_2max$, capillarization, mitochondrial respiratory capacity, and fiber size, plus a Type IIb to IIa fiber conversion as young individuals. Just as in young

FIGURE 3.5

Fiber type distribution and % change (△ area) in fiber type area in response to 10 months of vigorous endurance exercise training in men (♂) and women (♀). Drawn from Coggan, A. R., R. J. Spina, D. S. King, M. A. Rogers, M. Brown, P. M. Nemeth, and J. O. Holloszy. Skeletal muscle adaptations to endurance training in 60- to 70-yr-old men and women. J. Appl. Physiol. *72:1780–1786, 1992.* * (p<0.05) vs. pre-training ** (p<0.05) vσ = non-significant.*

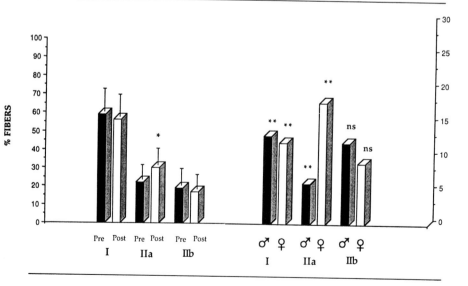

individuals, the adaptations that occur in response to vigorous endurance exercise training in older people are a function of the intensity and duration of the training stimulus. An exercise program that applies a training stimulus equivalent to that used in studies with young individuals will elicit similar relative changes in the morphology and metabolic capacity of the older individual's skeletal muscle.

Effect of Prolonged Endurance Training on Skeletal Muscle: Animal Studies
As in humans, aging in laboratory rats has been associated with a reduction in muscle mass. Interestingly, Fitts et al. [42] have shown that prolonged, voluntary wheel running in rats from the age of 6 to 28 months resulted in a 17% increase in the mass of the slow-twitch soleus muscle, while the fast-twitch extensor digitorum longus (EDL) muscle mass was reduced by about 20%. A lifetime of physical activity in these rats prolonged the isometric twitch duration by lengthening the one-half relaxation time of the soleus muscle but otherwise did not affect the contractile properties of either the soleus or EDL muscles. The authors concluded that rat skeletal muscle is fairly resistant to age-associated changes in function until very old age, i.e., older than 28 months of age.

Farrar et al. [39] found that 6 months of endurance exercise training increased state 3 respiration in subsarcolemmal mitochondria by 32% and 54% in 10- and 24-month-old Sprague-Dawley rats, respectively. Intermyofibrillar mitochondrial respiratory capacity increased by 24–27% in these two groups of rats. These results indicate that old rats have the capacity to adapt to the stress of prolonged endurance training that lasted for about one-fifth of their lifespan. This duration of exercise training corresponds to a training program lasting about 15 yr or so in the average human with a life span of about 74 yr. Similarly, Young et al. found that by both 9 and 24 months, SDH, CS, and β-HAD activity had increased by 20–40% in male Long-Evans rats that had commenced swim training at 6 months of age [142]. These results suggest that aging does not limit the adaptive capacity of aerobic metabolism in the skeletal muscle of rats subjected to chronic endurance training over a major portion of their life span [71].

Human Studies
We are not aware of any well-controlled, longitudinal human studies that have been performed to date to determine whether prolonged, vigorous endurance exercise training can maintain a high muscle respiratory capacity and capillary density over a period of years. However, several longitudinal studies have shown that chronic intense endurance exercise training can either reduce [115] or eliminate [113] the decline in $\dot{V}O_2max$ of master athletes over the span of 8 to 10 yr. Furthermore, Hagberg et al. have shown that the maximal estimated A-$\dot{V}O_2$ difference during exercise in master athlete distance runners who were matched on the basis of

training and performance with young runners is the same [58]. This indicates that there is no significant reduction in the oxygen extraction capacity of aged skeletal muscle. In this context, Coggan et al. [28] studied the histochemical and enzymatic characteristics of the gastrocnemius muscle of endurance-trained master athlete distance runners (63 ± 6 yr) and compared them with training and performance-matched young (26 ± 3 yr) runners (Table 3.2). While $\dot{V}o_2$max was 11% lower in the master athletes compared with the matched young runners, activities of β-HAD, CS, and SDH were 25 to 30% higher in these older runners indicating an enhanced muscle respiratory capacity. There were no significant differences in the glycolytic marker enzymes, PHOS or PFK, although total LDH activity was 46% lower in the master athletes. Coggan et al. also determined that the capillary/fiber ratio and number of capillaries in contact with each fiber were significantly greater in the master athletes compared with the matched young runners [28]. However, because the master athletes had larger Type I muscle fibers, capillary density was not different between the two groups. This seems to indicate that capillary supply in skeletal muscle can be maintained over a prolonged period of time. There was no difference in the percentage of Type I (59 vs. 60%), Type IIa (38 vs. 33%) or IIb (2 vs. 6%) muscle fibers between the master athletes and matched young runners, respectively; however, the master athletes' Type I fiber area was 34% greater than the matched young runners. Type II fiber area was not different between the groups. This selective hypertrophy of Type I muscle fibers also occurs in young individuals [48] and was probably due to the fact that the master athletes had been training longer than the matched young runners. One may hypothesize that the markedly increased muscle respiratory capacity and similar extent of muscle capillari-

TABLE 3.2
Skeletal Muscle Enzyme Activities and Capillarization in Master Athletes (MA) and Matched Young Runners (MYR)

	Master Athletes (N = 8)	Matched Young Runners (N = 8)	Δ
SDH	2.6 ± 0.6	2.0 ± 0.4*	30%
CS	6.0 ± 1.5	4.7 ± 0.8	28%
β-HAD	10.0 ± 1.8	8.0 ± 1.91*	25%
Capillaries/mm²	388 ± 93	367 ± 60	6%
Capillaries/fiber	2.4 ± 0.4	1.9 ± 0.4*	31%
Capillaries in contact with each fiber	5.9 ± 0.9	4.8 ± 0.8*	23%

SDH = succinate dehydrogenase; CS = citrate synthase; β-HAD = β-hydroxyacyl=coA dehydrogenase. Values are means ± SD in mol · kg protein^{-1} · h^{-1}.
*(p < 0.05) vs. master athletes.
Adapted from Coggan, A.R., R.J. Spina, M.A. Rogers, D.S. King, M. Brown, P.M. Nemeth, and J.O. Holloszy. Histochemical and enzymatic characteristics of skeletal muscle in master athletes. *J. Appl. Physiol.* 68:1896–1901, 1990.

zation in the master athletes compared with the matched young runners are due to the effects of vigorous endurance exercise training maintained for a prolonged period of time [63]. This notion is supported by the fact that the master athletes in this study had been running for an average of over 15 yr.

No vigorous endurance exercise training studies employing a progressive exercise stimulus for more than 12 months in duration have been conducted in humans. Limited evidence in animals and humans, however, suggests that not only can the respiratory capacity of skeletal muscle and its capillary supply be increased in older individuals but these adaptations that enhance functional capacity can be maintained over time if the duration and intensity of the exercise stimulus is adequate.

ADAPTABILITY OF OLDER INDIVIDUALS TO RESISTIVE TRAINING

A program of regular resistive training, carried out over an appropriate period of time, results in a myriad of physiological adaptations. Muscle hypertrophy and increases in strength, alterations in body composition, hormonal and neural adaptations, and changes in cardiovascular capacity have all been documented subsequent to various resistive training protocols [15, 35, 72, 111, 140, 141]. Up to the present, these adaptive responses have most frequently been shown in young men and women [102].

Skeletal Muscle Adaptations with Resistive Training: Young Individuals
An analysis of muscle strength improvements in young men and women summarized by Kraemer et al. [72] shows substantial increases after resistive training programs lasting between 9 and 24 weeks [15, 20, 95, 140]. Upper body strength in men increased by $21 \pm 10\%$ in 12 studies, while four studies in women showed a $28 \pm 8\%$ increase. Six studies conducted on lower body strength improvements with training in men showed a $27 \pm 23\%$ increase while four studies in women averaged a $35 \pm 12\%$ gain [72].

Considerable evidence indicates that skeletal muscle hypertrophy in humans is mediated by structural changes in muscle fibers. Resistive training increases the CSA of both Type I and Type II muscle fibers although the Type II fibers appear to be enlarged to a greater extent [51, 91]. The muscle hypertrophy is thought to be the result of an increase in the size and number of myofibrils, secondary to additional actin and myosin filaments, plus the addition of sarcomeres to the existing muscle fiber [90] rather than a cellular hyperplasia, although considerable controversy exists on this point [72]. In humans, the increase in size of the individual fibers translates into an increased CSA of the whole muscle. With computed tomography (CT) scans in young healthy men, Luthi et al. have shown that very heavy resistive exercise training increases CSA of vastus lateralis muscle by approximately 8%, most of the increase occurring during the second half of the training program [89]. High resistance/low repetition training protocols have generally produced a significant decrease in capillary density with no apparent changes in capillary/fiber ratio [131] while high repetition/low resistance training may effectively increase capillary supply [119]. The mitochondrial volume density appears to decrease with resistive training secondary to the hypertrophy of the muscle fiber [90].

Improvements in muscular strength are not only the result of structural changes in muscle but also are due to neural adaptations that typically account for strength gains during the early part of training [65, 101]. Neural adaptations that occur with resistive training include: *(a)* augmented neural drive to the skeletal muscle as evidenced by increased EMG activity; *(b)* increased motor unit recruitment and synchronization; and *(c)* improved coordination and learning [35].

Skeletal Muscle Adaptations with Resistive Training: Older Individuals
Early studies regarding the capacity of older people to adapt to resistive exercise indicated that 12 to 26 weeks of resistive exercise training elicited only minimal improvements in muscle strength of men and women between the ages of 60 and 75 yr (Table 3.3). Since that time, five reports in the literature have documented that, given an adequate training stimulus, older men and women show similar or greater strength gains compared to young individuals after resistive training [19, 25, 40, 47, 98].

Frontera et al. [47] trained the knee flexors and extensors of both legs in 12 men (66 ± 2 yr) for 12 weeks at 80% of 1 RM. In this study, the authors detected a weekly increment in muscle strength as measured by a 1-RM test that amounted to an improvement of 5%/day (Fig. 3.6A). This daily rate of strength gain compares favorably with the 4–6% increments observed in young men after an equivalent resistive training protocol [116] but is somewhat greater than other studies in older people [67, 101]. At the conclusion of 12 weeks of training, knee extensor and flexor strength (1 RM) had increased by over 100% and 200%, respectively. However, isokinetic strength increased by only 10% at slow angular velocities, and was unchanged at the faster speeds. CT scans of the thigh muscle before and after resistive training (Fig. 3.6B) showed that there was an 11% increase in muscle CSA, which was similar to the relative increase in area seen in young men after training [64, 89]. Furthermore, there was a substantial increase in Type I and Type II fiber area of 34% and 28%, respectively. In addition, strength training elicited a significant increase in muscle CS activity, capillary density, and

TABLE 3.3
Summary of Studies of Resistive Training in Older Individuals

Study	N	Gender	Age	Muscle	Type of Contractions	Training Frequency	Duration	% ↑ Strength	% ↑ CSA	% Δ Fiber Area I	II
Aniansson and Gustaysson (7)	12	M	72	Quadriceps	Concentric/eccentric	3×	12W	18			
Larsson (76)	6	M	59	Quadriceps	Concentric/eccentric (? sets/20 reps)	2×	15W	8(NS)		39	52
Aniansson et al. (9)	15	F	73	Quadriceps	Concentric/eccentric (elastic bands)	3×	26W	9			
Frontera et al. (47)	12	M	66 ± 2	Quadriceps	Concentric/eccentric (3 sets/8 reps)	3×	12W	107	11	34	28
Fiatarone et al. (40)	10	M3 F6	90 ± 1	Quadriceps	Concentric/eccentric (3 sets/8 reps)	3×	8W	174	15		
Brown et al. (19)	14	M	63 ± 3	Biceps Brachii	Concentric/eccentric (2–4 sets/10 reps)	3×	12W	48	17	14	30
Charette et al. (25)	13	F	69 ± 1	Quadriceps	Concentric/eccentric (3 sets/6 reps)	3×	12W	60		NS	20
Menkes et al. (98)	13	M	60 ± 2	Quadriceps	Concentric/eccentric (2 sets/15 reps)	3×	13W	41	8		

CSA = cross-sectional area; NS = non-significant; rep = repetitions.

FIGURE 3.6

A. *Time course of the dynamic strength improvement (1RM) of knee extensors (▲) and flexors (□). Results are means ± SE for 12 men, mean age 66 ± 2 yr.*

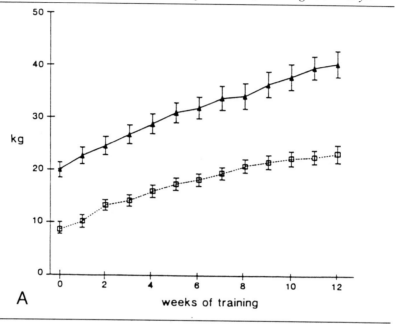

A

weeks of training

$\dot{V}O_2$max. Twenty-four-hour urinary excretion of 3-methyl-L-histidine was increased by 40% after resistive training, which suggests that the rate of myofibrillar protein turnover is accelerated as a consequence of vigorous resistive training [47]. Half of the men in this study were given a daily, protein calorie supplement (560 kcal/day) in addition to their ad libitum diet. CT scans showing greater gains in muscle for the protein supplement group and greater urinary creatinine excretion suggest that a change in total energy intake, or perhaps selected nutrients in the elderly beginning a strength training program can affect muscle hypertrophy. Older subjects exhibit a greater degree of exercise-induced muscle damage than young subjects do [41, 94], which may indicate a greater dietary protein requirement at the beginning of a training program.

Brown and co-workers [19] found that 12 weeks of progressive arm flexor training increased dynamic strength, as measured by 1 RM, by 48% in the trained arm with a 12% increase in the untrained control arm. CT scans before and after training showed a 17% increase in CSA of the elbow flexors of the trained arm but no significant change in the control arm. Type I and II fibers areas of the trained arm increased by 14% and

FIGURE 3.6

B. *Changes in thigh CSA* **(cm²)** *quantified by CT scans of the right and left leg pre-, mid-, and 12 weeks post-training in 12 men, mean age 66 ± 2 yr. (Reprinted with permission from Frontera, W. R., C. N. Meredith, K. P. O'Reilly, H. G. Knuttgen, and W. J. Evans. Strength conditioning in older men: skeletal muscle hypertrophy and improved function.* J. Appl. Physiol. *64(3):1038–1044, 1988). * (p<0.05) vs. pretraining.*

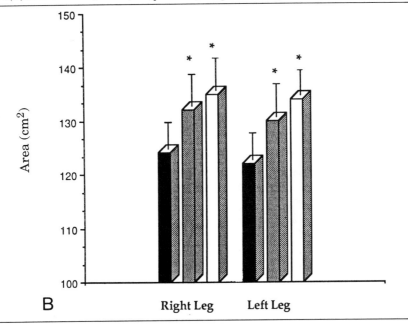

30%, respectively, while the percentage of distribution of Type I fibers in the biceps muscle was unchanged in the trained and untrained arm. This indicates a greater degree of hypertrophy in the Type II fibers, which is consistent with studies in young individuals [51, 91] but in contrast to the findings of Frontera et al. [47]. The 12% increase in dynamic strength of the control arm with no appreciable increase in size indicates that neural adaptations also occurred in response to resistive training in these older men [101]. The size and strength gains in the study by Brown et al. [19] were accompanied by an increase in muscular endurance so that the pretraining arm flexor 1 RM of the trained arm could be lifted an average of 14 times post-training compared with 7 times in the control arm. Furthermore, evoked twitch torque was not consistently increased in the trained arm compared with the control arm; thus, there appeared to be no improvement in the contractile property of the muscle. However, there was a significant increase in half-relaxation time that would theoretically prolong the twitch contraction and shift the force-velocity relationship to the left. The authors hypothesized that maximal tetanic tension of the muscle would therefore be developed at a lower motor unit firing frequency, which may impart a greater resistance to fatigue in the older mens' muscle after training [19].

One of the first studies to assess the capacity of older women to adapt to progressive resistive training was reported in 1991 by Charette et al. [25]. The women trained for 12 weeks with the training stimulus progressively increased from four to six sets at 65–75% of 1 RM. Increases in leg strength ranged from 28% (leg and hip extension) to 115% (leg flexion) indicating similar strength gains on the part of these older women as compared with older men and young individuals [15, 19, 20, 95, 140]. Type II fiber area increased 20% after training but there was no hypertrophy evident in the Type I muscle fibers. Most studies show that both Type I and Type II fibers increase in size after resistive training [19, 47, 126]. The extent of Type II fiber hypertrophy in these older women is similar to that observed in men [19, 47] but somewhat less than that of young resistive-trained women [126].

Recently, Klitgaard studied the effects of strength training on the contractile properties of old rat muscle and found that, while the muscle weights of the soleus and plantaris decreased significantly with age, 20 weeks of strength training somewhat counteracted the reduction in mass [69]. In addition, strength training neutralized the age-related decrease in twitch and tetanic tension and decreased both the time to peak tension and the half-relaxation time of the soleus and plantaris. These results have been interpreted to mean that resistive training carried out for a prolonged period during old age can have a positive effect on the contractile properties of skeletal muscle.

Resistive Training in the Very Old

In frail, institutionalized women and men, muscle strength is an important determinant of functional capacity, i.e., highly related to habitual walking speed. Recently, Bassey and co-workers [12, 13] found that leg extensor power is closely related to the speed of walking up stairs, to standing up from a chair, and to gait speed. Leg power, which represents a more dynamic measurement of muscle function may be a useful predictor of functional capacity in the very old.

The very old and frail elderly experience skeletal muscle atrophy of Type II fibers as a result of disuse, disease, undernutrition, and the effects of aging per se. In addition, the attendant muscle weakness that accompanies advanced age has been positively related to the risk of falling and fracture in these older individuals [120]. For this reason, Fiatarone and colleagues [40] studied the effects of high-intensity, progressive resistive training (Table 3.3) on quadriceps muscle strength in a group of institutionalized elderly men and women. Initial strength levels were extremely low in these subjects, with a mean 1 RM of 9 kg for the quadriceps. The absolute amount of weight lifted by the subjects during the training increased from 8 to 21 kg. The average increase in strength after 8 weeks of resistive training was $174 \pm 31\%$ and the mean increase in muscle CSA via CT scanning was $15 \pm 8\%$. The substantial increases in muscle size and strength were accompanied by clinically significant improvements in tandem gait speed, an index of functional mobility. Interestingly, repeat 1 RM testing in seven of the subjects after 4 weeks of no training showed that quadriceps strength had declined 32%. This study demonstrates that frail elderly men and women, well into the 10th decade of life, retain the capacity to adapt to progressive resistive exercise training with significant and clinically relevant muscle hypertrophy and increases in muscle strength. The results from the progressive, resistive training studies performed on young people, healthy free-living elderly, as well as the frail men and women mentioned above indicated that it is the intensity of the stimulus, not the underlying fitness or frailty of the individual, that determines the response to exercise training.

SUMMARY

There is an approximate 30% decline in muscle strength and a 40% reduction in muscle area between the second and seventh decades of life. Thus, the loss of muscle mass with aging appears to be the major factor in the age-related loss of muscle strength. The loss of muscle mass is partially due to a significant decline in the numbers of both Type I and Type II muscle fibers plus a decrease in the size of the muscle cells, with the Type II fibers showing a preferential atrophy. There appears to be no loss of glycolytic capacity in senescent skeletal muscle whereas muscle oxidative enzyme activity and muscle capillarization decrease by about 25%. Vigorous endurance exercise training in older people, where the stimulus is progressively increased, elicits a proliferation of muscle capillaries, an increase in oxidative enzyme activity, and a significant improvement in $\dot{V}O_2$max. Likewise, progressive resistive training in older individuals results in muscle hypertrophy and increased strength, if the training stimulus is of a sufficient intensity and duration. Since older individuals adapt to resistive and endurance exercise training in a similar fashion to young people, the decline in the muscle's metabolic and force-producing capacity can no longer be considered as an inevitable consequence of the aging process. Rather, the adaptations in aging skeletal muscle to exercise training may prevent sarcopenia, enhance the ease of carrying out the activities of daily living, and exert a beneficial effect on such age-associated diseases as Type II diabetes, coronary artery disease, hypertension, osteoporosis, and obesity.

ACKNOWLEDGMENTS

The authors thank Dr. James Hagberg and Dr. Ben Hurley for their critical comments and helpful suggestions during the preparation of this manuscript, along with the secretarial expertise of Dorothy O'Donnell.

REFERENCES

1. Andersen, P., and J. Henriksson. Capillary density of the quadriceps femoris muscle of man: adaptive response to exercise. *J. Physiol.* 270:677–680, 1977.
2. Andersen, P., and J. Henriksson. Training induced changes in the subgroups of human type II skeletal muscle fibers. *Acta Physiol. Scand.* 99:123–125, 1977.
3. Aniansson, A., G. Grimby, M. Hedberg, and M. Krotkiewski. Muscle morphology, enzyme activity and muscle strength in elderly men and women. *Clin. Physiol.* 1:73–86, 1981.
4. Aniansson, A., G. Grimby, M. Hedberg, A. Rundgren, and L. Sperling. Muscle function in old age. *Scand. J. Rehab. Med.* (Suppl) 6:43–49, 1978.
5. Aniansson, A., G. Grimby, E. Nygaard, and B. Saltin. Muscle fiber composition and fiber area in various age groups. *Muscle Nerve* 2:271–272, 1980.
6. Aniansson, A., G. Grimby, and A. Rundgren. Isometric and isokinetic quadriceps muscle strength in 70-year old men and women. *Scand. J. Rehab. Med.* 12:161–168, 1980.
7. Aniansson, A., and E. Gustavsson. Physical training in elderly men with specific reference to quadriceps muscle strength and morphology. *Clin. Physiol.* 1:87–98, 1981.
8. Aniansson, A., M. Hedberg, G.-B. Henning, and G. Grimby. Muscle morphology, enzymatic activity, and muscle strength in elderly men: A followup study. *Muscle Nerve* 9:585–591, 1986.
9. Aniansson, A., P. Ljungberg, A. Rundgren, and H. Weltequist. Effect of a training programme for pensioners on condition and muscular strength. *Arch. Gerontol. Geriatr.* 3:229–241, 1984.
10. Aniansson, A., C. Zetterberg, M. Hedberg, and P. V. Komi. Impaired muscle function with aging. A backward factor in the incidence of fractures of the proximal end of the femur. *Clin. Orthop. Relat. Res.* 191:193–200, 1984.
11. Apple, F. S., and M. A. Rogers. Skeletal muscle lactate dehydrogenase isozyme alterations in men and women marathon runners. *J. Appl. Physiol.* 61:477–481, 1986.
12. Bassey, E. J., M. J. Bendall, and M. Pearson. Muscle strength in the triceps surae and objectively measured customary walking activity in men and women over 65 years of age. *Clin. Sci.* 74:85–89, 1988.
13. Bassey, E. J., M. A. Fiatarone, E. F. O'Neil, M. Kelly, W. J. Evans, and L. A. Lipsitz. Leg extensor power and functional performance in very old men and women. *Clin. Sci.* 82:321–327, 1992.
14. Belanger, A. Y., and A. J. McComas. Extent of motor unit activation during effort. *J. Appl. Physiol.* 51:1131–1135, 1981.
15. Berger, R. A. Effect of varied weight training programs on strength. *Res Q* 33:168–181, 1962.
16. Borges, O., and B. Essén-Gustavsson. Enzyme activities in type I and II muscle fibers of human skeletal muscle in relation to age and torque development. *Acta Physiol. Scand.* 136:29–36, 1989.
17. Borkan, G. A., D. E. Hults, S. G. Gerzof, A. H. Robbins, and C. K. Silbert. Age changes in body composition revealed by computed tomography. *J. Gerontol.* 38:673–677, 1983.
18. Brooke, M. H., and K. K. Kaiser. Three "myosin adenosine triphosphase" systems: the

nature of their pH and sulphydryl dependence. *J. Histochem. Cytochem.* 18:670–672, 1970.

19. Brown, A. B., N. McCartney, and D. G. Sale. Positive adaptations to weight-lifting training in the elderly. *J. Appl. Physiol.* 69:1725–1733, 1990.

20. Brown C. H., and J. H. Wilmore. The effects of maximal resistance training on the strength and body composition of women athletes. *Med Sci Sports* 6:174–177, 1974.

21. Brown, W. F. A method for estimating the number of motor units in thenar muscles and the changes in motor unit count with ageing. *J. Neurol. Neurosurg. Psychiatry* 35:845–852, 1972.

22. Bruce, S. A., D. Newton, and R. C. Woledge. Effect of age on voluntary force and cross-sectional area of human adductor pollicis muscle. *Q. J. Exp. Physiol.* 74:359–362, 1989.

23. Campbell, M. J., A. J. McComas, and F. Petito. Physiological changes in aging muscle. *J. Neurol. Neurosurg. Psychiatry* 36:174–182, 1973.

24. Cartee, G. C., and R. P. Farrar. Comparison of muscle respiatory capacity and $\dot{V}o_2$max between young and old exercise-trained rats. *J. Appl. Physiol.* 63:257–261, 1987.

25. Charette. S. L., L. McEvoy, G. Pyka, C. Snow-Harter, D. Guido, R. A. Wiswell, and R. Marcus. Muscle hypertrophy response to resistance training in older women. *J. Appl. Physiol.* 70:1912–1916, 1991.

26. Coggan, A. R., R. J. Spina, D. S. King, M. A. Rogers, M. Brown, P. M. Nemeth, and J. O. Holloszy. Histochemical and enzymatic comparison of the gastrocnemius muscle of young and elderly men and women. *J. Gerontol. Biol. Sci.* 46B:71–76, 1992.

27. Coggan, A. R., R. J. Spina. D. S. King, M. A. Rogers, M. Brown, P. M. Nemeth, and J. O. Holloszy. Skeletal muscle adaptations to endurance training in 60- to 70-yr-old men and women. *J. Appl. Physiol.* 72:1780–1786, 1992.

28. Coggan, A. R., R. J. Spina, M. A. Rogers, D. S. King, M. Brown, P. M. Nemeth, and J. O. Holloszy. Histochemical and enzymatic characteristics of skeletal muscle in master athletes. *J. Appl. Physiol.* 68:1896–1901, 1990.

29. Cohn, S. H., D. Vartsky, S. Yasurura, A. Savitsky, I. Zanzi, A. Vaswani, and K. J. Ellis. Compartmental body composition based on total body potassium, and calcium. *Am. J. Physiol.* 239:E524–E530, 1980.

30. Cunningham, D. A., D. Morrison, C. L. Rice, and C. Cooke. Ageing and isokinetic plantar flexion. *Eur. J. Appl. Physiol.* 56:24–29, 1987.

31. Danneskiold-Samsoe, B., V. Kofod, J. Munter, G. Grimby, P. Schnohr, and G. Jensen. Muscle strength and functional capacity in 78–81 year old men and women. *Eur. J. Appl. Physiol.* 52:310–314, 1984.

32. Davies, C. T. M., D. O. Thomas, and M. J. White. Mechanical properties of young and elderly human muscle. *Acta Med. Scand. Suppl.* 711:219–226, 1986.

33. Davies, C. T. M., and M. J. White. Contractile properties of elderly human triceps surae. *Gerontology* 29:19–25, 1983.

34. Denis, C., J. C. Chatard, D. Dormois, M. T. Linossier, A. Geyssant, and J. Lacour. Effects of endurance training on capillary supply of human skeletal muscle of two age groups (20 and 60 years) *J. Physiol. Paris* 81:379–383, 1986.

35. Enoka, R. M. Muscle strength and its development: new perspectives. *Sports Med* 6:146–168, 1988.

36. Essén, B., E. Jansson, J. Henriksson, A. W. Taylor, and B. Saltin. Metabolic characteristics of fibre types in human skeletal muscle. *Acta Physiol. Scand.* 95:153–165, 1975.

37. Essén-Gustavsson, B., and O. Borges. Histochemical and metabolic characteristics of human skeletal muscle in relation to age. *Acta Physiol. Scand.* 126:107–114, 1986.

38. Evans. W. J. Exercise and muscle metabolism in the elderly. In *Nutrition and Aging.* New York: Academic Press, Inc., 1986, pp. 179–191.

39. Farrar, R. P., T. P. Martin, and C. M. Ardies. The interaction of aging and endurance

exercise upon the mitochondrial function of skeletal muscle. *J. Gerontol.* 36:642–647, 1981.

40. Fiatarone, M. A., E. C. Marks, N. D. Ryan, C. N. Meredith, L. A. Lipsitz, and W. J. Evans. High intensity strength training in nonagenarians. Effects on skeletal muscle. *JAMA* 263:3029–3034, 1990.

41. Fielding, R. A., C. A. Meredith, K. P. O'Reilly, W. R. Frontera, J. G. Cannon, and W. J. Evans. Enhanced protein breakdown following eccentric exercise in young and old men. *J. Appl. Physiol.* 71:674–679, 1991.

42. Fitts, R. H., J. P. Troup, F. A. Witzmann, and J. O. Holloszy. The effect of ageing and exercise on skeletal muscle function. *Mech. Ageing Dev.* 27:161–172, 1984.

43. Fleg, J. L., and E. G. Lakatta. Role of muscle loss in the age-associated reduction in $\dot{V}O_2$max. *J. Appl. Physiol.* 65:1147–1151, 1988.

44. Flynn, M. A., G. B. Nolph, A. S. Baker, W. M. Martin, and G. Krause. Total body potassium in aging humans: a longitudinal study. *Am. J. Clin. Nutr.* 50:713–717, 1989.

45. Frontera, W. R., V. A. Hughes, K. J. Lutz, and W. J. Evans. A cross-sectional study of muscle strength and mass in 45- to 78-yr-old men and women. *J. Appl. Physiol.* 71:644–650, 1991.

46. Frontera, W. R., C. N. Meredith, K. P. O'Reilly, and W. J. Evans. Strength training and determinants of $\dot{V}O_2$max in older men. *J. Appl. Physiol.* 68:329–333, 1990.

47. Frontera, W. R., C. N. Meredith, K. P. O'Reilly, H. G. Knuttgen, and W. J. Evans. Strength conditioning in older men: skeletal muscle hypertrophy and improved function. *J. Appl. Physiol.* 64:1038–1044, 1988.

48. Gollnick, P. D., R. B. Armstrong, B. Saltin, C. W. Saubert, W. L. Sembrowich, and R. E. Sheperd. Effect of training on enzyme activity and fiber composition of human skeletal muscle. *J. Appl. Physiol.* 34:107–111, 1973.

49. Gollnick, P. D., R. B. Armstrong, C. W. Saubert IV, K. Piehl, and B. Saltin. Enzyme activity and fiber composition in skeletal muscle of untrained and trained men. *J. Appl. Physiol.* 33:312–319, 1972.

50. Gollnick, P. D., and D. R. Hodgson. The identification of fiber types in skeletal muscle: a continual dilemma. K. B. Pandolf (ed). *Exercise and Sports Sciences Reviews* Vol 14, New York: Macmillan, 1986, pp. 81–104.

51. Gonyea, W. J., and D. Sale. Physiology of weight lifting exercise. *Arch Phys Med. Rehabil.* 63:235–237, 1982.

52. Green, H. J. Characteristics of aging human skeletal muscle. J. R. Sutton and R. M. Brook (eds.). *Sports Medicine for the Mature Athlete.* Indianapolis, IN: Benchmark Press, 1986. pp. 17–26.

53. Green, H. J., B. Daub, M. E. Houston, J. A. Thomson, I. Fraser, and D. Ranney. Human vastus lateralis and gastrocnemius muscles: a comparative histochemical and biochemical analysis. *J. Neurol. Sci.* 52:201–210, 1981.

54. Grimby, G. Physical activity and muscle training in the elderly. *Acta Med. Scand. Suppl.* 711:233–237, 1986.

55. Grimby, G., A. Aniansson, C. Zetterberg, and B. Saltin. Is there a change in relative muscle fibre composition with age? *Clin. Physiol.* 4:189–194, 1984.

56. Grimby, G., B. Danneskiold-Samsoe, K. Hvid, and B. Saltin. Morphology and enzymatic capacity in arm and leg muscles in 78–81 year old men and women. *Acta Physiol. Scand.* 115:125–134, 1982.

57. Grimby, G., and B. Saltin. The ageing muscle. *Clin. Physiol.* 3:209–218, 1983.

58. Hagberg, J. M., W. K. Allen, D. R. Seals, B. F. Hurley, A. A. Ehsani, and J. O. Holloszy. A hemodynamic comparison of young and older endurance athletes. *J. Appl. Physiol.* 58:2041–2046, 1985.

59. Hagberg, J. M., J. E. Graves, M. Limacher, D. R. Woods, S. H. Leggett, C. Cononie, J. J. Gruber, and M. L. Pollock. Cardiovascular responses of 70- to 79-yr old men and women to exercise training. *J. Appl. Physiol.* 66:2589–2599, 1989.

60. Harries, U. J., and E. J. Bassey. Torque-velocity relationships for the knee extensors in women in their 3rd and 7th decades. *Eur J. Appl. Physiol.* 60:187–190, 1990.

61. Heath, G. W., J. M. Hagberg, A. A. Ehsani, and J. O. Holloszy. A physiological comparison of young and older athletes. *J. Appl. Physiol.* 51:634–640, 1981.

62. Holloszy, J. O., and E. F. Coyle. Adaptations of skeletal muscle to endurance exercise and their metabolic consequences. *J. Appl. Physiol.* 56:831–838, 1984.

63. Houston, M. E., and H. J. Green. Skeletal muscle and physiologic characteristics of a world champion masters distance runner: a case study. *Int. J. Sports Med.* 2:47–49, 1981.

64. Hurley, B. F., R. A. Redmond, K. H. Koffler, A. Menkes, J. M. Hagberg, R. E. Pratley, J. W. R. Young, and A. P. Goldberg. Assessment of strength training effects on leg composition in older men using MRI. *Med. Sci. Sports Exerc.* 23:S108, 1991.

65. Ikai, M., and T. Fukunaga. A study on training effect on strength per unit cross-sectional area of muscle by means of ultrasonic measurement. *Eur. J. Appl. Physiol.* 28:173–180, 1970.

66. Jette, A. M., and L. G. Branch. The Framingham disability study: II. Physical disability among the aging. *Am. J. Public Health* 71:1211–1216, 1981.

67. Kaufman, T. L. Strength training effect in young and aged women. *Arch. Phys. Med. Rehabil.* 65:223–226, 1985.

68. Klein, C., D. A. Cunningham, D. H. Patterson, and A. W. Taylor. Fatigue and recovery contractile properties of young and elderly men. *Eur. J. Appl. Physiol.* 57:684–690, 1988.

69. Klitgaard, H., R. Marc, A. Brunet, H. Vandewalle, and H. Monod. Contractile properties of old rat muscles: effect of increased use. *J. Appl. Physiol.* 67:1401–1408, 1989.

70. Kohrt W. M., M. T. Malley, A. R. Coggan, R. J. Spina, T. Ogawa, A. A. Ehsani, R. E. Bourey, W. H. Martin, and J. O. Holloszy. Effects of gender, age, and fitness level on response of $\dot{V}O_2$max to training to 60–71 year olds. *J. Appl. Physiol.* 71:2004–2011, 1991.

71. Kovanen, V., and H. Suominen. Effects of age and life-time physical training on fibre composition of slow and fast skeletal muscles in rats. *Pflugers Arch.* 408:543–551, 1987.

72. Kraemer, W. J., M. R. Deschenes, and S. J. Fleck. Physiological adaptations to resistance exercise. *Sports Med.* 6:246–256, 1988.

73. Laforest, S., D. M. M. St-Pierre, J. Cyr, and D. Gayton. Effects of age and regular exercise on muscle strength and endurance. *Eur. J. Appl. Physiol.* 60:104–111, 1990.

74. Larsson, L. Histochemical characteristics of human skeletal muscle during ageing. *Acta Physiol. Scand.* 117:469–671, 1983.

75. Larsson, L. Morphological and functional characteristics of the ageing skeletal muscle in man. *Acta Physiol. Scand. Suppl.* 457:1–36, 1978.

76. Larsson, L. Physical training effects on muscle morphology in sedentary males at different ages. *Med. Sci. Sports Exerc.* 14:203–206, 1982.

77. Larsson, L., G. Grimby, and J. Karlsson. Muscle strength and speed of movement in relation to age and muscle morphology. *J. Appl. Physiol.: Respirat. Environ. Exercise Physiol.* 46:451–456, 1979.

78. Larsson, L., and J. Karlsson. Isometric and dynamic endurance as a function of age and skeletal muscle characteristics. *Acta Physiol. Scand.* 104:129–136, 1978.

79. Larsson, L., B. Sjodin, and J. Karlsson. Histochemical and biochemical changes in human skeletal muscle with age in sedentary males, age 22–65 years. *Acta Physiol. Scand.* 103:31–39, 1978.

80. Lennmarken, C., T. Bergman, J. Larsson, and L.-E. Larsson. Skeletal muscle function in man: force, relaxation rate, endurance and contraction time-dependence on sex and age. *Clin. Physiol.* 5:243–255, 1985.

81. Lexell, J., and D. Y. Downham. What is the effect of aging on type 2 muscle fibers? *J. Neurol. Sci.* 107:250–251, 1992.

82. Lexell, J. and D. Y. Downham. The occurrence of fiber type grouping in healthy human muscle: a quantitative study of cross-sectios of whole vastus lateralis from men between 15 and 83 years. *Acta Neuropathol.* 81:377–381, 1991.

83. Lexell, J., D. Downham, and M. Sjostrom. Distribution of different fibre types in human skeletal muscle: fibre type arrangement in m. vastus lateralis from three groups of healthy men between 15 and 83 years. *J. Neurol Sci.* 72:211–222, 1986.

84. Lexell, J., K. Hendriksson-Larsen, B. Winblad, and M. Sjostrom. Distribution of different fiber types in human skeletal muscles: effects of aging studied in whole muscle cross section. *Muscle Nerve* 6:588–595, 1983.

85. Lexell, J., and C. Taylor. Variability in muscle fibre areas in whole human quadriceps muscle. How much and why? *Acta Physiol. Scand.* 136:561–568, 1989.

86. Lexell, J., and C. Taylor. Variability in muscle fibre areas in whole human quadriceps muscle: how to reduce sampling errors in biopsy techniques. *Clin. Physiol.* 9:333–343, 1989.

87. Lexell, J., C. Taylor, and M. Sjostrom. What is the cause of the ageing atrophy? Total number, size and proportion of different fiber types studies in whole vastus lateralis muscle from 15- to 83-year-old men. *J. Neurol. Sci.* 84:275–294, 1988.

88. Lexell, J., and C. C. Taylor. Variability in muscle fiber areas in whole human quadriceps muscle: effects of increasing age. *J. Anat.* 174:239–249, 1991.

89. Luthi, J. M., H. Howald, H. Claasen, K. Rosler, P. Vock, and H. Hoppeler. Structural changes in skeletal muscle tissue with heavy-resistance exercise. *Int. J. Sports Med.* 7:123–127, 1986.

90. MacDougall, J. D. Morphological changes in human skeletal muscle following strength training and immobilization. Jones, N. L., et al. (eds.) *Human Muscle Power,* Champaign, IL: Human Kinetics Publishers, Inc. 1986, pp. 269–288.

91. MacDougall, J. D., G. C. B. Elder, D. G. Sale, J. R. Moroz, and J. R. Sutton. Effects of strength training and immobilization on human muscle fibers. *Eur. J. Appl. Physiol.* 43:25–34, 1980.

92. Maclennan, W. J., M. R. P. Hall, J. I. Timothy, and M. Robinson. Is weakness in old age due to muscle wasting? *Age Ageing* 9:188–192, 1980.

93. Makrides, L., G. J. H. Heigenhauser, and N. L. Jones. High-intensity endurance training in 20- to 30 and 60- to 70-yr-old healthy men. *J. Appl. Physiol.* 69:1792–1798, 1990.

94. Manfredi, T. G., R. A. Fielding, K. P. O'Reilly, C. N. Meredith, H. Y. Lee, and W. J. Evans. Serum creating kinase activity and exercise-induced muscle damage in older men. *Med. Sci. Sports Exerc.* 23:1028–1034, 1991.

95. Mayhew, J. L., and P. M. Grass. Body composition changes in young women with high intensity weight training. *Res Q* 45:433–440, 1974.

96. McComas, A. J., A. R. M. Upton, and R. E. P. Sica. Motoneuron disease and ageing. *Lancet* II: 1477–1480, 1973.

97. McDonagh, M. J. M., M. J. White, and C. T. M. Davies. Different effects of aging on the mechanical properties of arm and leg muscles. *Gerontology* 30:49–54, 1984.

98. Menkes, A. M., S. Mazel, R. A. Redmond, K. Koffler, C. R. Libanati, C. M. Gundberg, T. M. Zizic, J. M. Hagberg, R. E. Pratley, and B. F. Hurley. Strength training increases regional bone mineral density and bone remodeling in middle-aged and older men. *J. Appl. Physiol.* In press.

99. Meredith, C., W. Frontera, E. Fisher, V. Hughes, J. Herland, J. Edwards, and W. Evans. Peripheral effects of endurance training in young and old subjects. *J. Appl. Physiol.* 66:2844–2849, 1989.

100. Moller, P., J. Bergstrom, P. Furst, and K. Hellstrom. Effect of aging on energy-rich phosphagens in human skeletal muscle. *Clin. Sci.* 58:553–555, 1980.

101. Moritani, T., and H. A. DeVries. Neural factors versus hypertrophy in the time course of muscle strength gains. *Am. J. Phys. Med.* 82:521–524, 1979.

102. Moritani, T., and H. A. DeVries. Potential for gross muscle hypertrophy in older men. *J. Gerontol.* 35:672–682, 1980.
103. Murray, M. P., E. H. Duthie, S. T. Gambert, S. B. Sepic, L. A. Mollinger. Age-related differences in knee muscle strength in normal women. *J. Gerontol.* 40:275–280, 1985.
104. Novak, L. P. Aging, total body potassium, fat free mass, and cell mass in males and females between ages 18 and 85 years. *J. Gerontol.* 24:438–443, 1972.
105. Nygaard, E. Skeletal muscle fiber characteristics in young women. *Acta Physiol. Scand.* 112:299–304, 1981.
106. Nygaard, E., and J. Sanchez. Intramuscular variation of fiber types in the brachial biceps and the lateral vastus muscles of elderly men: how representative is a small biopsy sample? *Anat. Rec.* 203:451–459, 1982.
107. Örlander, J., and A. Aniansson. Effects of Physical training on skeletal muscle metabolism and ultrastructure in 70 to 75-year-old men. *Acta Physiol. Scand.* 109:149–154, 1980.
108. Örlander, J., K. H. Kiesling, L. Larsson, J. Karlsson, and A. Aniansson. Skeletal muscle metabolism and ultrastructure in relation to age in sedentary men. *Acta Physiol. Scand.* 104:249–261, 1978.
109. Parízkova, J. Body composition and exercise during growth and development. G. L. Rarick (ed.). *Physical Activity: Human Growth and Development.* New York: Academic Press, 1974.
110. Parízkova, J. E. Eiselt, S. Sprynarova, and M. Wachtlova. Body composition, aerobic capacity, and density of muscle capillaries in young and old men. *J. Appl. Physiol.* 31:323–325, 1971.
111. Petrofsky, J. S., R. L. Borse, and A. R. Lind. Comparison of physiological response of women and men to isometric exercise. *J. Appl. Physiol.* 38:863–868, 1975.
112. Poehlmann, E. T., and E. S. Horton. Regulation of energy expenditure in aging humans. *Ann. Rev. Nutr.* 10:255–275, 1990.
113. Pollock, M. L., C. Foster, D. Knapp, J. L. Rod, and D. H. Schmidt. Effect of age and training on aerobic capacity and body composition of master athletes. *J. Appl. Physiol.* 62:625–731, 1987.
114. Rikki, R., and S. Busch. Motor performance of women as a function of age and physical activity level. *J. Gerontol.* 41:645–649, 1986.
115. Rogers, M. A., J. M. Hagberg, W. H. Martin III, A. A. Ehsani, and J. O. Holloszy. Decline in Vo₂max with aging in master athletes and sedentary men. *J. Appl. Physiol.* 68:2195–2199, 1990.
116. Rutherford, O. M., C. A. Greig, A. J. Sargent, and D. A. Jones. Strength training and power output: transference effects in the human quadriceps muscle. *J. Sports Sci.* 4:101–107, 1986.
117. Sandler, R. B. Muscle strength assessments and the prevention of osteoporosis. *J. Am. Geriatr. Soc.* 37:1192–1197, 1989.
118. Sato, T., H. Akatsuka, K. Kuniyoshi, and Y. Tokoro. Age changes in size and number of muscle fibers in human minor pectoral muscle. *Mech. Ageing Dev.* 28:99–109, 1984.
119. Schantz, P. Capillary supply in hypertrophied human skeletal muscle *Acta Physiol. Scand.* 114:635–637, 1982.
120. Scheibel, A. Falls, motor dysfunction and correlative neurohistologic changes in the elderly. *Clin. Geriatr. Med.* 1:671–677, 1985.
121. Deleted in proof.
122. Seals, D. R., J. M. Hagberg, B. F. Hurley, A. A. Ehsani, and J. O. Holloszy. Endurance training in older men and women. I. Cardiovascular response to exercise. *J. Appl. Physiol* 57:1024–1029, 1984.
123. Silberman, M., S. Finkelbrand, A. Weiss, D. Gershon, and A. Reznick. Morphometric analysis of aging skeletal muscle following endurance training. *Muscle Nerve* 6:136–142, 1983.

124. Sjogaard, G. Muscle enzyme activity in relation to maximal oxygen uptake. *Acta Physiol. Scand.* 112:12A, 1981.
125. Sperling, L. Evaluation of upper extremity function in 70-year old men and women. *Scand. J. Rehabil. Med.* 12:139–144, 1980.
126. Stålberg, R., O. Borges, M. Ericcson, B. Essen-Gustavsson, P. Fawcett, L. Nordesjo, B. Nordgren, and R. Uhlin. The quadriceps femoris muscle in 20- 70-year-old subjects: relationship between knee extension torque, electrophysiological parameters, and muscle fiber characteristics. *Muscle Nerve* 12:382–389, 1989.
127. Stålberg, R., and P. R. W. Fawcett. Macro E.M.G. in healthy subjects of different ages. *J. Neurol. Neurosurg. Psychiatry* 45:870–878, 1982.
128. Staron, R. S., E. S. Malicky, M. J. Leonardi, J. E. Falkel, F. C. Hagerman, and G. A. Dudley. Muscle hypertrophy and fast fiber type conversions in heavy resistance-trained women. *Eur. J. Appl. Physiol.* 60:71–79, 1989.
129. Suominen, H., and E. Heikkinen. Enzyme activities in muscle and connective tissue of M. vastus lateralis in habitually training and sedentary 33 to 70-year-old men. *Eur. J. Appl. Physiol.* 34:249–254, 1975.
130. Suominen, H., E. Heikkinen, H. Liesen, D. Michel, and W. Hollmann. Effects of 8 weeks' endurance training on skeletal muscle metabolism in 56–70-year-old sedentary men. *Eur. J. Appl. Physiol.* 37:173–180, 1977.
131. Suominen, H., E. Heikkinen, and T. Parkatti. Effect of eight weeks physical training on muscle and connective tissue of the M. vastus lateralis in 69-year-old men and women. *J. Gerontol.* 32:33–37, 1977.
132. Tesch, P. A., A. Thorsson, and P. Kaiser. Muscle capillary supply and fiber type characteristics in weight and power lifters. *J. Appl. Physiol.* 56:35–38, 1984.
133. Tomlinson, B. E., and D. Irving. The numbers of limb motor neurons in the human lumbosacral cord throughout life. *J. Neurol. Sci.* 34:213–219, 1977.
134. Tomlinson, B. E., J. N. Walton, and J. J. Rebeiz. The effects of aging and cachexia upon skeletal muscle. A histopathological study. *J. Neurol. Sci.* 9:321–346, 1969.
135. Tomonaga, M. Histochemical and ultrastructural changes in senile human skeletal muscle. *J. Am. Geriatr. Soc.* 25:125–131, 1977.
136. Tzankoff, S. P., and A. H. Norris. Effect of muscle mass decrease on age-related BMR changes. *J. Appl. Physiol.* 43:1001–1006, 1977.
137. Tzankoff, S. P., and A. H. Norris. Longitudinal changes in basal metabolism in man. *J. Appl. Physiol.* 45:536–539, 1978.
138. Vandervoort, A. A., K. C. Hayes, A. Y. Belanger. Strength and endurance of skeletal muscle in the elderly. *Physiother. Can.* 38:167–173, 1986.
139. Vandervoort, A. A., and A. J. McComas. Contractile changes in opposing muscles of the human ankle joint with aging. *J. Appl. Physiol.* 61:361–367, 1986.
140. Wilmore, J. H. Alterations in strength, body composition, and anthropometric measurements consequent to a 10-week weight training program. *Med. Sci. Sports* 6:133–138, 1974.
141. Wilmore, J. H., R. B. Parr, R. N. Girandola, P. Ward, P. A. Vodak, T. J. Barstow, T. V. Pipes, G. T. Romero, and P. Leslie. Physiological alterations consequent to circuit weight training. *Med. Sci. Sports* 10:79–84, 1978.
142. Young, J. C., M. Chen, and J. O. Holloszy. Maintenance of adaptation of skeletal muscle mitochondria to exercise in old rats. *Med. Sci. Sports Exerc.* 15:243–246, 1983.
143. Young, A., M. Stokes, and M. Crowe. Size and strength of the quadriceps muscles of old and young women. *Eur. J. Clin. Invest.* 14:282–287, 1984.
144. Young, A., M. Stokes, and M. Crowe. The size and strength of the quadriceps muscles of old and young men. *Clin. Physiol.* 5:145–154, 1985.

4
Physiological Limiting Factors and Distance Running: Influence of Gender and Age on Record Performances

MICHAEL J. JOYNER, M.D.

INTRODUCTION

Results from competitive distance running events can provide valuable insight into several key areas of integrative physiology. First, world records and other marks by elite athletes offer a framework for the discussion of how various physiological factors interact as determinants of performance [13, 50, 52, 54, 58, 62, 84]. Such analysis can also serve as fuel for the never-ending speculation about just how fast the "ultimate" time for a given distance might be [50, 52, 73, 74, 86]. Second, the decline in performance in elite older athletes can be used to gain insight into the overall reduction in physiological function with advancing years. This approach may be especially useful since it can isolate the effects of aging from the confounding influences of decreased physical activity and degenerative diseases that are seen in some older individuals [11, 32, 38, 41, 78].

With this information as background, the overall purpose of this review is to examine the current state of human performance in a physiological context. Key questions addressed include:

1. Can the continued improvements in performance seen in younger men and women be explained on a physiological basis?
2. Is the rate of improvement leveling off?
3. When does the age-related decline in endurance performance begin?
4. What is the rate of decline in performance with aging?
5. What physiological factors might be responsible for the decline in performance seen in older elite athletes.

In discussing each of these issues, attempts will be made to identify areas were experimental data are lacking.

PERFORMANCES CONSIDERED

Most of the discussion of performances will focus on the 10,000-m and marathon (42,195 m) runs since a large database exists for comparison in younger and older athletes of both sexes [82, 92]. Occasionally, other performances will be considered when they illustrate an interesting point. The International Amateur Athletic Federation (IAAF) stipulates that official world records be set on a track, and refers to marks set on the road as "notable performances." The source for worldwide marks in open competition is the "Progression of World Best Performances and Official IAAF World Records" by zur Megede and Hymans [92]. Only records achieved prior to 1992 are used.

"Master" athletes will be defined as those over 40 yr old. Most of the age group records considered will come from TACSTATS/USA "Road Running Rankings" for 1990 [82]. This source provides a large and reliable database (primarily on U.S. citizens) that can be used to make valid comparisons across age groups. Other performances of interest by master athletes (and open competitors in their late 30s) have been culled from *Track and Field News* and *Runners World* magazines. The physiological data considered come from the scientific literature and books authored by international experts [4, 13, 59, 90].

PROGRESS OF HUMAN PERFORMANCE

Men have participated in organized competitions, over standard distances, with accurate time- and record-keeping for a little more than 100 years [86, 92]. In the past 20–30 years, similar competitions have become open to women. In both sexes, times continue to fall (Fig. 4.1, Table 4.1). Examples that highlight this ongoing improvement include:

1. In open men's competition, the pace for the current world best in the marathon (approximately 333 m · min^{-1}) is faster than the pace for the world-record 10,000-m run up to the late 1930s [92].
2. The current world best marathon for women (2:21.06) is faster than the men's mark was until 1952 [92].

A number of authors have analyzed the rates of decline in human performance over the years. Some have concluded that the decline is linear with time, while others have suggested that it is curvilinear and leveling off [59, 74, 86]. Additionally, the rate of decline in women is faster than that for men and has led to speculation about performances by women either equalling or "surpassing" those by men at some point in the future (Fig. 4.1 [86]).

There have also been remarkable performances by master athletes including a marathon best of 2:11.04 by a 41-yr-old man (Table 4.2). Such performances confirm laboratory investigations that suggest

FIGURE 4.1

Panel A *plots the change in average running velocity for the world record marathon* (**Mar.**) *and 1500 m distances against time for men.* **Panel B** *is a similar plot for times achieved by women.* **Panel C** *is a linear extrapolation of the lines from* **Panels A** *and* **B** *suggesting that if times for both men and women continue to improve at the same rate and in a linear manner, then the times by women will eventually equal and possibly surpass those by men.* (*Modified from Whipp, B. J., and S. A. Ward. Will women soon outrun men?* Nature *355:25, 1992.*)

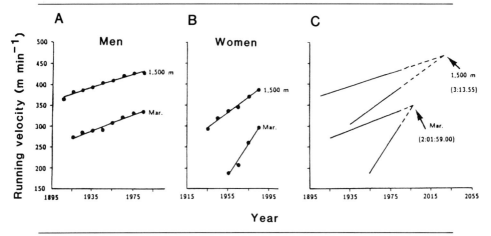

intense exercise training can reduce dramatically the decline in physiological function with aging [1–4, 23, 38, 41, 64, 71].

The possible determinants of these remarkable performances by younger or older athletes of both sexes will be discussed in the context of the physiological limiting factors in endurance exercise [50]. By focusing on the achievements of elite athletes, issues related to maximum human adaptability will be highlighted.

PHYSIOLOGICAL FACTORS THOUGHT TO LIMIT DISTANCE-RUNNING PERFORMANCE IN YOUNG MALES

Three physiological factors: maximal oxygen uptake ($\dot{V}O_2$max), the so-called "lactate threshold," and running economy appear to interact as determinants of distance running performance [1, 4, 11–14, 16, 22, 30, 40, 50, 53, 62, 75, 79, 90]. Many of the studies on these factors have been conducted in highly trained male runners successful in local but not national or international competitions. However, the data available in elite athletes of both sexes and all age groups also suggest that these

TABLE 4.1
Some Notable Distance Running Performances

Men						
10,000 m (Track)	31:40.0 George 1884	30:58.8 Bouin 1911	29:52.6 Mäki 1939	28:54.2 Zátopek 1954	27:39.4 Clarke 1965	27:08.23 Barrios 1989
Marathon	2:37:23 Siret 1908	2:29:39.2 Kolohmainen, A.W., 1912	2:18:40.2 Peters 1953	2:09:36.4 Clayton 1967	2:06:50 Densimo 1988	
Women						
10,000 m (Track)	35:30.5 Pigni 1970	34:01.4 Vahlensieck 1975	32:52.5* Shea 1979	31:35.3 Decker 1982	30:59.42 Kristiansen 1985	30:13.74 Kristiansen 1986
Marathon	2:55:22 Bonner 1971	2:49:40 Bridges 1971	2:38:19 Hanson 1975	2:27:32.6 Waitz 1979	2:21:06 Kristiansen 1985	

*Faster times had been run prior to this in "mixed" gender race.

TABLE 4.2
Some Notable Marks by Men and Women 35 Years of Age or Older

	Men			Women		
1500 m	3:33.91	Boit	36 yr	3:57.73	Puica	35 yr
Mile	3:55.19	Walker	38 yr	4:17.33	Puica	35 yr
	4:05.39	Waigwa	40 yr			
	4:30.6	Roberts	53 yr			
5000 m				15:15.2	Larrieu	35 yr
10,000 m	27:17.48	Lopes	37 yr	31:35.52	Larrieu	35 yr
	36:04	Jensen	65 yr	32:41.98	Palm	45 yr
Marathon	2:07:12	Lopes	38 yr	2:27:35	Larrieu	38 yr
	2:11:04	Campbell	41 yr	2:38:00	Palm	48 yr
	2:27:42	Green	55 yr	2:52:02	Irvine	54 yr
	2:38:46	Turnbill	60 yr			
	2:42:49	Davies	66 yr			

factors act as physiological determinants of performance in elite athletes [1, 12, 13, 19, 40, 60].

Maximal Oxygen Uptake

$\dot{V}O_2$max is thought to represent the maximum integrative ability of the body systems to transport oxygen from air to the active muscles where adenosine triphosphate (ATP) is generated via oxidative processes for muscle contractions [4, 13, 72, 75, 88, 90]. Values in healthy but sedentary 20- to 30-year-old males are usually in the range of 40–50 ml $\cdot$ kg^{-1} $\cdot$ min $^{-1}$ [2–4, 13, 88]. In elite endurance runners tested on the treadmill, values range from 68–70 ml $\cdot$ kg^{-1} $\cdot$ min^{-1} on the low side to approximately 85 ml $\cdot$ kg^{-1} $\cdot$ min^{-1} for an upper limit [4, 13, 14, 16, 59, 62, 63, 67, 69, 88]. The high values seen in elite endurance athletes probably represent the combination of prolonged intense training and genetic factors that result in more marked adaptations than normal to training. Bouchard and colleagues have reviewed the complex issues related to the genetics of $\dot{V}O_2$max in humans and concluded that "trainability" (i.e., the increase in $\dot{V}O_2$max in response to a standardized training program) appears to be, in large part, genetically determined [8].

There has been continuing controversy about whether $\dot{V}O_2$max in humans is limited by "central" (i.e., O_2 delivery) or peripheral factors in the active muscles [24, 72, 76]. If one takes the simple position that the muscle cannot extract what has not been delivered, then the conclusion is that the absolute highest $\dot{V}O_2$max achievable for any individual is set by the maximum O_2 flux (cardiac output $\times$ arterial oxygen content) at the aorta. This means that maximum cardiac output, the hemoglobin concentration of the blood, and the ability of the lung to oxygenate adequately the blood returning from the active muscles and other tissues are of paramount importance as determinants of $\dot{V}O_2$max [13, 28, 29, 51, 66, 85]. In this context, it appears that a large maximum stroke volume is the key adaptation that explains the high $\dot{V}O_2$max values in elite endurance athletes [72, 76, 85].

The concept of a central, O_2 delivery-dependent, limitation of $\dot{V}O_2$max is supported by experimental evidence that demonstrates maneuvers to either increase or decrease maximum O_2 flux cause directionally similar shifts in $\dot{V}O_2$max [28, 29, 66, 72, 85]. In contrast, it is possible to show that peripheral factors such as muscle mitochondrial content (or function) can be altered without having much effect on $\dot{V}O_2$max [21, 46, 47].

Of particular interest in the discussion of a central limitation of $\dot{V}O_2$max are the recent observations demonstrating that, during very heavy exercise (>80% $\dot{V}O_2$max) in some elite distance runners, the lung is unable to oxygenate fully the returning venous blood which results in arterial desaturation (SaO_2 = 86–92%) in a large percentage of such subjects. Such desaturation might decrease $\dot{V}O_2$max as much as 12–14% [24, 49]. This desaturation may limit $\dot{V}O_2$max in the affected individuals.

The reasons for the desaturation are complex, but center on several observations: *(a)* breathing occurs at a rate and depth that is limited by intrinsic mechanical factors in the lung; *(b)* ventilation/perfusion mismatch is increased, and *(c)* the high (>30 $1 \cdot min^{-1}$) cardiac outputs that speed the transit of red cells through the pulmonary capillaries limit the time for equilibration of alveolar and arterial O_2 tensions. Taken together, these arguments favor the concept that the heart and lungs limit $\dot{V}O_2$max in elite human endurance athletes [24, 49, 72, 76].

While $\dot{V}O_2$max represents the upper limit of "aerobic" performance, in most athletes the pace used in a 10,000-m run or marathon requires less than 100% of $\dot{V}O_2$max [1, 12–14, 16, 30, 62, 75, 79]. Studies conducted in good (but not world class) runners suggest that humans can run at speeds that require between 79 and 98% of $\dot{V}O_2$max during 10,000-m races and between 68% and 88% of $\dot{V}O_2$max during the marathon [30]. Similar conclusions are drawn from other studies at various distances [12–14, 16, 53, 79]. There have also been examples of champion runners who could sustain approximately 90% or more of their $\dot{V}O_2$max values for the marathon [13].

Lactate Threshold
Since $\dot{V}O_2$max is probably not sustained by most individuals over the entire course of a 10,000-m or marathon race, a key question is what factor(s) determines the fraction of $\dot{V}O_2$max that an individual can sustain for efforts between roughly 30 minutes and several hours? A number of studies suggest (based on blood samples) that the fraction of $\dot{V}O_2$max used in endurance races is somehow related to the accumulation of lactic acid in the active muscles [4, 16, 30, 53, 79]. In trained subjects, there is little or no increase in blood (or presumably muscle) lactate until a running speed that uses 60–85% of $\dot{V}O_2$max is reached [13, 14, 30]. This initial increase in blood lactate (Fig. 4.2) is followed by an exponential rise at faster running speeds [14, 30].

The phenomenon associated with and cause(s) of the changes in blood lactate have been described with a variety of terms, and the physiological events in active muscle that result in an increase in the blood lactate concentration during heavy exercise remain immersed in controversy [22]. An extensive discussion of this issue exceeds the scope of this review. However, the view that the rise in blood lactate is representative of inadequate oxygen delivery to the mitochondria in the active muscles is probably simplistic [22]. A more attractive explanation is that the increase in blood lactate is somehow reflective of a mismatch between the rate of pyruvate delivery to, and utilization by mitochondria in the otherwise "oxygenated" active muscles [46–48]. For the purposes of this review, the point at which there is a detectable (1–2 mMol) increase in the blood lactate concentration will be referred to as the "lactate threshold."

The essential concern from an applied point of view is that well-

FIGURE 4.2

An individual record of how blood lactate values change above resting as running speed and oxygen consumption increase. Note that there was little increase in blood lactate above resting values until the treadmill velocity exceeded 268 m·min⁻¹ and the oxygen consumption was above 50 ml·kg⁻¹·min⁻¹. (Reproduced with permission from Farrell, P. A., J. H. Wilmore, E. F. Coyle, J. H. Billing, and D. L. Costill. Plasma lactate accumulation and distance running performance. Med. Sci. Sports 11:338–344, 1979.)

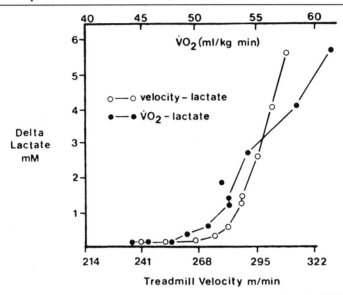

trained subjects can sustain a fraction of their V̇O₂max that is slightly above their lactate threshold for several hours, and that the lactate threshold is highly predictive of the fraction of V̇O₂max that can be sustained during shorter events as well [14, 30, 50, 53, 79]. The extremely high percentages of V̇O₂max that can be sustained by some elite athletes in marathon races is probably explained by their very high lactate threshold values [13].

Running Economy
The relationship between running speed and oxygen consumption (in ml · kg⁻¹ · min⁻¹) has been termed running economy. It can differ among individuals so that two hypothetical runners with identical V̇O₂max values may require different amounts of O₂ to run the same submaximal speed [12, 13, 16, 19, 20, 60, 63] (Fig. 4.3).

The oxygen cost to run progressively faster speeds appears to increase linearly when this issue is studied using relatively slow speeds in both average subjects and competitive runners on the treadmill at speeds up

FIGURE 4.3

*The relationship between running speed and oxygen consumption for individuals with "low," "average," and "high values" for running economy is demonstrated. Individuals with low running economy curves achieve substantially less running speed than individuals with high values for a given $\dot{V}O_2$. The high and low curves were generated using linear regression equations for the two most economical and two least economical individuals studied by Conley and Krahenbuhl [12, and Krahenbuhl, personal communication]. The "average" running economy curve was generated using the mean values from these data [12]. These curves were then extrapolated to higher running speeds, and individual examples (**triangles**) of excellent running economy values were plotted at high speed in elite athletes [Daniels, unpublished observations] to confirm that linear extrapolation of the data collected at lower speeds by Conley was justified. (For more details, see Joyner [50].)*

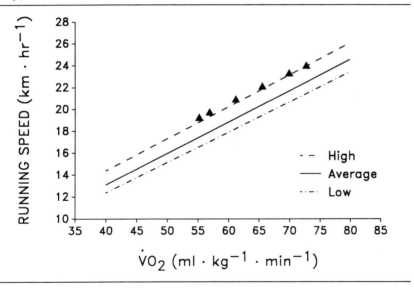

to approximately 320 m·min^{-1} [12, 13, 37, 59, 63]. While a few studies and anecdotal data suggest that the increase remains linear at faster speeds, there has been little systematically collected data at running speeds ≥20 km·hr^{-1} that would have relevance to competitive efforts by elite athletes. There is also little information on how the O_2 cost of actual overground running differs from treadmill running at higher speeds because of factors like wind resistance [18, 50]. Finally, most measurements of running economy have been made during brief treadmill runs, so there is little information on how any upward drift in $\dot{V}O_2$max over time might alter running economy during several hours of exercise [50].

Integration of Factors

In groups of subjects with widely differing $\dot{V}O_2$max values, a strong correlation between performance and $\dot{V}O_2$max exists. The relationship between $\dot{V}O_2$max and performance is much weaker in subjects with more homogeneous $\dot{V}O_2$max values [12, 13, 30, 59, 63]. The current concept is that the lactate threshold determines (or is related to) the fraction of $\dot{V}O_2$max that can be sustained by an individual in events lasting beyond 10–15 minutes, and that this value interacts with running economy to determine the actual running speed in competition [13, 30, 40, 50]. The so-called running speed at lactate threshold appears to be highly predictive of distance running performance at events including the 10,000-m run and marathon [1, 11–13, 30, 50, 53, 79].

This interaction explains how a subject with relatively "low" $\dot{V}O_2$max values for elite runners can remain competitive with those whose $\dot{V}O_2$max values are 80–85 ml·kg^{-1}·min^{-1} or more. The individuals with "low" $\dot{V}O_2$max values usually do not reach their lactate threshold until 85–90% of $\dot{V}O_2$max. They also generally have excellent running economy values. These concepts are illustrated by the fact that at 5000-m and 10,000-m, the performances of Frank Shorter ($\dot{V}O_2$max of ~70 ml·kg^{-1}·min^{-1}) are virtually identical to those of Steve Prefontaine ($\dot{V}O_2$max ~85 ml·kg^{-1}·min^{-1}) [13, 59, 63]. Shorter was known to have excellent running economy values and probably also had a very high lactate threshold [13, 63].

If $\dot{V}O_2$max, lactate threshold, and running economy interact as discussed, then it should be possible to predict an "optimal" time for the marathon if the same individual possessed exceptional values for all three variables, and race conditions were otherwise ideal. This means that for an individual with a very high $\dot{V}O_2$max value (84 ml·kg^{-1}·min^{-1}), a lactate threshold at 85% of $\dot{V}O_2$max, and an excellent running economy curve, the predicted optimal marathon time would be about 1:57, an improvement of roughly 9 min in comparison to the current world best [50]. This calculation leads to several conclusions: *(a)* there are additional poorly understood limiting factors in truly elite athletes; *(b)* exceptional values for one of the limiting factors might preclude exceptional values in another (i.e., $\dot{V}O_2$max and running economy?); and *(c)* there is a relative lack of systematically collected lactate threshold and running economy data in truly elite athletes running at fast (>20 km·hr^{-1}) but submaximal speeds during both treadmill and overground running.

PHYSIOLOGICAL IMPROVEMENT OVER THE LAST 50–100 YEARS?

Can improvement in any one or all three of these factors explain the improvements in performance in men over the last 100 years? Robinson,

Edwards, and Dill, working at the Harvard fatigue laboratory, observed very high $\dot{V}O_2$max values in elite runners in the 1930s [69]. A value of 82 $ml \cdot kg^{-1} \cdot min^{-1}$ was observed in Donald Lash who was one of the first men to run 2 miles in less than 9 min and held the world record for that distance at the time he was studied. They also noted values in the 75-$ml \cdot kg^{-1} \cdot min^{-1}$ range in several individuals [67, 69]. Based on recent studies demonstrating that brief but very intense training can elicit and maintain large changes in $\dot{V}O_2$max, it would appear reasonable to assert that the training programs used by elite athletes of the 1930s probably allowed the runners studied by Robinson to achieve their individual genetically limited $\dot{V}O_2$max values [33, 42–45, 67, 69, 91]. These data also make it seem unlikely that large improvements in $\dot{V}O_2$max are responsible for the 10% (or more) improvements in the world records for 10,000 m and the marathon since the 1930s.

In the 1960s, Saltin and Åstrand observed similar $\dot{V}O_2$max values to those reported by Robinson in elite runners [75]. They speculated that the factor(s) responsible for the improvement in performance by elite world-class runners from the 1930s to the 1960s was probably related to an improved ability to sustain a high fraction of $\dot{V}O_2$max in competition and to better technique [75]. This view is consistent with how training has evolved in this century. Initially, there was little year-round training, and not even daily training during the competitive season [91]. From 1900 to about 1960, there was a steady increase in the frequency, intensity, and duration of training so that, by the late 1950s or early 1960s, it was not uncommon for athletes to average 2 hr of training (some of it very intense) per day on a year-round basis. Since that time, the training programs used by top athletes have not changed dramatically [91].

These changes in training methodology are consistent with the observation that the mitochondrial adaptations in skeletal muscle that probably cause the lactate threshold to increase to the high values seen in elite athletes are maximized with 1.5–2.0 hr of daily training [27, 46, 47]. Therefore, it would appear reasonable to speculate that training-induced mitochondrial adaptations appear to have allowed athletes to sustain higher percentages of their $\dot{V}O_2$max values in competition as a result of improved lactate threshold values. These adaptations would seem to explain much of the improvement in performance from the 1930s to the 1960s [75].

This view is supported by the lactate threshold and running economy values first observed in elite competitors from the 1960s [13, 14, 16]. These data suggest that there have been no dramatic improvements in these factors over the last 20–30 yr since the currently used approaches to training emerged. However, the improvements in performance for both the 10,000 m and marathon have both been only about 2% since this time.

If champion human athletes have been training "as hard as possible" and, hence, have maximized their training-induced physiological adaptations (i.e., $\dot{V}O_2$max, lactate threshold) since the early 1960s, and if running economy is only minimally altered by training, why have world records continued to fall? One explanation is that synthetic tracks and better footwear have contributed to the improved performances. Although there are few hard data to support this contention, there is evidence to suggest that the design and composition of running tracks can improve competitive performance by about 2–3% [55, 56]. If the current synthetic surfaces and shoes offer an advantage of this magnitude, the last world records set on natural tracks (i.e., cinder or clay) in the middle 1960s came remarkably close to matching the current world marks if they are "corrected" by about 2% for the different surfaces (Table 4.3). This interpretation supports the contention that physiological improvement by record holders in the last 25 yr has probably been minimal.

Competitive Opportunities

A variety of sociological factors have probably contributed to the improvements in world record performance in men over the last 30 yr. First, beginning with Alain Mimoun (a native of Algeria who competed for France) at Melbourne in 1956, and Abeke Bikila (Etheopia) in 1960 at Rome, there has been the emergence of competitive opportunities for individuals from the so-called "developing countries." Their contribution is highlighted by the success of East Africans in the Olympic games. Second, the financial rewards to those successful in international competition have increased dramatically.

These factors mean that more potential record setters have the opportunity, motivation, and means to train and to compete (full time) beyond their early 20s into their 30s. This increases the number of top-class athletes that can be drawn to selected races and enhance the competitive atmosphere, contribute to the early pace, share the burden of overcoming wind resistance, and generally improve the chances for a record in current competitions.

An example of how these sociological factors might improve performance can be seen by comparing results of the 1969 Antwerp marathon in which Derek Clayton set a world best of 2:08:33, with the results of the 1988 Rotterdam marathon that produced a world best of 2:06:50 for Belayneh Densimo. The second place finisher in the 1969 race was almost 3 minutes behind in comparison to a gap of only 17 seconds between first and second in 1988. The tenth place time in 1969 was 2:22:13 vs. 2:12:42 in 1988. There were no finishers from the developing nations in the top 12 in 1969. Seven of the 12 finishers, including the first four who all broke 2:10, were from developing countries in the 1988 Rotterdam race [92].

TABLE 4.3
Comparison of World Records* on "Natural" and Synthetic Track Surfaces

Surface	1500 m	1 Mile	3000 m	5000 m	10,000 m
Natural	3:33.1 Ryun, 1967	3:51.1 Ryun, 1967	7:39.6 Keino, 1966	13:16.6 Clarke, 1966	27:39.4 Clarke, 1965
Synthetic	3:29.46 Aouita, 1985	3:46.32 Cram, 1985	7:29.45 Aouita, 1989	12:58.39 Aouita, 1987	27:08.23 Barrios, 1989
Improvement	1.7%	2.1%	2.2%	2.3%	1.9%

*Records set before 1992.

Doping

It is possible that the use of banned substances may have contributed to improved performances by some distance runners. In endurance competition, much attention has been focused on autologous transfusions of red blood cells to athletes or "blood-doping," and the more recent related use of synthetic erythropoietin [28, 29, 66, 87]. Both approaches are effective in increasing $\dot{V}O_2$max and, possibly, performance in fit subjects [87]. However, neither technique has been extensively studied in truly elite athletes.

In any case, it is impossible to say what effect (if any) these procedures have had on world records because of a lack of reliable information. The success of athletes from developing countries and the formidable logistical challenge that blood-doping might present to these individuals makes it seem less likely that blood-doping has had a major impact on international competitions. Additionally, the previously stated argument that the record holders from the middle 1960s are as physiologically gifted as those today suggests a minimal impact. It can only be hoped that this is the case.

Performances by Women

The IAAF did not sanction races for women that were longer than 1000 m until 1967 when the 1500 m and mile were recognized. The 10,000-m event was not added until 1981. It is unclear when the IAAF first began to acknowledge the women's marathon, but the event was not contested in the Olympics until 1984 [92]. When "pre-IAAF" times are considered, the time span available to analyze women's records should probably be limited to the last 20–25 yr because of insufficient opportunities for women to compete at almost every level. In the last 20 yr, the record for 10,000 m has dropped from 35:00.4 in 1975 to the current mark of 30:13.74 set by Ingird Kristiansen in 1986. The marathon best has fallen from 2:46:36 (set by Gorman in 1973) to 2:21:06 (also by Kristiansen in 1985). Based on these improvements, it is clear that, in the recent past, world records for women have fallen at a much faster rate than for men (Fig. 4.1, Table 4.1). An interesting issue is whether this improvement is due primarily to physiological or sociological factors (or both), and whether the rate will continue.

When historical performances for women and men are plotted against time (in years), several authors have concluded that performances are advancing at a linear rate (see Fig. 4.1 [74, 86]). Others can view similar data and conclude that the rate of improvement is subtly curvilinear and may be leveling off [59]. If care is not taken, it is possible to imply that the reason for the continued "linear" improvement is due to "physiological" improvement while ignoring the previously discussed sociological and other factors that might be contributing to improved performance. This is especially possible when evaluating trends in running performance by women who, unlike men, experienced a dramatic increase in the severity of their training regimens and opportunities to compete *at about the same time*. This experience contrasts with the more gradual changes in training and competitive opportunities previously discussed for men. These issues will be discussed below.

Physiologically Limiting Factors in Women
There was little information on the physiological determinants of running performance in women until the 1970s. The currently available data, while limited in comparison to those available on men, suggests that $\dot{V}O_2$max, lactate threshold, and running economy interact in women as determinants of performance in a manner similar to that in men [13, 15, 19, 60, 88]. The areas where information is particularly lacking for women in comparison with men are on the relationship among the lactate threshold, running economy, and performance.

By the middle 1970s, at least a few women runners who were studied had $\dot{V}O_2$max values approaching 70 ml·kg^{-1}·min^{-1}, with values up to 77 ml·kg^{-1}·min^{-1} seen in a cross-country skier [4, 25, 88]. These values are near the upper limit of those currently observed. However, the best early studies (1970s) on groups of elite female runners suggested that the average $\dot{V}O_2$max value in these groups was 58–60 ml·kg^{-1}·min^{-1} [19, 60, 89]. Subsequent studies indicated that $\dot{V}O_2$max values in elite female athletes are approximately 67 ml·kg^{-1}·min^{-1} [60]. Individual values of 73–77 ml·kg^{-1}·min^{-1} seem to be near the upper limit reported for women runners [13, 59, 60]. These values are about 10–15% lower than the average value of 77 ml·kg^{-1}·min^{-1} and highest value of 84–85 ml·kg^{-1}·min^{-1} seen in comparable groups of men [59, 88].

When absolute (l·min^{-1}) values for $\dot{V}O_2$max are considered in elite runners, they are much lower (3.15 vs. 5.19 l·min^{-1}) in women than in men [60, 63]. This should not be surprising since the women are much smaller than the men and, therefore, probably have smaller stroke volumes and lower cardiac outputs during peak exercise. Additionally, the hemoglobin concentrations in elite female runners are lower [26, 57].

The current explanation of the gender differences in $\dot{V}O_2$max among elite runners when expressed relative to body weight is 2-fold. First, elite females have more (14% vs. 5%) body fat than men [35, 65, 89]. Much of the difference in $\dot{V}O_2$max disappears when it is expressed relative to lean body weight [60, 80]. Second, the hemoglobin concentration of elite female runners in 5–10% lower in women than in men [26, 57, 85].

Lactate Threshold
The mitochondrial adaptations in the skeletal muscles of highly trained male and female runners appear similar [15, 31]. These adaptations are thought to play a key role in explaining the very high lactate threshold values observed in elite athletes and other trained runners [46, 47].

While comprehensive studies relating lactate values to performance similar to those by Costill [14, 16] and Farrell et al. [30] have not been conducted on female athletes, there is no reason to believe that values for the lactate threshold will be lower in women than in men. It is interesting to wonder if some of the extremely high anecdotal values seen in men for the lactate threshold (90% of $\dot{V}O_2$max) will also be seen in women.

Running Economy
The average oxygen cost to run a given speed (241 m·min^{-1}) by groups of elite male and female runners appears to be similar [12, 13, 60, 63]. This comparison requires some extrapolation because the running speeds used in the best study to date on women [60] differ from those used in the studies of men (230 and 248 m·min^{-1} for women vs. 241, 268, 295, and 322 m·min^{-1} in men) [12, 63]. Additionally, the range of values observed within a group of female athletes also appears to be similar and probably explains much of the difference in performance observed among women with high $\dot{V}O_2$max values [12, 60].

Of note are the fairly complete running economy data available on Grete Waitz, the dominant female marathon runner of the late 1970s and early 1980s. Her running economy values at speeds from 215–295 m·min^{-1} are almost identical to those recorded by Derek Clayton and other male athletes noted for their excellent running economy values [12, 13, 50, 63]. This is further evidence that running economy values for elite male and female runners are similar and probably play the same role in determining success in distance running performance. As is the case for men, there are few reported data for elite women at very fast speeds during both treadmill and overground running.

Integration of Factors
When reviewing the current information about how the three key factors thought to limit human performance interact in women, it appears that although comprehensive data is lacking, they probably operate in the same manner in women and in men. The major physiological reason that would appear to "explain" the slower records by women than men is probably the lower $\dot{V}O_2$max values observed in women. However, this conclusion relies on average data and ignores the fact that a number of female athletes have $\dot{V}O_2$max values that are as *high or higher* than champion male runners! If such a value occurred in a women with excellent running economy and a high lactate threshold, it is easily conceivable that the world best marathon for women could fall to at least several minutes under 2:20, and that the world record for 10,000 m might drop below 30 minutes. Such times would certainly seem feasible based on currently available data and concepts [13, 50, 60].

However, the same caution required in concluding that there is substantial "physiological" room for improvement in record performance by elite male athletes should also be applied to women [50]. If, for example, an exceptional value for $\dot{V}O_2$max somehow precludes outstanding values for either running economy or the lactate threshold, then the marked improvements speculated about would be less likely to occur [50]. It should be remembered that while a number elite male and female runners have similar $\dot{V}O_2$max values, these values are at the low end of the elite range for men versus the upper end of the elite range for women. If an excellent value for one of the limiting factors is mutually exclusive with another, this means that it might be more likely for some of the males with $\dot{V}O_2$max values in the low range for men to have outstanding running economy and lactate threshold values and, therefore, faster times in competition than a female competitor with the same $\dot{V}O_2$max [50].

Competitive Opportunities
The rapid improvement in distance running performance by women over the last 20 yr would appear to represent the synergistic effects of both physiological improvement and enhanced competitive opportunities occurring at the same time for women in contrast to the more gradual experience of men. The rapid physiological improvement probably resulted from the fact that women were quick to adopt training programs similar to those developed by men through trial and error over many years. These improvements were magnified by improved competitive opportunities and a larger talent pool.

Additionally, most of the improvements in distance running times by women have been achieved by competitors from the developed countries. This means that, in some respects, the situation for women is similar to what it was for men before the emergence of runners from the developing countries in the 1960s. Recently though, women from East Africa have started to make their presence known in international competition. It is likely that these athletes will contribute to the continued improvement in performance by women.

It is also tempting to speculate that women from the developing countries will continue to improve since it is now more socially acceptable for young girls to participate in sports. Such participation could enhance any long-term adaptations that might occur during growth and development and contribute to improved performances in the future. It is unclear, however, if such changes will overcome the negative societal trends toward inactivity and obesity by children in the developed countries, particularly in the U.S. [90].

Will distance running records set by women ever match or exceed those by men (Fig. 4.4 and 4.5) [86]? The previously discussed data indicate that, at least for men, and possibly for women, there has been little physiological improvement among champions since the adoption of prolonged intense daily training regimens. If this is the case, then it is unlikely that records will continue to fall at a linear rate [59, 74, 86]. A

FIGURE 4.4

The record running pace for women and men in races ranging from 1500 m to the marathon in the middle 1980s is plotted. The differences in record performance by men and women are fairly constant across a wide range of endurance running events. (Reproduced with permission from Costill, D. L. Inside Running: Basics of Sports Physiology. *Indianapolis, IN: Benchmark, 1986, pp. 1–189.)*

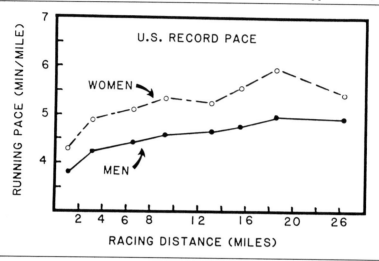

closer look at the data shows that all of the world records for distance races (more than 1500 m) by women were set before 1986, whereas a number of men's records have improved since then. These observations would seem to make it less likely that men's and women's records will converge in the near future. However, sociological factors may be more likely to lead to further marked improvements in women.

Performances by Older Elite Athletes

A number of notable marks by athletes in their late 30s or older are listed in Table 4.2. When the best times by citizens (of both sexes) of the United States for the 10,000 m (road courses) and marathon are plotted against age, it appears that the rate of decline in performance with aging is slight until the late 30s (Figs. 4.6 and 4.7). Thereafter performance appears to fall at the rate of between 6–9% per decade until the late 50s when it accelerates further. The decline in records by women appears to be greater than that for men. It is likely that this reflects the fact that there are fewer women engaged in master's competition than men, and that many more of the men have probably been active and engaged in competitive sports throughout life.

A similar rate of decline in performance also appears to occur when all

FIGURE 4.5

The distribution of performances for men and women in a 15-km race is shown. While a large number of women achieve faster times than men, the sex-based differences seen when record performances are considered (Fig. 4.4) are also evident when larger groups of nonelite performers are considered. (Reproduced with permission from Costill, D. L. Inside Running: Basics of Sports Physiology. *Indianapolis, IN: Benchmark, 1986, pp. 1–189.*

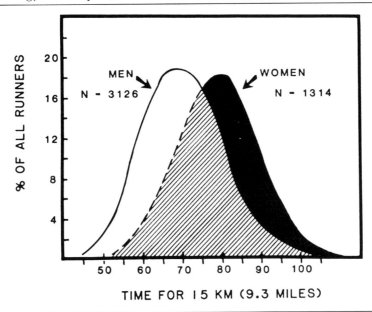

TIME FOR 15 KM (9.3 MILES)

finishers of endurance competitions are considered, indicating that it applies to highly trained (but non-elite) competitors in the older age groups ([6, 7] and Fig. 4.8). These and other performances (many by athletes in their 50s and 60s), along with physiological data, clearly suggest that the rate of decline in performance in well-trained aging endurance athletes is probably less than the frequently cited 9–10% per decade drop in $\dot{V}O_2$max seen in sedentary subjects [2–4, 9, 10, 23, 25, 32, 36, 38, 39, 63–65, 78, 81].

Physiological Factors and Aging
  $\dot{V}O_2$MAX. The study of how the physiological factors that limit endurance running performance decline with age has focused primarily on measurements of $\dot{V}O_2$max [2–4, 23, 32, 36, 41, 67–69, 81]. Large population-based studies are difficult to apply to highly motivated athletes because most study "normal" older subjects, and the decline in $\dot{V}O_2$max observed reflects both the effects of aging per se and any changes in habitual physical activity and body composition that are

FIGURE 4.6

*Year-by-year age record performances in 10,000-m road races by U.S. citizens. The **left panel** demonstrates that, in men, the decline in record time with age appears to be about 6% per decade until the middle or late 50s. Thereafter, the rate of decline appears to accelerate. In women, the average rate of decline with aging appears to be closer to 9% per decade into the late 50s. However, some of the individual values suggest a rate of decline similar to that seen in men. After age 60 yr, the rate of decline in women appears to be substantially greater than that for men. It is unclear if this apparent faster decline in women has a biological basis, or is merely the result of sociological factors that have limited the participation of women (in comparison with men) in distance running competitions. (Data from* TACSTATS/USA Road Running Rankings, *1990.)*

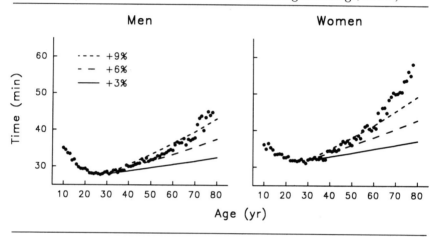

FIGURE 4.7.

Year-by-year U.S. age record performances in the marathon for men and women. These data confirm the observation made in Figure 4.6. (Data from TACSTATS/USA Road Running Rankings, *1990.)*

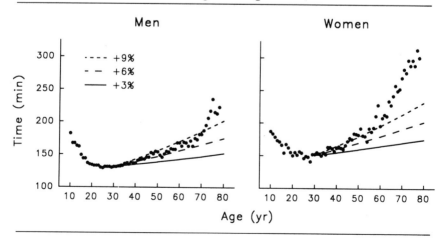

FIGURE 4.8
The increase in either running (**closed circles**) *or cross-country skiing* (**open circles**) *times during two long distance races is shown. The results are the relative time it took competitors in various age groups to complete the courses in comparison with the average time for the fastest age group. These data suggest that the decline in performance among well-trained, but nonelite competitors is also 6–7% per decade. This value is similar to the decline in performance seen when only record performers are considered. (Reproduced with permission from Böttiger, L. E. Regular decline in physical working capacity with age.* Br. Med. J. *3:270–271, 1973.)*

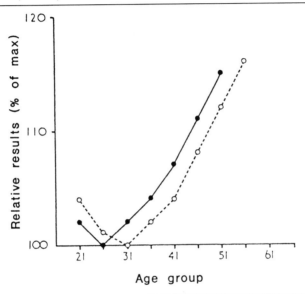

frequently associated with aging [9, 10, 32, 41, 81]. In general, these studies suggest that $\dot{V}O_2$max falls at the rate of about 9–10% per decade beginning at age 30 yr in healthy but sedentary older subjects of both sexes. For the general population, cross-sectional studies may underestimate the rate of decline because it is likely that only more vigorous and disease-free subjects volunteer to be tested [81]. In longitudinal studies of athletes who stop training, a similar decline is seen [67].

The factors responsible for the age-related decline in $\dot{V}O_2$max in inactive subjects are complex and controversial. It is likely that a reduction in maximum cardiac output because of a decline in maximum heart rate and stroke volume plays a major role [34, 38, 41, 81]. While there is some evidence to suggest that maximum cardiac output is maintained in older subjects [70], this observation has not been confirmed by other studies [34, 81]. Additionally, there is no reason to expect that the well-established relationship between maximum cardiac output and $\dot{V}O_2$max seen among other populations does not also occur with aging. There is also probably a modest decline in peripheral oxygen extraction [34, 81]. Age-related increases in body weight and body fat also contribute to the decline in $\dot{V}O_2$max when it is expressed relative to body weight [81]. Some have also argued that the loss of lean body tissue plays a role [5, 32]. It is unclear how changes in total body hemoglobin that can alter $\dot{V}O_2$max in younger subjects might affect $\dot{V}O_2$max in older individuals [4, 85].

The rate of decline in $\dot{V}O_2$max in sedentary subjects first noted many years ago appears to be substantially greater than the rate of decline in performance seen in older athletes [6, 7]. These observations suggested that training might limit some of the age-related decline in $\dot{V}O_2$max. This possibility was supported by observations of high $\dot{V}O_2$max values in at least some older athletes, and observations that the $\dot{V}O_2$max fell less in more active subjects followed in longitudinal studies [9, 23, 36]. Additionally, one of the champion runners followed by Robinson continued moderately hard training into his 50s [67, 69, Wilt, personal communication]. Fred Wilt, who ran 4:08 for the mile, and is a noted authority on the history of distance running training, did not "retire" from competition until age 36. He then continued to train vigorously 5 days/week, frequently running repeat 200-m intervals (Wilt, personal communication). His $\dot{V}O_2$max fell from 4.7 $1 \cdot min^{-1}$ in his early 20s to 4.4 $1 \cdot min$ in his middle 50s. This type of limited duration but intense training is thought to be capable of maintaining $\dot{V}O_2$max at or near its upper limit [33, 42–45].

Subsequent well controlled cross-sectional and longitudinal studies of older elite distance runners have been conducted demonstrating that the fall in $\dot{V}O_2$max with aging can be blunted by about one-half (i.e., to 5% per decade [see Fig. 4.9]) with continued hard training [41, 64, 71]. The primary reason for the decline appears to be an age-related reduction in maximum heart rate that causes a decline maximum cardiac output [36, 39, 41, 61, 68]. It appears that highly trained aging subjects are able to maintain their stroke volume, peripheral oxygen extraction, and body composition at or near the levels they possessed in their 20s and 30s [41, 64, 71]. Continued training may also limit the age-related decline in maximum heart rate [71].

Some have speculated that the pulmonary factors which cause arterial desaturation during heavy exercise that might limit $\dot{V}O_2$max in some younger athletes might become more common in older athletes due to age-related deterioration of pulmonary function [49]. However, the preliminary evidence to date suggests that these events are no more common in older than younger subjects primarily because of a decreased metabolic demand and, therefore, of pulmonary ventilation in the older athletes [49]. Additionally, it is possible that the pulmonary system might impair performance (not $\dot{V}O_2$max) in some older subjects because of

FIGURE 4.9

The decline in $\dot{V}O_2$max vs. age for a variety of groups is plotted. The **top line** *shows the decline in $\dot{V}O_2$max among older participants in orienteering [36]. The* **two bottom lines** *are examples of the rate of decline among individuals who were either sedentary as young adults or champion runners who stopped training. The cluster of* **open circles** *labeled* **"Masters Athletes"** *in the upper right-hand corner were obtained in highly trained older champions and demonstrate that the $\dot{V}O_2$max values in these individuals are substantially higher than any other group of older subjects. These data form the basis for the observation that prolonged intense endurance exercise training by older individuals can reduce dramatically the decline in $\dot{V}O_2$max with aging. (A variety of data sources were used in the construction of this figure, see Heath et al. [41] for details.)*

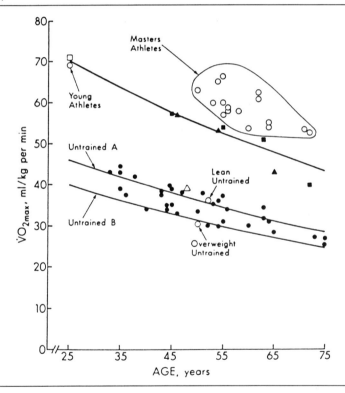

age-related increases in the oxygen cost of breathing during exercise that result from an increase in physiological dead space. This means that a larger percentage of O_2 consumption during exercise would be used by the ventilatory muscles and unavailable to the other exercising muscles [49, 61].

In summary, it appears that continued prolonged intense endurance exercise training by older male subjects limits the age-related decline in $\dot{V}O_2$max by roughly one-half to 5% per decade beginning at age 30 yr (or perhaps not until the late 30s in some individuals). There are almost no data on this issue in older female athletes.

Lactate Threshold

As is the case with younger competitors, master athletes probably do not run 10,000-m and marathon races at speeds that require $\dot{V}O_2$max. In older subjects, there is some evidence that the absolute $\dot{V}O_2$max at which the lactate threshold occurs remains constant or only declines minimally with aging. This means that the lactate threshold as a percentage of $\dot{V}O_2$max may increase somewhat with aging [1, 11]. If the lactate threshold changes in this way, then such alterations would serve to maintain performance in the face of declines in $\dot{V}O_2$max. Such a mechanism could explain the continued world class performances of some individuals in open competition into their late 30s and early 40s.

This possibility is consistent with observations that suggest that training preserves the mitochondrial adaptations in skeletal muscles that are thought to play a key role in regulating lactate production in contracting skeletal muscles [11]. It also appears that the normal mitochondrial adaptations to training can be made in older subjects [79]. These data indicate that either continued training or the initiation of training by older humans can prevent or eliminate the age-related decline in skeletal muscle oxidative capacity [83]. They also indicate that the decline in muscle oxidative capacity with aging results from inactivity and not from advancing years.

Running Economy

There are few data on the extent of running economy changes with aging in well-trained older athletes. The currently available information culled from various sources and reports of oxygen uptake at various stages of treadmill exercise protocols suggests that aging per se does not alter the oxygen cost to perform a given treadmill workload [1, 11, 78]. This issue needs further study to determine what effect (if any) the increased oxygen cost of breathing during exercise might have on running economy [61].

Integration of Factors

Elite older (male) endurance athletes can remain competitive in open competition at the highest international levels until their middle or late 30s, with a few individuals remaining competitive until their early 40s. The current concept is that the normal age for peak performance for distance running occurs during the late 20s or early 30s [77]. That some individuals are able to achieve very high levels of performance later in life probably reflects some combination of genetic variability (i.e., they are "slow" agers), natural ability, and continued hard training.

In the early stages of aging, any declines in $\dot{V}O_2$max may have little impact on performance because of the maintenance of the lactate threshold at the same absolute workload (i.e., running speed). Later on it appears $\dot{V}O_2$max declines at rate (5%) per decade beginning in the 30s and that this rate is slightly less than the decline in performance (6–7%). It is unclear if these rates of decline will be lower in individuals who were champions in their 20s who continue to train intensely and compete at a high level throughout life.

It is not clear why the decline in performance appears to be slightly greater than the fall in $\dot{V}O_2$max with aging. It is possible that, even among the most competitive runners, there might be an age-related decline in the frequency, intensity, and duration of training due to a combination of the inevitable reduction in physiological factors along with orthopedic or motivational considerations. This means that although older competitors may be far more active than the average individuals of the same age, they might be marginally less active than they once were. In follow-up studies of master athletes it appears that there might be at least some reduction in absolute training intensity [64, 71]. This might explain the slightly faster decline in performance and the further slowing seen beginning in the seventh decade of life. Another possibility is that the oxygen cost of achieving a given alveolar ventilation increases with aging due to age-related increases in dead space. If this occurred, it could result in a respiratory muscle steal syndrome, and limit performance since a higher fraction of total body $\dot{V}O_2$ would be used by the respiratory as opposed to locomotor muscles [49, 61]. These issues will only be resolved by continued studies on elite older runners including longitudinal evaluations of aging champion athletes who remain highly competitive.

Based on the simple evaluation of the decline in record performance (Figs. 4.6 and 4.7), it appears that similar events might occur in older women. However, as is the case for younger elite females, there are much fewer (almost no) data on elite older female athletes. Studies on these individuals are especially needed to determine if lifelong exercise training is as effective in reducing the age-related decline in physiological function in women as men.

CONCLUSIONS

Based on the previously discussed information, the following conclusions appears to be justified:

1. The improvement in performance by men in open competition probably resulted from progressive increases in $\dot{V}O_2$max as a result of changes in training from the late 1800s to the 1930s. From the 1930s

to the 1960s, performance improved because training programs changed in a manner that allowed the top athletes to sustain a greater fraction of their $\dot{V}O_2$max in competition. There is little evidence to suggest that current record holders have physiologically improved over the last 25–30 yrs. It is likely that improvement since the 1960s represents the combination of better tracks and equipment along with enhanced competitive opportunities for a larger fraction of the world's population.

2. The rapid improvement in performance by women over the last 20 yr seems to have resulted from the rapid emergence of improved competitive opportunities and harder training regimens at roughly the same time. If lifelong competitive opportunities for women (throughout the world) continue to increase, records by women may continue to improve at a faster rate than those by men for some time. Some elite female runners clearly have $\dot{V}O_2$max values and running economy curves comparable to those of world class male runners. If these women are able to train in a manner that allows them to develop very high lactate threshold values, it is likely that women will run (at a minimum) 2:20 for the marathon and well under 30:00 minutes for 10,000 m.

3. The concept that there is physiological "room" for dramatic improvements in distance running performance in both men and women should be viewed with caution. This approach is useful primarily because it highlights the relative lack of information on how $\dot{V}O_2$max, running economy, and lactate threshold (or some other poorly understood factor) interact in truly elite runners of both sexes (particularly women) as determinants of distance running performance.

4. In older humans, endurance training can blunt or eliminate the changes in $\dot{V}O_2$max, body composition, and muscle oxidative capacity seen in sedentary subjects as they age. In older competitors, the decline in performance with aging appears to be (at best) 6–7% per decade for men up to their late 50s. This rate of decline is probably slightly greater than the decline in $\dot{V}O_2$max in these individuals. These reductions are substantially less than those observed in the normal sedentary population. When considered in the context of the higher baseline values at the "onset" of aging in trained subjects, they indicate that prolonged intense endurance training throughout life allows the performance of older humans to surpass that of a majority of the younger population. Similar trends in performance are seen in older women, but there are much fewer (almost no) data on such women and few if any have had lifetime opportunities to compete in sports. Cross-sectional and longitudinal studies of elite female athletes as they age are needed to fill this gap. A key question is whether the decline in physiological function and competitive

performance with aging will be even less as larger numbers of athletes who were highly trained in their 20s continue truly vigorous exercise programs throughout life?

ACKNOWLEDGMENTS

Mrs. Catherine Nelson provided expert secretarial assistance. Mrs. Kathy Street prepared the figures. Dr. Bruce Johnson provided valuable criticism and discussion. The author would also like to thank Professor Jack H. Wilmore for his continued encouragement and friendship over the last 15 yr.

REFERENCES

1. Allen, W. K., D. R. Seals, B. F. Hurley, A. A. Ehsani, and J. M. Hagberg. Lactate threshold and distance-running performance in young and older endurance athletes. *J. Appl. Physiol.* 58:1281–1284, 1985.
2. Åstrand, I. Aerobic work capacity in men and women with special reference to age. *Acta Physiol. Scand.* 49:1–92, 1960.
3. Åstrand, I., P.-O. Åstrand, I. Hallbäck, and Å. Kilbom. Reduction in maximal oxygen uptake with age. *J. Appl. Physiol.* 35:649–654, 1973.
4. Åstrand, P.-O., and K. Rodahl. *Textbook of Work Physiology*, 2nd ed. New York: McGraw-Hill, 1977, pp. 1–681.
5. Booth, F. W. $\dot{V}o_2$max limits (letter). *J. Appl. Physiol.* 67:1299–1300, 1989.
6. Böttiger, L. E. Physical working capacity and age. ("Vasaloppet"). *Acta Med. Scand.* 190:359–362, 1971.
7. Böttiger, L. E. Regular decline in physical working capacity with age. *Br. Med. J.* 3:270–271, 1973.
8. Bouchard, C., F. T. Dionne, J.-A. Simoneau, and M. R. Boulay. Genetics of aerobic and anaerobic performances. *Exerc. Sport Sci. Rev.* 20:27–58, 1992.
9. Bruce, R. A. Exercise, functional aerobic capacity, and aging—another viewpoint. *Med. Sci. Sports Exerc.* 16:8–13, 1984.
10. Buskirk, E. R., and J. L. Hodgson. Age and aerobic power: the rate of change in men and women. *Fed. Proc.* 46:1824–1829, 1987.
11. Coggan, A. R., R. J. Spina, M. A. Rogers, et al. Histochemical and enzymatic characteristics of skeletal muscle in master athletes. *J. Appl. Physiol.* 68:1896–1901, 1990.
12. Conley, D. L., and G. S. Krahenbuhl. Running economy and distance running performance of highly trained athletes. *Med. Sci. Sports Exerc.* 12:357–360, 1980.
13. Costill, D. L. *Inside Running: Basics of Sports Physiology.* Carmel, IN: Benchmark Press, 1986, pp. 1–189.
14. Costill, D. L. Metabolic responses during distance running. *J. Appl. Physiol.* 28:251–255, 1970.
15. Costill, D. L., W. J. Fink, M. Flynn, and J. Kirwan. Muscle fiber composition and enzyme activities in elite female distance runners. *Int. J. Sports Med.* 8:103–106, 1987.
16. Costill, D. L., H. Thomason, and E. Roberts. Fractional utilization of the aerobic capacity during distance running. *Med. Sci. Sports* 5:248–252, 1973.
17. Cureton, K. J., and P. B. Sparling. Distance running performance and metabolic responses to running in men and women with excess weight experimentally equated. *Med. Sci. Sports Exerc.* 12:288–294, 1980.

18. Daniels, J., P. Bradley, N. Scardina, P. Van Handel, and J. Troup. Aerobic responses to submax and max treadmill and track running at sea level and altitude (Abstract). *Med. Sci. Sports Exerc.* 17:187, 1985.
19. Daniels, J., G. Krahenbuhl, C. Foster, J. Gilbert, and S. Daniels. Aerobic responses of female distance runners to submaximal and maximal exercise. *Ann. N.Y. Acad. Sci.* 301:726–733, 1977.
20. Daniels, J. T. A physiologist's view of running economy. *Med. Sci. Sports Exerc.* 17:332–338, 1985.
21. Davies, K. J. A., J. J. Maguire, G. A. Brooks, P. R. Dallman, and L. Packer. Muscle mitochondrial bioenergetics, oxygen supply, and work capacity during dietary iron deficiency and repletion. *Am. J. Physiol.* 242:E418–E427, 1982.
22. Davis, J. A. Anaerobic threshold: review of the concept and directions for future research. *Med. Sci. Sports Exerc.* 17:6–18, 1985.
23. Dehn, M. M., and R. A. Bruce. Longitudinal variations in maximal oxygen intake with age and activity. *J. Appl. Physiol.* 33:805–807, 1972.
24. Dempsey, J. A. Is the lung built for exercise? *Med. Sci. Sports Exerc.* 28:143–155, 1986.
25. Drinkwater, B. L. Women and exercise: physiological aspects. *Exerc. Sport Sci. Rev.* 12:21–51, 1984.
26. Durstine, J. L., R. R. Pate, P. B. Sparling, G. E. Wilson, M. D. Senn, and W. P. Bartoli. Lipid, lipoprotein, and iron status of elite women distance runners. *Int. J. Sports Med.* 8:119–123, 1987.
27. Dudley, G. A., W. M. Abraham, and R. L. Terjung. Influence of exercise intensity and duration on biochemical adaptations in skeletal muscle. *J. Appl. Physiol.* 53:844–850, 1982.
28. Ekblom, B., and B. Berglund. Effect of erythropoietin administration on maximal aerobic power. *Scand. J. Med. Sci. Sports* 1:88–93, 1991.
29. Ekblom, B., A. N. Goldberg, and B. Gullbring. Response to exercise after blood loss and reinfusion. *J. Appl. Physiol.* 33:175–180, 1972.
30. Farrell, P. A., J. H. Wilmore, E. F. Coyle, J. E. Billing, and D. L. Costill. Plasma lactate accumulation and distance running performance. *Med. Sci. Sports* 11:338–344, 1979.
31. Fink, W. J., D. L. Costill, and M. L. Pollock. Submaximal and maximal working capacity of elite distance runners. Part II. Muscle fiber composition and enzyme activities. *Ann. N.Y. Acad. Sci.* 301:323–327, 1977.
32. Fleg, J. L., and E. G. Lakatta. Role of muscle loss in the age-associated reduction in $\dot{V}o_2$max. *J. Appl. Physiol.* 65:1147–1151, 1988.
33. Gorostiaga, E. M., C. B. Walter, C. Foster, and R. C. Hickson. Uniqueness of interval and continuous training at the same maintained exercise intensity. *Eur. J. Appl. Physiol.* 63:101–107, 1991.
34. Granath, A., B. Jonsson, and T. Strandell. Circulation in healthy old men, studied by right heart catheterization at rest and during exercise in supine and sitting position. *Acta Med. Scand.* 176:425–446, 1964.
35. Graves, J. E., M. L. Pollock, and P. B. Sparling. Body composition of elite female distance runners. *Int. J. Sports Med.* 8:96–102, 1987.
36. Grimby, G., and B. Saltin. Physiological analysis of physically well-trained middle-aged and old athletes. *Acta Med. Scand.* 179:513–526, 1966.
37. Hagan, R. D., T. Strathman, L. Strathman, and L. R. Gettman. Oxygen uptake and energy expenditure during horizontal treadmill running. *J. Appl. Physiol.* 49:571–575, 1980.
38. Hagberg, J. M. Effect of training on the decline of $\dot{V}o_2$max with aging. *Fed. Proc.* 46:1830–1833, 1987.
39. Hagberg, J. M., W. K. Allen, D. R. Seals, B. F. Hurley, A. A. Ehsani, and J. O. Holloszy. A hemodynamic comparison of young and older endurance athletes during exercise. *J. Appl. Physiol.* 58:2041–2046, 1985.

40. Hagberg, J. M., and E. F. Coyle. Physiological determinants of endurance performance as studied in competitive racewalkers. *Med. Sci. Sports Exerc.* 15:287–289, 1983.
41. Heath, G. W., J. M. Hagberg, A. A. Ehsani, and J. O. Holloszy. A physiological comparison of young and older endurance athletes. *J. Appl. Physiol.* 51:634–640, 1981.
42. Hickson, R. C., H. A. Bomze, and J. O. Holloszy. Linear increase in aerobic power induced by a strenuous program of endurance exercise. *J. Appl. Physiol.* 42:372–376, 1977.
43. Hickson, R. C., C. Foster, M. L. Pollock. T. M. Galassi, and S. Rich. Reduced training intensities and loss of aerobic power, endurance, and cardiac growth. *J. Appl. Physiol.* 58:492–499, 1985.
44. Hickson, R. C., C. Kanakis, Jr., J. R. Davis, A. M. Moore, and S. Rich. Reduced training duration effects on aerobic power, endurance, and cardiac growth. *J. Appl. Physiol.* 53:225–229, 1982.
45. Hickson, R. C., and M. A. Rosenkoetter. Reduced training frequencies and maintenance of increased aerobic power. *Med. Sci. Sports Exerc.* 13:13–16, 1981.
46. Holloszy, J. O., and E. F. Coyle. Adaptations of skeletal muscle to endurance exercise and their metabolic consequences. *J. Appl. Physiol.* 56:831–838, 1984.
47. Holloszy, J. O., M. J. Rennie, R. C. Hickson, R. K. Conlee, and J. M. Hagberg. Physiological consequences of the biochemical adaptations to endurance exercise. *Ann. N.Y. Acad. Sci.* 301:441–450, 1977.
48. Hurley, B. F., J. M. Hagberg, W. K. Allen, et al. Effect of training on blood lactate levels during submaximal exercise. *J. Appl. Physiol.* 56:1260–1264, 1984.
49. Johnson, B. D., and J. A. Dempsey. Demand vs. capacity in the aging pulmonary system. *Exerc. Sport Sci. Rev.* 19:171–210, 1991.
50. Joyner, M. J. Modeling: Optimal marathon performance on the basis of physiological factors. *J. Appl. Physiol.* 70:683–687, 1991.
51. Kanstrup, I.-L., and B. Ekblom. Blood volume and hemoglobin concentration as determinants of maximal aerobic power. *Med. Sci. Sports Exerc.* 16:256–262, 1984.
52. Khosla, T. Unfairness of certain events in the Olympic games. *Br. Med. J.* 4:111–113, 1968.
53. LaFontaine, T. P., B. R. Londeree, and W. K. Spath. The maximal steady state versus selected running events. *Med. Sci. Sports Exerc.* 13:190–192, 1981.
54. Lloyd, B. B. World running records as maximal performances. Oxygen debt and other limiting factors. *Circ. Res.* XX, XXI:I-218–226, 1967.
55. McMahon, T. A., and P. R. Greene. Fast running tracks. *Sci. Am.* 239:148–163, 1978.
56. McMahon, T. A., and P. R. Greene. The influence of track compliance on running. *J. Biomech.* 12:893–904, 1979.
57. Martin, R. P., W. L. Haskell, and P. D. Wood. Blood chemistry and lipid profiles of elite distance runners. *Ann. N.Y. Acad. Sci.* 301:346–360, 1977.
58. Mognoni, P., C. Lafortuna, G. Russo, and A. Minetti. An analysis of world records in three types of locomotion. *Eur. J. Appl. Physiol.* 49:287–299, 1982.
59. Noakes, T. D. *Lore of Running.* Champaign, IL: Leisure Press, 1991, pp. 1–804.
60. Pate, R. R., P. B. Sparling, G. E. Wilson, K. J. Cureton, and B. J. Miller. Cardiorespiratory and metabolic responses to submaximal and maximal exercise in elite women distance runners. *Int. J. Sports Med.* 8:91–95, 1987.
61. Patrick, J. M., E. J. Bassey, and P. H. Fentem. The rising ventilatory cost of bicycle exercise in the seventh decade: a longitudinal study of nine healthy men. *Clin. Sci.* 65:521–526, 1983.
62. Péronnet, F., and G. Thibault. Mathematical analysis of running performance and world running records. *J. Appl. Physiol.* 67:453–465, 1989.
63. Pollock. M. L. Submaximal and maximal working capacity of elite distance runners. Part I: Cardiorespiratory aspects. *Ann. N.Y. Acad. Sci.* 301:310–322, 1977.
64. Pollock, M. L., C. Foster, D. Knapp, J. L. Rod, and D. H. Schmidt. Effect of age and

training on aerobic capacity and body composition of master athletes. *J. Appl. Physiol.* 62:725–731, 1987.

65. Pollock, M. L., L. R. Gettman, A. Jackson, J. Ayres, A. Ward, and A. C. Linnerud. Body composition of elite class distance runners. *Ann. N.Y. Acad. Sci.* 301:361–370, 1977.

66. Robertson, R. J., R. Gilcher, K. F. Metz, et al. Hemoglobin concentration and aerobic work capacity in women following induced erthyrocythemia. *J. Appl. Physiol.* 57:568–575, 1984.

67. Robinson, S., D. B. Dill, R. D. Robinson, S. P. Tzankoff, and J. A. Wagner. Physiological aging of champion runners. *J. Appl. Physiol.* 41:46–51, 1976.

68. Robinson, S., D. B. Dill, S. P. Tzankoff, J. A. Wagner, and R. D. Robinson. Longitudinal studies of aging in 37 men. *J. Appl. Physiol.* 38:263–267, 1975.

69. Robinson, S., H. T. Edwards, and D. B. Dill. New records in human power. *Science* 85:409–410, 1937.

70. Rodeheffer, R. J., G. Gerstenblith, L. C. Becker, J. L. Fleg, M. L. Weisfeldt, and E. G. Lakatta. Exercise cardiac output is maintained with advancing age in healthy human subjects: Cardiac dilatation and increased stroke volume compensate for a diminished heart rate. *Circulation* 69:203–213, 1984.

71. Rogers, M. A., J. M. Hagberg, W. H. Martin, III, A. A. Ehsani, and J. O. Holloszy. Decline in $\dot{V}O_2$max with aging in master athletes and sedentary men. *J. Appl. Physiol.* 68:2195–2199, 1990.

72. Rowell, L. B. *Human Circulation Regulation During Physical Stress.* New York: Oxford University Press, 1986, pp. 1–416.

73. Rumball, W. M. and C. E. Coleman. Analysis of running and the prediction of ultimate performance. *Nature* 228:184–185, 1970.

74. Ryder, H. W., H. J. Carr, and P. Herget. Future performance in footracing. *Sci. Am.* 234:109–119, 1976.

75. Saltin, B., and P.-O. Åstrand. Maximal oxygen uptake in athletes. *J. Appl. Physiol.* 23:353–358, 1967.

76. Saltin, B., and S. Strange. Maximal oxygen uptake: "old" and "new" arguments for a cardiovascular limitation. *Med. Sci. Sports Exerc.* 24:30–37, 1992.

77. Schulz, R., and C. Curnow. Peak performance and age among superathletes: track and field, swimming, baseball, tennis, and golf. *J. Gerontol.: Psychol. Sci.* 43:113–120, 1988.

78. Seals, D. R., B. F. Hurley, J. Schultz, and J. M. Hagberg. Endurance training in older men and women. II. Blood lactate response to submaximal exercise. *J. Appl. Physiol.* 57:1030–1033, 1984.

79. Sjödin, B., and I. Jacobs. Onset of blood lactate accumulation and marathon running performance. *Int. J. Sports Med.* 2:23–26, 1981.

80. Sparling, P. B., and K. J. Cureton. Biological determinants of the sex difference in 12-minute run performance. *Med. Sci. Sports Exerc.* 15:218–223, 1983.

81. Stamford, B. A. Exercise and the elderly. *Exerc. Sport Sci. Rev.* 16:341–379, 1988.

82. *TACSTATS/USA Road Running Rankings,* 1990. The National Center for Long Distance Running & Race Walking Records & Research, Santa Barbara, CA.

83. Trounce, I., E. Byrne, and S. Marzuki. Decline in skeletal muscle mitochondrial respiratory chain function: possible factor in ageing. *Lancet* 1:637–639, 1989.

84. Ward-Smith, A. J. A mathematical theory of running, based on the first law of thermodynamics, and its application to the performance of world-class athletes. *J. Biomech.* 18:337–349, 1985.

85. Warren, G. L., and K. J. Cureton. Modeling the effect of alterations in hemoglobin concentration on $\dot{V}O_2$max. *Med. Sci. Sports Exerc.* 21:526–531, 1989.

86. Whipp, B. J., and S. A. Ward. Will women soon outrun men? *Nature* 355:25, 1992.

87. Williams, M. H., S. Wesseldine, T. Somma, and R. Schuster. The effect of induced erythrocythemia upon 5-mile treadmill run time. *Med. Sci. Sports Exerc.* 13:169–175, 1981.

88. Wilmore, J. H. The assessment of and variation in aerobic power in world class athletes as related to specific sports. *Am. J. Sports Med.* 12:120–127, 1984.

89. Wilmore J. H., C. H. Brown, and J. A. Davis. Body physique and composition of the female distance runner. *Ann. N.Y. Acad. Sci.* 301:764–776, 1977.

90. Wilmore, J. H., and D. L. Costill. *Training for Sport and Activity. The Physiological Basis of the Conditioning Process.* 3rd Ed. Dubuque, IA: Wm. C. Brown Publishers, 1988, pp. 1–420.

91. Wilt, F. *How They Train. Vol. II: Long Distances.* 2nd Ed. Track and Field News, 1973, pp. 1–126.

92. zur Megede, E., and R. Hymans. *Progression of World Best Performances and Official IAAF World Records.* Monaco: International Athletic Foundation, 1991, pp. 1–705.

5
Exercise and Inhibition of Glucocorticoid-Induced Muscle Atrophy

ROBERT C. HICKSON, Ph.D.

JANE R. MARONE, M.D.

INTRODUCTION

Glucocorticoids have widespread functions in the body. At physiological levels, they are involved in maintaining glucose production from protein, facilitating fat metabolism, supporting vascular responsiveness, and modulating central nervous system (CNS) functions. They also influence the immune system, protein turnover, renal function, and may be responsible for initiating parturition [48]. Excessive levels of glucocorticoids, either from diseases such as Cushing's syndrome, clinical treatment of inflammatory diseases, or experimental administration can promote tissue catabolism and atrophy by simultaneously accelerating the rate of protein breakdown and amino acid efflux and decreasing the rate of protein synthesis [58]. In recent years, members of this laboratory have examined the catabolic effects of glucocorticoids on muscle tissue with particular emphasis on the prevention of this process through exercise training. The purpose of this review is to discuss these findings in skeletal muscle and their implications for future research, as well as to present a brief overview of the mechanism through which glucocorticoids function.

MECHANISM OF ACTION

In the classic model of steroid-hormonal control, cellular metabolism is regulated directly at the level of the gene rather than through a second messenger system. Since the steroid is lipid soluble, it is able to diffuse through the target cell membrane and into the cytosol where it binds to a receptor protein. The binding of the hormone to the receptor causes a transformation, or activation, of the hormone-receptor complex, which enables the receptor to take on DNA-binding capabilities. The complex then passes into the nucleus and binds to DNA resulting in altered RNA transcription [53]. Thus, it appears that the steroid receptor plays a pivotal role in ultimately influencing the translation of cellular proteins.

RECEPTOR PROTEIN—STRUCTURE AND FUNCTIONS

The glucocorticoid receptor (GR) protein can be divided into three functional domains (Fig. 5.1). The C-terminal region (domain A) is involved in steroid binding, which promotes transformation, or activation, of the hormone-receptor complex. The central core (domain B) is involved in DNA binding; it is thought that steroid specificity of the receptor protein with regard to DNA interaction is conferred here. The amino terminal region (domain C) comprises approximately 50% of the protein and has a less well-defined function (19, 35, 49, 53].

DOMAIN A—STEROID BINDING AND TRANSFORMATION. In the unactivated or untransformed state, the glucocorticoid receptor exists as an oligomer consisting of three components—one molecule of steroid-binding protein and two molecules of a 90-kDa heat shock protein (hsp-90s), each of which is bound to the hormone-binding region of the receptor [27]. The possibility of yet a fourth component is suggested by Rexin et al. [103] who performed cross-linking experiments to identify the association of a 59-kDa protein with one of the hsp-90s in receptors isolated from mouse lymphoma cells. The steroid-binding domain itself consists of a hydrophobic region with two cysteines and one methionine residue located at the center of this region. Binding of the steroid appears to involve these sites of interaction [18].

Studies examining the transformation of the receptor determined that

FIGURE 5.1

Functional domains of the glucocorticoid receptor.

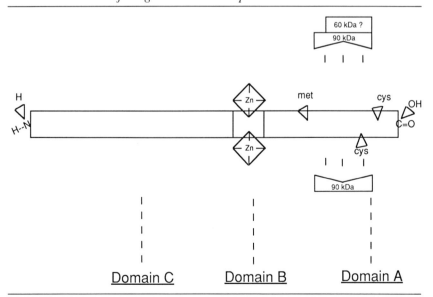

cleavage of the C-terminal region resulted in constitutive binding of the receptor to DNA [35, 50, 65]. This suggested that steroid binding unmasked a preexisting functional DNA-binding domain and that the steroid was not necessary for DNA binding once activation had occurred [33, 35, 50, 98]. Later work indicated that activation of the receptor involves the dissociation of the hsp-90s in response to steroid binding, resulting in a reduction in molecular size of the oligomer from a molecular radius (Mr) of 300,000 to a Mr of 94,000–100,000. The hsps are thought to be a stabilizing factor in steroid binding [89, 92, 98]; binding of the steroid to the receptor occurs $100\times$ more readily in the presence of the hsp-90 than in its absence [92].

Other factors appear to be necessary for transformation to occur. Sulfhydryl groups, most likely from cysteine residues within the steroid-binding pocket [90], appear to be essential in maintaining the receptor in steroid-binding form [98, 122]. Thiol oxidation of these groups inhibits both steroid and DNA binding [117]. Several studies have suggested that dephosphorylation of the receptor protein is necessary for activation to occur [98]; however, direct measurements of radioactively labeled phosphorus (^{32}P) in activated and unactivated receptors indicate that this is not a factor [123].

DOMAIN B—DNA BINDING. The DNA-binding domain of the receptor is located at the central core of the receptor protein [107]. Although its main function involves recognition of appropriate DNA nucleotides, in the human GR, there also appears to be a sequence of residues essential for inducing transcription from a glucocorticoid responsive promoter [65]. This domain is a short, highly conserved region with not less than 80% homology among species [1]. There are two repeat units of basic residues and a cysteine-rich motif [19, 35, 49]; eight of these cysteine residues tetrahedrally coordinate two zinc ions in a zinc-finger configuration [44, 56]. Alterations of the amino acid sequence within this region can completely abolish receptor function [49].

Binding regions of the DNA contain no promoter activity, but as for other steroid hormones, they behave as enhancer elements whose activity is strictly hormone dependent and who act in *cis* either upstream or downstream from the promotor site [10, 53]. Exactly how the activated receptor binds to DNA is not completely understood, but evidence suggests that after dissociation of the hsp-90s, the activated receptor forms a dimer that interacts with guanine residues in two sequential major grooves of DNA double helix in a head-to-head orientation [110, 125]. Recognition of the appropriate DNA sequence by the receptor may involve amino acids in proximity to one of the zinc ions [28].

DOMAIN C. The N-terminus, domain C, encompasses approximately one-half of the protein. Its amino acid structure is not highly conserved and the exact function remains unclear. It appears to be the immunodominant region and may be involved in modulating enhancer function [1] and/or DNA binding [35]. Deletions or mutations of this region will decrease transcription rate by 90–95% [35, 49, 65]. More recently, Eriksson and Wrange [34] have suggested that this domain may affect the steric arrangement of the DNA-binding domains of the receptor dimer thereby promoting specificity of binding of the activated receptor to the DNA response elements.

Glucocorticoid Regulation
As mentioned previously, glucocorticoids are believed to influence transcription primarily by interacting with enhancer or regulatory elements upstream or downstream from the promotor regions [10, 53]. However, there must exist a mechanism to regulate the glucocorticoids once they are inside the cell. Recent evidence indicates that at least some of this regulation occurs at transcriptional, post-transcriptional, or post-translational levels of the receptor protein itself (for review, see [16]). Several studies provide evidence that exposure of cells to glucocorticoids both in vitro [15, 95] and in vivo [71] is correlated with a decrease in glucocorticoid receptor mRNA from 40–95%. Conversely, the removal of the glucocorticoid stimulus in vivo may increase the level of receptor mRNA [71]. Rosewicz at al. [105] performed nuclear run-on experiments and showed a 50% decrease in the transcription rate of mRNA in cells exposed to glucocorticoids; no difference in the half-life of receptor mRNA was found. Receptor protein levels in cells exposed to glucocorticoids parallel the mRNA changes; a 50% reduction in the amount of receptor protein was seen in cells exposed to dexamethasone, leading the authors to conclude that there is an actual reduction in receptor protein production, rather than a transformation to the unactivated form of the receptor [15]. Thus, the general mechanisms through which glucocorticoids operate hormonally to influence transcription and ultimately translation of cellular proteins may, in fact, be the same mechanism through which they control their own receptor production.

EXERCISE AND INHIBITION OF MUSCLE ATROPHY

Four exercise and contractile activity model systems have been used to study the prevention of the muscle atrophy associated with excessive levels of glucocorticoids. These are: functional overload, resistance exercise, endurance exercise, and in vitro cell culture stimulation. Functional overload involves severing the tendons (tenotomy) from synergistic muscles or by partially or completely removing the synergistic muscles (ablation or myectomy). Following the surgical procedures, the remaining or intact synergistic muscle(s) undergoes a "compensatory overload" on a full-time basis and increases in mass. Resistance or strength exercise involves performing repetitions and sets (number of work intervals) by a specific muscle group or groups at a prescribed relative intensity. This form of exercise can result in muscle enlargement, but increased mass is not always a universal effect. Endurance exercise such as treadmill running does not increase muscle mass or strength to any great extent but develops aerobic energy-generating systems in skeletal muscle. Intermittent repetitive mechanical stimulation of skeletal muscle cell cultures is a new procedure that offers potential for examining atrophy inhibition by contractile activity in an in vitro model [21].

Effectiveness of Exercise and Contractile Activity Programs in Attenuating Loss of Muscle Mass
Comparisons of types of contractile activity and the degree of atrophy prevention are given in Table 5.1. Contractile activity as a model of atrophy prevention was initially studied over 20 years ago. Using the tenotomy model, Goldberg and Goodman [51] observed 58% less atrophy in the overloaded plantaris muscles after cutting the gastrocnemius tendon than in the corresponding control plantaris muscles following cortisone treatment. A greater inhibition of glucocorticoid-related muscle mass loss is found following functional overload by synergist ablation. After removal of most of the gastrocnemius and soleus muscles, Kurowski et al. [77] observed 90% less atrophy in plantaris muscles following 7 days of cortisone acetate injections. In these two studies, both types of functional overload and glucocorticoids were initiated simultaneously.

However, if functional overload is implemented and the muscle is allowed to attain a steady-state of muscle enlargement, a somewhat

TABLE 5.1
Contractile Activity Prevention of Glucocorticoid-induced Muscle Atrophy

Type of Activity	Experimental Conditions (Onset of Activity and/or Hormone)	Relative Atrophy Prevention (%)
Tenotomy	Simultaneously	Approximately 60
Synergist ablation	Simultaneously	90
Synergist ablation	After muscle enlarged	7
Resistance training (rats)	Simultaneously	46
Resistance training (humans)	Clinically stable renal transplant patients receiving hormone therapy	9–44
Endurance training (10–11 days)	Simultaneously	25–60
Endurance training (3–4 months)	After muscle trained	25–100
Endurance training (10–11 days)	While muscles are atrophying	23–40
Mechanical stimulation (in vitro)	Simultaneously	65

different response is observed. When plantaris muscles were allowed to enlarge for at least 30 days, a sufficient time to attain maximal growth, the hypertrophied state of the muscle was not maintained when glucocorticoids were given. Over the 7-day hormone period, the rates of decline in hypertrophied and control muscles were similar, although 7% of the total enlargement still remained in the overloaded group. These findings suggested that the resistance to glucocorticoids by functional overload was limited to the normal range of plantaris muscle mass in that the previously enlarged muscles returned to the same range (from 391 ± 8 to 304 ± 10 mg), but were not lower than the muscles of controls (284 ± 7 mg) not receiving steroids.

Resistance training in animals and humans has been shown to be successful in attenuating or reversing the glucocorticoid-associated muscle atrophy (Table 5.1). Based on the data of Gardiner et al. [46], we estimate that about 46% of gastrocnemius muscle wasting was prevented in rats who participated in lifting weights by using trunk and hindlimb muscles. Horber et al. [67–69] employed isokinetic (cyclex) training in clinically stable renal transplant patients receiving prednisone therapy. They found improved muscle function by isokinetic measurements and increased thigh girth and thigh muscle area between 9% and 44% as performed by computer tomography and compared with healthy matched controls (Table 5.1).

Programs of endurance running are also capable of preventing glucocorticoid-mediated muscle atrophy. In the first of these studies to determine whether endurance exercise was effective against muscle atrophy from glucocorticoids, male rats were trained by treadmill running up to $110–112 \text{ min} \cdot \text{day}^{-1}$ for 12 weeks [59]. Additionally because of the possibility that androgens were involved in inhibiting glucocorticoid-related events, the effects of removing most of the endogenous androgens were studied by employing trained and sedentary castrated rats. The running program prevented between one-fourth and one-half of the muscle wasting in the fast-twitch gastrocnemius and plantaris muscles. For certain muscle comparisons, the relative loss of mass with hormone treatment was greater in the castrated group than in the intact group. Total protein concentration ($\text{mg} \cdot \text{g}^{-1}$) was unchanged by glucocorticoid treatment, and the hormone injections did not interfere with the exercise-induced increases in citrate synthase and myoglobin in mixed plantaris or red muscle types [59]. With functional or compensatory overload as well as resistance training, sparing of muscle mass may involve a "growth vs. atrophy" antagonism within the same muscle since both fast-twitch and slow-twitch fibers increase in size during the overload period and fast-twitch fibers initially atrophy from glucocorticoids. With endurance running, there is little or no increase in muscle mass. This suggested the possibility that the cellular and molecular basis of atrophy prevention could be dictated by the type of exercise.

In several subsequent investigations, endurance training was used in studying the effects of exercise in attenuating the muscle atrophy response [62, 63]. In these experiments, hormone treatments were begun only after some training level was reached. We then studied whether being previously trained offered an advantage over starting out on an exercise program. This was based on the reasoning that endurance-trained muscles, which have an increased capacity for aerobic metabolism, were perhaps better suited to stop the atrophying process. These results, which were obtained after initiating an endurance running program for 90 min · day^{-1} and glucocorticoid treatment simultaneously for 11 consecutive days, produced muscle atrophy prevention of 25% in gastrocnemius and 60% in plantaris muscles [23]. These values were in the same range of muscle sparing as obtained from studies of endurance-trained rats [59, 62, 63]. In the 11-day glucocorticoid-treated runners, citrate synthase activities increased 37% in gastrocnemius and 60% in plantaris muscles [23]. By comparison, citrate synthase levels in plantaris muscles of the 12-week runners were increased 80–100% [59]. This difference in aerobic metabolism capacity does not appear to be a factor in atrophy prevention, and the results solidified the concept that prior endurance training was not a prerequisite to atrophy prevention.

Recently, studies have been conducted to evaluate whether starting a regular endurance exercise program is a deterrent to a developing state of muscle atrophy [40]. Exercise (running 90 min/day) was introduced after 4 days of steroid treatment, when the animals had already lost approximately 10% of their muscle mass and were in a progressive catabolic state. For those who began the exercise program following the initial 4 days of glucocorticoid treatment, there were 23% and 36% less atrophy in quadriceps and plantaris muscles, respectively. This level of protection is consistent with that observed in the other studies when exercise was initiated simultaneously with glucocorticoid administration or when an endurance training regimen of at least 12 weeks was used before 11 days of hormone treatment [23, 59, 62, 63]. When compared with the decline in muscle mass from the 4-day time point in sedentary animals, the daily exercise prevented 28% and 45% of the atrophy in quadriceps and plantaris muscle mass, respectively. Based on the fiber-type composition of quadriceps muscles [3], it is estimated that fast-twitch red fibers comprise approximately 27% of the total fiber population. Consequently, the relative atrophy prevention observed is similar to the proportion of fast-twitch red fibers present, and is consistent with the observation that atrophy sparing occurs to a greater extent in muscle types that are highly recruited by endurance running programs. Similar comparisons apply for the plantaris muscle. In humans receiving hormone therapy for various diseases, illnesses, and disorders, beginning an exercise program that includes endurance-type activities can prove to be an important therapeutic countermeasure to the muscle atrophy accompanying steroid excess.

Preliminary studies indicate that repetitive mechanical stimulation of cultured myotubes can attenuate loss of muscle fiber diameter and protein content in dexamethasone-treated cells [21]. This in vitro model may have value in helping elucidate the regulation of muscle atrophy prevention by contractile activity.

Glucocorticoid and Exercise Effects on Skeletal Muscle Fiber Types
Glucocorticoid-mediated atrophy is selective for fast-twitch fibers and, particularly, for white regions of muscle [47, 51, 59, 106, 113]. In the rat, muscles with a large percentage of fast-twitch fibers like the whole quadriceps, gastrocnemius, and plantaris undergo atrophy, while muscles that are predominantly slow-twitch (such as the soleus) are resistant to atrophy. In attempting to understand the fiber-type specificity of exercise in inhibiting the muscle wasting associated with excessive levels of glucocorticoids, Falduto et al. [36] studied the effects of hormone treatment and an 11-day exercise program on Type IIA and IIB fibers, as determined by histochemical staining for myofibrillar ATPase with alkaline and acid preincubation in both a deep (Type I, 13%; Type IIA, 24%; and Type IIB, 63%) and a superficial (all Type II) area of plantaris muscles. On a regional basis, 11 days of cortisol-acetate (CA) treatment (100 mg · kg^{-1} body weight) resulted in less atrophy in the deep than in the superficial portions. Across regions, Type IIA fibers were less susceptible to atrophy than IIB fibers. Type I fibers were unchanged by hormone treatment, and the percentage of Type IIA fibers in the superficial region was three-fold higher (27% vs. 9%) following cortisol-acetate treatment. In the deep region, the exercise program prevented 100% and 67% of the atrophy in Types IIA and IIB, respectively. The running program prevented 50% and 40% atrophy in Types IIA and IIB fibers, respectively, in the superficial region. These results also indicated that the fast-twitch fibers most frequently recruited by the running program exhibit the highest degree of glucocorticoid resistance.

Glucocorticoid Receptor as a Regulatory Site in Atrophy Prevention
In attempting to identify a possible mechanism of contractile activity in preventing muscle atrophy, several parameters of glucocorticoid-receptor binding; namely, receptor capacity, binding affinity, and binding specificity have been examined. In response to functional overload, several studies [37, 60, 77] have shown glucocorticoid receptor-binding capacity, generally measured using [^{3}H]dexamethasone or [^{3}H]triamcinolone acetonide as the labeled ligand, increases between 50% and 100% in hypertrophied plantaris muscles (Table 5.2). Receptor-binding affinity, as measured by dissociation constants (kd), and binding specificity, as determined by competition of receptors for

TABLE 5.2
Androgen and Glucocorticoid Receptor Binding and Receptor Activation in
Overloaded-Hypertrophied and in Endurance-Trained Skeletal Muscles

	Overload		Endurance Training	
Variable	[³H]R 1881 Binding	[³H]Triamcinolone Acetonide or [³H]Dexamethasone Binding	[³H]R 1881 Binding	[³H]Triamcinolone Acetonide or [³H]Dexamethasone Binding
Receptor capacity	40–71% increase	50–100% increase	No change	No change
Binding affinity	No change	No change	No change	No change
Binding specificity	No change	No change	No change	No change
Receptor activation (DNA-cellulose binding DEAE-cellulose chromatography)	No change	No change	No change (predicted)	No change (predicted)

various glucocorticoids, remained unchanged in hypertrophied muscles [77]. The increased glucocorticoid receptor-binding levels in hypertrophied muscles suggest that a greater hormonal effect is possible. In support of this conclusion, the inability of hypertrophied muscles to maintain increased muscle mass in the wake of excessive glucocorticoids may be directly related to this increased glucocorticoid-receptor capacity [60]. In general, somewhat higher values of glucocorticoid-receptor binding have been observed in overloaded as compared with control animals receiving hormone treatment [77]; however, there is marked down-regulation of the receptor by 90% or more by steroid administration. Consequently, the significance of this observation is unknown. These results are summarized in Table 5.2.

The effects of endurance running on glucocorticoid-receptor binding are somewhat different than that observed following functional overload (Table 5.2). In the exercise studies, mixed and fiber-type specific muscle regions were studied. The highest glucocorticoid-receptor binding values are found in slow-twitch red muscles (50–55 fmoles · mg protein-$^{-1}$) lowest in fast-twitch white muscles (20–25 fmoles · mg protein^{-1}), and intermediate in whole gastrocnemius (28–32 fmoles · mg protein^{-1}) and fast-twitch red muscles (approximately 40 fmoles · mg protein $^{-1}$ [62]). However, endurance running over 13–18 weeks had little effect on the [³H]triamcinolone acetonide cytosol binding in the gastrocnemius muscle or any of the fiber types (Table 5.2). Yet, when rats are exercised for only 11 days [23], a small (25%) consistent increase in [³H]triamcinolone acetonide binding by all muscle types has been observed. The significance of this latter finding is not yet clear and may represent a transient effect appearing during the early stages of an endurance exercise program. The fact that glucocorticoid binding levels are lowest in fast-twitch white muscle and highest in slow-twitch red muscle is paradoxical, since the former is the fiber type most highly susceptible to atrophy and the latter is the fiber type most resistant to atrophy. These observations offer the possibility that other factors in addition to receptor content contribute to the glucocorticoid and exercise responses.

Depletion-repletion rates of glucocorticoid receptors were examined when sedentary controls and runners were given a single intraperitoneal injection of cortisol while at rest [62]. Faster receptor repletion was observed at 2 hours after hormone injection in slow-twitch red and fast-twitch red muscles of the runners, but other time points were not markedly different. The accelerated repletion kinetics in the red muscle types of the trained animals suggest that the residence time of the steroid-receptor complex within the nuclei is reduced and/or that there is an increased reprocessing of the cytoplasmic form of the receptor. Glucocorticoid effects may possibly be attenuated by exercise, in part, by alterations in receptor dynamics.

Activation or transformation of the steroid-receptor complex is a process associated with both conformational changes and an increased ability to translocate from the cytoplasm into nuclei, and bind to DNA [111]. Among the conformational changes, two forms of the activated glucocorticoid receptor (termed binders II and IB according to the nomenclature of Litwack and colleagues [80, 85, 96] appear during elution from anion exchange chromatography columns after thermal activation. Controversy existed, however, as to whether the IB peak (wash fraction of DEAE cellulose columns) is a separate receptor or a proteolytic product of binder II. For example, several tissues are known to exhibit a predominance of one form of the activated receptor over the other [2, 8, 84]. Furthermore, the distribution of activated receptors was found to be specific in various muscle fiber types, with heart and slow-twitch soleus muscles containing approximately equal content of binders II and IB, whereas mixed muscle and fast-twitch white fiber types contain proportionally more binder IB than binder II [26]. On the other hand, the major form in rat kidney, binder IB, is absent when receptor preparation contains sodium molybdate and the activated IB form reacts with monoclonal antibody BUGR-1, which was raised against rat liver glucocorticoid receptor (predominantly binder II) [32]. In addition, multiple glucocorticoid receptor genes have not been found.

The presence of increased numbers of glucocorticoid receptors in enlarged muscle cells prompted our investigation regarding several aspects of glucocorticoid-receptor activation [37]. Specifically, the first purpose was to quantify the extent of activation in hypertrophied vs. normal or control muscles. Since overloaded muscles have the capacity to spare some of the atrophy caused by excess glucocorticoids [51, 60, 77], it was thought that one of the possible mechanisms would be through a reduced capacity for receptor activation. Second, because of the increased receptor binding and the relative differences in binder II and binder IB in various muscle types, we determined whether the distribution of the activated steroid-receptor complexes was shifted toward that observed in heart and slow-twitch muscles [26]. In plantaris muscles hypertrophied by functional overload, several functional and biochemical changes toward a slow-twitch muscle have been shown to occur [37]. On the basis that hypertrophied muscles are assuming certain biochemical and contractile characteristics of slow-twitch fibers, it was anticipated that the activated receptor distribution would shift to the profiles observed in slow fibers. However, in view of the limited capacity of hypertrophied plantaris muscles to resist atrophy from glucocorticoids [60], a shift in this direction would disprove any potential relationship between the receptor distribution and the muscles' response to steroid administration.

These results showed that the increased [^{3}H]triamcinolone acetonide binding in hypertrophied vs. control muscles (125 vs. 79 fmol $\cdot$ mg^{-1} protein) was not related to any changes in ability to bind to DNA based on binding to DNA-cellulose [37]. DEAE-cellulose chromatography of activated receptors revealed higher activated binding forms in hypertrophied muscles than in control muscles, which was consistent with the increased receptor binding, but the relative distribution of activated binding forms remained unchanged [37]. Despite the observed fast- to slow-twitch biochemical transformations by functionally enlarged plantaris muscles, there was no shift in activated receptor distribution toward that found in glucocorticoid-resistant muscles such as soleus. This observation is consistent with the results that hypertrophied plantaris muscles are not capable of resisting atrophy from glucocorticoids to the same extent as nonoverloaded slow-twitch soleus muscles [59, 63]. An increase in the binder II form of the receptor without a corresponding ability to resist muscle atrophy would have implied a lack of relationship with the activated receptor forms and the muscles' response to administered hormone. Moreover, the inability of hypertrophied muscles to resist atrophy is consistent with the fact that neither the percentage of activated receptors nor the activated receptor profiles from DEAE-cellulose columns were changed.

Although Falduto et al. [37] observed no effects of skeletal muscle hypertrophy induced by functional overload on glucocorticoid receptor activation, these experiments were performed in vitro. Previous studies have established the time dependency of activation in several tissues of animals [25, 85]. As a further step, in vivo activation during treadmill running was examined [22]. Immediately before running or remaining sedentary, adrenalectomized rats were given an intraperitoneal injection (50 μCi $\cdot$ 100 g^{-1} body weight) of [^{3}H]triamcinolone acetonide. Exercise did not alter the rate or extent of receptor activation as measured by DNA-cellulose binding in any whole muscle or muscle type studied (Fig. 5.2). Additionally, the time courses of DEAE-cellulose chromatography elution profiles of unactivated and activated [³H]triamcinolone acetonide receptor complexes in fast-twitch red (deep quadriceps) muscles are shown in Figure 5.3. In these chromatography profiles, the unactivated form of the receptor is the predominant form observed before steroid administration (0-time point) and elutes at approximately 250 mM potassium phosphate (KP). The unactivated peak appears at fractions 26–40 on each panel of the figure. There were small or no activated peaks seen for binder II (fractions 18–24), which eluted at 50–100 mM KP. Binder IB is also present in small amounts in the wash fractions (1–10) prior to adding the KP gradient to the columns. By 5 min after injection (5-min panel of Fig. 5.3), there was a decrease in the unactivated forms and increases in activated forms. At 30, 60, and 90 min, the unactivated form progressively declined to barely detectable levels. The radioactivity of the activated forms increased and then decreased during this time frame (30–90 min), indicating down-regulation and/or nuclear translocation of receptors. There were no differences during the 90 min of exercise in DEAE-cellulose steroid-receptor complex elution profiles between the runners and sedentary controls. Similar data were obtained for whole gastrocnemius, slow-twitch red, fast-twitch white, and heart muscles. These results indicated that glucocorticoid receptor activation occurs at a rate that is independent of both fiber type and delivery of steroid to working muscles during exercise.

In conclusion, although some changes in glucocorticoid binding were seen in response to certain types of contractile activity, the receptor-binding and receptor-activation studies have not provided definitive clues as to whether the exercise effects are directed at the glucocorticoid receptor. It is possible that these methods are not sensitive enough to evaluate glucocorticoid receptor changes by exercise or that exercise is altering molecular events beyond the receptor activation step.

Is Muscle Atrophy Prevention by Exercise Mediated by the Anticatabolic Actions of Androgens?

Androgens and their synthetic derivatives (collectively termed androgenic-anabolic steroids) represent another class of steroid hormones. They have actions opposing those of glucocorticoids in that they can increase protein synthesis and promote total body and muscle growth [72, 76]. The ability of these compounds to exert their effects through inhibition of glucocorticoid functioning remains a potential alternative mechanism of action [81, 88]. In attempting to elucidate the potential anticatabolic and/or antiglucocorticoid action of androgens, several aspects of hormone functioning should be considered: the requirement

FIGURE 5.2

DNA-cellulose binding in various muscles or muscle regions of exercising (**RUN**) *and sedentary* (**SED**) *rats after in vivo [³H]triamcinolone acetonide administration. Values are means ± SE for three or four observations per point. The* **0-min** *values were obtained from tissues, the cytosols of which were labeled in vitro. From Czerwinski, S. M., and R. C. Hickson, Glucocorticoid receptor activation during exercise in muscle.* J. Appl. Physiol. *68:1615–1620, 1990. with permission from the American Physiological Society.*

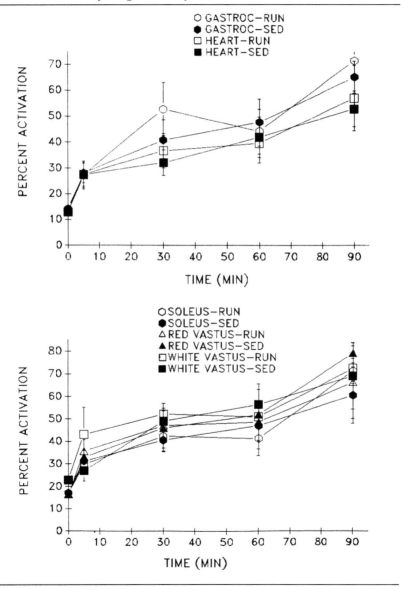

FIGURE 5.3

DEAE-cellulose chromatography of unactivated and activated [³H]triamcinolone acetonide-receptor complexes in fast-twitch red (deep quadriceps) muscles of exercising **(RUN)** *and sedentary* **(SED)** *rats after in vivo [³H]triamcinolone acetonide administration. Unactivated form of receptor eluted 200–300 mM potassium phosphate* **(KP)**; *"classical" activated form (binder II) eluted 50–100 mM KP; wash fraction (binder IB) eluted before KP gradient (fraction 1–10). The 0-min time point was obtained as described in legend of Figure 5.2. From Czerwinski, S. M., and R. C. Hickson. Glucocorticoid receptor activation during exercise in muscle.* J. Appl. Physiol. *68:1615–1620, 1990. With permission from the American Physiological Society.*

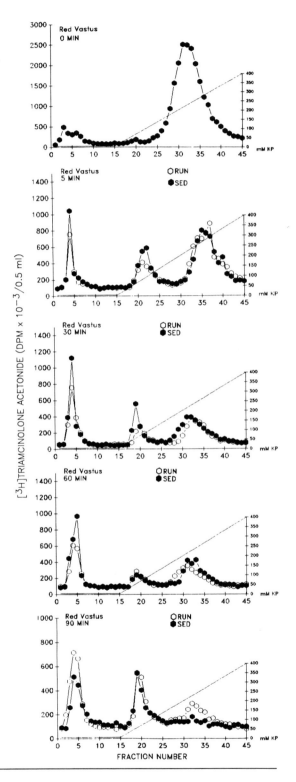

of steroid-receptor interaction in initiating hormone events; the ability of androgenic-anabolic steroids to exert antiglucocorticoid action by binding to the glucocorticoid receptor in vitro and in vivo; androgen interaction with DNA sequences corresponding to hormone-responsive elements on inducible genes; and physiological effects of androgenic-anabolic steroids as anticatabolic agents.

STEROID-RECEPTOR INTERACTION REQUIREMENT. With steroid-sensitive tissues, hormone actions require ligand-receptor binding, receptor activation, followed by binding of the activated receptor to specific DNA sequences. Steroid-receptor binding appears as an essential first step in hormone action. As one example, Konagaya et al. [74] have demonstrated the importance of glucocorticoid-receptor interaction with the use of the synthetic glucocorticoid antagonist RU 38486 in skeletal muscle. Administration of RU 38486 blocked glucocorticoid binding to its receptor and attenuated the muscle atrophy associated with glucocorticoid administration [74].

POTENTIAL ANDROGENIC-ANABOLIC STEROID BINDING TO GLUCO-CORTICOID RECEPTORS. The results of in vitro and in vivo binding specificity studies of various androgen and anabolic steroid competitors for the glucocorticoid receptor have been reviewed previously [58]. In general, in vitro competition experiments have shown a low affinity of androgens and anabolic steroids for glucocorticoid receptor binding, although exceptions were also found. For competition studies performed in vivo, a consistent positive interaction of androgenic-anabolic steroid binding to glucocorticoid receptors has not been observed [58].

TRANSCRIPTIONAL INTERFERENCE OF GLUCOCORTICOID ACTION BY ANDROGENIC-ANABOLIC STEROIDS. Besides their potential for binding to the glucocorticoid receptor, there is a possibility that androgenic-anabolic steroids can directly or indirectly inhibit glucocorticoid action at the gene level. Different steroid hormones are able to regulate the same set of genes. DNA sequences, termed hormone regulatory or response elements (HRE), are found in inducible proteins mostly upstream from the start of transcription [9, 11]. For the glucocorticoid receptor, a 15-mer consensus glucocorticoid response element (GRE) sequence has been identified from a variety of DNA binding sites [9, 11] (Fig. 5.4). However, the GRE does not have exclusive specificity for the glucocorticoid receptor. Recent evidence indicates that the GRE is able to mediate induction by other steroid hormones including androgens. This has been shown in the mouse mammary tumor virus, long-term repeat, and in the rat tyrosine aminotransferase gene [20, 31, 55]. Further, androgen induction of transcription at the GRE is inhibited by androgen receptor antagonists [20]. The physiological consequences of several steroids functioning through the same HRE are unknown as yet. However, when the same gene may be modified by both androgens and glucocorticoids

FIGURE 5.4

Model of androgen-anabolic steroid inhibition of glucocorticoid action at the GRE. From Hickson, R. C., S. M. Czerwinski, M. T. Falduto, and A. P. Young. Glucocorticoid antagonism by exercise and androgenic-anabolic steroids. Med. Sci. Sports Exerc. *22:331–340, 1990. With permission from Williams & Wilkins.*

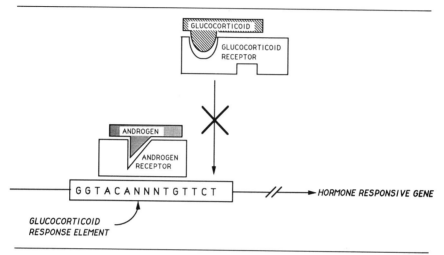

in different ways, a plausible mechanism of glucocorticoid inhibition by androgenic-anabolic steroids exists through the HRE (Fig. 5.4).

ANDROGENIC-ANABOLIC STEROIDS AS POTENTIAL ANTIGLUCOCORTI-COID AGENTS. A lack of consistency is apparent regarding the role of androgens or anabolic steroids in retarding the muscle atrophy associated with high-dosage glucocorticoids. Capaccio et al. [17] did not see any androgen prevention of gastrocnemius muscle wasting from cortisol acetate (20 mg · kg^{-1}) treatment in slowly growing (>300 g), intact, female rats. These animals were pretreated with testosterone acetate at double the cortisol-acetate dosage 2 hr before the cortisol acetate injections over a 12-day period. In contrast, Danhaive and Rousseau [29] reported that RU 486 (RU 38486), testosterone, and trenbolone all were affective in attenuating corticosterone-induced retardation of body weight gain in gastrocnemius, extensor digitorum longus, and soleus muscles of young, rapidly growing (>100 g), adrenalectomized rats. In both studies, under appropriate conditions (using intact females and gonadectomized males + estradiol (E$_2$), androgenic-anabolic steroids increased total body and muscle growth independent of glucocorticoid treatment. Danhaive and Rousseau [29] claim that androgens can behave as antiglucocorticoids because of their ability to diminish glucocorticoid-modulated liver tyrosine aminotransferase activity. However, this was demonstrated in a nonmuscle tissue, where androgenic actions may differ from those in muscle. The tyrosine aminotransferase gene has not been found in skeletal muscle. Further, androgenic-anabolic steroids were ineffective competitors of glucocorticoid-receptor binding in the same study [29]. Thus, the mechanism of muscle sparing by androgenic-anabolic steroids remains obscure. The use of rapidly growing vs. slowly growing animals may be important because, in the former case, androgens may not be retarding atrophy but inhibiting a glucocorticoid-mediated reduction in growth rate.

ANDROGEN RECEPTOR BINDING IN RESPONSE TO FUNCTIONAL OVER-LOAD AND ENDURANCE TRAINING. As summarized in Table 5.2, androgen receptor content increases by 40–80% in hypertrophied plantaris muscles following removal of synergistic muscles [13, 61, 64, 77]. Receptor-binding affinities and binding specificities remain unchanged in the enlarged muscles [61, 77]. With glucocorticoid treatment, androgen receptor binding was not significantly reduced (0.91 ± 0.07 (vehicle-treated) vs. 0.80 ± 0.10 (hormone-treated) fmol $\cdot$ mg^{-1} protein) in control muscles but was markedly lower (1.27 ± 0.10 (vehicle-treated) vs. 0.56 ± 0.22 (hormone-treated) fmoles $\cdot$ mg^{-1} protein) in overloaded muscles [77]. Thus, in control muscles or those not overloaded, glucocorticoids do not appear to be functioning through the androgen receptor, but the reduction in androgen receptor binding by glucocorticoids in the hypertrophied muscles suggests the possibility of interference of androgen functioning. Nevertheless, since androgen receptor content is low in plantaris muscles, about one-thirtieth of glucocorticoid receptor levels, the impact of significant changes in androgen receptor binding is still uncertain. Further, the ligand employed in these studies to bind androgen receptors, [^{3}H]methyltrinolone (R1881), also binds to glucocorticoid-binding sites at high or near-saturating concentrations of labeled ligand in muscle [78]. While steps were taken to separate both androgen and glucocorticoid components of receptor binding [77, 78], some caution in the glucocorticoid interaction of androgen receptor binding is warranted.

With endurance training, the androgen receptor represented a mechanism of interference because a bout of exercise can elevate blood androgen levels [75, 115, 124]. Potential increased androgen receptor binding resulting from regular exercise would suggest an enhanced anticatabolic potential for sparing muscle from atrophy. Nonetheless, androgen cytosol-binding capacity, binding affinities, and binding specificities remained unchanged by endurance training [63] (Table 5.2). Therefore, at the binding level, endurance training does not appear to exert any influence on androgen-related events in altering the progression of muscle atrophy. Transient elevations in blood and muscle testosterone levels as well as androgen receptor content have been observed following a single bout of swimming exercise [121]. The impact of these responses is currently unknown.

Candidate Genes in the Regulation of Atrophy and Prevention of Atrophy by Exercise

While the molecular basis for the hormone-induced muscle wasting and the exercise-induced resistance to atrophy remains unresolved, a model has been proposed to explain the therapeutic effects of exercise [38]. The model stipulates that the hormonal induction of a set of genes contributes in producing atrophy and that exercise attenuates expression of a subset of these genes.

GLUTAMINE SYNTHETASE (GS). The GS enzyme, which catalyzes the ATP-dependent condensation of glutamic acid and ammonia to form the amino acid glutamine, is glucocorticoid inducible in skeletal muscle [83, 87]. Moreover, skeletal muscle is a major site of glutamine synthesis as glutamine comprises over 50% of the total amino acid pool [42] and this quantity cannot be accounted for by the proportion of glutamine in major muscle proteins, which is 5–7% [73]. During catabolic conditions, skeletal muscle releases glutamine at a high rate [4, 102] and transport of glutamine accounts for approximately 25–30% of the total amino acid efflux during glucocorticoid-mediated muscle atrophy [86]. These observations imply increased glutamine biosynthesis during muscle wasting. Further, with glucocorticoid administration, the level of glutamine in muscle tissue declines [91] even though GS expression increases [87]. Consequently, the hormonal induction of GS in skeletal muscle appears to have physiological relevance to the overall process of atrophy and atrophy prevention, and study of GS provided an initial test of the atrophy prevention model.

In the first investigation, the effects of a 12- to 16-week endurance training program on whole plantaris muscles were evaluated [38]. The running program prevented 52% of the atrophy found in muscles of sedentary animals. Hydrocortisone 21-acetate administration produced 2.4- and 5.9-fold increases in plantaris muscle glutamine synthetase and mRNA respectively. Endurance training diminished basal levels of GS expression to approximately 60% of the values observed in sedentary controls. The exercise program also produced a similar effect in plantaris muscles of glucocorticoid-treated rats as enzyme activity was reduced to 79% (4.56/5.79) and mRNA was reduced to 62% (3.57/5.94) of those in sedentary controls. These data established that exercise and glucocorticoids do in fact exert opposing effects on the expression of GS enzyme activity and GS mRNA in skeletal muscle.

GS expression has recently been examined in the three types of skeletal muscle with the goal of determining whether the suppression of glucocorticoid-induced up-regulation is a generalized response seen in all fiber types, perhaps resulting from some systemic alteration, or in fact, is uniquely localized to fiber types that are known to be primarily recruited during endurance running [39]. GS enzyme activity (nmol · hr^{-1} mg protein^{-1}) in the basal state was 106 ± 16, 74 ± 10, and

43 ± 3 for fast-twitch white (superficial quadriceps), fast-twitch red (deep quadriceps) and slow-twitch red fibers (soleus) respectively. Hormone treatment produced a 2.3- to 2.7-fold increase in GS enzyme activity in all fiber types (Fig. 5.5). Endurance running of both vehicle- and glucocorticoid-treated animals reduced enzyme activities in fast-twitch red fibers that were 35% (26/74) and 56% (107/191) of those in their respective sedentary controls. In slow-twitch red fibers of CA-treated trained animals, GS enzyme activity was significantly reduced to 70% (68/97) of that seen in the sedentary animals receiving hormone treatment. The exercise program had no significant effect on GS enzyme levels in fast-twitch white fibers.

GS mRNA levels, when normalized to poly (A) + RNA, followed the same pattern as enzyme activity. In relative values, GS mRNA was highest in fast-twitch white (5.4 ± 1.3), intermediate in fast-twitch red (1.7 ± 0.2), and lowest in slow-twitch red fibers (arbitrarily set = 1.0). Glucocorticoid treatment induced mRNA content three- to fourfold in all fiber types (Fig. 5.5). Endurance training of vehicle- and glucocorticoid-treated rats diminished GS mRNA levels in fast-twitch red fibers to 70% (1.21/1.7) and 54% (3.7/6.9) of the values for their respective sedentary controls. The mRNA content in the other fiber types was not significantly different between trained and sedentary groups.

These results show that the absolute levels of GS enzyme activity and mRNA are in accord with the susceptibility of a fiber type to atrophy. Further, the relationship of GS expression among fiber types was maintained following glucocorticoid treatment. Nevertheless, these observations might suggest that the glucocorticoid induction in the atrophy-resistant slow-twitch fibers contradicts the relationship of GS expression and susceptibility to atrophy. This does not appear to be the case; however, because our contention is that the absolute level of GS expression is related to atrophy from glucocorticoids. The small absolute increases in GS enzyme activity and mRNA seen with glucocorticoid treatment are not associated with any degree of atrophy in the slow-twitch muscle type. The lack of atrophy in this fiber type suggests the glucocorticoid-induced level of GS was still below some threshold level at which atrophy occurs. Further evidence for the relationship between atrophy and absolute GS expression was obtained by the fact that the hormone-induced levels of GS mRNA and enzyme activity in the slow-twitch fibers are the same or less than those of fast-twitch red or white fibers from vehicle-treated sedentary animals, where there is no ongoing atrophy at these activities. Moreover, the finding that the highest levels of GS induction were in fast-twitch white fibers is also consistent with this interpretation.

When performed at intensities similar to those currently used, adaptations to endurance training, particularly those involving mito-chondrial protein increases and substrate utilization during exercise, are

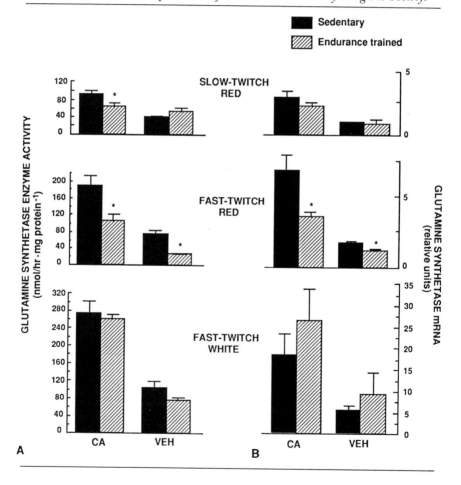

FIGURE 5.5

*GS activity (**A**) and GS mRNA (**B**) in three muscle types after **CA** or **VEH** treatments. Animals were either endurance trained or sedentary. Values are means ± SE from six separate experiments. GS mRNA/poly(A) + RNA for each muscle is expressed relative to **slow-twitch red** vehicle sedentary value = 1.0 *Significantly different from respective sedentary value, p < 0.05. Note different axis for fast-twitch white mRNA values. From Falduto, M. T., A. P. Young, and R. C. Hickson. Exercise inhibits glucocorticoid-induced glutamine synthetase expression in red skeletal muscles. Am. J. Physiol. 262 (Cell Physiol. 31): C214–C220, 1992, with permission from the American Physiological Society.*

seen primarily in the red muscle types [5–7, 66]. The training protocol employed in the fiber-type study [39], which included periodic running at a faster speed, may have also increased respiratory capacity in white muscle types, but the absolute and relative increases are still generally much higher in the red fibers [66]. The fiber-type data, which show that exercise diminished the basal and glucocorticoid-stimulated increases in GS enzyme activity and mRNA content in fast-twitch red fibers and GS activity in hormone-treated slow-twitch fibers, are consistent with the red fiber-type responses to exercise. The fact that the different slow-twitch red and fast-twitch white fiber populations appear very similar in having a limited or absent GS response to exercise in the basal or hormone-induced states does not, in fact, alter the conclusion about fiber recruitment. There was no exercise effect on GS under basal conditions in the slow-twitch red fibers possibly because these values have reached some lower limit. Exercise may not provide a sufficient stimulus to cause a further reduction to these already low GS activities in the slow-twitch red fibers. On the other hand, fast-twitch white fibers display the highest GS levels and are highly susceptible to atrophy. The training protocol, even with intermittent faster running, probably still did not provide enough contractile activity in this fiber type to induce a reduction in GS levels.

Additional studies have examined whether glutamine synthetase expression is related, at least in part, to changes in muscle mass and altered muscle contractile activity. First, in the situation where a state of ongoing muscle atrophy was antagonized by the initiation of an exercise program [40], further GS induction by glucocorticoids was stopped. In these studies, GS enzyme activity and mRNA were threefold higher in the deep quadriceps muscles (fast-twitch red fibers) following 4 days of glucocorticoid treatment. Daily endurance running (90 min/day for 11 days) completely interfered with further hormonal induction (to five-fold) of enzyme activity and mRNA levels. These experiments continue to substantiate that the relationship of glutamine synthetase, muscle atrophy, and endurance exercise still exists under a different experimental system.

Second, the issue whether denervation, which is associated with a reduction in contractile activity, would up-regulate GS expression was also examined [39]. Denervation of the tonically active soleus muscle resulted in a 2.6-fold elevation of GS enzyme activity and GS mRNA to a smaller extent (50%). These results add support to the hypothesis that the concomitant reduction of contractile activity following denervation has some role in GS expression. However, it is possible that other intracellular alterations may have contributed to this response. The fact that GS enzyme levels in denervated soleus muscles were up-regulated but did not reach levels of atrophying fast-twitch muscles of glucocorticoid-treated animals indicated that other mechanisms, besides the glucocorticoid influences, participate in the atrophy associated with denervation in this muscle.

Third, experiments were undertaken to determine whether GS expression is down-regulated by increased contractile activity associated with functional overload [41]. Overloaded plantaris muscles were 70% heavier than control muscles. GS enzyme activity and intramuscular glutamine concentration remained unchanged. However, plantaris muscles of overloaded animals contained only 30% as much GS mRNA as that observed in control animals.

The degree of inhibition of GS mRNA was greater in overloaded plantaris muscles than that previously seen in plantaris or deep quadriceps muscles after endurance training [38, 39]. This response may be associated with the continuous nature of the overload stimulus in comparison with the intermittent nature of the endurance-training stimulus. Moreover, a selective increase in ribosomal RNA in hypertrophied muscle could potentially decrease the proportion of all mRNAs within the total RNA pool and provide a simple explanation for the reduction in GS mRNA. There was no difference in the relative proportion of poly A+ RNA in hypertrophied muscles relative to controls. Thus, based on hybridization of the total RNA samples to oligo $(dT)_{16}$, this explanation is not tenable. Further, there was a 38% increase in the concentration of total RNA in hypertrophied muscles compared with controls. Therefore, GS mRNA in overloaded muscle, when expressed per mg of tissue, is 41% of the control level. To verify further that GS mRNA was reduced by overload in relation to other cellular RNAs, the level of β-myosin heavy-chain mRNA was quantified. β-myosin heavy-chain mRNA in overloaded muscle was 3.5 ± 0.4 times higher than in control muscles. The increase in β-myosin heavy-chain mRNA in overloaded plantaris muscles supports the concept that down-regulation of GS mRNA occurs even though there are increases in other cellular RNAs. Consequently, as was the case with endurance training [38, 39], these results indicate that functional overload results in a specific decrease in the amount of GS mRNA relative to all mRNAs.

Several general factors may contribute to the nonuniform GS enzyme activity responses to the different types of increased contractile activity (overload vs. endurance training). First, the dynamics of muscle metabolism are quite different during overload and endurance training. During functional overload, there is an increased synthesis of noncontractile as well as contractile proteins [52, 93]. Protein degradation is also enhanced during compensatory growth [52]. With endurance training, mitochondrial proteins primarily exhibit increased synthesis rates, and changes in total protein or contractile protein synthesis cannot be detected as a chronic adaptation to training [14, 24, 30, 120]. It is possible that the increased rates of general protein turnover and/or synthesis during overload provide a signal to maintain or to augment GS enzyme activity independent of the diminution of GS mRNA. Secondly, there are little or no increases in muscle mass following endurance-training regimens as compared with the marked hypertrophy observed following overload [38, 57, 61, 63, 64]. Thus, another possibility contributing to the disparity between GS mRNA and GS enzyme activity responses between overload and endurance running could be that muscle growth per se induces a stimulus that increases GS enzyme activity and counterbalances the reduction in GS mRNA mediated by increased contractile activity.

Intramuscular glutamine concentrations were considered to have a role in regulating GS expression during functional overload. Glutamine decreases GS enzyme activity without altering GS mRNA when added to cultured cells [43, 108, 118] and is thought to act by specifically increasing the turnover of the GS enzyme [45]. Therefore, the similar plantaris muscle glutamine concentrations between overloaded and control groups are consistent with the lack of change in enzyme activity between groups. Intramuscular concentrations of glutamine are also directly related to rates of muscle protein synthesis [70, 82, 102]. In this regard, these data also indicate that the increased protein synthetic rates found over this time frame in hypertrophied muscles [52, 93] are not associated with increased glutamine levels. Thus, if glutamine is involved in the regulation of GS enzyme activity or protein synthetic capacity of hypertrophied muscle, then other components of the process, such as transport of glutamine from the muscle or intracellular compartmentalization of the amino acid or enzyme, may be involved; but this possibility has not been tested at this time.

The underlying biochemistry that explains how GS enzyme activity is maintained in the overloaded state despite a 70% reduction in GS mRNA is not known. Direct alterations in the rates of GS enzyme biosynthesis and/or turnover are possible, as is a posttranslational modification that alters enzyme activity. Alternatively, there may be multiple pools of GS mRNA that make different contributions to the total level of GS enzyme protein. These putative pools might be affected in a different manner by functional overload. Based on the data presented; however, a precise unequivocal mechanism is not yet known.

MYOSIN HEAVY CHAINS. Changes in muscle protein turnover by glucocorticoids are mediated, to a large extent, by impaired protein synthesis as determined from measurements of total muscle proteins [94, 101, 116]. This approach, however, does not identify glucocorticoid influences on individual proteins, some of which may be up-regulated and others down-regulated. The identification of a specific protein that is down-regulated by glucocorticoids and follows the same pattern as observed for total muscle mass can permit a more sensitive and precise analysis of glucocorticoid functioning and of exercise in altering glucocorticoid effects.

Myosin, a contractile protein, is the most abundant of all muscle cell proteins and is the major component of the thick filaments. In its native state, myosin is a polymorphic molecule that exists in one of several isoforms in rodent hindlimb muscles, with the isomyosin composition specific to fiber type [119]. The ATPase activity of myosin appears related to the isozyme composition of the muscle types [119]. The isozymes are the result of the differences in the makeup of the myosin heavy chains (MHC) and myosin light chains. Several investigations have found that the myosin molecule is glucocorticoid responsive in skeletal muscle. Cortisol acetate treatment alters native myosin isoform profiles [79], whereas dexamethasone injections result in reduced MHC synthesis [112].

The fact that MHC are down-regulated and follow the same pattern as total muscle mass provided the background for study of myosin as a potential candidate in the glucocorticoid regulation of individual proteins associated with muscle catabolism and in the exercise-induced interference of glucocorticoid functioning. In these experiments, protein synthesis measurements were performed by constant infusion of [^{3}H]leucine. Fractional synthesis rates of MHC were determined from the leucyl-tRNA precursor pool, which was similar in all groups (range 2.85 ± 0.32 to 3.51 ± 0.43 dpm/pmol). Endurance running (90 min/day for 11 consecutive days) prevented 30% of the plantaris muscle mass loss as the result of cortisol acetate treatment. MHC synthesis rates (% /day) in plantaris muscles of sedentary animals were reduced by glucocorticoid treatment to 65% (6.2/9.5) of the rates observed in vehicle-treated sedentary rats and reduced to 45% (6.2/13.0) of that in the vehicle-treated exercised group. Exercise did not alter this depression of MHC synthesis. The combination of exercise and glucocorticoid treatment reduced the calculated MHC breakdown rate (%/day) to 80% ($-8.0/ -10.1$) of the rate resulting from hormone treatment alone and 60% ($-8.0/-13.3$) of the rate resulting from exercise alone. These results show that endurance exercise did not reverse the glucocorticoid inhibition of MHC synthesis in muscle but may act through reducing MHC breakdown. Additional studies on MHC are needed to establish clearly glucocorticoid and exercise regulation of this molecule.

AMINOTRANSFERASES. The participation of additional known glucocorticoid-responsive amino acid-synthesizing enzymes in other tissues also has been investigated in muscle. Based on previous studies in some rat tissues, the activities of alanine aminotransferase and aspartate aminotransferase enzymes and the mRNA for cytosolic aspartate aminotransferase were induced after the administration of glucocorticoids [97, 114]. In addition, besides glutamine, alanine is the second most predominant amino acid in muscle and in plasma [42]. It is an important glucoconeogenic precursor in liver and, like glutamine, is released during catabolic conditions from muscle at a high rate [91]. In human muscle, endurance training elevates aspartate aminotransferase activity by approximately 50% [109]. In a preliminary report [40], both enzyme activities were found to remain unchanged by glucocorticoid treatment in a muscle region containing fast-twitch red fibers. Other data (unpublished) also show that both aminotransferase enzyme activities were not hormone inducible in a muscle region containing primarily fast-twitch white fibers.

Endurance exercise for 11 days increased aspartate aminotransferase activity in fast-twitch red fibers by approximately 30% in the hormone-treated runners [40]. Glucocorticoid treatment suppressed cytosolic aspartate aminotransferase (cAspAT) mRNA by 30% and 50% after 4 and 15 days, respectively. Exercise stimulated basal cAspAT mRNA content twofold and completely abolished the hormone-mediated mRNA suppression. Alanine aminotransferase mRNA analyses were not performed, since a cloned fragment, complementary to alanine aminotransferase mRNA has not been isolated. The absence of any consistent hormone-mediated effects on the activities of both enzymes suggests that these genes are not involved in the steroid regulation of muscle atrophy or atrophy prevention. Whether changes in mRNA alone contribute to muscle atrophy is unclear. However, enzyme activity measured in vitro may not reflect the in vivo state of the enzyme. In any case, the regulation of cAspAT mRNA by exercise may serve as an important model toward understanding how muscle contractile activity counteracts hormone-induced, down-regulated gene expression.

BRANCHED-CHAIN α-KETO ACID DEHYDROGENASE (BCKAD). BCKAD is a multisubunit complex similar to pyruvate dehydrogenase, which is located on the inner surface of the mitochondrial membrane. The enzyme is regulated by phosphorylation and is considered to be rate-limiting for branched-chain amino acid metabolism in muscle [12]. BCKAD is activated by glucocorticoids acutely within a few hours and chronically over several days [12]. Insulin administration can partially block the glucocorticoid-mediated activation of BCKAD [12]. The effects of exercise and glucocorticoids on this enzyme have not been studied.

FUTURE DIRECTIONS

Endurance and strength exercise and other forms of increased contractile activity have been shown to be effective in retarding the progression of muscle atrophy associated with high circulating levels of glucocorticoids. With the use of one or more of these models, further experiments are needed to determine whether exercise produces a generalized response through the glucocorticoid receptor. This possibility is attractive, because it implies that the expression of an entire network of glucocorticoid-inducible genes should be attenuated by endurance training.

The effect of exercise on glutamine synthetase in the presence and absence of hormone raises the possibility that increased contractile activity is capable of diminishing the expression of a subset of glucocorticoid-inducible genes, and at regulatory steps that are beyond steroid-receptor binding and activation. Alternative transcription factors can also serve an obligatory function in mediating basal as well as glucocorticoid-inducible expression of certain genes such as glutamine synthetase. The chicken glutamine synthetase gene has been cloned in the laboratory of Dr. A. Young [100]. It confers glucocorticoid-inducible expression with a single GRE located approximately 2 kb upstream from the transcription start point [99]. The gene is inducible in mouse L6 muscle cells (unpublished, Dr. Young's laboratory). Recent unpublished studies by his laboratory have shown that the gene contains a sequence comprising the core of a cyclic AMP response element (CRE) [104], and is also contained within an activating transcription factor (ATF) binding site [54], which is 9 nt upstream from the GRE. The ATF/CRE site is a critical constituent of many cellular promoters and many transcription factors exert their effects by binding at ATF/CRE sites [54, 104]. These data further raise the importance of studying whether glucocorticoid inducibility of glutamine synthetase requires the interaction between a transcription factor binding at the ATF/CRE site and glucocorticoid-receptor binding at the GRE. The opposing effects of glucocorticoids and exercise on the glutamine synthetase and cAspAT mRNAs suggest that a common transcription factor may be responsible for the glucocorticoid and exercise effects on these genes. Consequently studies are needed to examine whether exercise affects the amount or activity of one or more transcription factors and whether a subset of genes require this factor for basal and hormone-inducible expression. Additionally, investigations should examine whether cyclic AMP is the cellular signal that transmits the effect of endurance training on glutamine synthetase.

The importance of glutamine as a modifier of glutamine synthetase expression and muscle cell metabolism has been cited previously. However, the role of this and other amino acid substrates in atrophy prevention require further attention.

ACKNOWLEDGMENTS

The assistance of Kathy Kozik is greatly appreciated.

This research was supported by NIH Grants AM26408, K04 AM01100, and AR39496, by a Grant-in-Aid from the American Heart Association with funds contributed, in part, by the American Heart Association, Florida Affiliate, and by a Grant-in-Aid from the American Heart Association of Metropolitan Chicago.

REFERENCES

1. Alexis, M. N. Glucocorticoids: new insights into their molecular mechanisms. *TIPS* 8:10–11, 1987.
2. Andrews, G. K. Glucocorticoid receptors in murine visceral yolk sac and liver during development. *J. Steroid Biochem.* 23:437–443, 1985.
3. Armstrong, R. B., and R. O. Phelps. Muscle fiber type composition of rat hindlimb. *Am. J. Anat.* 171:259–272, 1984.
4. Babij, P., H. S. Hundal, M. J. Rennie, and P. W. Watt. Effects of corticosteroid on glutamine transport in rat skeletal muscle (Abstract). *J. Physiol. Lond.* 347:35P, 1986.
5. Baldwin, K. M., G. H. Klinkerfuss, R. L. Terjung, P. A. Mole', and J. O. Holloszy. Respiratory capacity of white, red, and intermediate muscle: adaptive response to exercise. *Am. J. Physiol.* 222:373–378, 1972.
6. Baldwin, K. M., J. S. Reitman, R. L. Terjung, W. W. Winder, and J. O. Holloszy. Substrate depletion in different types of muscle and in liver during prolonged running. *Am. J. Physiol.* 225:1045–1050, 1973.
7. Baldwin, K. M., W. W. Winder, and J. O. Holloszy. Adaptation of actomyosin ATPase in different types of muscle to endurance exercise. *Am. J. Physiol.* 229:422–426, 1975.
8. Bastl, C. P., C. A. Barnett, T. J. Schmidt, and G. Litwack. Glucocorticoid stimulation of sodium absorption in colon epithelia is mediated by corticosteroid IB receptor. *J. Biol. Chem.* 259:1186–1195, 1984.
9. Beato, M. Gene regulation of steroid hormones. *Cell* 56:335–344, 1989.
10. Beato, M. Induction of transcription by steroid hormones. *Biochim. Biophys. Acta* 910:95–102, 1987.
11. Beato, M., J. Arnemann, G. Chalepakis, E. Slater, and T. Willmann. Gene regulation by steroid hormones. *J. Steroid Biochem.* 27:9–14, 1987.
12. Block, K. P., and M. G. Buse. Glucocorticoid regulation of muscle branched-chain amino acid metabolism. *Med. Sci. Sports Exerc.* 22:316–324, 1990.
13. Boissonneault, G., J. Gagnon, M. A. Ho-Kim, and R. R. Tremblay. Lack of effect of anabolic steroids on specific mRNA's of skeletal muscle undergoing compensatory hypertrophy. *Molec. Cell Endocrinol.* 51:19–24, 1987.
14. Booth, F. W., and J. O. Holloszy. Cytochrome c turnover in rat skeletal muscles. *J. Biol. Chem.* 252:416–419, 1977.
15. Burnstein, K. L., D. L. Bellingham, C. M. Jewell, F. E. Powell-Oliver, and J. A. Cidlowski. Autoregulation of glucocorticoid receptor gene expression. *Steroids* 56:52–58, 1991.
16. Burnstein, K. L., and J. A. Cidlowski. At the cutting edge. The downside of glucocorticoid receptor regulation. *Molec. Cell Endocrinol.* 83:C1–C8, 1992.
17. Capaccio, J. A., T. T. Kurowski, S. M. Czerwinski, R. T. Chatterton, Jr., and R. C. Hickson. Testosterone fails to prevent skeletal muscle atrophy from glucocorticoids. *J. Appl. Physiol.* 63:328–334, 1987.
18. Carlstedt-Duke, J., P-E., Stromstedt, B. Persson, E. Cederlund, J.-A. Gustafsson, and H. Jornvall. Identification of hormone-interacting amino acid residues within the steroid-binding domain of the glucocorticoid receptor in relation to other steroid hormone receptors. *J. Biol. Chem.* 263:6842–6846, 1988.
19. Carlstedt-Duke, J., P.-E. Stromstedt, O. Wrange, T. Bergman, J.-A. Gustafsson, and H. Jornvall. Domain structure of the glucocorticoid receptor protein. *Proc. Natl. Acad. Sci. USA* 84:4437–4440, 1987.
20. Cato, A. C. B., D. Henderson, and H. Ponta. The hormone response element of the mouse mammary tumor virus DNA mediates the progestin and androgen induction of transcription in the proviral long terminal repeat region. *EMBO J.* 6:363–368, 1987.
21. Chromiak, J. A., and H. H. Vanderburgh. Intermittent mechanical stretch-relaxation of cultured skeletal muscle reduces glucocorticoid-induced atrophy. *Med. Sci. Sports Exerc.* (Abstract) 23:S3, 1991.

22. Czerwinski, S. M. and R. C. Hickson. Glucocorticoid receptor activation during exercise in muscle. *J. Appl. Physiol.* 68:1615–1620, 1990.
23. Czerwinski, S. M., T. G. Kurowski, T. M. O'Neill, and R. C. Hickson. Initiating regular exercise protects against muscle atrophy from glucocorticoids. *J. Appl. Physiol.* 63:1504–1510, 1987.
24. Czerwinski, S. M., T. T. Kurowski, M. T. Falduto, R. Zak, and R. C. Hickson. Myosin heavy chain turnover and glucocorticoid deterence by exercise in muscle. *J. Appl. Physiol.* 67:2311–2315, 1989.
25. Czerwinski, S. M., E. E. McKee, and R. C. Hickson. Glucocorticoid receptor activation in isolated perfused rat hearts. *Am. J. Physiol.* 256 (*Cell Physiol.* 25): C219–C225, 1989.
26. Czerwinski-Helms, S. M., and R. C. Hickson. Specificity of activated glucocorticoid receptor expression in heart and skeletal muscle types. *Biochem. Biophys. Res. Commun.* 142:322–328, 1987.
27. Dalman, F. C., L. C. Scherrer, L. P. Taylor, H. Akil, and W. B. Pratt. Localization of the 90-kDA heat shock protein-binding site within the hormone-binding domain of the glucocorticoid receptor by peptide competition. *J. Biol. Chem.* 266:3482–3490, 1991.
28. Dahlman-Wright, K., A. Wright, J.-A. Gustafsson, and J. Carstedt-Duke. Interaction of the glucocorticoid receptor DNA-binding domain with DNA as a dimer is mediated by a short segment of five amino acids. *J. Biol. Chem.* 266:3107–3112, 1991.
29. Danhaive, P. A. and G. G. Rousseau. Evidence for sex-dependent anabolic response to androgenic steroids mediated by muscle glucocorticoid receptors in the rat. *J. Steroid Biochem.* 29:575–581, 1988.
30. Davis, T. A., I. E. Karl, E. D. Tegtmeyer, D. F. Osborne, S. Klahr, and H. R. Harter. Muscle protein turnover: effects of exercise training and renal insufficiency. *Am. J. Physiol.* 248(Endocrinol. Metabol. 11):E337–E345, 1985.
31. Denison, S. H., A. Sands, and D. J. Tindall. A tyrosine aminotransferase glucocorticoid response element also mediates androgen enhancement of gene expression. *Endocrinology* 124:1091–1093, 1989.
32. Eisen, L. P., R. W. Harrison, and J. M. Harmon. Immunochemical characterization of the rat kidney glucocorticoid receptor. *J. Biol. Chem.* 261:3725–3731, 1986.
33. Eisen, L. P., M. E. Reichman, E. G. Thompson, B. Gametchu, R. W. Harrison, and H. J. Eisen. Monoclonal antibody to the rat glucocorticoid receptor. Relationship between the immunoreactive and DNA-binding domain. *J. Biol. Chem.* 260:11805–11810, 1985.
34. Eriksson, P., and O. Wrange. Protein-protein contacts in the glucocorticoid receptor homodimer influence its DNA binding properties. *J. Biol. Chem.* 265:3535–3542, 1990.
35. Evans, R. M. The steroid and thyroid hormone receptor superfamily. *Science* 240:889–895, 1988.
36. Falduto, M. T., S. M. Czerwinski, and R. C. Hickson. Glucocorticoid-induced muscle atrophy prevention by exercise in fast-twitch fibers. *J. Appl. Physiol.* 69:1058–1062, 1990.
37. Falduto, M. T., S. M. Czerwinski, T. T. Kurowski, and R. C. Hickson. Glucocorticoid-receptor activation in hypertrophied skeletal muscle. *J. Appl. Physiol.* 63:2048–2052, 1987.
38. Falduto, M. T., R. C. Hickson, and A. P. Young. Antagonism by glucocorticoids and exercise on expression of glutamine synthetase in skeletal muscle. *FASEB J.* 3:2623–2628, 1989.
39. Falduto, M. T., A. P. Young, and R. C. Hickson. Exercise inhibits glucocorticoid-induced glutamine synthetase expression in red skeletal muscles. *Am. J. Physiol.* 262 (*Cell Physiol.* 31):C214–C220, 1992.
40. Falduto, M. T., A. P. Young, and R. C. Hickson. Interruption of ongoing glucocorticoid-induced muscle atrophy and glutamine synthetase induction by exercise. *Med. Sci. Sports Exerc.* (Abstract) 24:S3, 1992.

41. Falduto, M. T., A. P. Young, G. Smyrniotis, and R. C. Hickson. Reduction of glutamine synthetase mRNA in hypertrophied skeletal muscle. *Am. J. Physiol.* (Regulatory Integrative Comp. Physiol 31) 262:R1131–R1136, 1992.

42. Felig, P. Amino acid metabolism in man. *Annu. Rev. Biochem.* 44:933–955, 1975.

43. Feng, G., S. K. Shiber, and S. R. Max. Glutamine regulates glutamine synthetase expression in skeletal muscle cells in culture. *J. Cell Physiol.* 145:376–380, 1990.

44. Freedman, L. P., B. F. Luisi, Z. R. Korszum, R. Basavappa, P. B. Sigler, and K. R. Yamamoto. The function and structure of the metal coordination sites within the glucocorticoid receptor DNA binding domain. *Nature* 334:543–546, 1988.

45. Freikopf-Cassel, A., and R. G. Kulka. Regulation of the degradation of ^{125}I-labeled glutamine synthetase introduced into cultured hepatoma cells by erythrocyte ghost mediated injection. *FEBS Lett.* 128:63–66, 1981.

46. Gardiner, P. F., B. Hibl, D. R. Simpson, R. R. Roy, and V. R. Edgerton. Effects of a mild weight-lifting program on the progress of glucocorticoid-induced atrophy in rat hindlimb muscles. *Pfluegers Arch.* 385:147–153, 1980.

47. Gardiner, P. F., and V. R. Edgerton. Contractile responses of rat fast and slow muscles to glucocorticoid treatment. *Muscle Nerve* 2:274–281, 1979.

48. Genuth, S. M. The endocrine system. In Berne, R. M. and M. N. Levy, eds. *Physiology,* 2nd Ed. St. Louis: C. V. Mosby Co., 1988, pp. 950–982.

49. Giguere, V., S. M. Hollenberg, M. G. Rosenfeld, and R. M. Evans. Functional domains of the human glucocorticoid receptor. *Cell* 46:645–652, 1986.

50. Godowski, P. J., S. Rusconi, R. Miesfeld, and K. R. Yamamoto. Glucocorticoid receptor mutants that are constitutive activators of transcriptional enhancement. *Nature* 325:365–368, 1987.

51. Goldberg, A. L., and H. M. Goodman. Relationship between cortisone and muscle work in determining muscle size. *J. Physiol. (Lond.)* 200:667–675, 1969.

52. Goldspink, D. F., P. J. Garlick, and M. A. MacNurlan. Protein turnover measured in vivo and in vitro in muscles undergoing compensatory growth and subsequent denervation atrophy. *Biochem. J.* 210:89–98, 1983.

53. Gustafsson, J.-A., J. Carlstedt-Duke, L. Poellinger, S. Okret, A.-C. Wikstrom, M. Bronnegard, M. Gillner, Y. Dong, K. Fuxe, A. Cintra, A. Harfstrand, and L. Agnati. Biochemistry, molecular biology, and physiology of the glucocorticoid receptor. *Endocrine Rev.* 8:185–234, 1987.

54. Hai, T., F. Liu, W. J. Coukos, and M. R. Green. Transcription factor ATF cDNA clones: an extensive family of leucine zipper proteins able to selectively form DNA-binding hetrodimers. *Genes Dev.* 3:2083–2090, 1989.

55. Ham, J., A. Thomson, M. Needham, P. Webb, and M. Parker. Characterization of response elements for androgens, glucocorticoids and progestins in mouse mammary tumor virus. *Nucleic Acids Res.* 16:5263–5276. 1988.

56. Hard, T., E. Kellenbach, R. Boelens, B. A. Maler, K. Dahlman, L. P. Freedman, J. Carlstedt-Duke, K. R. Yamamoto, J.-A. Gustafsson, and R. Kaptein. Solution structure of the glucocorticoid receptor DNA-binding domain. *Science* 249:157–160, 1990.

57. Harms, S. J., and R. C. Hickson. Skeletal muscle mitochondria and myoglobin, endurance, and intensity of training. *J. Appl. Physiol.* 54:798–802, 1983.

58. Hickson, R. C., S. M. Czerwinski, M. T. Falduto, and A. P. Young. Glucocorticoid antagonism by exercise and androgenic-anabolic steroids. *Med. Sci. Sports Exerc.* 22:331–340, 1990.

59. Hickson, R. C., and J. R. Davis. Partial prevention of glucocorticoid-induced muscle atrophy by endurance training. *Am. J. Physiol.* 241 (*Endocrinol. Metabol.* 4:):E226–E232, 1981.

60. Hickson, R. C., T. M. Galassi, J. A. Capaccio, and R. T. Chatterton, Jr. Limited resistance of hypertrophied skeletal muscle to glucocorticoids. *J. Steroid Biochem.* 24:1179–1183, 1986.

61. Hickson, R. C., T. M. Galassi, T. T. Kurowski, D. G. Daniels, and R. T. Chatterton Jr.

Skeletal muscle cytosol [³H]Methyltrienolone receptor binding and serum androgens: effects of hypertrophy and hormonal state. *J. Steroid. Biochem.* 19:1705–1712, 1983.

62. Hickson, R. C., T. T. Kurowski, G. H. Andrews, J. A. Capaccio, and R. T. Chatterton, Jr. Glucocorticoid cytosol binding in exercise-induced sparing of muscle atrophy. *J. Appl. Physiol.* 60:1413–1419, 1986.

63. Hickson, R. C., T. T. Kurowski, J. A. Capaccio, and R. T. Chatterton, Jr. Androgen cytosol binding in exercise-induced sparing of muscle atrophy. *Am. J. Physiol.* 247 (*Endocrinol. Metabol.* 10):E597–E603, 1984.

64. Hickson, R. C., T. T. Kurowski, T. M. Galassi, D. G. Daniels, and R. J. Chatterton, Jr. Androgen cytosol binding during compensatory overload-induced skeletal muscle hypertrophy. *Can. J. Biochem. Cell Biol.* 63:348–354, 1985.

65. Hollenberg, S. M., V. Giguere, P. Segui, and R. M. Evans. Colocalization of DNA-binding and transcriptional activation functions in the human glucocorticoid receptor. *Cell* 49:39–46, 1987.

66. Holloszy, J. O., and F. W. Booth. Biochemical adaptations to endurance exercise in skeletal muscles. *Annu. Rev. Physiol.* 38:273–291, 1976.

67. Horber, F. F., H. Hoppeler, J. R. Scheidegger, B. E. Grunig, H. Howald, and F. J. Frey. Impact of physical training on the ultrastructure of midthigh muscle in normal subjects and in patients treated with glucocorticoids. *J. Clin. Invest.* 79:1181–1190, 1987.

68. Horber, F. F., J. R. Scheidegger, B. E. Grunig, and F. J. Frey. Evidence that prednisone-induced myopathy is reversed by physical training. *J. Clin Endocrinol. Metabol.* 61:83–88, 1985.

69. Horber, F. F., J. R. Scheidegger, B. E. Grunig, and F. J. Frey. Thigh muscle mass and function in patients treated with glucocorticoids. *Eur. J. Clin. Invest.* 15:302–307, 1985.

70. Jepson, M. M., P. C. Bates, P. Broadbent, J. M. Pell, and D. J. Millward. Relationship between glutamine concentration and protein synthesis in rat skeletal muscle. *Am. J. Physiol.* 255:E166–E172, 1988.

71. Kalinyak, J. E., R. I. Dorin, A. R. Hoffman, and A. J. Perlman. Tissue-specific regulation of glucocorticoid receptor mRNA by dexamethasone. *J. Biol. Chem.* 262:10441–10444, 1987.

72. Kochakian, C. D. Regulation of muscle growth by androgens. In E. J. Briskey, R. G. Cassens, and J. C. Trautman (eds.). *Physiology and Biochemistry of Muscle as a Food.* Madison, WI: University of Wisconsin Press, 1966, pp. 81–112.

73. Kominz, D. R., A. Hough, P. Symonds, and K. Lak. The amino composition of actin, myosin, tropomyosin and the meromyosins. *Arch. Biochem.* 50:148–159, 1954.

74. Konagaya, M., P. A. Bernard, and S. R. Max. Blockade of glucocorticoid-receptor binding and inhibition of dexamethasone-induced muscle atrophy in the rat by RU38486, a potent and selective glucocorticoid antagonist. *Endocrinology* 119:375–380, 1986.

75. Kraemer, W. J. Endocrine responses to resistance exercise. *Med. Sci. Sports Exerc.* 20:S152–S157, 1988.

76. Kruskemper, H. L. *Anabolic Steroids.* New York: Academic Press, 1968.

77. Kurowski, T. T., R. T. Chatterton, Jr., and R. C. Hickson. Countereffects of compensatory overload and glucocorticoids in skeletal muscle: androgen and gluco-corticoid cytosol receptor binding. *J. Steroid Biochem.* 21:137–145, 1984.

78. Kurowski, T. T., J. A. Capaccio, R. T. Chatterton, Jr., and R. C. Hickson. Depletion of [³H]methyltrienolone cytosol binding in glucocorticoid-induced muscle atrophy. *Proc. Soc. Expr. Biol. Med.* 178:215–221, 1985.

79. Kurowski, T. T., R. Zak, and R. C. Hickson. Development of glucocorticoid-induced growth and atrophy in heart and skeletal muscle. *J. Cell Biol.* (Abstract) 105:11A, 1987.

80. Litwack, G., and S. Rosenfield. Liver cytosol corticosteroid binder IB, a new binding protein. *J. Biol. Chem.* 250:6799–6850, 1975.

81. Loeb, J. N. Corticosteroids and growth. *N. Engl. J. Med.* 295:547–552, 1976.
82. MacLennan, P. A., R. A. Brown, and M. J. Rennie. A positive relationship between protein synthetic rate and intracellular glutamine concentration in perfused rat skeletal muscle. *FEBS Lett.* 215:187–191, 1987.
83. Magnuson, S. R., and A. P. Young. Murine glutamine synthetase: cloning, developmental regulation, and glucocorticoid inducibility. *Dev. Biol.* 130:536–542, 1988.
84. Markovic, R. D., H. Eisen, L. G. Parchman, C. A. Barnett, and G. Litwack. Evidence for a physiological role of corticosteroid binder IB. *Biochemistry* 19:4556–4564, 1980.
85. Markovic, R. D., and G. Litwack. Activation of liver and kidney glucocorticoid-receptor complexes occurs in vivo. *Arch. Biochem. Biophys.* 202:374–379, 1980.
86. Marliss, E. B., T. T. Aok. T. Pozefsky, A. S. Most, and G. F. Cahill. Muscle and splanchnic glutamine and glutamate metabolism in postabsorptive and starved man. *J. Clin. Invest.* 50:814–817, 1971.
87. Max, S. R., J. Mill, K. Mearow, M. Konagaya, Y. Konagaya, J. W. Thomas, C. Banner, and L. Vitkovic. Dexamethasone regulates glutamine synthesis expression in rat skeletal muscles. *Am. J. Physiol.* 255 (*Endocrinol. Metabol.* 18): E397–E403, 1988.
88. Mayer, M., and F. Rosen. Interaction of anabolic steroids with glucocorticoid receptor sites in rat muscle cytosol. *Am. J. Physiol.* 229:1381–1386, 1975.
89. Meshinchi, S., J. F. Grippo, E. R. Sanchez, E. H. Bresnick, and W. B. Pratt. Evidence that the endogenous heat-stable glucocorticoid receptor stabilising factor is a metal component of the untransformed receptor complex. *J. Biol. Chem.* 263:16809–16817, 1988.
90. Meshinchi, S., G. Matic, K. A. Hutchison, and W. B. Pratt. Selective molybdate-directed covalent modification of sulfhydryl groups in the steroid-binding versus the DNA-binding domain of the glucocorticoid receptor. *J. Biol. Chem.* 265:11643–11649, 1990.
91. Muhlbacher, F., C. R. Kapadia, M. F. Colpoys, R. J. Smith, and D. W. Wilmore. Effects of glucocorticoids on glutamine metabolism in skeletal muscle. *Am. J. Physiol.* 247(Endocrinol. Metabol. 10):E75–E83, 1984.
92. Nemoto. T., Y. Ohara-Nemoto, M. Denis, and J.-A. Gustafsson. The transformed glucocorticoid receptor has a lower steroid-binding affinity than the nontransformed receptor. *Biochemistry* 29:1880–1886, 1990.
93. Noble, E. G., Q. Tang, and P. B. Taylor. Protein synthesis in compensatory hypertrophy of rat plantaris. *Can. J. Physiol. Pharmacol.* 62:1178–1182, 1984.
94. Odedra, B. R., P. C. Bates, and D. J. Millward. Time course of the effect of catabolic doses of corticosterone on protein turnover in rat skeletal muscle and liver. *Biochem. J.* 214:617–627, 1983.
95. Okret, S., L. Poellinger, Y. Dong, and J.-A. Gustafsson. Down-regulation of glucocorticoid receptor mRNA by glucocorticoid hormones and recognition by the receptor of a specific binding sequence within a receptor cDNA clone. *Proc. Natl. Acad. Sci. USA* 83:5899–5903, 1986.
96. Ohl, V. S., M. Mayer, B. C. Sekula, and G. Litwack. Receptor properties of corticosteroid binder IB. *Arch. Biochem. Biophys.* 217:162–173, 1982.
97. Pave'-Preux, M., N. Ferry, J. Bouget, J. Hanoune, and R. Barouki. Nucleotide sequence and glucocorticoid regulation of the mRNAs for the isoenzymes of rat aspartate aminotransferase. *J. Biol. Chem.* 263:17459–17466, 1988.
98. Pratt, W. B. Transformation of glucocorticoid and progesterone receptors to the DNA-binding state. *Cell Biochem.* 35:51–68, 1987.
99. Pu, H., and A. P. Young. Glucocorticoid-inducible expression of a glutamine synthetase-CAT-encoding fusion plasmid after transfection of intact chicken retinal explant cultures. *Gene* 89:259–263, 1990.
100. Pu, H., and A. P. Young. The structure of the chicken glutamine synthetase-encoding gene. *Gene* 81:169–175, 1989.
101. Rannels, S. R., and L. S. Jefferson. Effect of glucocorticoids on muscle protein

turnover in perfused rat hemicorpus. *Am. J. Physiol.* 238 (*Endocrinol. Metabol.* 1):E564–E572, 1980.

102. Rennie, M. J., P. A. MacLennan, H. S. Hundal, B. Weryk, K. Smith, P. M. Taylor, C. Egan and P. W. Watt. Skeletal muscle glutamine transport, intramuscular glutamine concentration and muscle-protein turnover. *Metabolism* 38:47–51, 1989.

103. Rexin, M., W. Busch, and V. Gehring. Protein components of the non-activated glucocorticoid receptor. *J. Biol. Chem.* 266:24601–24605, 1991.

104. Roesler, W. J., G. R. Vandenbark, and R. W. Hanson. Cyclic AMP and the induction of eukaryotic gene transcription. *J. Biol. Chem.* 263:9063–9066, 1988.

105. Rosewicz, S., A. R. McDonald, B. A. Maddux, I. D. Goldfine, R. L. Miesfeld, and C. D. Logsdon. Mechanism of glucocorticoid receptor down-regulation by glucocorticoids. *J. Biol. Chem.* 263:2581–2584, 1987.

106. Roy, R. R., P. F. Gardiner, D. R. Simpson, and V. R. Edgeton. Glucocorticoid-induced atrophy in different fiber types of selected rat jaw and hindlimb muscles. *Arch. Oral Biol.* 28:639–643, 1983.

107. Rusconi, S., and K. R. Yamamoto. Functional dissection of the hormone and DNA binding activities of the glucocorticoid receptor. *EMBO J.* 6:1309–1315, 1987.

108. Sandrasagra, A., G. Patejunas, and A. P. Young. Multiple mechanisms by which glutamine synthetase levels are controlled in murine tissue culture cells. *Arch. Biochem. Biophys.* 266:522–531, 1988.

109. Schantz, P. G., B. Sjöberg, and J. Svedenhag. Malate-aspartate and alpha-glycerophosphate shuttle enzyme levels in human skeletal muscle: methodological considerations and effect of endurance training. *Acta Physiol. Scand.* 128:397–407, 1986.

110. Scheidereit, C., H. M. Westphal, C. Carlson, H. Bosshard, and M. Beato. Molecular model of the interaction between the glucocorticoid receptor and the regulatory elements of inducible genes. *DNA* 5:383–391, 1986.

111. Schmidt, T. J., and G. Litwack. Activation of the glucocorticoid-receptor complex. *Physiol. Rev.* 62:1131–1192, 1982.

112. Seene, T., and K. Alev. Effect of glucocorticoids on the turnover rate of actin and myosin heavy and light chains on different types of skeletal muscle fibers. *J. Steroid Biochem.* 22:767–771, 1985.

113. Seene, T., and A. Viru. The catabolic effects of glucocorticoids on different types of skeletal muscle fibers and its dependence upon muscle activity and interaction with anabolic steroids. *J. Steroid Biochem.* 16:349–352, 1982.

114. Segal, H. L., and Y. S. Kim. Glucocorticoid stimulation of the biosynthesis of glutamic-alanine transaminase. *Proc. Natl. Acad. Sci. USA* 50:912–918, 1963.

115. Shangold, M. M. Exercise and the adult female: hormonal and endocrine effects. In R. L. Terjung (ed.). Exercise and Sports Sciences Reviews. Lexington, KY: Heath, 1984, pp. 53–79.

116. Shoji, S., and R. J. T. Pennington. The effects of cortisone on protein breakdown and synthesis in rat skeletal muscle. *Molec. Cell Endocrinol.* 6:159–169, 1977.

117. Silva, C. M., and J. A. Cidlowski. Direct evidence for intra- and intermolecular disulfide bond formation in the human glucocorticoid receptor. *J. Biol. Chem.* 264:6638–6647, 1989.

118. Smith, R. J., S. J. Larson, S. E. Stred, and R. P. Durschlag. Regulation of glutamine synthetase and glutamine activities in cultured skeletal muscle cells. *J. Cell Physiol.* 120:197–203, 1984.

119. Swynghedauw, B. Developmental and functional adaptation of contractile proteins in cardiac and skeletal muscles. *Physiol. Rev.* 66:710–771, 1986.

120. Tapscott, E. G., Jr., G. J. Kasperek, and G. L. Dohm. Effect of training on muscle protein turnover in male and female rats. *Biochem. Med.* 27:254–259, 1982.

121. Tchaikovsky, V. S., J. V. Astratenkova, and O. B. Basharina. The effect of exercises

on the content and reception of the steroid hormones in rat skeletal muscle. *J. Steroid Biochem.* 24:251–253, 1986.

122. Tierugroj, W., S. Meshinchi, E. R. Sanchez, S. E. Pratt, J. F. Grippo, A. Holmgren, and W. B. Pratt. The role of sulfhydryl groups in permitting transformation and DNA binding of the glucocorticoid receptor. *J. Biol. Chem.* 262:6992–7000, 1987.

123. Tierugroj, W., E. R. Sanchez, P. R. Housley, R. W. Harrison, and W. B. Pratt. Glucocorticoid receptor phosphorylation, transformation, and DNA binding. *J. Biol. Chem.* 262:17342–17349, 1987.

124. Vogel, R. B., C. A. Books, C. Ketchum, C. W. Zauner, and F. T. Murray. Increase of free and total testosterone during submaximal exercise in normal males. *Med. Sci. Sports Exerc.* 17:119–123, 1985.

125. von der Ahe, D., J. Rnoir, T. Buchou, E. Baulieu, and M. Beato. Receptors for glucocorticosteroid and progesterone recognize distinct features of a DNA regulatory element. *Proc. Natl. Acad. Sci. USA* 83:2817–2821, 1986.

6
Sport and Socialization

JAY COAKLEY, Ph.D

Early research on socialization and sport was typically grounded in widespread concerns about who participated in sports, how they became involved, why they participated, and how they were changed by participation. Those who asked these questions were often associated with organized sport programs, and they usually had vested interests in recruiting new participants into their programs and promoting programs by linking participation in them to positive developmental outcomes. The social and behavioral scientists who actually did the research on socialization often responded to these concerns. Researchers were also interested in discovering whether sport was a unique context for human experience and whether there was any truth to pervasive beliefs that participation in sports builds character and shapes people in positive ways.

Research on socialization and sport has continued to focus on these concerns, but in recent years new questions have been asked about sport participation as a social process linked to the larger social world in which it occurs. These questions focus on why sport experiences take the forms they take; how sport experiences are mediated by gender, class, and race relations; how sport participation is tied to identity and identity formation processes; why sport participation choices are made by people at various points in their lives; and what connections exist between participation choices and the cultural, social, political, and economic contexts in which people live their lives. These questions are closely tied to changes in socialization theory and the methodological approaches used by social scientists. These changes are used to frame much of this review of the literature on socialization and sport.

CONCEPTUAL APPROACHES TO SOCIALIZATION

Although the topic of socialization has been investigated in sociology, psychology, and anthropology, most research on socialization and sport has been grounded in sociological approaches. Research in psychology has focused primarily on personality characteristics among athletes and, more recently, on relationships among sport participation and moral development [210], competence motivation, and achievement motiva-

169

tion [18]. Psychologists interested in sport research have given much more attention to questions about motivation and performance than to questions about socialization.

Research in anthropology has generally focused on the role of play, games, and sports in helping people adapt to and internalize values in their society or group. Most often this research has been done in hunting and gathering and agricultural societies or in special contemporary cultural groups, such as Native Americans [9]. Rather than focusing on socialization in particular, anthropologists have been more concerned with the connection between general cultural patterns and the normative structure of play and games within a particular group or society [152, 200, 201].

Sociological research is usually based on a conception of socialization as a dual process of social interaction and social development. Through this dual process people not only learn who they are and how they are connected to the world around them, but they also learn the orientations that serve as a basis for behavior and social organization in that world. Socialization occurs through people's social relationships and is the basis for the development of their understanding of how social life is organized, maintained, and changed.

Sociological research has traditionally focused on the relationship between socialization and: *(a)* identity and self-development; *(b)* role selection and role performance through the life cycle; *(c)* systems of social control; and *(d)* factors such as social class, gender, and other background characteristics that mediate the learning of orientations and values [23]. Much of this research has tried to identify how people are shaped by social forces and external social constraints. Research before the early 1960s was often based on deterministic models in which people were characterized as passive learners "molded" and "shaped" by "society" [128, 213]. These studies were designed to identify socialization "outcomes" experienced by people who were exposed to certain social influences or who took on certain roles in existing social systems [86]. They were based on the assumption that socialization simply involved an "internalization" of normative influences in a person's environment.

This "socialization-as-internalization" approach has been widely criticized for ignoring the content and dynamics of the social relationships through which socialization occurs. Focusing on the product of socialization leads researchers to overlook the processes that constitute the core of socialization itself. Missed, therefore, are the tensions, negotiations, misunderstandings, and resistances that characterize the social relationships associated with a person's entry into and participation in a particular sphere of the social world. By ignoring these factors the person "being socialized" is seldom seen by researchers as an active agent, as someone with self-reflective abilities and creative potential, as someone seeking autonomy and affirmation of identities, as someone who is not simply a passive learner.

Critiques of socialization theory and research have led many social scientists to move from a "socialization-as-internalization" approach to a "socialization-as-interaction" approach [128, 213]. In this latter approach, human beings are assumed to be active, self-reflective decision makers who define situations and act on the basis of their decisions. It is also assumed that socialization is a lifelong process characterized by reciprocity and the interplay of the self-concepts, goals, and resources of all those involved in social interaction. Finally, the socialization-as-interaction approach assumes that identities, roles, and social organization are social constructions emerging from social relations that reflect the distribution of power and resources within a particular cultural setting.

In general, socialization research in sociology has shifted from an emphasis on the internalization of social norms to an emphasis on the processes through which human beings are themselves involved in the creation of social and cultural formations, and how those formations serve as parameters for social relations, action, and identity development. The interactionist approaches that inform an increasing amount of the socialization research focus attention on social relations and social action rather than social learning, and on identity formation rather than individual responses to the social environment.

OVERVIEW OF RESEARCH ON SOCIALIZATION AND SPORT

Research on socialization and sport has reflected these changes in mainstream sociology. But it should be noted that the socialization-as-internalization approach has not been abandoned in the sociology of sport. Some studies continue to use this model. They involve cross-sectional, and a few longitudinal, statistical comparisons of the experiences and characteristics of so-called "athletes" (i.e., those who participate in selected organized sport programs) with the experiences and characteristics of so-called "nonathletes" (i.e., those who do not participate in selected programs). The goal of these studies is usually to identify: *(a)* sources of social influence and other factors that lead a person to participate in sport, and *(b)* the developmental outcomes of participation itself.

Increasingly common since the early-1980s have been studies based on the socialization-as-interaction model and variations of this model. These studies have attempted to do two things: *(a)* uncover the meanings and dynamics underlying the process of sport involvement and the social relationships associated with involvement, and *(b)* understand sport participation as an integral part of the social and cultural context in which it occurs. The following sections in this review provide an overview of socialization as it has been studied and discussed in the sociology of sport. Emphasis is placed on changes in the conceptual and methodological approaches used and on the findings of some of the more recent examples of socialization research.

A survey of the literature shows there is no shortage of reviews and critiques of socialization and sport [2, 25, 27, 28, 52, 60–63, 67, 81, 89, 90, 106, 113, 118, 119, 121, 122, 129, 130, 162, 180, 183, 195, 197, 204]. This topic has been a central concern among those who study sport. In this overview, I use these past reviews as a starting point and attempt to document how research on socialization and sport has emerged and changed as there has been a shift from studies using internalization models to studies using interactionist models.

Overviews of socialization and sport have traditionally been organized to cover the following three topics: *(a)* socialization into sport (dealing with the initiation and continuation of sport participation); *(b)* socialization out of sport (dealing with the termination of sport participation); and *(c)* socialization through sport (dealing with sport participation and social development). Although these topics reflect research questions asked by those who favored internalization approaches to socialization, using them as an organizational framework for this discussion does not preclude a review of more current research based on interactionist models.

Socialization Into Sport: Who Participates and How They Become Involved
Much of the research done on socialization into sport has been inspired by a 1973 paper by Kenyon and McPherson [90]. The paper outlined a "social role-social system" model designed to guide subsequent research on this topic. This model emphasized that those who entered and performed "sport roles" (including athletes at all levels of competition, spectators, coaches, and sport administrators) went through a social learning process that was shaped and mediated by three sets of factors: *(a)* the physical and psychological attributes of the learners; *(b)* the encouragement and rewards received by learners, and the opportunities they had to practice or rehearse sport roles; and *(c)* the various social systems (such as family, peer group, school, and community) in which learners developed personal values and orientations.

Although Kenyon and McPherson did not ignore the interactional nature of socialization, their model seems to have encouraged researchers to emphasize a socialization-as-internalization approach in which those being socialized are assumed to be shaped by external social forces, especially in the form of encouragement and reinforcement coming from "significant others" in their lives (such as parents, other family members, friends, teachers, and coaches). Critics of the social role-social system model argue that it is inherently deterministic and precludes a consideration of the person being socialized as an active, creative, and even resistant agent in the socialization process [204]. Others argue that the model itself is not deficient, but that those using it have simply failed to utilize research designs that uncover and highlight interaction processes [52, 67].

Regardless of this debate, much of the research utilizing the social role-social system model has involved the use of quantitative data collection methods in which subjects have been asked to outline their sport participation histories, including references to influential events and people. Findings from these studies have been mixed, but they generally indicate the following: *(a)* Socialization into sports occurs in connection with support and encouragement coming from significant others [64, 98, 102, 103, 112, 115, 161, 188, 190, 193]. *(b)* The influence exerted by others and the importance of various social systems in the socialization process vary by *gender* [48, 59, 60, 64, 69, 102, 161, 188, 190], *socioeconomic status* [63, 78, 79, 104, 209], *race* [68, 76, 135], *age* [20, 156, 184], *place of residence (rural vs. urban)* [21], *type of sport program (community vs. school sponsored)* [20], and *culture* [66, 214]. *(c)* Being socialized into sport generally depends on a person's self-evaluation of athletic abilities [50, 94, 98, 151]. *(d)* Sport participation by one person often occasions socialization experiences for others. For example, parents often learn to provide the systematic support in response to the demands of their children's sport participation [7, 77, 186].

Apart from these general findings, this research provides little information about specific differences between those who become involved in sport and those who do not [211], and it says little about the social contexts in which participation decisions occur and in which participation is maintained on a day-to-day basis. Those who base research on interactionist models generally focus attention on the ways in which sport participation decisions are integrated into the lives of the people making them; how gender, class, race, and ethnic relations mediate those decisions; how participation decisions are tied to identity formation processes; how the meanings underlying sport participation are created and maintained through social relationships among partici- pants themselves; and how sport participation often takes the form of a "career" characterized by shifting activities, orientations, commitments, identities, and relationships [22, 30, 34, 37, 39, 49, 53, 54, 70, 144, 153, 168, 169, 198, 199, 203]. The major findings of research based on interactionist models are highlighted through the following summaries of three studies.

INTERACTIONIST STUDIES.   *Donnelly and Young Study.* Donnelly and Young [39] used an interactionist model to examine ethnographic, observational, and interview data on the subcultures of climbers and rugby players. Their analysis led to the creation of a model in which socialization into sport is characterized as a highly problematic, long-term process of identity construction and confirmation. According to the model, becoming a climber or rugby player involves more than receiving encouragement and rewards from significant others and being exposed to opportunities to rehearse climbing and rugby roles. Instead, it involves a combination of long-term processes through which individuals acquire knowledge about the sport, become associated with a sport group, learn the norms and expectations shared by group members, and earn the acceptance of group members in a way that, over time, confirms and reconfirms their identity as a climber or rugby player. In other words, socialization into sport is not marked by a single decision or event, or the influence of a particular person or set of persons. Instead, it involves an extended interactive process through which individuals come to identify themselves as athletes as they become accepted members of sport groups or subcultures.

Stevenson Study. Stevenson [198, 199] used an interactionist approach to examine the initial stages of international athletes' careers in sport. In-depth interviews indicated that socialization into sport involves processes of sponsored recruitment and the development of commitment to participation. Young people are introduced to sports through important relationships in their lives and then their participation in specific sport activities is sponsored through those relationships as the young people receive specific forms of support and encouragement. However, continued participation in sport depends on the development of commitments grounded in factors such as participants' assessments of their success potential, the formation of a "web of personal relationships" connected with their participation, and the development of personal reputations and identities as athletes. Overall, being socialized into sport involves altering personal priorities, making choices, and engaging in active, self-reflexive efforts to develop desired identities as athletes and to elicit confirmation of those identities through important social relationships. The socialization into sport process itself is problematic in that it does not lead to "once and for all time" decisions. Social support cannot be taken for granted, resources may disappear, and new opportunities may lead to alterations in priorities. In other words, a person does not simply "*get socialized* into sport."

Coakley and White Study. Coakley and White [30] used an interactionist model to guide their study of sport participation decisions made by a sample of British adolescents growing up in a working class area east of London. In-depth interviews with 34 young men and 26 young women indicated that sport participation is the result of decisions mediated by past experiences in sport and physical activities, conclusions about how sport participation might facilitate the achievement of personal development goals, a desire to develop and display competence, support from significant others, access to resources, and general social and cultural forces. In the lives of the young people, sport participation occurs to the extent that they decide it will help them extend control over their lives, make a smooth transition into adulthood, and present themselves to the rest of the world as competent human beings. Young women are less likely than young men to see sport participation having these effects in their lives. Therefore, the process of socialization into sport is much different for them.

The young people in this study were not passive learners in the socialization into sport process. They actively negotiated participation decisions in light of how they saw participation fitting with the rest of their lives including their concepts of selves and what they wanted for themselves as they moved from adolescence to adulthood. Participation in sport shifted over time depending on access to opportunities, changes in young people's lives, and changes in the way they saw themselves and their connections to the world in which they lived.

The Coakley and White study also suggests that people make choices to participate in sport for different reasons at different points in their lives. This is consistent with theories on development and aging that indicate the life cycle is not only characterized by patterned developmental tasks, but that it is subject to definition and redefinition in light of socially constructed meanings attached to age at different historical points in time. Furthermore, sport participation decisions at all points during the life course are tied to the perceived cultural importance of sport and the links among involvement, general social acceptance, and the achievement of personal goals. This suggests that studies of socialization into sport need to take into account the ways in which sport participation patterns are connected to changes and transitions normally occurring through life.

These examples of research based on interactionist models are not intended to illustrate that past research based on internalization models has been fruitless. In fact, those using interactionist approaches have used studies based on internalization models to inform their data collection and interpretive analyses. This will continue to occur although there seem to be limits on the usefulness of studies based on internalization models and using research designs that cannot capture the reciprocity in social relationships or the conscious, self-reflection that underlies behavioral choices made my those involved in the socialization process [112].

In summary, studies based on interactionist models have clearly indicated that sport participation is grounded in decision-making processes involving a combination of self-reflection and social reaffirmation and acceptance. This process of decision making is never totally completed; instead, it occurs over and over through time and is mediated by the social and cultural contexts in which people live. Therefore, decisions about participation are tied to gender, class, race, and age relations as well as to political, economic, social, and cultural factors. People who participate in sport regularly change their priorities and redefine who they are and how they are connected to the world; this is also important in the following discussion of the literature on socialization out of sport.

Socialization Out of Sport: Terminating Sport Participation

Research on termination of sport participation is difficult to characterize in terms of the conceptual approaches and methodologies used. Studies have focused on numerous issues including the relationships among participation turnover rates and the structures of sport programs, the attributes and experiences of those who terminate sport participation, the dynamics of transitions out of sport roles, the termination of participation in highly competitive sport contexts as a form of retirement or even as a form of 'social death,' and the connection between declining rates of participation and the process of aging. Putting this research into historical context helps explain why "socialization out of sport" became a popular topic in the 1970s and 1980s.

ATTRITION. Before the early 1970s attrition in sports had not been identified as a research issue because organized sport programs had grown at such a rapid pace during the 1950s and 1960s. The problem during those years was simply providing enough opportunities for everyone, especially for children. But during the 1970s, several factors caused people to take note of attrition [111]. In the first place, there were enough different sport programs that young people could pick and choose, switch, and stop and start their participation in ways they could never do in the past. This created patterns of participation that some adults defined as problematic since adults often become nervous when the behavior of young people is based on self-reflection rather than conformity to adult expectations. Second, baby boom cohorts in the 13-year-old and younger categories started to become smaller at the same time that those administering youth sport programs became sensitive to the local political and financial clout that came with ever-growing numbers of participants; without political clout, it was difficult to ensure continued access to public facilities, and without financial clout, it was difficult to maintain access to private facilities. Third, there were growing interests in the cultivation of elite athletes and the maintenance of a "feeder" system through which skilled athletes could be produced and "graduated" to higher levels of competition. These interests were fueled by those who wanted to draw from expanded pools of athletes to field "winners" on interscholastic, international, and professional teams. Finally, beliefs about the value of sport participation for development and health among people of all ages were rapidly expanding in western industrial countries. Therefore, combined concerns about socializing children through sport, maintaining control over the socialization process, producing high-performance athletes, and promoting social and physical development made everyone from parents to community leaders to social scientists more aware of "attrition as a problem."

ADMINISTRATION OF PROGRAMS. Some of the research in the first wave of studies on attrition from sport programs was also informed by a unique collection of critical analyses and exposés of sport that appeared around 1970 [45, 46, 83, 92, 123, 167, 175]. Descriptions of oppressively administered sport programs and autocratic, command-style coaches led some social scientists to become sensitive to the possibility that people who had been socialized into sport discontinued participation because of problems with the programs themselves. Many of the early studies and discussions of attrition in sport programs, especially in children's programs, focused on this possibility [11, 58, 136, 137, 163]. Rather than developing theories about socialization out of sport, these treatments of attrition were designed to critique programs and challenge those who controlled them to make changes. At the same time, there was also a growing awareness that sport termination cases might also be tied to issues of exploitation and alienation. The emerging sense that athletes in elite amateur and professional sports were victims of exploitation and that highly specialized, long-term sport participation itself could be a socially alienating experience opened the academic door for explorations of "athletic retirement" and the personal fates of former athletes [74, 75, 82, 90, 99, 117, 155].

A number of studies from the mid-1970s to the present have called direct attention to the following facts: *(a)* Attrition from particular sport programs does not always mean dropping out of all sports forever [58, 88, 94, 122, 140], nor does it mean that all connections to sport are severed [35]. *(b)* Withdrawing from sport often involves shifting priorities and may be positively related to social development [3, 17, 30, 36, 88, 202]. *(c)* Retirement from sport is not always tied to victimization or to a decrease in life satisfaction [3, 4, 35, 71, 100, 150, 202]. *(d)* Terminating participation is often associated with exposure to new and challenging opportunities [3, 65, 88, 91, 185].

In light of these studies and related discussions [26, 117, 120], the literature soon reflected the fact that terminating sport participation involves complex processes integrally linked to social development, identity formation, shifts in personal priorities, changes in social support, success experiences in sport, access to opportunities in and out of sport, gender relations, and the life course and social definitions of age. The following examples of selected studies are used to illustrate some of these connections.

Brown Study. Brown [17] used a conceptual framework based on a combination of social learning theory, reference group theory, role theory, symbolic interactionism, and exchange theory to study withdrawal from sport roles. Brown's statistical analysis of questionnaire data collected from former and current competitive female swimmers suggests that withdrawing from an important sport role involves a relatively extended desocialization process through which there is a gradual divestment of commitment to and identification with the role. This desocialization process is not initiated or driven by any single factor. More accurately, it is tied to choices made by the young women themselves as they shift their time and attention to alternatives to swimming and start to identify themselves in new ways. Although family and peers are important in the withdrawal process, the data suggest that their influence reinforced rather than initiated or shaped choices made by the young women. This indicates that young people do not simply get socialized out of sport; instead, leaving sport occurs when young people actively change social participation patterns and make conscious efforts to distance themselves from a role that has lost relative importance in their lives. Other research has consistently documented this pattern for both men and women, adolescents and adults, and for athletes in individual and team sports [3, 35, 88, 202].

Greendorfer and Blinde Study. Greendorfer and Blinde [65] used survey data from 1123 men and women who were former intercollegiate athletes (at a major American university) to examine what happens when people "retire" from a visible and demanding sport role to which they had been strongly committed for a relatively long period of time. The intent of the study was to test the applicability of conceptual frameworks grounded in either social gerontology (retirement theories) or a combination of life course developmental theory and role theory. Their data indicated the following: *(a)* When long-term participation in a highly visible and demanding sport role is terminated, people often shift involvement to other sport settings and other roles in sport. *(b)* Interest in participating in specific sport roles shifts over time as there are changes in anticipated rewards, involvement opportunities, and priorities assigned to nonsport interests, activities, and goals. *(c)* Terminating participation in a demanding sport role is followed by a certain sense of loss, along with a realization that there are new opportunities to do things that there was no time to do in the past.

On the basis of these findings, Greendorfer and Blinde concluded that the end of intercollegiate sport participation is not a terminal event in a person's sport biography; it marks a change, but it cannot be conceptually or methodologically treated as a discrete event that simply happens to a person. They also noted that studying so-called retirement from high performance sport calls for the use of conceptual and theoretical frameworks focusing on transition, process, and the reprioritization of interests among those experiencing the change. They concluded that there is a need for data collection techniques that reveal information on how athletes themselves interpret and react to their sport involvement and to the experience of leaving sport. This conclusion has been reaffirmed in Allison and Meyer's [3] study of former players in women's professional tennis and Swain's [202] study of male athletes who had retired from a variety of professional sports.

Coakley Study. Coakley [24] used an interactionist approach to study the origins of burnout among high performance adolescent athletes. Data from 15 in-depth interviews with young athletes who were identified as cases of burnout led to the conclusion that, contrary to stress-based models, burnout is more accurately conceptualized as a social problem than as a personal affliction. This is because burnout is grounded in the way high performance sport is organized rather than in an athlete's inability to cope with the stress created by the demands of training and competition. Coakley found that burnout occurs when young athletes become disempowered to the point that sport participation is seen as interfering with personal development and gaining meaningful control over their lives. In other words, the origin of burnout is not chronic stress; instead, it is the social processes and social relations that *(a)* interfere with a young person developing desired identities apart from the identity of athlete, and *(b)* preclude establishing the autonomy and independence that are so important in the lives of adolescents. Overall, Coakley's data strongly support the idea that burnout is related more to an institutionalized powerlessness than to personal flaws in coping skills among athletes themselves. The stress associated with burnout among adolescent athletes is simply a correlate of their lack of control over the conditions of their own sport participation. As this lack of control becomes internalized, it leads to chronic stress and other symptoms commonly listed in clinical descriptions of burnout. This suggests that burnout is a unique form of transition in young athletes' lives and that effectively dealing with it over the long run depends on empowering athletes and changing the social organization of the sport contexts in which athletes train and compete.

In summary, the phenomenon of changing or terminating sport participation seems to be tied to the same kinds of processes that underlie the initiation of participation. Just as people do not simply "get socialized into sport," neither do they simply "get socialized out of sport." Sport participation, changes in participation, and "nonparticipation" are all grounded in decision-making processes tied to the lives, life courses, and social worlds of those involved. In fact, it is possible for so-called sport participants, nonparticipants, and "drop-outs" to give the same reason for their different participation statuses (e.g., "my parents pressured me"). This "reason" can only be understood in context, and contexts are social constructions that change over time and in connection with social and cultural factors that transcend the immediate control of individuals.

SELECTION PROCESSES. It should be mentioned that research on socialization into and out of sport has tended to ignore the pervasive and pernicious "selection processes" that exist in many organized sport programs, especially high performance programs. In many cases, the socialization process is complemented by selection processes based on criteria defined by adults. When young people possess characteristics that coaches and other participation gatekeepers define as noteworthy and valuable, they are selected into programs; when they do not, they are cut out. In other words, socialization is tied to selection, and ignoring this fact makes it difficult to understand sport participation. Furthermore, the existence of selection processes must be taken into account when attempting to understand the consequences of sport participation. This brings the discussion to the next topic.

Socialization Through Sport: Consequences of Sport Participation
The belief that sport builds character has its origins in the class and gender relations of mid-19th century England. Although the history of beliefs about the consequences of sport participation varies by country, the notion that sport produces positive socialization effects has been widely accepted across western industrial societies, especially England, Canada, and the United States. For nearly a century the validity of these beliefs was taken for granted and promoted by those associated with organized competitive sports in these countries. It was not until the 1950s that people began to use research to subject the belief to a systematic test [97, 106].

Most of the studies done from the 1950s through the 1970s were atheoretical, correlational analyses presenting statistical comparisons of the attributes of "athletes" and "nonathletes." Because only a handful of the studies used longitudinal, pretest/post-test designs, research findings were usually qualified in light of questions about "socialization effects" (i.e., what attributes were actually "caused" by sport participation) versus "selection effects" (i.e., what attributes were initially possessed by those who chose to play organized sports or were selected to play by coaches and program managers).

McCormack and Chalip [113] have criticized much of the correlational research on socialization through sport by pointing out that studies have been based on two faulty assumptions. First, researchers have assumed that sport invariably offers all participants the same unique experiences, and that those experiences are strong enough to influence people's characters and orientations. Second, researchers have assumed that sport participants passively internalize "moral lessons" inherently contained in the sport experience, and that these lessons are not readily passed on through other activities or settings. These assumptions led researchers to overlook several important factors: (*a*) Sport itself is a social construction and offers an infinite array of potential socialization experiences. (*b*) Sport participation takes on meaning only within the context of the experiences and social relations of those involved. (*c*) The personal implications of sport participation are integrated into people's lives through general processes of social relations. *(d)* Sport is a site for human agency, resistance, and the transformation of social relations as well as cultural reproduction.

Due to these oversights, correlational research based on internalization models has generated a long list of contradictory and confusing findings often leading to the conclusion that the effects of sport participation are negligible. However, this is not to say that this research should be ignored. Actually, it has enhanced our knowledge of socialization through sport in several respects. First, studies have provided extensive quantitative data on the attributes and behavior rates of those who participate in certain types of sport programs and those who do not. Second, the findings of these studies provide a basis for asking questions and raising issues that can inform interpretive studies based on interactionist and other dynamic socialization models. Because of these contributions, it is helpful to review correlational research on the topics that have elicited the most attention over the years.

ACADEMIC ACHIEVEMENT AND ASPIRATIONS. It has been relatively easy to obtain data on sport participation and academic achievement and aspirations simply by adding the variable of interscholastic or varsity sport participation to larger studies of students and student life. Most of these data come from studies of American high school students although there are a few studies of the academic achievement of college student-athletes compared with their peers who do not participate on intercollegiate teams [126]. Studies of high school students generally indicate that when socioeconomic status is controlled, students who participate on high school teams have slightly better grade point averages and slightly higher educational aspirations than peers who do not play.

When the research reporting a positive relationship between varsity sport participation and grades/academic aspirations is grouped together [72, 73, 87, 114, 138, 142, 147, 149, 166, 184, 187, 190–192, 212], it suggests that academic benefits occur when sport participation brings student-athletes prestige that leads peers and significant others to treat them more seriously as students [29]. Therefore, when participation occurs in a "low profile" sport, when athletes are only mediocre performers, when participation does not attract attention in the form of academic support, and when important relationships in the participant's life do not change in connection with participation, academic benefits are rare or nonexistent. This may explain why some studies have not found a positive relationship between sport participation and academic achievement and aspirations [80, 124, 126, 146, 177, 179]. After all, it stands to reason that relationships are primary vehicles for change when it comes to academic matters. Thus, when sport participation causes young people to be noticed by those who can positively influence their academic lives, changes are likely. Unfortunately, correlational research does not capture the dynamics of the processes underlying such changes.

There is now a need for interpretive studies on the way sport participation among students is integrated into their lives. Attention should be given to relationships with parents, friends, teachers, coaches, and others who might be sources of certain types of support in the lives of student-athletes. Do these people serve as advocates, exemplars, or role models? Are they concerned with growth and achievement in realms other than sport? How do they alter a young person's access to the resources and experiences needed to perform well in school and move on to other educational challenges? How do these relationships take shape in light of gender and the social class and racial backgrounds of the students? How are the decisions made by student-athletes informed by their connections with others?

SOCIAL AND OCCUPATIONAL MOBILITY. Correlational analyses of career success and social mobility patterns among former athletes and nonathletes have not supported the popular belief that being an athlete creates attributes, connections, or reputations facilitating achievement in nonsport activities. In fact, former athletes as a group do not have career success or failure patterns any different from those of peers who did not participate in interscholastic sports in high school and/or college [10, 41, 42, 72–74, 84, 105, 134, 138, 143, 159, 174, 181, 191, 196]. Again, this suggests the need for interpretive research. Future studies need to focus on how sport participation is connected with the following issues: *(a)* completing degrees, developing job-related skills, and acquiring information about how the world apart from sport is organized and operates; *(b)* receiving consistent social, emotional, and material support for *overall* growth and development from significant others; *(c)* developing social networks extending beyond sport and sport organizations; and *(d)* expanding personal and social experiences and identities having little or nothing to do with sport.

These issues, suggested by correlational analyses, provide good leads for interpretive studies of sport participation and occupational mobility [26, 29]. Although it has been suggested that many sport experiences shared by athletes do not lead to the development of skills needed for social mobility and career success [205], future studies should identify the ways in which sport experiences can be integrated into athletes' lives and serve as links to work histories and occupational careers apart from sport [189].

DEVIANT BEHAVIOR. Research has also tested popular beliefs about sport keeping young people "off the streets" and out of trouble. The findings of correlational analyses based on data from American high school students are somewhat confusing and difficult to interpret, but they generally indicate that rates of deviance among "athletes" are similar to or lower than rates among so-called "nonathletes." This pattern seems to hold across societies, for both males and females, for those from all racial and social class backgrounds, and across sports [19, 95, 145, 164, 170–173, 178, 194, 206]. However, these analyses provide little information on the dynamics of socialization processes related to the deviant behavior-sport participation connection.

However, there are several correlational studies utilizing pretest/post-test designs that provide very useful leads about how sport participation may be connected to deviant behavior rates. For example, Trulson [207] studied the effects of three carefully designed sport participation programs on the characteristics of 34 young men (13–17 years old) classified as juvenile delinquents. After 6 months of participation in the programs (1-hour sessions three times per week) the young men assigned to a *traditional* Tae Kwon Do training course had decreased scores on measures of aggression and increased scores on measures of personality adjustment, while comparable counterparts assigned to a "modern" Tae Kwon Do course, or a course in which they jogged, and played basketball and football did not show similar "improvements." Notably, participation in traditional Tae Kwon Do was grounded in a philosophy emphasizing nonviolence, respect for self and others, fitness and self-control, self-confidence, and responsibility; explicit emphasis on these factors was not a part of the other two participation experiences.

Another longitudinal study [194] using national data collected in five waves from 2000 young men from the time they were high school sophomores until they were 24 years old focused on the long-term relationship between rates of delinquency and participation in all forms of organized sports. Statistical analysis identified no sport participation effects in the sample as a whole, but there was an interesting pattern that emerged when race was controlled. Whites participating in organized sports had lower delinquency rates than white nonparticipating counterparts, while the opposite was true for blacks. Over time, however, the rates of deviance among blacks participating in organized sports declined below their black counterparts. This suggests that selection processes associated with organized sport participation are tied to patterns of race relations, and that race relations mediate experiences in sport and consequences of participation.

Interpretive research based on interactionist models of socialization is now needed to explore selection processes in sport [38] and the dynamics of specific sport experiences and the ways those experiences are connected with gender, class, and race relations when it comes to their implications for rates of deviant behavior.

POLITICAL ORIENTATIONS. The belief that sport participation social-izes young people to "fit into" established social systems attracted considerable attention during the 1960s and 1970s [141, 148, 165]. The possibility that sport participation served social control functions by producing compliant, conforming, and politically conservative people was unsettling among those committed to bringing about social change in society [46, 83, 167, 175].

Correlational research during this period generally discovered that high school and college sport participation in the United States was associated with personal and political conservatism and a lack of political awareness [132, 148, 165], although this pattern was not reported in Canadian studies [141]. More recent studies of Canadian university students shows that athletes tend to be slightly more conservative on social and economic policy issues than peers not involved in organized sports, but these differences do not seem to be related to political behavior [56]. Studies of high school and college coaches in the U.S. also report unique patterns of political attitudes [160]. Unfortunately, none of these studies provide information on why athletes and nonathletes might have different political attitudes, or why coaches' attitudes differ from those held by adults in other occupations; nor do they provide information on how those differences are related to sport participation itself. Research on these issues remains to be done.

INDIVIDUAL CHARACTER TRAITS AND MORAL DEVELOPMENT. In sport psychology, there is a long history of research dealing with the personality traits [31, 101, 208], but these studies focus on selection and performance issues rather than socialization issues. Few studies have actually examined the relationship between sport participation and the formation of character or personality traits. The research that comes closest is work done on moral development, aggression, and prosocial versus antisocial behaviors. The research on moral development done by Bredemeier and her colleagues [11–15, 210] suggests that sport is a unique context for moral decision making, and that under most circumstances sport experiences are negatively associated with moral reasoning and moral development. The only exception is when sport has been intentionally organized to encompass experiences designed to promote moral development [16, 154].

Other research suggests that prosocial behaviors such as sharing and helping are negatively associated with most sport participation, while antisocial behaviors such as aggression are positively associated with participation [5, 6, 43, 55, 93, 116, 176, 182]. For example, research by Kleiber and Roberts [93] led to the conclusion that an emphasis on competition can dominate interpersonal relationships to the point that the potential for sport participation to encourage prosocial behaviors is subverted. Kleiber and Roberts also suggest that the display of prosocial interpersonal orientations such as cooperation, sharing, helping, empathy, and altruism may be undermined when the display of individual traits such as independence, achievement, motivation, courage, and perseverance is emphasized in a sport program. A similar experimental study [57] involving the use of field methods found that reinforcement strategies used to increase sportsperson-like behaviors among 12-year-old boys on recreational sport teams were more effective in reducing antisocial behaviors than in promoting prosocial behaviors. It was also found that when prosocial behaviors are learned in a particular sport setting, they do not appear to carry over to other settings, even other sport settings. Dubois' [40, 43] longitudinal study of values changes among 8- to 10-year-old boys and girls in competitive and instructional soccer leagues found that over the course of a single season scores increased on measures of the importance of winning, fitness, sportspersonship, and relationships with fellow participants, although these changes varied by type of program and gender.

An absence of data on the actual experiences of the children across different activity spheres, on the meanings assigned to those experiences by the children, and on the ways those experiences are integrated into the lives of the children makes it difficult to explain the ways in which socialization effects occur in connection with sport participation. There is still a need for interpretive research to explore the connection between the dynamics of how such behaviors are socially constructed in sport and then how individuals may use them to inform behavior in other settings. However, it is very difficult to begin to discuss so-called "carryover" from sport to other settings until more is known about what occurs in the sport participation process itself and how identities are constructed in connection with participation. People may identify themselves as athletes, but the attributes associated with that identity are not automatically applied to other settings. The possibility that identities are situation specific [107–110] raises many questions about the connection between the behaviors engaged in during sport participation and those engaged in during other activities.

More recently, there has been an increase in interpretive studies of the socialization consequences of sport participation. These studies, based on interactionist and other dynamic models, and using qualitative data, have built on and extended what has been found in correlational analyses. They have also been informed by a broader range of questions about sport experiences and the ways those experiences are integrated into people's lives. For the purpose of summarizing this research, six examples have been chosen for review.

Moral Socialization and Sport Participation: Fine's Study [5] of Little Leaguers. Fine used an interactionist approach in his study of 10 Little League teams in five different leagues. Data were collected over 3 years through participant observations and informal conversations and interviews. In his observations and analysis, Fine gave detailed attention to the specific situations in which children are exposed to the normative guidelines for behavior in sport. His findings indicate that moral socialization through sport is a complex process through which young people redefine and transform the idealized rules and moral lessons offered by adults into concerns that fit their own immediate needs, primarily needs for acceptance among peers. Peer acceptance is achieved through efforts to "be a man" in a traditional moral sense. This leads preadolescent boys to choose behaviors that express autonomy and to establish distance between themselves and anyone defined as weak and submissive, i.e., girls and younger children. Since being identified with girls or younger children interferes with being defined as "men," the boys on youth teams tend to mimic stereotypical models of traditional masculinity. This tendency is seldom discouraged by coaches because it can be used to motivate the boys to play in aggressive ways. This process leads to the reproduction of a masculinity grounded in displays of toughness and dominance, and to expressions of disdain for females and any boys seen as unable to fend for themselves or unwilling to engage in daring or bold behaviors.

Fine also found that boys seldom accept at face value the moral messages stressed by coaches and parents. But their resistance to and transformation of moral messages is difficult for many adults to detect because the Little League players quickly learn to present themselves in ways that express and reaffirm the "moral truths" proclaimed by coaches and other adults; they also learn that to avoid sanctions when caught violating rules, they must use particular expressions of "moral rhetoric" that will appease adults. This does not mean that these preadolescent boys simply ignore the moral talk offered by adults or see it as useless, but it does indicate that this moral talk is transformed by the boys to fit their own definitions of the situation. Furthermore, these boys evaluate what adults say by comparing it to what adults do. When there are contradictions, the boys raise questions about the credibility of those adults and the moral lessons they proclaim. This does not mean that the boys overtly reject the values of the adults who control the sport programs, but it does mean that they question them and take the liberty of creatively adapting adult values to fit their own lives.

Fine's study illustrates that socialization through sport is an inherently problematic process. It does not happen according to some prescribed recipe. Instead, it emerges out of a combination of the concerns of those who control sport structures and the concerns of the participants, even when the participants are children. Even when participants lack formal power relative to those who control sport structures, they do not simply internalize the values of the organizers and controllers; instead, they interpret and transform those values in light of tasks and issues important in their lives and in the peer or subcultural groups in which they seek acceptance.

Self and Sport Participation: Adler and Adler's [1] Study of Intercollegiate Athletes. Adler and Adler also used an interactionist approach in their decade-long study of the "structure and dynamic processes" [1, p. 28] of the selves of men on a high-profile college basketball team. Through a combination of observation, participant observation, and both formal and informal in-depth interviews with athletes, coaches, and others associated with the basketball program, the Adlers collected data on how the self-concepts of intercollegiate student-athletes changed in connection with their sport participation. The major finding in the Adlers' research is that young men on high-profile intercollegiate teams are likely to become so engulfed in their athlete roles that they make adjustments and compromises in their academic lives. This role engulfment involves increasing commitments to identities based exclusively on sport participation. These commitments are consistently and ardently reinforced by coaches, students, fans, community members, and teammates. Thus, being an athlete becomes a "master status" for these young men, and the athletic subculture becomes the context in which they set goals, evaluate themselves, and define their identities. The Adlers point out that role engulfment among intercollegiate athletes reflects the role specialization that commonly occurs in highly institutionalized and rationalized social contexts, such as American society.

Although the Adlers suspected that intercollegiate athletes learned something about the importance of focusing their attention on specific tasks and delaying gratification in the process, they found nothing to suggest that these lessons would be applied in settings apart from sport. This may be due to the fact that role engulfment involves a heightened salience of a situation-specific identity that seems unique and unrelated to other identities and contexts. However, the process of role engulfment is itself problematic. For example, research on women intercollegiate athletes did not seem to be characterized by the same exclusive commitments to athletic identities and revisions in academic standards and goals [127].

Normalization of Pain and Injury in Sport: Curry's Study [32] of the Sport Career of an Amateur Wrestler. Curry examined biographical data on the sport career of an amateur wrestler. The case study data were collected through three 2-hour interviews over a 2-month period. These interviews followed several years of observing the wrestling team on which this young man (in his early 20s) participated. Curry's analysis clearly outlines the socialization process through which many athletes come to define pain and injury as normal parts of their sport experiences. For example, this young wrestler initially learned to define pain and injury as a routine part of sport participation simply by observing other wrestlers and interacting with people connected to the sport. As he progressed to higher levels of competition, he became increasingly aware of how the endurance of pain and injury are commonplace among fellow athletes and former athletes who are now coaches. Over time, this young man learned the following in connection with his wrestling career: to "shake off" minor injuries, to see special treatment for minor injuries as a form of coddling, to express desire and motivation by playing while injured or in pain, to avoid using injury or pain as excuses for not practicing or competing, to use physicians and trainers as experts whose roles were to keep him competing when not healthy, to see pain-killing anti-inflammatory drugs as necessary performance-enhancing aids, to commit himself to the idea that all athletes must pay a price as they strive for excellence, and to define any athlete (including himself) unwilling to pay the price or to strive for excellence as morally deficient. Finally, through a combination of injuries to his spine and knees, and repeated injuries that disfigured his ears ("cauliflower ear" is common among long time wrestlers), he became a role model for younger wrestlers.

The socialization experiences associated with this young man's wrestling career clearly illustrate what has been described as the "sport ethic" [85]. By adopting the sport ethic, young athletes learn to define sacrifice, risk, pain, and injury as the price one must pay to be accepted as an athlete in competitive sports. In many sport groups, the normative guidelines of the sport ethic become the criteria used to evaluate oneself and others as athletes and to gain status among peers. When these guidelines are accepted uncritically, athletes often overconform to them to the point that they jeopardize the health and physical well-being of themselves and others: and they do this in the name of duty, honor, loyalty, and self-respect. This point has also been documented in other research on sport socialization [47, 131, 157, 158].

Sport Rituals and Socialization in the Culture of a Community: Foley's Ethnography [53, 54] of a Small Texas Town. Foley used field methods (observation, participant observation, and informal and formal interviews) over a 2-year period to study sports as a socialization process within the community life of a small town. Popular culture theory was used to view the socialization process from a broad, holistic perspective. In particular, Foley's goal was to examine the extent to which sport served as a site for cultural practices through which community members might resist and transform the capitalist, racial, and patriarchal order that defined social life in the small town. Foley found that sport in general and high school football in particular were important examples of community rituals that partially constituted a general socialization process in the social life of the town. These rituals were especially critical in the socialization of young people and the overall preservation of the status system in the local adolescent subculture. The ritual of high school football in particular seemed to encompass uniquely the lives of adults as well as young men and women.

Although Foley set out to examine sport as a site for progressive practices challenging the dominance of those few who controlled capital resources in the town, he found few examples. Resistance and counter-hegemonic cultural practices did occur, but they produced few effects beyond specific individuals and immediate situations. This led Foley to conclude that sport is best described as an outdated, traditional force, at least in the life of the small town he studied.

Foley's work indicates that socialization through sport is not limited to small group or subcultural settings; it also occurs in connection with the economic, political, and cultural systems that make up the everyday culture of a community. Although sport as a process of socialization offers possibilities for forms of transformative resistance, Foley discovered that sport rituals generally reproduced forms of social inequality in race, class, and gender relations. Ethnographic research done by Eder and Parker [44] in a racially mixed high school in a medium-size community in the U.S. midwest support Foley's findings: highly visible extracurricular activities such as varsity sports and cheerleading reproduce gender inequities in the peer culture of the school. Other research indicates that this process has occurred through history [133] and across cultural settings [22, 96].

Sport Participation and the Social Construction of Masculinity: Messner's Study [125] of the Lives of Male Athletes. Messner used a form of critical feminism to study the ways in which masculinities were socially constructed in connection with men's athletic careers. Open-ended in-depth interviews were conducted with 30 former athletes from different racial and social class backgrounds to discover how gender identities develop and change as men interact with the socially constructed world of sports. The men in Messner's study began their first sport experiences with already gendered identities; in fact, their emerging identities during childhood were associated with their initial attraction to sport. They did not enter sports as blank slates ready to be "filled in" with culturally approved masculine orientations and behaviors. As athletic careers progressed, these men constructed orientations, relationships, and experiences "consistent with the dominant values and power relations of the larger gender order" [125, p. 150–151]. Furthermore, their masculinity was based on *(a)* limited definitions of public success, *(b)* relationships with men in which bonds were shaped by homophobia and misogyny [33], and *(c)* a willingness to use their bodies as tools of domination regardless of consequences for health or general well-being. This not only influenced their public presentations of self and their relationships with women, but it engendered a continuing sense of insecurity about issues related to "manhood."

Messner also found that "sport does not simply and unambiguously reproduce men's existing power and privilege" [125, p. 151]. His interviews revealed significant tensions in the sport-masculinity connection. These tensions were related to three factors. First, sport participation brought many of the men temporary public recognition but discouraged formation of needed intimate relationships; it also enabled them to develop physical competence, but it frequently led to chronic health problems. Second, since the social construction of masculinity is tied to opportunities and constraints in a man's social world, sport careers took different forms depending on the sexual preferences and the racial and class backgrounds of the men. Third, the involvement and success of women in sport raised serious questions for those who had learned that becoming a man necessarily involved detaching themselves from all things female.

Messner's research indicates that sport participation is a process through which men enhance their public status, create nonintimate bonds of loyalty with each other, perpetuate patriarchal relationships with women, and construct masculinity in a way that privileges some men over others. This process is sometimes challenged by participants, but transformations of sport and sport experiences are difficult to initiate. Messner also calls attention to the fact that gender is a social construction and that sport offers a fruitful site for exploring the formation of gender identities. This has also been noted in Palzkill's research [139] on women in elite, amateur sport.

Transformation of Sport Structures and Experiences: Birrell and Richter's Study [8] of Women's Recreational Softball. Birrell and Richter used feminist theory informed by interactionist and cultural studies approaches to examine the way in which sport was socially constructed by selected women involved in recreation slow-pitch softball leagues in two communities. Intensive interviews and observations over 4 years focused on the ways feminist consciousness might inform and structure women's sport experiences, the interpretation of those experiences, and the integration of the experiences into women's lives. Birrell and Richter reported that the women in their study were concerned with developing and expressing skills, playing hard, and challenging opponents, but that they wanted to do these things without adopting orientations characterized by an overemphasis on winning, power relationships between players and coaches, social exclusion and skill-based elitism, an ethic of risk and endangerment, and the derogation of opponents. In other words, the women attempted to create sport experiences that were "process oriented, collective, supportive, inclusive, and infused with an ethic of care" [8, p. 408].

Birrell and Richter found that creating an alternative to a "masculinist hegemony and dominant, male-sustained definition of sport" was not something that occurred without struggle. Transformations of the teams and the games played came slowly over the 4-year research period, but they did come. This provided the women with not only a sense of satisfaction and enjoyable sport experiences, but also a reaffirmation of collective feminist consciousness and feelings of political empowerment.

Birrell and Richter's research illustrates that sport is not so much a product as it is a process of invention [8, p. 397]. This invention process is grounded in the consciousness and collective reflection of the participants themselves, and it is shaped by conversations about experiences, feelings, decisions, behaviors, accounts of and responses to incidents, and a combination of individual and collective conclusions about the connection between sport and the lives of the participants. In other words, not only is sport a social construction, but so too are the consequences of participation.

In summary, these six examples of what occurs in connection with sport participation illustrate that participation itself is a social process and, as such, has emergent qualities that reflect the interests of those involved and the context in which it occurs. This means that it makes much more sense to frame discussions of socialization through sport in terms of human agency, cultural practices, struggle, power relations, and social construction than it does to frame them in terms of specific outcomes manifested through measurable changes in the character traits of athletes and former athletes. Research on sport participation and what happens in connection with it is important because sport is highly visible, heavily promoted, and organized in ways that often support long-standing systems of power and privilege. Research is also important, however, because sport can be the site of human agency, resistance, struggle, and transformation. An awareness of this can effectively inform an understanding of how sport is organized, how it is played, what it means, and what implications it has for participants, even those simply watching. It is expected that future research will build on this awareness and focus even more attention on the voices of those involved in sport and what those voices say about participation, its meaning, and its consequences.

CONCLUSION

This overview is framed in terms of major changes in the conceptual and methodological approaches used to study socialization. Until the late 1970s, internalization models were used to guide socialization research. Those using such models assumed that human beings were passive learners "socialized into, out of, and through sport." Since then, a growing number of social scientists have realized that sport as well as sport experiences are social constructions and that interactionist research models are needed to capture the dynamics of socialization processes.

The use of interactionist models has been informed by an awareness that sport and sport participation are parts of larger processes of social relations encompassing gender, class, race, ethnicity, and sexual orientations. Since sport itself is part of general social and cultural formations, it cannot be separated from the economic and political practices that often constrain people's choices and activities, nor can it be separated from human agency and processes of resistance and transformation. This means that socialization cannot be approached in terms of unreflexive responses to specific events, relationships, and external forces. Socialization research has also begun to take into account the fact that sport participation and the termination of participation are choices informed by identity and social relations, and that participation itself is a socially constructed process mediated by power relations and the consciousness and collective reflection of participants.

Socialization research based on interactionist models has not only uncovered the dynamics of differing social realities in sport, but it has begun to contextualize those realities so we can better understand how sport practices are connected to larger social and cultural formations.

REFERENCES

1. Adler, P. A., and P. Adler. *Backboards and blackboards: College athletes and role engulfment.* New York: Columbia University Press, 1991.
2. Allison, M. T. Sport, culture and socialization. *Int. Rev. Sociol. Sport* 17:11–37, 1982.
3. Allison, M. T., and C. Meyer. Career problems and retirement among elite athletes: the female tennis professional. *Sociol. Sport J* 5:212–222, 1988.
4. Arviko, I. Factors influencing the job and life satisfaction of retired baseball players. Unpublished Master's Thesis, University of Waterloo, Ontario, 1976.
5. Barnett, M., and J. Bryan. Effects of competition with outcome feedback on children's helping behavior. *Dev. Psychol.* 10:838–842, 1974.
6. Berkowitz, L. Sports, competition, and aggression. In I. Williams and L. Wankel (eds.). *Fourth Canadian symposium on psychology of learning and sport.* Ottawa: University of Ottawa Press, 1972, pp. 321–326.
7. Berlage, G. I. Children's sports and the family. *ARENA Rev.* 6:43–47, 1982.
8. Birrell, S., and D. M. Richter. Is a diamond forever? Feminist transformations of sport. *Women's Studies Int. Forum* 10:395–409, 1987.
9. Blanchard, K., and A. Cheska. *The anthropology of sport.* South Hadley, MA: Bergin & Garvey Publishers, Inc. 1985.
10. Braddock, J. Race, sports and social mobility: a critical review. *Soc. Symp.* 30:18–38, 1980.
11. Bredemeier, B. J. Moral reasoning and perceived legitimacy of intentionally injurious acts. *J. Sport Psychol.* 7:110–124, 1985.
12. Bredemeier, B. J. The moral of the youth sport story. In E. W. Brown and C. F. Banta (eds.). *Competitive sports for children and youth.* Champaign IL: Human Kinetics, 1988, pp. 285–296.
13. Bredemeier, B. J. The relationship between children's legitimacy judgments and their moral reasoning, aggression tendencies, and sport involvement. *Sociol. Sport J.* 4:48–60, 1987.
14. Bredemeier, B. J., and D. L. Shields. Moral growth among athletes and nonathletes: a comparative analysis of females and males. *J. Genet. Psychol.* 147:7–18, 1986.
15. Bredemeier, B. J., D. L. Shields, M. R. Weiss, and B. A. B. Cooper. The relationship of sport involvement with children's moral reasoning and aggression tendencies. *J. Sport Psychol.* 8:304–318, 1986.
16. Bredemeier, B. J., M. R. Weiss, D. L. Shields, and R. Shewchuk. Promoting moral growth in a summer sport camp: the implementation of theoretically grounded instructional strategies. *J. Moral Educ.* 15:212–220, 1986.
17. Brown, B. A. Factors influencing the process of withdrawal by female adolescents from the role of competitive age group swimmer. *Sociol. Sport J.* 2:111–129, 1985.
18. Brustad, R. J. Integrating socialization influences into the study of children's motivation in sport. *J. Sport Exerc. Psychol.* 14:59–77, 1992.

19. Buhrmann, H. G. Athletics and deviancy: an examination of the relationship between athletic participation and deviant behavior of high school girls. *Rev. Sport Leisure* 7:119–128, 1977.

20. Butcher, J. Longitudinal analysis of adolescent girls' participation in physical activity. *Social. Sport J.* 2:130–143, 1985.

21. Carlson, R. The socialization of elite tennis players in Sweden: an analysis of the players' backgrounds and development. *Sociol. Sport J.* 5:241–256, 1988.

22. Carrington, B., T. Chivers, and T. Williams. Gender, leisure and sport: a case-study of young people of South Asian descent. *Leisure Studies* 6:265–279, 1987.

23. Clausen, J. A. A historical and comparative view of socialization theory and research. In J. A. Clausen (ed.). *Socialization and society*. Boston: Little, Brown & Co., 1968, pp. 18–72.

24. Coakley, J. Burnout among adolescent athletes: A personal failure or social problem? *Sociol. Sport J.* 9:271–285, 1992.

25. Coakley, J. Children and the sport socialization process. In D. Gould and M. R. Weiss (eds.). *Advances in pediatric sport sciences* (Vol. 2, Behavioral Issues). Champaign, IL: Human Kinetics, 1987, pp. 43–60.

26. Coakley, J. Leaving competitive sport: retirement or rebirth? *Quest* 35:1–11, 1983.

27. Coakley, J. Socialization and sport. R. Singer, M. Murphey, and L. K. Tennant (eds.). *Handbook on research in sport psychology*. New York: Macmillan, 1993, pp. 571–586.

28. Coakley, J. Socialization and youth sports. In C. R. Rees and A. W. Miracle (eds.). *Sport and social theory*. Champaign, IL: Human Kinetics, 1986, pp. 135–143.

29. Coakley, J. *Sport in society*. St. Louis: Times Mirror/Mosby, 1990.

30. Coakley, J., and A. White. Making decisions: gender and sport participation among British adolescents. *Sociol. Sport J.* 9:20–35, 1992.

31. Cratty, B. J. *Psychology in contemporary sport*. Englewood Cliffs, NJ: Prentice Hall, 1989.

32. Curry, T. J. A little pain never hurt anyone: athletic career socialization and the normalization of sport injury. Presented at the Gregory Stone Symposium, Las Vegas, February, 1992.

33. Curry, T. J. Fraternal bonding in the locker room: a profeminist analysis of talk about competition and women. *Sociol. Sport J.* 8:119–135, 1991.

34. Curry, T. J., and O. Weiss. Sport identity and motivation for sport participation: a comparison between American college athletes and Austrian student sport club members. *Sociol. Sport J.* 6:257–268, 1989.

35. Curtis, J. E., and R. Ennis. Negative consequences of leaving competitive sport? Comparative findings for former elite-level hockey players. *Sociol. Sport J.* 5:87–106, 1988.

36. Curtis, J., and P. White. Age and sport participation: decline in participation with age or increased specialization with age? In N. Theberge and P. Donnelly (eds.). *Sport and the sociological imagination*. Ft. Worth: Texas Christian University Press, 1984, pp. 273–294.

37. Deem, R. *All work and no play: the sociology of women and leisure*. Philadelphia: Open University Press, 1986.

38. Donnelly, P. Athletes and juvenile delinquents: a comparative analysis based on a review of literature. *Adolescence* 16:415–432, 1981.

39. Donnelly, P., and K. Young. The construction and confirmation of identity in sport subcultures. Sociol. Sport J. 5:223–240, 1988.

40. Dubois, P. E. Gender differences in value orientation toward sports: a longitudinal analysis. *J. Sport Behavior* 13:3–14, 1990.

41. Dubois, P. E. Participation in sport and occupational attainment: an investigation of selected athlete categories. *J. Sport Behav.* 2:103–114, 1979.

42. Dubois, P. E. Participation in sports and occupational attainment: a comparative study. *Res. Q.* 49:28–37, 1978.

43. Dubois, P. E. The effects of participation in sport on the value orientations of young athletes. *Sociol. Sport J.* 3:29–42, 1986.

44. Eder D., and S. Parker. The cultural production and reproduction of gender: the effect of extracurricular activities on peer-group culture. *Sociol. Educ.* 60:200–213, 1987.
45. Edwards, H. *Sociology of sport.* Homewood, IL: The Dorsey Press, 1973.
46. Edwards, H. *The revolt of the black athlete.* New York: The Free Press, 1969.
47. Ewald, K., and R. M. Jiobu. Explaining positive deviance: Becker's model and the case of runners and bodybuilders. *Sociol. Sport J.* 2:144–156.
48. Fagot, B. I. Teacher and peer reactions to boys' and girls' play styles. *Sex Roles* 11:691–702, 1984.
49. Faulkner, R. Coming of age in organizations: a comparative study of career contingencies and adult socialization. *Sociol. Work Occup.* 1:131–173, 1974.
50. Feltz, D. L., and L. Petlichkoff. Perceived competence among interscholastic sport participants and dropouts. *Can. J. Appl. Sport Sci.* 8:231–235, 1983.
51. Fine. G. A. *With the boys: Little League baseball and preadolescent culture.* Chicago: University of Chicago Press, 1987.
52. Fishwick, L., and S. Greendorfer. Socialization revisited: a critique of the sport-related research. *Quest* 39:1–9, 1987.
53. Foley, D. E. *Learning capitalist culture.* Philadelphia: University of Pennsylvania Press, 1990a.
54. Foley, D. E. The great American football ritual: reproducing race, class, and gender inequality. *Sociol. Sport J.* 7:111–135, 1990b.
55. Gelfand, D., and D. Hartman. Some detrimental effects of competitive sports on children's behavior. In R. Magill, M. J. Ash, and F. L. Smoll (eds.). *Children in sport: a contemporary anthology.* Champaign, IL: Human Kinetics, 1978, pp. 165–174.
56. Gelinas, M. The relationship between sport involvement and political attitudes and behaviours. M. A. Thesis, University of Waterloo, Ontario, 1988.
57. Giebink, M. P., and T. L. McKenzie. Teaching sportsmanship in physical education and recreation: an analysis of interventions and generalization effects. *J. Teaching Phys. Educ.* 4:167–177, 1985.
58. Gould, D., D. Feltz, T. Horn, and M. R. Weiss. Reasons for discontinuing involvement in competitive youth swimming. *J. Sport Behav.* 5:155–165, 1982.
59. Greendorfer, S. L. Childhood sport socialization influences on male and female track athletes. *ARENA Rev.* 3:39–53, 1979b.
60. Greendorfer, S. L. Differences in childhood socialization influences on women involved in sport and women not involved in sport. In M. Krotee (ed.). *The dimensions of sport sociology.* New York: Leisure Press, 1979a, pp. 59–72.
61. Greendorfer, S. L. Gender bias in theoretical perspectives: the case of female socialization into sport. *Psychol. Women Q.* 11:327–347, 1987.
62. Greendorfer, S. L. Shaping the female athlete: the impact of the family. In M. A. Boutilier and L. SanGiovanni, *The sporting woman.* Champaign, IL: Human Kinetics, 1983, pp. 135–156.
63. Greendorfer, S. L. Social class influence on female sport involvement. *Sex Roles* 4:619–625, 1978.
64. Greendorfer, S. L. The role of socializing agents on female sport involvement. *Res. Q.* 48:304–310, 1977.
65. Greendorfer, S. L., and E. M. Blinde. "Retirement" from intercollegiate sport: theoretical and empirical considerations. *Sociol. Sport J.* 5:101–110, 1985.
66. Greendorfer, S. L., E. M. Blinde, and A. M. Pellegrini. Differences in Brazilian children's socialization into sport. *Int. Rev. Sociol. Sport* 21:51–64, 1986.
67. Greendorfer, S. L., and T. Bruce. Rejuvenating sport socialization research. *J. Sport Soc. Issues* 15:129–144, 1991.
68. Greendorfer, S. L., and M. Ewing. Race and gender differences in children's socialization into sport. *Res. Q. Exerc. Sport* 52:301–310, 1981.

69. Greendorfer, S. L., and J. H. Lewko. The role of family members in sport socialization of children. *Res. Q.* 49:146–152, 1978.

70. Gruneau, R. S. Elites, class and corporate power in Canadian sport: some preliminary findings. In F. Landry and W. A. R. Orban (eds.). *Sociology of sport: sociological studies and administrative, economic and legal aspects of sport and leisure.* Miami, FL: Symposia Specialists, 1978, pp. 201–242.

71. Haerle, R. Career patterns and career contingencies of professional baseball players. In D. Ball and J. Loy (eds.). *Sport and social order.* Reading, MA: Addison-Wesley, 1975, pp. 457–519.

72. Hanks, M. Race, sexual status and athletics in the process of educational achievement. *Social Sci. Q.* 60:482–496, 1979.

73. Hanks, M., and B. K. Eckland. Athletics and social participation in the educational attainment process. *Sociol. Educ.* 49:271–294, 1976.

74. Hare, N. A study of the black fighter. *Black Scholar* 3:2–9, 1971.

75. Harris, D. S., and D. S. Eitzen. The consequences of failure in sport. *Urban Life* 7:177–188, 1971.

76. Harris, O. Athletics and academics: contrary or complimentary activities. In G. Jarvie (ed.). *Sport, racism and ethnicity.* New York: Falmer Press, 1991, pp. 124–149.

77. Hasbrook, C. H. Reciprocity and childhood socialization into sport. In L. Vander Velden and J. H. Humphrey (eds.). *Psychology and sociology of sport: Current selected research.* New York: AMS Press., 1986, pp. 135–147.

78. Hasbrook, C. H. The sport participation-social class relationship among a selected sample of female adolescents. *Sociol. Sport J.* 4:37–47, 1987.

79. Hasbrook, C. H. The sport participation-social class relationship: some recent youth sport participation data. *Sociol. Sport J.* 3:154–159, 1986.

80. Hauser, W. J., and L. B. Lueptow. Participation in athletics and academic achievement: a replication and extension. *Sociol. Q.* 19:304–309, 1978.

81. Helanko, R. Sports and socialization. *Acta Sociol.* 2:229–240, 1957.

82. Hill, P., and B. Lowe. The inevitable metathesis of the retiring athlete. *Int. Rev. Sport Sociol.* 4:5–29, 1974.

83. Hoch, P. *Rip off the big game.* Garden City, NY: Doubleday & Co., 1972.

84. Howell, F. M., Miracle, A. W., and Rees, C. R. Do high school athletics pay? The effects of varsity participation on socioeconomic attainment. *Sociol. Sport J.* 1:15–25, 1984.

85. Hughes, R. H., and J. Coakley. Positive deviance among athletes: the implications of overconformity to the sport ethic. Sociol. Sport J. 8:307–325, 1991.

86. Inkeles, A. Social structure and socialization. In D. A. Goslin (ed.). *Handbook of socialization theory and research.* Chicago: Rand McNally, 1969, pp. 615–632.

87. Jerome, W., and J. C. Phillips. The relationship between academic achievement and interscholastic participation: a comparison of Canadian and American high schools. *CAHPER J.* 37:18–21, 1971.

88. Johns, D. P., K. J. Lindner, and K. Wolko. Understanding attrition in female competitive gymnastics: applying social exchange theory. *Sociol. Sport J.* 7:154–171, 1990.

89. Kenyon, G. The use of path analysis in sport sociology with reference to involvement socialization. *Int. Rev. Sport Sociol.* 5:191–203, 1970.

90. Kenyon, G., and B. D. McPherson. Becoming involved in physical activity and sport: a process of socialization. In G. L. Rarick (ed.). *Physical activity: Human growth and development.* New York: Academic Press, 1973, pp. 303–332.

91. Kidd, B., and J. Mcfarland. *The death of hockey.* Toronto: New Press, 1972.

92. Kleiber, D., S. L. Greendorfer, E. Blinde, D. Samdahl. Quality of exit from university sports and life satisfaction in early adulthood. *Sociol. Sport J.* 4:28–36, 1987.

93. Kleiber, D., and G. Roberts. The effects of sport experience in the development of social character: an exploratory investigation. *J. Sport Psychol.* 3:114–122, 1981.

94. Klint, K. A., and M. R. Weiss. Perceived competence and motives for participating in youth sports: a test of Harter's Competence Motivation Theory. *J. Sport Psychol* 9:55–65, 1987.

95. Landers, D. M., and D. M. Landers. Socialization via interscholastic athletics: its effects on delinquency. *Sociol. Educ.* 51:299–303, 1978.

96. Leaman, O., and B. Carrington, Athleticism and the reproduction of gender and ethnic marginality. *Leisure Studies* 4:205–218, 1985.

97. Lee, M. J. Moral and social growth through sport: the coach's role. In G. Gleeson (ed.). *The growing child in competitive sport.* London: Hodder & Stoughton, 1986, pp. 248–255.

98. Leonard, W. M. Socialization into an avocational subculture. *J. Sport Behav.* 14:169–188, 1991.

99. Lerch, S. Athletic retirement as social death: an overview. In N. Theberge and P. Donnelly (eds.). *Sport and the sociological imagination.* Fort Worth: Texas ·Christian University Press, 1984, pp. 259–272.

100. Lerch, S. The adjustment to retirement of professional baseball players. In S. L. Greendorfer and A. Yiannakis (eds.). *Sociology of sport: diverse perspectives.* West Point, NY: Leisure Press, 1981, pp. 138–148.

101. LeUnes, A. D., and J. R. Nation. *Sport psychology.* Chicago: Nelson-Hall, 1989.

102. Lewko, J. H., and M. E. Ewing. Sex differences and parental influence in sport involvement of children. *J. Sport Psychol.* 2:63–68, 1980.

103. Lewko, J. H., and S. L. Greendorfer. Family influences in sport socialization of children and adolescents. In F. L. Smoll, R. A. Magill, and M. J. Ash (eds.). *Children in sport.* Champaign, IL: Human Kinetics Publishers, Inc., 1988, pp. 287–300.

104. Loy, J. W. Social origins and occupational mobility of a selected sample of American athletes. *Int. Rev. Sport Sociol.* 7:5–23, 1972.

105. Loy, J. W. The study of sport and social mobility. In G. S. Kenyon (ed.). *Sociology of sport.* Chicago: The Athletic Institute, 1969, pp. 101–119.

106. Loy, J. W., and A. G. Ingham. Play, games, and sport in the psychosocial development of children and youth. In G. L. Rarick (ed.). *Physical activity: human growth and potential.* New York: Academic Press, 1973, pp. 257–302.

107. Marsh, H. W. Verbal and math self-concepts: an internal/external frame of reference model. *Am. Educ. Res. J.* 23:129–149, 1986.

108. Marsh, H. W., and N. Peart. Competitive and cooperative physical fitness training programs for girls: effects on physical fitness and multidimensional self-concepts. *J. Sport Exerc. Psychol.* 10:390–407, 1988.

109. Marsh, H. W., G. E. Richards, and J. Barnes. Multidimensional self-concepts: the effect of participation in an Outward Bound program. *J. Personal. Social Psychol.* 50:195–204, 1986.

110. Marsh, H. W., I. D. Smith, M. Marsh, and L. Owens. The transition from single-sex to coeducational high schools: effects on multiple dimensions of self-concept and on academic achievement. *Am Educ. Res. J.* 25:237–269, 1988.

111. Martens, R. *Joy and sadness in children's sports.* Champaign, IL: Human Kinetics Publishers, 1978.

112. Martin, D. E., and R. A. Dodder. Socialization experiences and level of terminating participation in sports. *J. Sport Behav.* 14:113–128, 1991.

113. McCormack, J. B., and L. Chalip. Sport as socialization: a critique of methodological premises. *Social Sci. J.* 25:83–92, 1988.

114. McElroy, M. Sport participation and educational aspirations: an explicit consideration of academic and sport value climates. *Res. Q.* 40:241–248, 1979.

115. McGuire, J., and D. L. Cook. The influence of others and the decision to participate in youth sports. *J. Sport Behav.* 6:9–16, 1983.

116. McGuire, J., and M. Thomas. Effects of sex, competence and competition on sharing behavior in children. *J. Personal. Soc. Psychol.* 32, 490–494, 1975.

117. McPherson, B. Retirement from professional sport: the process and problems of occupational and psychological adjustment. *Sociol. Symp.* 30:126–143, 1980.
118. McPherson, B. D. Socialization into and through sport. In G. Luschen and G. H. Sage (eds.). *Handbook of social science of sport.* Champaign, IL: Stipes, 1981, pp. 246–273.
119. McPherson, B. D. Socialization theory and research: toward a "new wave" of scholarly inquiry in a sport context. In C. R. Rees and A. W. Miracle (eds.). *Sport and social theory.* Champaign, IL: Human Kinetics Publishers, Inc., 1986, pp. 111–134.
120. McPherson, B. D. Sport participation across the life cycle: a review of the literature and suggestions for future research. *Sociol. Sport J.* 1:213–230, 1984.
121. McPherson, B. D., and B. Brown. The structure, processes, and consequences of sport for children. In F. L. Smoll, R. A. Magill, and M. J. Ash (eds.). *Children in sport.* Champaign, IL: Human Kinetics, 1988, pp. 265–286.
122. McPherson, B. D., L. N. Guppy, and J. P. McKay. The social structure of the game and sport milieu. In J. G. Albinson and G. M. Andrews (eds.). *Child in sport and physical activity.* Baltimore: University Park Press, 1976, pp. 161–200.
123. Meggyesy, D. *Out of their league.* New York: Paperback Library, 1971.
124. Melnick, M. J., B. E. Vanfossen, and D. F. Sabo. Developmental effects of athletic participation among high school girls. *Sociol. Sport J.* 1:22–36, 1988.
125. Messner, M. A. *Power at play: sports and the problem of masculinity.* Boston: Beacon Press, 1992.
126. Messner, M. A., and D. Groisser. Intercollegiate athletic participation and academic achievement. In A. O. Dunleavy, A. W. Miracle, and C. R. Rees (eds.). *Studies in the sociology of sport.* Fort Worth: Texas Christian University Press, 1982, pp. 257–270.
127. Meyer, B. B. From idealism to actualization: the academic performance of female collegiate athletes. *Sociol. Sport J.* 7:44–57, 1990.
128. Musgrave. P. W. *Socializing contexts: the subject in society.* Boston: Allen & Unwin, 1987.
129. Nixon, H. L. II. An exploratory study of the effects of encouragement and pressure on the sports socialization of males and females. In S. L. Greendorfer and A. Yiannakis (eds.). *Sociology of sport: diverse perspectives.* West Point, NY: Leisure Press, 1981, pp. 83–94.
130. Nixon, H. L. II. Rethinking socialization and sport. *J. Sport Soc. Issues* 14:33–47, 1990.
131. Nixon, H. L. II. Accepting the risks and pain of sports injuries: understanding the nature of "consent" to play. Presented at the North American Society for the Sociology of Sport Conference, Milwaukee, 1991.
132. Ogilvie, B. C., and T. A. Tutko. Sport: if you want to build character, try something else. *Psychol. Today* 5:60–63, 1971.
133. O'Hanlon, T. Interscholastic athletics, 1900–1940: shaping citizens for unequal roles in modern industrial states. *Educ. Theory* 30:89–103, 1980.
134. Okihiro, N. Extracurricular participation, educational destinies and early job outcomes. In N. Theberge and P. Donnelly (eds.). *Sport and the sociological imagination.* Fort Worth: Texas Christian University Press, 1984, pp. 334–349.
135. Oliver, M. Race, class and the family's orientation to mobility through sport. *Sociol. Symp.* 30:62–86, 1980.
136. Orlick, T. D. The athletic dropout—a high price of efficiency. *CAHPER J.* (November/December): 21–27, 1974.
137. Orlick, T. D., and C. Botterill. *Every kid can win.* Chicago, IL: Nelson-Hall, 1975.
138. Otto, L. B., and D. F. Alwin. Athletics, aspirations and attainments. *Sociol. Educ.* 42:102–113, 1977.
139. Palzkill, B. Between gymshoes and high-heels—the development of a lesbian identity and existence in top class sport. *Int. Rev. Sociol. Sport* 25:221–233, 1990.
140. Patriksson, G. Theoretical and empirical analyses of drop-outs from youth sport in Sweden. Presented at the ICHPER World Conference, Vancouver, 1987.
141. Petrie, B. M. The political attitudes of Canadian university students: a comparison

between athletes and non-athletes." Presented at the AAHPERD Conference, Minneapolis, 1973.

142. Picou, J. S. Race, athletic achievement and educational aspiration. *Sociol. Q.* 19:429–438, 1978.

143. Picou, J. S., V. McCarter, and F. M. Howell. Do high school athletics pay? Some further evidence. *Sociol. Sport J.* 2:72–76, 1985.

144. Prus, R. Career contingencies: examining patterns of involvement. In N. Theberge and P. Donnelly (eds.). *Sport and the sociological imagination.* Fort Worth: Texas Christian University Press, 1984, pp. 297–317.

145. Rankin, J. H. Social factors and delinquency: interactions by age and sex. *Sociol. Soc. Res.* 64:420–434, 1980.

146. Rees, C. R., F. M. Howell, and A. W. Miracle. Do high school sports build character? A quasi-experiment on a national sample. *Soc. Sci. J.* 27:303–315, 1990.

147. Rehberg, R. A., and M. Cohen. Athletes and scholars: an analysis of the compositional characteristics of these two youth culture categories. *Int. Rev. Sport Sociol.* 10:91–106, 1975.

148. Rehberg, R. A., and Cohen, M. Political attitudes and participation in extra-curricular activities with special emphasis on interscholastic athletics. Presented at Sport and Social Deviancy Conference, SUNY-Brockport, 1971.

149. Rehberg, R. A., and W. E. Schafer. Participation in interscholastic athletics and college expectations. *Am. J. Sociol.* 73:732–740, 1968.

150. Reynolds, M. The effects of sports retirement on the job satisfaction of the former football player. In S. L. Greendorfer and A. Yiannakis (eds.). *Sociology of sport: Diverse perspectives.* West Point, NY: Leisure Press, 1981, pp. 127–137.

151. Roberts, G. C., D. A. Kleiber, and J. L. Duda. An analysis of motivation in children's sport: the role of perceived competence in participation. *J. Sport Psychol.* 3:206–216, 1981.

152. Roberts, J. M., and B. Sutton-Smith. Child training and game involvement. *Ethnology* 1:166–185, 1962.

153. Robins, D. Sport and youth culture. In J. Hargreaves (ed.). *Sport, culture and ideology.* Boston: Routledge & Kegan Paul, 1982, pp. 136–151.

154. Romance, T. J., M. R. Weiss, and J. Bockoven. A program to promote moral development through elementary school physical education. *J. Teaching Phys. Educ.* 5:126–136, 1986.

155. Rosenberg, E. Athletic retirement as social death: Concepts and perspectives. In N. Theberge and P. Donnelly (eds.). *Sport and the sociological imagination.* Fort Worth: Texas Christian University Press, 1984, pp. 245–258.

156. Rudman, W. J. Age and involvement in sport and physical activity. *Sociol. Sport J.* 6:228–246, 1989.

157. Sabo, D. F. Pigskin, patriarchy, and pain. *Changing men: issues in gender, sex and politics* 16:24–25, 1986.

158. Sabo, D. F., and J. Panepinto. Football ritual and the social reproduction of masculinity. In M. A. Messner and D. F. Sabo (eds.). *Sport, men, and the gender order.* Champaign, IL: Human Kinetics Books, 1990, pp. 115–126.

159. Sack, A., and R. Theil. College football and social mobility: a case study of Notre Dame football players. *Sociol. Educ.* 52:60–66, 1979.

160. Sage, G. H. An occupational analysis of the college coach. In D. W. Ball and J. W. Loy (eds.). *Sport and social order.* Reading, MA: Addison-Wesley Publishing Company, 1975, pp. 391–456.

161. Sage, G. H. Parental influence and socialization into sport for male and female intercollegiate athletes. *J. Sport Soc. Issues* 4:1–13, 1980.

162. Sage, G. H. Socialization and sport. In G. H. Sage (ed.). *Sport and American society.* Reading, MA: Addison-Wesley, 1980, pp. 133–142.

163. Sapp, M., and J. Haubenstricker. Motivation for joining and reasons for not

continuing in youth sport programs in Michigan. Presented at American Alliance for Health, Physical Education, Recreation and Dance Conference, Kansas City, 1978.

164. Schafer, W. E. Some social sources and consequences of interscholastic athletics: the case of participation and delinquency. In G. Kenyon (ed.). *Aspects of contemporary sport sociology.* Chicago, IL: The Athletic Institute, 1969, pp. 29–44.

165. Schafer, W. E. Sport, socialization and the school. Presented at the Third Annual Symposium of the Sociology of Sport, Waterloo, Ontario, 1971.

166. Schafer, W. E., and J. M. Armer. Athletes are not inferior students. *Trans-action* 6:21–26, 61–62, 1968.

167. Scott, J. *The athletic revolution.* New York: The Free Press, 1971.

168. Scott, L. Career contingencies: the social construction of continuing involvements in women's intercollegiate basketball. Presented at the North American Society for the Sociology of Sport Conference, Toronto, 1982.

169. Scraton, S. "Boys muscle in where angels fear to tread"—girls' subcultures and physical activities. In J. Horne, D. Jary, and A. Tomlinson (eds.). *Sport, leisure and social relations.* New York: Routledge & Kegan Paul (Sociological Review Monograph 33), 1987, pp. 160–186.

170. Segrave, J. Do organized sports programs deter delinquency? *J. Phys. Educ. Recreation Dance* 57:16–17, 1986.

171. Segrave, J., and D. Chu. Athletics and juvenile delinquency. *Rev. Sport Leisure* 3:1–24, 1978.

172. Segrave, J., and D. N. Hastad. Delinquent behavior and interscholastic athletic participation. *J. Sport Behav.* 5:96–111, 1982.

173. Segrave, J., C. Moreau, and D. N. Hastad. An investigation into the relationship between ice hockey participation and delinquency. *Sociol. Sport J.* 2:281–298, 1985.

174. Semyonov, M. Sport and beyond: ethnic inequalities in attainment. *Sociol. Sport J.* 1:358–365, 1984.

175. Shaw, G. *Meat on the hoof.* New York: St. Martins Press, 1972.

176. Silva, J. The perceived legitimacy of rule violating behavior in sport. *J. Sport Psychol.* 5:438–448.

177. SIRLS Sport & Leisure Database. Annotated bibliography: Sport and academic achievement. *Sociol. Sport J.* 3:87–94, 1986.

178. SIRLS Sport & Leisure Database. Annotated bibliography: Sport and deviance. *Sociol. Sport J.* 4:91–98, 1987.

179. SIRLS Sport & Leisure Database. Annotated bibliography: High school sport. *Sociol. Sport J.* 5:390–398, 1988.

180. SIRLS Sport and Leisure Database. Annotated bibliography: Socialization in sport. *Sociol. Sport J.* 6:294–302, 1989.

181. SIRLS Sport & Leisure Database. Annotated bibliography: Sport and social mobility. *Sociol. Sport J.* 7:95–102, 1990.

182. Smith, M. *Violence and sport.* Toronto: Butterworths, 1983.

183. Snyder, E. E. Aspects of socialization in sports and physical education. *Quest* 14:1–7, 1970.

184. Snyder, E. E. High school athletes and their coaches: educational plans and advice. *Sociol. Educ.* 45:313–325, 1972.

185. Snyder, E. E., and L. Baber. A profile of former college athletes and nonathletes: leisure activities, attitudes towards work, and aspects of satisfaction with life. *J. Sport Behav.* 2:211–219, 1979.

186. Snyder, E. E., and D. A. Purdy. Socialization into sport: parent and child reverse and reciprocal effects. *Res. Q. Exerc. Sport* 53:263–266, 1982.

187. Snyder, E. E., and E. Spreitzer. Correlates of sport participation among adolescent girls. *Res. Q.* 47:804–809, 1976.

188. Snyder, E. E., and E. Spreitzer. Family influence and involvement in sports. *Res. Q.* 44:249–255, 1973.

189. Snyder, E. E., and E. Spreitzer. High school athletic participation as related to college attendance among Black, Hispanic, and White males. *Youth Soc.* 21:390–398, 1990.

190. Snyder, E. E., and E. Spreitzer. Socialization comparisions of adolescent female athletes and musicians. *Res. Q.* 49:342–350, 1978.

191. Spady, W. G. Lament for the letterman: effects of peer status and extra curricular activities on goals and achievement. *Am. J. Sociol.* 75:680–702, 1970.

192. Spreitzer, E. E., and M. Pugh. Interscholastic athletics and educational expectations. *Sociol. Educ.* 46:171–182, 1973.

193. Spreitzer, E., and E. E. Snyder. Socialization into sport: an exploratory path analysis. *Res. Q.* 47:238–245, 1976.

194. Stark, R., L. Kent, and R. Finke. Sports and delinquency. In M. Gottfredson and T. Hirshi (eds.). *Positive criminology.* Beverly Hills, CA: Sage Publications, 1987, pp. 115–124.

195. Stevenson, C. L. College athletics and "character": the decline and fall of socialization research. In D. Chu, J. O. Segrave, and B. J. Becker (eds.). *Sport and higher education.* Champaign, IL: Human Kinetics, 1985, pp. 249–266.

196. Stevenson, C. L. Institutionalization and college sport. *Res. Q.* 47:1–8, 1976.

197. Stevenson, C. L. Socialization effects of participation in sport: a critical review of the research. *Res. Q.* 46:287–301, 1975.

198. Stevenson, C. L. The athletic career: some contingencies of sport specialization. *J. Sport Behav.* 13:103–113, 1990.

199. Stevenson, C. L. The early careers of international athletes. *Sociol. Sport J.* 7:238–253, 1990.

200. Sutton-Smith, B. *The folkgames of children.* Austin, TX: University of Texas Press, 1972.

201. Sutton-Smith, B., and J. M. Roberts. The cross-cultural and psychological study of games. In G. Luschen (ed.). *The cross-cultural analysis of sport and games.* Champaign, IL: Stipes Publishing Co., 1970, pp. 100–108.

202. Swain, D. A. Withdrawal from sport and Schlossberg's model of transitions. *Sociol. Sport J.* 8:152–160, 1991.

203. Talbot, M. Beating them at our own game? Women's sport involvement. In E. Wimbush and M. Talbot (eds.). *Relative freedoms: women and leisure.* Philadelphia: Open University Press, 1988, pp. 102–114.

204. Theberge, N. On the need for a more adequate theory of sport participation. *Sociol. Sport J.* 1:26–35, 1984.

205. Thomas, C. E., and K. L. Ermler. Institutional obligations in the athletic retirement process. *Quest* 40:137–150, 1988.

206. Thorlindsson, T. Sport participation, smoking, and drug and alcohol abuse among Icelandic youth. *Sociol. Sport J.* 6:136–143, 1989.

207. Trulson, M. E. Martial arts training: a novel "cure" for juvenile delinquency. *Hum. Relat.* 39:1131–1140, 1986.

208. Vealey, R. S. Sport personology: a paradigmatic and methodological analysis. *J. Sport Exerc. Psychol.* 11:216–235, 1989.

209. Watson, G. G. Games, socialization and parental values: social class differences in parental evaluation of Little League baseball. *Int. Rev. Sociol. Sport* 12:17–48, 1977.

210. Weiss, M. R., and B. J. L. Bredemeier. Moral development in sport. *Exerc. Sport Sci. Rev.* 18:331–378, 1990.

211. Weiss, M. R., and A. Knoppers. The influence of socializing agents on female intercollegiate volleyball players. *J. Sport Psychol.* 4:267–279, 1982.

212. Wells, R. H., and J. S. Picou. Interscholastic athletes and socialization for educational achievement. *J. Sport Behav.* 3:119–128, 1980.

213. Wentworth, W. M. *Context and understanding: an inquiry into socialization theory.* New York: Elsevier, 1980.

214. Yamaguchi, Y. A cross-national study of socialization into physical activity in corporate settings: the case of Japan and Canada. *Sociol. Sport J.* 4:61–77, 1987.

7
Orthostasis: Exercise and Exercise Training

G. GEELEN, Ph.D.

J. E. GREENLEAF, Ph.D.

INTRODUCTION

Since humans have evolved in a 1-G environment with the brain at the end of a linear hydrostatic column, adaptation to the upright posture is a continuing problem. The daily requirement for stimulation of the physiological system to maintain brain perfusion to counteract the tendency for blood pressure to decrease has not been resolved. Normal, ambulatory people on earth spend approximately 8 hr/day sleeping in the horizontal body position where considerable body movement occurs, and about 16 hr/day in the sitting, standing, and ambulatory modes. It is uncertain whether the 8 hr horizontal to 16 hr/day upright posture ratio is optimal, but many years of trial and error suggest it is. There is continuing discussion concerning the portion of the 16 hr that should be devoted to physical exercise; what mode, intensity, and duration of time should be devoted to the performance of exercise training, and whether there is a positive or negative interaction between maintenance of the upright posture (brain perfusion) via muscular movement and exercise training. While ambulatory earth-bound people alternate sitting and standing body positions frequently and "decondition" during sleep for about 8 hr/day, the horizontal to upright postural adaptive mechanism is stimulated daily. On the other hand, the deconditioning (adaptation) interval for astronauts in microgravity has varied between a few days to 1 yr and it is uncertain whether the 8 hr/16 hr ratio is optimal for them. Some hospitalized or nursing home patients spend years in bed, and one man in Laurel Springs, North Carolina has remained in bed continuously since 1932 [2]; he had not sat up since 1942 nor rolled over since 1960. Clearly, postural adaptation is not necessary for life, but it surely is necessary for mobility.

The word orthostatic, derived from the Greek word *statos*—verbal of *histanai* to cause to stand—is defined: "of, relating to, or caused by erect posture" [43]. The word orthostasis is also often used in reference to physiological responses induced by lower body negative pressure (LBNP) and head-to-foot (+ Gz) acceleration. In this review, orthostasis will refer only to standing or head-up tilted (HUT) postures. Orthostatic tolerance is the time a subject can tolerate standing or head-up suspension, when the physiological system can no longer compensate for the stress, resulting in *presyncopal symptoms* and subsequent fainting, i.e., the actual point of *orthostatic tolerance*. For humane reasons, the time to onset of presyncopal symptoms should generally be used as tolerance.

Evidence is accumulating that suggests that while some responses to tilting, LBNP, and slow-onset +Gz acceleration may be qualitatively similar (for example, all three stressors cause blood stagnation in the legs and ultimately lead to partial and then to complete loss of consciousness), their cardiovascular and hormonal response patterns and fainting mechanisms may not be similar quantitatively [45, 118, 124]. Thus, it should not be assumed that data and conclusions obtained from studies of these three gravitational stressors can be interchanged without definitive evidence that comparable stress has been induced. Also, a clear distinction must be made between effects of a treatment (exercise) and a condition (trained or untrained) on physiological responses or tolerance: the former (responses) should not be used to define the latter (tolerance) until cause and effect has been established.

There is evidence suggesting that endurance-trained athletes fail to maintain adequate blood pressure responses when exposed to gravitational challenges: HUT or standing [9, 11, 63, 75, 107, 109, 110], LBNP [69–71, 105], but apparently there are no reports of adverse responses to +Gz acceleration [35, 59, 60, 61, 120, 121]. Conversely, there are findings indicating that a period of aerobic endurance training has no deleterious effect on *tolerance* to upright tilting [19, 45, 46], to LBNP [19, 20, 36, 67], or to +Gz acceleration [3, 21, 28, 29, 44, 45, 114, 120, 122]. The propensity for muscular and presumably fit men to faint when presented with a stressful situation is not a new observation [34].

Because some exercise-trained athletes have exhibited "adverse" changes in some gravitational stress responses and tolerances, a few investigators [108] have concluded—possibly incorrectly—that the changes were due only to the exercise-training procedures without measuring orthostatic responses before training, and considering other possible contributing factors such as hereditary predisposition.

Because of these divergent responses, some essential questions arise. *(a)* Is the reported enhancement of fainting in some endurance-trained subjects due to environmental factors; i.e., physiological adaptations of the blood pressure control system to their continual, intermittent exercise training, or to a primary or modifying influence of hereditary factors that separate "athletes" from nonathletes? *(b)* Is gravitational intolerance a characteristic of untrained subjects with high hereditary aerobic capacity (peak oxygen uptake), or is it a function of the exercise-training process itself? *(c)* Do presyncopal and syncopal responses to these three gravitational stressors (HUT, LBNP, +Gz acceleration) occur via the same or similar mechanisms? Can tolerance to one be equated or compared directly with tolerances of the other two? *(d)* Can physiological responses occurring prior to the presyncopal state be used to predict the point of tolerance? *(e)* Does deconditioning, induced by reducing or ceasing exercise training or by prolonged exposure to water immersion or bed rest, modify the incidence of presyncopal signs and symptoms in untrained or endurance-trained subjects?

Reviews by Harrison [48], Convertino [12], Ebert and Barney [25], and Tipton [116] have discussed some aspects of the problem: hopefully the present review will add further insights.

The purpose for this paper is to review evidence and discuss possible mechanisms concerning the effect of various levels of exercise training in athletes and nonathletes on control of blood pressure as it relates to the fainting response in the head-up posture (orthostasis), with relevant findings from LBNP and + Gz acceleration studies.

SUPPORT FOR THE HYPOTHESIS THAT ORTHOSTATIC INTOLERANCE IS ASSOCIATED WITH AEROBIC CAPACITY

Cross-sectional Studies

Observations from both space missions and ground-based simulations of microgravity (immersion and bed rest) have suggested the hypothesis that endurance-trained athletes may be less tolerant to gravitational stress, i.e., they may have lower orthostatic tolerance. From the 1973 Skylab 4 mission, higher heart rates, lower pulse pressures (Table 7.1) [115], and greater incidence of presyncopal symptoms in response to LBNP application in flight were observed in the scientist pilot and pilot whose aerobic capacities ($\dot{V}O_2max$) were 49 and 47 ml·min^{-1}·kg^{-1}, respectively, than in the commander who had a somewhat lower $\dot{V}O_2max$ of 40 ml·min^{-1}·kg^{-1} [55, 78]. Compared with the commander's responses, there were greater vascular compliances in the scientist pilot and pilot [115]: essentially similar observations were made postflight. These findings suggested that moderately intensive endurance training by the scientist pilot and pilot in flight were associated with decreased LBNP tolerance, although tolerance was not measured; results of ground-based studies supported this concept. Reduced total body water and hypovolemia in the astronauts in flight and immediately after landing could partially explain their reduced LBNP tolerance. Stegemann and associates [107–110] have observed significantly greater incidences of presyncopal symptoms to HUT in athletes and trained men after 4 to 8 hr of head-out water immersion. Reduced total body water and hypovolemia in the astronauts and immersed subjects could contribute to their reduced gravitational tolerances. Luft et al. [69, 71] reported that LBNP tolerance (to presyncope) decreased by 42% in five

TABLE 7.1
Differences Between Mean In-flight Values for Heart Rate and Blood Pressure of the Skylab 4 Crewmen During Rest and 50 mm Hg Phase of LBNP from Corresponding Mean Values During Preflight Tests

	Commander	Scientist Pilot	Pilot
Resting control			
Heart rate (bpm)	+7.8*	+13.3*	+11.3*
Systolic blood pressure (mm Hg)	+1.8	+2.5	+1.0
Diastolic blood pressure (mm Hg)	−5.6*	−2.0	−2.5
Pulse pressure (mm Hg)	+7.4*	+4.5*	+3.4
Mean arterial pressure (mm Hg)	−3.2*	−0.5	−1.3
Stressed—50 mm Hg:			
Heart rate (bpm)	+12.2*	+36.7*	+26.7*
Systolic blood pressure (mm Hg)	+6.2*	+10.9*	−1.6
Diastolic blood pressure (mm Hg)	−1.0	−4.8	+1.3
Pulse pressure (mm Hg)	+7.1*	+6.1	−2.8
Mean arterial pressure (mm Hg)	−1.5	−6.8*	+0.3

*$P < 0.05$ by Student's paired t-test.

trained runners ($\bar{X}$ cycle ergometer $\dot{V}O_2max$ = 50 ml·min^{-1}·kg^{-1}) compared to that of five untrained men ($\dot{V}O_2max$ = 34 ml·min^{-1}·kg^{-1}). In addition, more blood shifted into the runners' lower limbs during LBNP suggesting greater venous compliance. Klein et al. [62] reviewed responses of athletes and nonathletes exposed to altitude, acceleration, orthostasis, simulated weightlessness, and spaceflight. They derived from the data of Luft et al. [71] a significant inverse relationship ($r = -0.60$) between $\dot{V}O_2max$ and LBNP tolerance, together with a significant positive relationship ($r = 0.72$) between $\dot{V}O_2max$ and lower limb compliance. Later, Luft et al. [69] studied 37 athletes (13 endurance runners, 12 weight-lifters, 12 swimmers) and 10 nonathletes, whose mean $\dot{V}O_2max$ were 51, 39, 35, and 35 ml·min^{-1}·kg^{-1}, respectively. Tolerance to progressive LBNP was significantly less in the 13 runners than in all 34 nonrunners combined. Moreover, heart rate increased less and changes in leg volume (venous compliance) were larger during LBNP in the runners when compared with all other groups. They concluded that it was the exercise training-induced high aerobic capacity that caused the lower LBNP tolerance, but indices of aerobic capacity ($\dot{V}O_2max$) were not measured before training. The suggested mechanism was an increase in leg compliance, together with increased cardiac parasympathetic tone, which limited the cardioacceleration required to maintain venous return.

Stegemann et al. [108] compared systemic blood pressure responses in 25 young, highly trained athletes with those in 25 young, untrained students by changing transmural pressure in the carotid artery with an upper body pressure dome. Because the curve relating carotid artery transmural pressure and mean arterial blood pressure was significantly flatter in the athletes (Fig. 7.1), they concluded that "endurance training obviously reduces the effectiveness of the blood pressure control system"; but blood pressure responses were not measured before training (see section on arterial baroreflex control). Mangseth and Bernauer [78] subjected four highly fit endurance-trained athletes ($\dot{V}O_2$max = 67 ml·min^{-1}·kg^{-1}) and four other normally fit nonendurance-trained subjects ($\dot{V}O_2$max = 53 ml·min^{-1}·kg^{-1}) to 30 min of HUT. All highly fit men fainted ($\tilde{X}$ tolerance = 17 min) while all normally fit subjects tolerated 30 min of tilt. Since systolic volume decreased by 43% in both groups upon tilt, cardiac output decreased more in nonfainters (-18.5%) than in fainters (-6.7%), and these responses took place without inordinate leg blood pooling, syncope did not appear to be the result of decreased stroke volume or cardiac output. Rather, a fundamental difference in regulation of total peripheral resistance was suggested between the fainters and nonfainters. These results are interesting because orthostatic intolerance occurred in extremely fit subjects and not in normally fit subjects suggesting perhaps an hereditary factor, which engenders high endurance capacity, is somehow related to low orthostatic tolerance. Charles and Richardson [11] demonstrated differences between runners and nonrunners in their responses to thoracic blood volume changes elicited by 10° HUT or head-down tilts (HDT). Since mean arterial and pulse pressures were not affected by either HUT or HDT, decreased effectiveness of cardiopulmonary baroreceptors was implicated.

From an extensive study of subjects with varying levels of training and $\dot{V}O_2$max, Levine et al. [65] found that decreased tolerance to LBNP was not a simple linear function of aerobic capacity and that $\dot{V}O_2$max was a poor estimation of LBNP tolerance; a more complex interaction of stroke volume, maximal leg conductance, and baroreflex function appears to be an important factor in the mechanism of tolerance. They proposed a new nonbaroreceptor hypothesis to explain the apparent reduced (nonsignificant) orthostatic tolerance in "athletes" ($\dot{V}O_2$max >60 ml·min^{-1}·kg^{-1} vs. nonathletes ($\dot{V}O_2$max <45 ml·min^{-1}·kg^{-1}) [66]. The basis for the hypothesis was that athletes had steeper ventricular function and flatter diastolic-pressure curves over the physiological range of filling pressures when exposed to LBNP and after rapid infusion of isotonic saline. The athletes always had greater stroke volumes in response to all changes in blood volumes and cardiac filling pressures, and their pressure-volume curve shifted downward to the right suggesting greater ventricular diastolic chamber compliance and distensibility as a result of chronic training-induced increase in central blood volume. Thus, without incorporating basic factors for blood pressure regulation, e.g., baroreflex control of heart rate and peripheral

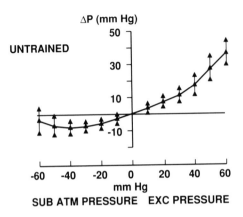

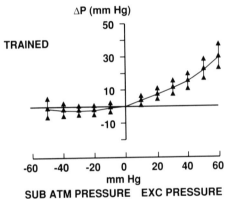

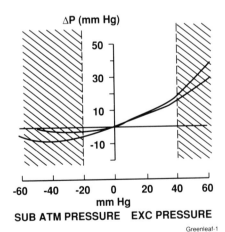

Greenleaf-1

FIGURE 7.1

Responses of mean arterial blood pressures to subatmospheric (**SUB ATM PRESSURE**) *and excessive atmospheric dome pressures* (**EXC PRESSURE**) *(referenced to atmospheric pressure) in untrained* (**top panel**) *and trained* (**middle panel**) *subjects.* **Arrows** *indicate* ± *SD.* **Bottom panel** *presents* **shaded areas** *where the superimposed curves are different (P<0.05). Redrawn and reprinted with permission of Stegemann, J., A. Busert, and D. Brock. Influence of fitness on the blood pressure control system in man.* Aerospace Med. *45:45–48, 1974.*

resistance, Levine et al. [66] proposed that stroke volume might be an important independent factor not controlled by the autonomic nervous system, and that exercise training modifies diastolic properties of the heart, which can be mechanical, autonomic-independent causes of orthostatic intolerance. Again, since their measurements were not taken before training, it cannot be determined if these responses in the athletes were due to training.

Thus, findings from cross-sectional studies [55, 78] suggest: that endurance training in astronauts during exposure to microgravity causes decreased LBNP tolerance (that was not measured); that endurance-trained runners and athletes had lower LBNP and orthostatic tolerances than comparable less-trained or untrained subjects [69, 71, 75]; and that aerobic capacity was inversely related to LBNP tolerance [62]. The usual, untenable, explanation was that the exercise training-induced elevation of aerobic capacity was related to or caused the decreased tolerance despite the fact that aerobic capacity was not measured before and occasionally not after training. An equally plausible explanation for decreased tolerance in endurance-trained subjects is that they have an hereditary predisposition that allows them to run but not to stand. The only way to answer this question is to measure aerobic capacity and gravitational tolerance before and after a period of exercise training.

SUPPORT FOR THE HYPOTHESIS THAT ORTHOSTATIC INTOLERANCE IS NOT ASSOCIATED WITH AEROBIC CAPACITY

Cross-sectional Studies

Early in this century it was suggested that athletic training may result in better circulatory adjustments to standing [22, 117]. Hyman [53] indicated that 280 "well-conditioned" athletes showed little variation or deviation, but chiefly positive changes, to the four phases of blood pressure responses comprising the Postural Mean Blood Pressure Index (blood pressure recorded after 1 min standing, after 3 min supine, immediately after, then after 1 min of standing up quickly). This index was always negative when the test was applied to 411 nonathletic but "normal" students. The influence of physical fitness on gravitational tolerance was measured, using 20 min of 90° passive HUT or $+Gz$ tolerance, on 12 highly fit athletes ($\dot{V}O_2max = 65$ ml·min^{-1}·kg^{-1}) and 12 healthy, sedentary students ($\dot{V}O_2max = 44$ ml·min^{-1}·kg^{-1}) [59, 60]. HUT and $+Gz$ tolerances were almost identical: with HUT, there were 5 of 12 fainters among the athletes and 4 of 12 in the controls and, with the exception of heart rate, which was 22% lower in the athletes during tilt; the responses of blood and pulse pressures during tilt in the nonfainters were essentially the same in both groups. Thus, neither orthostatic tolerance nor acceleration tolerance was related to the level of aerobic capacity, and there was no significant correlation between the orthostatic and acceleration tolerances. In a following study, Klein et al. [61] completed their previous work by having highly trained athletes and nonathletes undergo submaximal and maximal loading tests: orthostasis during a 20-min 90° passive HUT, acceleration, hypoxia, exercise, and exercise in hypoxia. Again, the number of fainters and responses of blood and pulse pressures in the two groups during tilting showed only minor differences. These data did not support the hypothesis of deterioration in tolerance to tilting in highly-trained athletes. Shvartz [96] studied responses to 20-min passive 70° HUT performed after "endurance training" in 17 young men. Five subjects fainted but it appeared that nonfainters performed better than fainters on all exercise tests, particularly in the number of sit-ups and push-ups; the latter was significantly correlated with good orthostatic adjustment. Thus, these results suggested that the condition of the abdominal muscles was an important factor for prevention of orthostatic intolerance. Then Shvartz and Meyerstein [102] showed that among 34 average-fit subjects tested for their response to a 20-min passive 70° HUT, the four subjects who fainted and the nonfainters all had similar $\dot{V}O_2$max (44 ml·min^{-1}·kg^{-1}). Later, Shvartz et al. [100] tested responses to 20-min standing against a wall (i.e., a test approximately equivalent to 70° HUT with a foot support) in 12 high-fit subjects ($\dot{V}O_2$max = 57–65 ml·min^{-1}·kg^{-1}) and in 16 untrained young men, before and after bouts of exercise of increasing duration and/or load. Before exercising, under basal conditions, the high-fit group withstood the orthostatic test better than the untrained: none of the them fainted but 3 of 16 untrained subjects did. Average blood pressure responses were similar in both groups while average heart rate responses during the 20-min HUT were significantly lower in the high-fit than in the untrained group (82 ± 8 vs 92 ± 12 bpm, respectively). Comparing responses to a 10-min HUT control test before immersion, Stegemann et al. [109] found no differences in heart rate and blood pressure changes in four trained vs. four untrained subjects. Most of these cross-sectional studies were not designed to measure presyncopal tolerance; nevertheless, in most of them, some subjects fainted.

From these cross-sectional studies it was shown that: (a) there were approximately as many fainters in trained as in untrained subject groups [59, 60]; (b) that fainters and nonfainters had similar $\dot{V}O_2$max [102]; (c) that some highly trained athletes withstood tilting better than untrained subjects [53, 100] before exercise under basal or resting conditions; and (d) that +Gz tolerance was unchanged in high-fit subjects and there were no significant correlations between +Gz tolerance and $\dot{V}O_2$max or HUT tolerance [60, 61].

Longitudinal Studies

SHORT-TERM TRAINING 1–42 DAYS). Allen et al. [1] observed increased tolerance to passive HUT in three subjects, including twins, after 3–6 weeks of training regimens utilizing graduated abdominal and trunk exercises, or badminton, rope skipping, and abdominal exercises. The three subjects who were "tiltboard" fainters before training, withstood the 20-min 70° passive HUT after training. Beetham and Buskirk [7] compared the responses to "passive" tilting (4-min 70° HUT on a tilt-table with a footboard) in sedentary subjects (control), subjects given 3 weeks of rigorous physical training (running), and subjects who were physically trained and heat acclimated (alternately walking 30 min on a treadmill and resting 30 min for 4 hr/day at 48.8°C dry bulb temperature [DBT]). Cardiovascular responses to tilting were measured before and after the subjects were dehydrated. There was no effect of training and/or heat acclimation on $\dot{V}O_2$max. Physical training with or without acclimation resulted in essentially constant systolic blood pressures and similar increases in diastolic blood pressures. Dehydration increased diastolic blood pressure and heart rate responses and induced presyncopal symptoms during tilt in two of the 14 subjects.

After observing longer tilt-tolerance in subjects after heat acclimation [102], Shvartz et al. [103] investigated whether such orthostatic improvement was the result of repeated tilting in the heat, exercise training, or both when compared with a heat-rest acclimation treatment without exercise. Eighteen young unacclimated and untrained Bantu men were allocated into three groups. All were submitted first to a 70° HUT test at 21°C (DBT) using foot supports for 20 min unless presyncope occurred; then to a second HUT (33.9°C DBT, 32.2°C wet-bulb temperature [WBT]) following either 4 hr training at 21°C DBT, 4 hr training 33.9°C DBT, or 4 hr resting at 33.9°C DBT. On 8 consecutive days exercise was block stepping at 12 steps/min, with block height adjusted to give each subject a moderate load of 35 watts. Repeated tilting alone in the heat failed to improve orthostatic responses. Exercise training in the thermoneutral environment improved orthostatic responses; an even greater improvement in the group who trained in the heat over the other groups was obvious, with no fainting episodes and lower heart rate and higher blood pressure responses during the second tilt test following training. These results suggest that exercise training or heat acclimation alone results in enhanced orthostatic responses, and that the two exercise training procedures combined act additively [103]. To clarify the reasons for improved orthostasis after training and heat acclimation, Shvartz et al. [99] measured passive HUT responses in fainters and nonfainters before and after 8 days of exercise training; cycling at 50% of $\dot{V}O_2$max for 2 hr/day either at 40°C DBT (n=5, acclimation group) or at 24°C DBT (n=5, control group). Of the five subjects who improved their responses after training (disappearance of dizziness and stabilized heart rate and blood pressure), two were acclimated, and three were controls. Improvement in orthostatic responses, especially in the nonfainters, was explained mainly by increased post-tilt plasma volume following exercise training and acclimation. Orthostasis-induced increases in plasma renin activity (PRA) and vasopressin (PVP) were attenuated by 50% and 75%, respectively, after training; the decreased PVP appeared to be a result of hypervolemia.

Convertino et al. [18] compared cardiovascular and hormonal responses to a maximum of 60 min of 60° passive HUT in 8 moderately fit young men ($\dot{V}O_2$max = 55 ml·min^{-1}·kg^{-1}) before and after 8 days of exercise training consisting of cycling for 2 hr/day at a load of 65% $\dot{V}O_2$max. Training increased $\dot{V}O_2$max by 8% (P<0.05), decreased resting heart rate (P<0.05), and increased resting plasma volume by 12.2% (P<0.05) with no change in red cell volume (RCV). Orthostatic tolerance was unchanged from 40 ± 5 min before to 47 ± 3 min after training. The post-training tilting blood pressures and PRA and PVP responses were unchanged compared with pretraining, while heart rate increased less (77 ± 3 after vs. 86 ± 4 bpm before training). More importantly, plasma volume (PV) decreased significantly during HUT as a consequence of the significant increases in PV induced by training, even though the percentage of changes in PV was similar.

On the same 10 subjects (six women aged 21–23 yr; four men aged 21–38 yr; $\dot{V}O_2$max = 47 and 64 ml·min^{-1}·kg^{-1}, respectively) Greenleaf et al. [45] compared the effect of 12 days of exercise-heat acclimation on orthostatic (70° passive HUT to presyncope) and +Gz acceleration (0.5 G·min^{-1} linear ramp to grayout) tolerances. Training consisted of 2 hr/day cycle ergometer exercise at 49% of peak $\dot{V}O_2$ for the women, and 44% for the men in 40°C DBT and 42% relative humidity (rh). Exercise-heat acclimation resulted in similar unchanged acceleration tolerances in both women and men, while there was a two-fold increase in tilt tolerance post-training in the men (from 30 min before to 54 min after, P<0.05) but no significant change in the women (from 34 to 40 min) (Fig. 7.2). However, men and women showed essentially similar training-induced resting hypervolemia (women = +11%, men = +12%), blood pressure changes, and shifts in PV and electrolytes during HUT or acceleration. While there were similar vasoactive hormone responses (except for PVP) in the women and men during HUT before and after training, differences in the magnitudes and patterns of responses of PRA, plasma catecholamines, and PVP at the point of tolerance during tilting and acceleration indicated that responses to tilting should not be used to predict responses during acceleration unless it can be verified that comparable stimuli were applied. These results again emphasize that exercise training in the heat can have beneficial effects on orthostatic tolerance but not on +Gz acceleration tolerance.

INTERMEDIATE-TERM TRAINING (6–11 WEEKS). Three studies were designed to examine effects of 7-week training on orthostatic responses

FIGURE 7.2

Mean (±SE) pre- and postacclimation acceleration **(upper panel)** *and orthostatic* **(lower panel)** *tolerances, and terminal (presyncopal) heart rates and systolic/diastolic blood pressures in the six women (22 ± 1 yr) and four men (27 ± 8 yr).* **Numbers inside bars** *are heart rates* **(above)** *and systolic blood pressure/diastolic blood pressure* **(below). A, B** *is P<0.05 from preacclimation A and/or B values. Reprinted with permission of Greenleaf, J. E., P. J. Brock, D. Sciaraffa, A. Polese, and R. Elizondo. Effects of exercise-heat acclimation on fluid, electrolyte, and endocrine responses during tilt and +Gz acceleration in women and men.* Aviat. Space Environ. Med. 56:683–689, 1985.

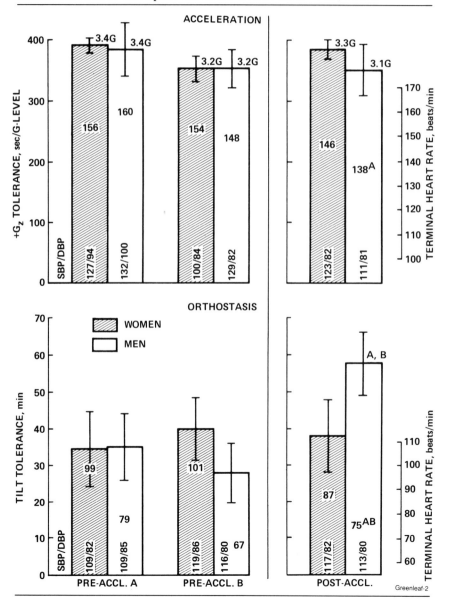

Greenleaf-2

or tolerance. First, 33 young men were placed into three groups [98]. Two groups were subjected to a 7-week training program of two 30 min/week sessions: the first group performed mainly bench stepping with the legs, which raised heart rate from 76 to 168 bpm; and the second group performed mainly pull-ups and dips with the arms, which raised heart rate from 74 to 144 bpm. The third group (control) remained sedentary. Orthostatic responses were determined before and after 5 min of 90° passive HUT, followed by 5 min standing after a short interval supine. Both exercise groups displayed better orthostatic responses standing and only the arm-training group showed improved responses during tilt. The interesting finding was that upper body training may be more effective than lower body training. Second, Kilbom [57] tested orthostatic tolerance (8 min of standing against a wall) in three groups of women (24–56 yr of age) before and after cycle training at 70% of $\dot{V}O_2$max two to three times/week for 7 weeks. After training heart rate decreased significantly, and blood pressures and $\dot{V}O_2$max increased significantly in the young and middle-aged groups. No subject fainted during the stand test before or after training. Third, Pawelezyk et al. [82] subjected five women and five men ($\bar{X}$ age 23 yr) to 7 weeks of training with 50 min sessions four times/week at 70% of $\dot{V}O_2$max with leg exercise. Since a slight but significant decrease (by 3.4 mm Hg) in systolic blood pressure was noted after training, it was concluded that control of blood pressure during 10 min of orthostasis may be altered by endurance training.

LONG-TERM TRAINING (3–8 MONTHS). Five studies have been conducted to assess effects of long-term training on orthostatic responses and tolerance. In 1968 Shvartz [97] reported that three months of heavy apparatus training improved orthostatic response in 10 young men during 10 min standing at attention, mainly by a rise in systolic blood pressure and a smaller decrease in pulse pressure; no such changes were observed in a control group of seven young subjects. Sheldahl et al. [95] investigated effects of 6 months' supervised endurance training ($\Delta\dot{V}O_2$max from 33 to 44 ml·kg^{-1}·min^{-1}, P<0.05) on the response to 3–5 min of HUT (angle not indicated) in seven middle-aged and five older, healthy men. With HUT, there was no change in heart rate, systolic blood pressure, diastolic blood pressure, cardiac index, or total peripheral resistance before and after training. Thus, in middle-aged men, responses to short-term HUT are unchanged with long-term training.

Länsimies and Rauhala [64] studied 85 healthy men (43 ±3 yr) receiving similar dietary instructions for the half-year study period. After a 2-month familiarization period, they were allocated into training and nontraining groups. After a 4-month aerobic training period, there were no changes in orthostatic responses to 10 min of HUT. Subjects with greater increases in $\dot{V}O_2$max after training had similar orthostatic responses as those with lesser increases; $\dot{V}O_2$max was similar in those with lesser or greater orthostatic responses; and the changes in orthostatic responses were not related to the changes in $\dot{V}O_2$max. Thus, there was no significant relationship between orthostatic responses and changes or absolute levels of maximal oxygen uptake.

The fourth investigation determined the effect of 6 months of moderately intense aerobic training for 1 hr/day, 3 days/week on orthostatic tolerance before and after 6 hr of water immersion (34.5°C) deconditioning [46]. The group session exercise-training frequency and intensity increased to nearly maximal intensity during the last 3 months ($\Delta\dot{V}O_2$max from 39.3 to 47.8 ml·min^{-1}·kg^{-1}, P<0.05). Before and after training, the subjects were tested at 60° HUT with foot-support for up to 90 min. The five male subjects (27–42 yr) wore a lower body positive pressure garment inflated to 50 mm Hg around the legs and abdomen. The suit was then deflated during the last 60 min of tilt or until presyncopal signs intervened. None of the subjects fainted during the orthostatic tolerance tests before or after immersion. There were no significant changes in tilt tolerances after training or after immersion: pretraining control tolerance was 74 ± 16 min and post-training tolerance was 74 ± 16 min (postimmersion tolerance was 44 ± 13 min) (Fig. 7.3, *upper panel*). In both pretraining tolerance tests, four subjects had a tolerance of 90 min, while one subject had a tolerance of 9 and 10 min, respectively. Hypovolemic levels were not significantly different (Fig. 7.3. *lower panel*). Fluid, electrolyte, and endocrine responses were essentially the same during both tilts. Thus, increased aerobic capacity resulting from 6 months of moderately intense physical training does not change orthostatic tolerance. On the other hand, Raven and Stevens [86] trained seven young male subjects aerobically for 8 months ($\Delta\dot{V}O_2$max = +23%, P<0.05) and found a significant decrease in LBNP tolerance, measured with the cumulative stress index (CSI = torr × min), after a rapid fall in blood pressure and presyncopal signs occurred. Conversely, Convertino et al. [20] found that 10 weeks of sitting ergometer endurance training at 70–80% of $\dot{V}O_2$max resulted in increased LBNP tolerance (progressive 3-min decompression steps of − 10 mm Hg from − 20 mm Hg to tolerance) from 747 ± 61 to 958 ± 88 torr × min (Δ = +28%, P<0.05). These results emphasize that tolerance to LBNP should not be compared directly with HUT tolerance, and that physiological responses leading to syncope with these two procedures may be different.

Among the 14 longitudinal studies where the effect of training on orthostatic tolerance was determined from physiological response to HUT or standing, only five were designed so the subjects could reach presyncope (tolerance) [18, 45, 46, 99, 103]. In none of those five studies, where exercise training lasted from 8 days to 3 weeks, were orthostatic responses different or tolerances decreased during 60–70° HUT or standing. On the contrary, Shvartz et al. [103] and Greenleaf et al. [45]

FIGURE 7.3

Mean (±SE) tilt tolerance and change in plasma volume before (**control**) *and after immersion in the pre- and post-training (6 month) conditions.* *P<0.05 from the corresponding control value. Reprinted with permission of Greenleaf, J. E., E. R. Dunn, C. Nesvig, L. C. Keil, M. H. Harrison, G. Geelen, and S. E. Kravik. Effect of longitudinal physical training and water immersion on orthostatic tolerance in men.* Aviat. Space Environ. Med. *59:152–159, 1988.*

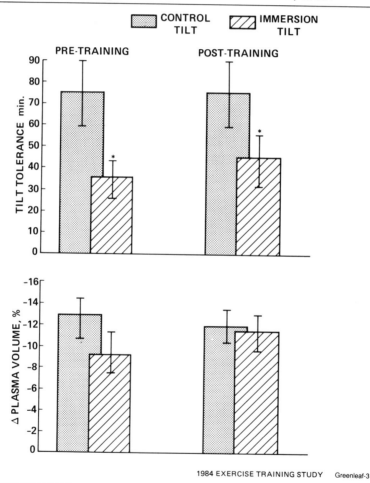

reported increased orthostatic tolerances in men but not in women after 8–10 days of aerobic training, and Convertino et al. [18] showed a nonsignificant trend toward an increased orthostatic tolerance after 8 days of training. When training lasted for 7 weeks, only Pawelezyk et al. [82] reported a significant decrease of 3.4 mm Hg in average systolic blood pressure over 10 min of HUT, with no changes in diastolic blood pressure, peripheral pulse, and greater compensatory increases in heart rate. Hormonal adaptation to vigorous aerobic exercise training occurred within 3 weeks, while cardiac adaptation continued for at least 5 weeks [123, 124]. As emphasized by Raven and Stevens [86]:. . . . "specific adaptations may occur within the blood pressure regulating system over months of training which are not manifest in the 1- to 7-week training studies." But the findings indicate that, after 4–6 months of training, there were no significant changes in orthostatic or acceleration tolerances.

The spectrum of physiological responses to gravitational stimuli in the longitudinal studies precludes any definitive statements or conclusions regarding the mechanism(s) of presyncope or syncope. But the preponderance of evidence indicates no significant reduction in tolerance due to exercise training [1, 18, 44, 46, 56, 101].

MECHANISMS OF ORTHOSTATIC HYPOTENSION

The following section is a discussion of possible mechanisms of blood pressure control to gain insight as to how endurance training may be related to "impaired" orthostatic responses.

Endurance-Training Effects

Endurance training has three well-known effects: *(a)* it increases plasma volume acutely and perhaps chronically, and it is associated with decreases in *(b)* resting heart rate and *(c)* in blood pressure chronically [116]. The important role of blood volume in cardiovascular adjustments to orthostasis is well established. The propensity to faint increases as blood volume decreases [8, 18, 48] whether because of hemorrhage, dehydration, or plasma redistribution as occurs during standing, HUT, LBNP, or +Gz acceleration. Endurance-trained people usually have greater plasma volumes, and thus greater blood volumes per kg of body weight due to greater lean body mass, as compared with comparable untrained people [13, 15, 18, 50, 81]. This acute hypervolemia may also function as a protective factor against orthostatic intolerance. But there is evidence that plasma volume was unchanged after 6 months of training [46]. However, chronically increased central blood volume and central venous pressure can result in continuous stimulation of cardiopulmonary baroreceptors [17], perhaps inducing a resetting, resulting in decreased sensitivity. In addition, chronic hypervolemia may adversely affect distensibility of vascular smooth muscle, especially in capacitance vessels in highly trained people. Both decreased baroreceptor sensitivity and impaired smooth muscle action could affect syncope.

A second chronic effect of endurance training is reduction in resting heart rate, which appears to be mainly the consequence of increased vagal parasympathetic activity [4, 37, 91], and also reduction in cardiac sympathetic activity [27, 91]. Any exercise training-induced modification of the balance between these two components of the autonomic nervous system may put endurance-trained athletes at a disadvantage, since it likely limits compensatory cardioacceleration during tilting or perturbations induced by nitroprusside and phenylephrine [58]. But, on the other hand, their probable hypervolemia can facilitate increased stroke volume, which would augment cardiac output during orthostasis.

The third chronic effect is decrease in resting systolic and (mainly) diastolic blood pressures [18, 57, 76, 111, 113, 116]. The evidence for the mechanism of this decreased pressure suggests interactions among exercise-induced hypovolemia and increases in PVP and especially in PRA [49], which will be discussed later.

Arterial Baroreflex Control of Heart Rate and Blood Pressure

CROSS-SECTIONAL STUDIES. In 1974, Stegemann et al. [108] reported the first evidence that arterial baroreflex regulation of blood pressure was less sensitive in endurance-trained athletes when compared with that of untrained subjects. Their blood pressure control systems were tested by randomly changing the transmural pressure from -60 to $+60$ mm Hg in the carotid artery by means of a sealed pressure dome around the neck and head of the subjects who were breathing air. The blood pressure and heart rate responses to changes in transmural pressure were measured at 3 min after the onset of the stimulus so that modulation of the carotid baroreflex response by the action or interaction of aortic or cardiopulmonary baroreceptors, as well as other reflexes (e.g., somatic), had had time to intervene. The heart rate, reflex blood pressure, and mean arterial blood pressure changes during dome pressure changes were significantly less responsive in the highly trained athletes (Fig. 7.1). Also, with decreasing transmural (dome) pressure, the heart rate of the athletes increased much less than that of the controls indicating attenuated compensatory response to the stress. The pressure compensatory system was much more effective in response to a decrease than to an increase in pressure. While Stegemann et al. concluded that the less responsive (flatter) blood pressure response curve in the athletes indicated reduced effectiveness of the blood pressure control system, an alternative interpretation could be that a flatter (less responsive) curve could indicate increased effectiveness; that is, a lesser response to the stimuli and better physiological adjustment. Raven et al. [85], Paweleczyk et al. [83], and Smith et al. [104–106) compared responses with hypotensive (graded LBNP) and hypertensive (phenylephrine infusion) stimuli in endurance exercise-trained athletes, in resistive exercise-trained athletes, and in untrained subjects. The overall response to LBNP was consistent; an attenuated increase in heart rate in the endurance-trained, compared with both the resistive exercise-trained and the untrained subjects, suggested attenuated baroreflex sensitivity only in the endurance-trained group. The slope of the heart rate-blood pressure regression during phenylephrine infusion was also modified somewhat in the endurance-trained group. These findings were confirmed in 10 men after being endurance trained for 4 weeks [58]. Although not as definitive as the LBNP responses, they agreed with the suggestion by Stegemann et al. [108] of a nonlinear relationship between blood pressure and heart rate during extended perturbations of external pressure. However, when acute hypotensive stimuli were applied to the carotid baroreceptors with the neck collar technique and LBNP, carotid baroreceptor regulation of heart rate and blood pressure were unimpaired in moderately fit competitive swimmers ($\dot{V}O_2$max = 56 ml·min^{-1}·kg^{-1}) when compared with nine untrained men ($\dot{V}O_2$max = 42 ml·min^{-1}·kg^{-1}); but carotid baroreflex control of forearm vascular resistance was impaired in the swimmers [30]. Fiocchi and associates [32, 33] conducted two studies and found divergent results. In the first study [33], 24 male cyclists (ages 16–60 yr), who had been involved in touring for more than 7 yr, were given eight intensities of neck suction. Carotid baroreflex sensitivity (maximal R-R interval prolongation within the first 5 sec after stimulation) showed no significant relationship with basal heart rate, blood pressure, or peak oxygen uptake. However, in the second study [32], Fiocchi et al. showed that baroreflex sensitivity was significantly increased in 11 distance runners (10 ± 6 ms/mm Hg) compared with that in 12 age-matched untrained controls (7 ± 4 ms/mm Hg). Barney and collegues conducted two baroreflex responsiveness studies: one with seven young athletes and seven untrained men ($\dot{V}O_2$max = 62 and 47 ml·min^{-1}·kg^{-1}, respectively [5]); and the other with 11 high-fit and nine sedentary men ($\dot{V}O_2$max = >53 and 34–43 ml·min^{-1}·kg^{-1}, respectively [4]). They found that: *(a)* resting vagal cardiac activity was greater in the athletes and fit men; *(b)* neck suction/pressure stimuli elicited greater R-R interval changes in the athletes and fit men; and *(c)* respiratory sinus arrhythmia and baroreflex slope were increased in the fit compared with the sedentary subjects indicating increased baroreflex sensitivity. Since reflex control of heart rate was not decreased in the athletes at specific intensities of carotid stimuli, deficient baroreflex control of the heart appeared an unlikely mechanism for explaining possible orthostatic intolerance.

LONGITUDINAL STUDIES. Seals and Chase [92] trained 11 men (ages 45–68 yr) with a 30-week jogging program at an intensity of 68% and 81% of the heart rate reserve ($\Delta\dot{V}O_2$max from 31.6 to 41.0 ml·min^{-1}·kg^{-1}) to determine if endurance training would affect baroreflex control of heart rate and limb vascular resistance. These were the first available data on carotid baroreflex responsiveness indicating that prolonged endurance training does *not* alter arterial baroreflex control or heart rate; i.e., it did not evoke changes in chronotropic responsiveness to either carotid baroreflex stimulation or inhibition (using neck suction or pressure) or to nonspecific unloading of the arterial baroreceptors (LBNP >20 mm Hg). These findings might be explained by the decreasing resting cardiac vagal tone observed with aging, which agrees with the authors' observation of substantially lower heart rate variability in their middle-aged men compared with that of younger men. On the other hand, Kingwell et al. [58] found that moderately intensive cycle endurance training ($\Delta \dot{V}O_2$max = 13%) did not change reflex baroreceptor sensitivity in the presence of functioning vagus and sympathetic nerves. But the vagal response was reduced significantly after sympathetic blockade with propranolol. Maximal tachycardic response to decreased blood pressure after training was reduced significantly from 106 to 97 bpm. Since this attenuation did not occur after propranolol, a sympathetic mechanism was apparently involved. Thus, exercise training decreased the sympathetic contribution to reflex tachycardia resulting from blood pressure reduction, and reduced the vagal response to baroreflex sensitivity.

These findings from cross-sectional studies, and particularly from the two longitudinal studies, indicate no appreciable change in baroreflex sensitivity in endurance-trained athletes, resistive-trained athletes, fit competitive swimmers, touring cyclists, or in men trained for 4 and 30 weeks.

Cardiopulmonary Baroreflex Control of Vascular Resistance
FOREARM VASCULAR RESISTANCE (FVR). Attenuation of cardiopulmonary baroreceptor action in humans, particularly the ventricular baroreceptors, triggers intensive arteriolar but minimal venous forearm vasoconstriction [31]. Low-pressure baroreceptors exert prolonged action on forearm resistance vessels, while they have minor influence on the splanchnic circulation. Conversely, arterial baroreceptors have only minor influence on limb vascular resistance but play a major role for control of splanchnic resistance [74].

Results from cross-sectional studies indicate that low levels of LBNP (−5 to −20 mm Hg) decrease cardiac filling and central venous pressures significantly without modifying arterial pulse pressure, mean arterial pressure, arterial dP/dt, or heart rate. The resulting unloading of low-pressure baroreceptors induces mainly forearm vasoconstriction [25, 104]. Mack et al. [72] reported decreased FVR in response to graded low levels of LBNP (zero to −20 mm Hg) in six moderately fit ($\dot{V}O_2$max = 57.0 ml·min^{-1}·kg^{-1}) vs. five unfit ($\dot{V}O_2$max = 38.5 ml·min^{-1}·kg^{-1}) subjects. Conversely, Takeshita et al. [112] observed that −10 mm Hg

LBNP reduced central venous pressures similarly in a group of athletes and nonathletes, but induced greater forearm vasoconstriction in the athletes. Similar increases in FVR induced by LBNP to -40 mm Hg or application of neck pressure were observed in swimmers and nonswimmers [30]. However, when both stimuli (LBNP plus neck pressure) were applied simultaneously, the increase in FVR was attenuated more in the trained than in the untrained subjects. Ebert and Barney [25] suggest "there may be some inhibitory or antagonistic effect of the central processing of afferent neural input during the simultaneous unloading of both low-and high-pressure baroreceptors in the trained athletes."

Results from longitudinal studies suggest different mechanisms. After a mild 4-month exercise-training regimen in middle-aged men, Jingu [54] reported that cardiopulmonary control of FVR increased in response to -10 mm Hg LBNP. Vroman et al. [119] found no change in the FVR response to -10 mm Hg LBNP after endurance training in young subjects, while -40 mm Hg decreased FVR markedly. In contrast, FVR and the vasoconstrictor response were attenuted markedly at each level of LBNP (-10, -20, -30 mm Hg) after a vigorous 30-week training program ($\Delta \dot{V}O_2$max $= 31.6$ to 41.0 ml·min^{-1}·kg^{-1}) in middle-aged men [92]. After 10 weeks of cycling training (70% of $\dot{V}O_2$max), Mack et al. [73] also found decreased cardiopulmonary baroreflex control of FVR to graded LBNP (0 to -20 mm Hg). Since increase in total peripheral resistance (TPR) per unit reduction in central venous pressure and ability to maintain blood pressure during LBNP after training were unchanged, the longer training period may have decreased both FVR *and* TPR, or the decrease in low-pressure baroreceptor-mediated vasocontriction in the forearm following training may have been offset by an increase in arterial baroreceptor-mediated vasoconstriction. In any case, modification of cardiopulmonary baroreflex function was correlated (r $= 0.65$) with the training-induced increase in blood volume [73]. Thus, the hypervolemia that accompanies training could have contributed to the reduction in cardiopulmonary baroreflex control of FVR because less vasoconstriction would be required to maintain pressure with the expanded blood volume. This may be an advantage of training because a greater vasoconstrictive reserve would be available to compensate for greater reductions in venous pressure.

TOTAL PERIPHERAL RESISTANCE (TPR). Carotid baroreceptors and, to a lesser extent, cardiopulmonary baroreceptors participate in control of TPR [74]. Increases in FVR and TPR occurred when subjects were subjected to -60 mm Hg LBNP for 10 min, to 10 min of active standing, or to passive 80–90° HUT [39]. Charles and Richardson [11] compared the effects of 10° HUT or HDT for 10 min each (maneuvers that presumably acted only on the cardiopulmonary baroreceptors since there were no significant changes in blood or mean arterial pressures) in six runners and in five sedentary men. Differences in the runners' forearm blood flow and resistance suggested that TPR may fall periodically with orthostatic stress. The decreased ability to maintain TPR with training may be caused by reduced peripheral sympathetic tone and effectiveness of the cardiopulmonary baroreceptors, which may be linked to the hypervolemia induced by training.

TPR increased less during LBNP (>40 mm Hg) in endurance-trained athletes ($\dot{V}O_2$max = 70 ml·min^{-1}·kg^{-1}) than in resistance-trained, average fit, or nonathletes [84, 105]. There was no change in TPR in women during LBNP between 0 and −40 mm Hg, but TPR decreased when they became hypotensive [52]. Seals and Chase [92] also found in middle-aged men a marked decrease in their TPR to −30 mm Hg after 30 weeks of intense training. Convertino [14] reported no change in TPR during LBNP after 10 weeks of training despite reduced cardiopulmonary baroreceptor control of FVR. Thus, when endurance-trained humans became hypotensive during LBNP stress, thereby unloading the arterial barorecptors, the findings imply unchanged or decreased peripheral vascular resistance, which may contribute to decreased tolerance.

Lower Extremity Compliance

Gravitational stress, induced by standing, HUT, LBNP, or +Gz acceleration, results in an immediate stagnation (pooling) of blood in the lower extremities. If venous compliance (the amount of displacement per unit of applied force) is increased preferentially in trained athletes, the net result would be greater decreases in venous return, stroke volume, and cardiac output. Thus, investigators have measured the amount of blood "pooled" in the legs of athletes and nonathletes, mainly during LBNP using strain gauge plethysmography, impedence plethysmography, and computed tomography scanning [82]. The results were inconsistent. Luft et al. [71] found that the rate of calf volume change, as a function of LBNP level (compliance), was increased significantly in five runners when compared with that in five sedentary controls. Hudson [51] and Smith and Raven [106] also found significant increases in calf circumference (volume) in fit men ($\dot{V}O_2$max = 43.5–62.0 ml·min^{-1}·kg^{-1}) compared with sedentary controls ($\dot{V}O_2$max = 38.8 ml·min^{-1}·kg^{-1}). Increased *peak* fluid accumulation was found in the calf and total leg, but after 8 days of training there was no change in the *mean* rate of fluid accumulation in the legs during 60° HUT, which did not affect orthostatic tolerance [18]. Leg fluid accumulation and peak LBNP levels were highly correlated (r = 0.91) [18], so subjects who tolerated greater pooling displayed greater LBNP tolerance [90]. But Mansegth and Bernauer [75], Raven et al. [84], and Raven and Smith [85] were unable to detect differences in leg compliance between fit and unfit subjects. Because the amount of leg muscle mass was highly correlated (negatively) with leg compliance, it was suggested that larger muscle mass restricts fluid accumulation in veins [16]. This negative mass-compliance relationship could explain why some endurance-trained runners with relatively smaller leg muscle masses have lower orthostatic or LBNP tolerance than others with larger leg muscle masses.

Orthostasis and Vasoactive Hormonal Interactions
The first line of defense against an orthostatic challenge involves autonomic nervous system response within seconds after application of the stimulus; there is baroreflex-mediated withdrawal of vagal tone and activation of the sympathetic system. Muscle sympathetic nerve activity correlates highly with changes in arterial blood pressure, limb vascular resistance, and venous plasma norepinephrine concentration [26, 93]. Maintenance of blood pressure during prolonged standing, HUT, LBNP, or +Gz acceleration requires secretion of vasoactive enzymes and hormones; first norepinephrine (NE), then PRA, and finally PVP [10, 23, 24, 41, 77, 79, 80, 87–89, 94]. However, the stimuli for hormonal release vary with each system. The NE response is immediate and almost maximal within 5 min, while significant increases in PRA-angiotensin or PVP require the stimulus to be applied longer. Unloading cardiopulmonary baroreceptors alone, by application of nonhypotensive levels of LBNP (< -20 mm Hg) that decrease central venous pressure but do not change arterial pulse pressure or heart rate, does not increase PRA [77] or PVP significantly [41, 87]. Concomitantly, there is a reflex increase in plasma NE and FVR [41]. These observations suggest that selective unloading of low-pressure baroreceptors does not increase PRA or PVP in the presence of physiological tonic inhibition of the high-pressure baroreceptors. However, unloading of both cardiopulmonary and arterial baroreceptors during prolonged standing, HUT, or under higher (-20 to -40 mm Hg) levels of LBNP results in substantial increases in PRA and PVP concentration [12, 74, 77, 87]. These inhibitory effects of cardiopulomary baroreceptor loading are difficult to achieve when starting from a basal or resting condition [40]. On the other hand, the magnitude of the increased PVP response to orthostatic hypotension has been proposed as a test of the integrity of the afferent limb of the baroreflex [26]. These findings do not exclude an influence of cardiopulmonary baroreceptor stimuli on PRA or PVP secretion, since sustained loading or cardiopulmonary baroreceptors (head-out water immersion, HDT, LBNP) is accompanied in some instances by sustained decreases in plasma NE, PRA, and PVP.

Vasoactive hormones are intimately involved in controlling blood volume and pressure during orthostasis. Convertino et al. [15] suggested that daily exercise training for 8 days stimulated PRA and PVP to facilitate salt and water conservation, which may have contributed to the training-induced hypervolemia. Sather et al. [89] found no differences in plasma NE, PRA, or PVP concentrations at -50 mm Hg LBNP in subjects with high or low tolerance to LBNP, suggesting that higher tolerance subjects release the same amounts of vasoactive hormones at lower percentages of their maximal LBNP tolerance. However, at peak (syncopal) levels of LBNP, their higher tolerance group had significantly greater PRA and PVP concentrations than the low-tolerance group, indicating perhaps greater hormonal reserve capacity in the former group. This high reserve capacity is particularly evident when plasma PVP concentration rose to >500 pg/ml at the point of syncope (Greenleaf, personal observation).

Dehydration increases plasma concentrations of vasoactive hormones and accentuates the physiological responses to orthostasis [7, 47, 48]. Induction of dehydration has been proposed as a means of identifying potentially orthostatically intolerant subjects. Before standing or HUT, resting supine systolic blood pressure was significantly lower and PRA significantly higher in those dehydrated subjects who became orthostatically intolerant earliest [49]; that is, induction of a pre-HUT stressor reduces subsequent orthostatic capacity. But the large increases in PVP observed in dehydrated subjects upon standing often occur in response to the severity of presyncopal symptoms rather than to the orthostatically induced changes in blood pressure [6, 24, 48].

From two cross-sectional studies: (a) middle-aged men with low orthostatic tolerance had, together with a low basal PRA, an attenuated PRA response when subjected to LBNP [42]; (b) and in average fit subjects the higher LBNP tolerant group ($\dot{V}O_2$max = 46.8 ml·min^{-1}·kg^{-1}) had significantly higher PRA and PVP concentrations at the presyncopal point than the lower tolerant group ($\dot{V}O_2$max = 43.1 ml·min^{-1}) [89] suggesting that magnitude of hormonal response may be proportional to tolerance time and independent of aerobic capacity.

Hormonal parameters were measured in three of the 13 longitudinal studies discussed earlier whose findings showed no deleterious effect of training on orthostatic tolerance. Shvartz et al. [99] found that PRA and PVP increased significantly during HUT before and after 8 days of training, but significantly less in the post-training tilt in the previously determined nonfainters; decreases were 15-fold for PRA and five-fold for PVP. Convertino et al. [18] noted similar PRA and PVP responses upon 60° HUT in men with essentially similar tolerances before and after 8 days of training; and PRA and PVP increased with the duration of HUT in the same way before and after 6 months of training, reaching similar concentrations at the point of tolerance [46]. Thus, post-training hormonal responses to standing or HUT were not influenced by training but were proportional to the time required to reach orthostatic tolerance.

If orthostatic tolerance were reduced after training, what could be possible contributions of altered hormonal responses? Training-induced hypervolemia could induce chronic stimulation of cardiopulmonary receptors resulting in their decreased responsiveness, particularly to unloading. However, as mentioned previously, unloading of these receptors has little or no effect on PRA and PVP secretion until concomitant unloading of arterial baroreceptors occurs. Lower PRA levels at rest after training [38, 68] could affect the balance between parasympathetic and sympathetic function toward increased sympathetic activity (greater PRA reserve), which could increase tolerance via central and peripheral vascular mechanisms.

SUMMARY

There are two major problems here that are not independent. One is the more practically oriented problem of determining the effect of various modes of exercise training on gravitational tolerances, i.e., the point of syncope (unconsciousness) usually estimated from the time of appearance of presyncopal signs and symptoms. The other is more theoretical and concerns the mechanism of blood pressure failure that results in syncope. In many experimental designs these two problems or purposes have been intermingled, with equivocal results.

Exercise Training and Gravitational Tolerance
One major experimental design flaw is that tolerance levels of subjects have been assumed from changes in some vital signs (usually heart rate and blood pressure) without measurement of tolerance or use of a transfer function that relates changes in the vital signs with changes in tolerance. A basic design premise seems to be that measurement of changes of vital signs will somehow lead to an understanding of the mechanism controlling the relationship between blood pressure and tolerance.

Other reasons for some disparate results between studies arise from use of terms like athletes vs. nonathletes and trained vs. untrained without accepted measurements that define these adaptive states physiologically. Is only the level of peak or maximal oxygen uptake sufficient to define the trained state? Are those with higher $\dot{V}O_2$max necessarily in higher trained states? If a training program increased $\dot{V}O_2$max in one person from 3 to 4 liters/min and from 3.5 to 4.0 liters/min in another, are the two in an equally trained state? Are they in an equally trained state as an untrained person with a genetically determined sedentary $\dot{V}O_2$max of 4 liters/min? Since 10–15% of the general population are genetic premature fainters, test subject populations should be tested for this trait. Do those endurance-trained "athletes" who faint prematurely when trained also faint more quickly when deconditioned like normal, sedentary people subjected to water immersion, prolonged bed rest, or prolonged microgravity? The genetic predisposition hypothesis has not been tested; fraternal twins could be studied.

A practical question is whether astronauts should engage in intensive endurance-exercise training before or during flight? There is sufficient evidence to conclude that orthostatic (tilt) and $+Gz$ (head-to-foot) acceleration tolerances are not exacerbated by normal exercise training programs. It may be prudent not to select highly endurance-trained athletes as shuttle pilots without intensive orthostatic testing to be certain they are not premature fainters.

Mechanism of Blood Pressure Failure

The section headings; baroreflex control, vascular peripheral resistance TPR, extremity compliance, and vasoactive hormones suggest some important factors involved in the control of blood pressure and its failure. Various combinations of these factors have been utilized and applied to the practical problem. It is clear that a more encompassing approach will be necessary to understand this mechanism fully. While intensive analyses of traditional cardiovascular measurements have contributed significantly, the major part of the control mechanism probably resides in the neuroendocrine system. Modification of mechanical properties of the heart may be important. It is anticipated that significant progress will occur when test subject state is better defined physiologically, and more direct measurements of nerve function and interaction of the atriopeptins, urodilatin, endothelin, and other as yet undiscovered enzymes and hormones are applied to this problem, to aid in understanding the fine balance between parasympathetic and sympathetic control of blood pressure.

ACKNOWLEDGMENTS

The authors thank our collaborators on studies cited in this chapter, Drs. V. A. Convertino and C. M. Tipton for their critical reviews, and A. J. Hardesty for preparation of the manuscript. This work was supported by NASA Task 199–18–12–07.

REFERENCES

1. Allen, S. C., C. L. Taylor, and V. E. Hall. A study of orthostatic insufficiency by the tiltboard method. *Am. J. Physiol.* 143:11–20, 1945.
2. Associated Press. Puzzling illness keeps man in bed 50 years. *San Jose Mercury,* May 26, 1982, p. 12A.
3. Balldin, U. I., K. Myhre, P. A. Tesch, U. Wilhelmsen, and H. T. Andersen. Isometric abdominal muscle training and G tolerance. *Aviat. Space Environ. Med.* 56:120–124, 1985.
4. Barney, J. A., T. J. Ebert, L. Groban, P. A. Farrell, C. V. Hughes and J. J. Smith. Carotid baroreflex responsivensss in high-fit and sedentary young men. *J. Appl. Physiol.* 65:2190–2194, 1988.
5. Barney, J. A., T. J. Ebert, L. Groban, and J. J. Smith. Vagal-cardiac activity and

carotid-to-cardiac baroreflex resposes in trained and untrained men. *Fed. Proc.* 44:818, 1985.

6. Baylis, P. H., and D. A. Heath. The development of a radioimmunoassay for the measurment of human plasma arginine vasopressin. *Clin. Endocrinol.* 7:91–102, 1977.

7. Beetham, W. P., Jr., and E. R. Buskirk. Effects of dehydration, physical conditioning and heat acclimatization on the response to passive tilting. *J. Appl. Physiol.* 13:465–468, 1958.

8. Bergenwald, L., U. Freyschuss, and T. Sjöstrand. The mechanism of orthostatic and haemorrhagic fainting. *Scand. J. Clin. Lab. Invest.* 37:209–216, 1977.

9. Boening, D., H.-V. Ulmer, U. Meier, W. Skipka, and J Stegemenn. Effects of a multi-hour immersion on trained and untrained subjects: I. Renal function and plasma volume. *Aerospace Med.* 43:300–305, 1972.

10. Brown, J. J., D. L. Davies, A. F. Lever, D. McPherson, and J. I. S. Robertson. Plasma renin concentration in relation to changes in posture. *Clin. Sci.* 30:279–284, 1966.

11. Charles, J. B., and D. R. Richardson. Differences in response to central blood volume shifts between aerobic conditioned and unconditioned subjects. *Aerospace Med. Assoc. Preprints,* 1981, p. 317–318.

12. Convertino, V. A. Aerobic fitness, endurance training, and orthostatic intolerance. *Exerc. Sport Sci. Rev.* 15:233–259, 1987.

13. Convertino, V. A. Blood volume: its adaptation to endurance training. *Med. Sci. Sports Exerc.* 23:1338–1348, 1991.

14. Convertino, V. A. Endurance exercise training: conditions of enhanced hemodynamic responses and tolerance to LBNP. *Med. Sci. Sports Exerc.* 1993. In press.

15. Convertino, V. A., P. J. Brock, L. C. Keil, E. M. Bernauer, and J. E. Greenleaf. Exercise training-induced hypervolemia: role of plasma albumin, renin, and vasopressin. *J. Appl. Physiol.* 48:665–669, 1980.

16. Convertino, V. A., D. F. Doerr, J. F. Flores, G. W. Hoffler, and P. Buchanan. Leg size and muscle functions associated with leg compliance. *J. Appl. Physiol.* 64:1017–1021, 1988.

17. Convertino, V. A., G. W. Mack, and E. R. Nadel. Elevated central venous pressure: a consequence of exercise training-induced hypervolemia? *Am. J. Physiol.* 260:R273–R277, 1991.

18. Convertino, V. A., L. D. Montgomery, and J. E. Greenleaf. Cardiovascular responses during orthostasis: effect of an increase in V_{O_2}max. *Aviat. Space Environ. Med.* 55:702–708, 1984.

19. Convertino, V. A., T. M. Sather, D. J. Goldwater, and W. R. Alford. Aerobic fitness does not contribute to prediction of orthostatic intolerance. *Med. Sci. Sports Exerc.* 18:551–556, 1986.

20. Convertino, V. A., C. A. Thompson, D. L. Eckberg, J. M. Fritsch, G. W. Mack, and E. R. Nadel. Baroreflex responses and LBNP tolerance following exercise training. *Physiologist* 33:S40–S41, 1990.

21. Cooper, K. H., and S. Leverett, Jr. Physical conditioning versus +Gz tolerance. *Aerospace Med.* 37:462–465, 1966.

22. Crampton, C. W. The gravity resisting ability of the circulation; its measurement and significance (blood ptosis). *Am. J. Med. Sci.* 160:721–731, 1920.

23. Davies, R., M. L. Forsling, and J. D. H. Slater. The interrelationship between the release of renin and vasopressin as defined by orthostasis and propranolol. *J. Clin. Invest.* 60:1438–1441, 1977.

24. Davies, R., J. D. H. Slater, M. L. Forsling, and N. Payne. The response of arginine vasopressin and plasma renin to postural change in normal man, with observations on syncope. *Clin. Sci. Mol. Med.* 51:267–274, 1976.

25. Ebert, T. J., and J. A. Barney. Physical fitness and orthostatic tolerance. J. J. Smith (ed). *Circulatory Response to the Upright Posture.* Boca Raton, FL: CRC Press, 1990, p. 47–63.

26. Eckberg, D. L., R. F. Rea, O. K. Andersson, T. Hedner, J. Pernow, J. M. Lundberg,

and B. G. Wallin. Baroreflex modulation of sympathetic activity and sympathetic neurotransmitters in humans. *Acta Physiol. Scand.* 133:221–231, 1988.

27. Ekblom, B., A. Kilbom, and J. Soltysiak. Physical training, bradycardia, and autonomic nervous system. *Scand. J. Clin. Lab. Invest.* 32:251–256, 1973.

28. Epperson, W. L., R. R. Burton, and E. M. Bernauer. The influence of differential physical conditioning regimens on simulated aerial combat maneuvering tolerance. *Aviat. Space Environ. Med.* 53:1091–1097, 1982.

29. Epperson, W. L., R. R. Burton, and E. M. Bernauer. The effectiveness of specific weight training regimens on simulated aerial combat maneuvering G tolerance. *Aviat. Space Environ. Med.* 56:534–539, 1985.

30. Falsetti, H. L., E. R. Burke, and J. Tracy. Carotid and cardiopulmonary baroreflex control of forearm vascular resistance in swimmers. *Med. Sci. Sports Exerc.* 15:183, 1983.

31. Ferguson, D. W., M. D. Thames, and A. L. Mark. Effects of propranolol on reflex vascular responses to orthostatic stress in humans. Role of ventricular baroreceptors. *Circulation* 67:802–807, 1983.

32. Fiocchi, R., R. Fagard, J. Staessen, L. Vanhees, and A. Amery. Atrioventricular block induced in an athlete by carotid baroreceptor stimulation. *Am. Heart J.* 109:1102–1104, 1985.

33. Fiocchi, R, R. Fagard, L. Vanhees, R. Grauwels, and A. Amery. Carotid baroreflex sensitivity and physical fitness in cycling tourists. *Eur. J. Appl. Physiol.* 54:461–465, 1985.

34. Flaubert, G. *Madame Bovary.* New York: Oxford University Press, Inc., First American Edition, 1949. 403 p. First published: Paris 1857.

35. Forster, E. M., and J. E. Whinnery. Dynamic cardiovascular response to +Gz stress in aerobically trained individuals. *Aviat. Space Environ. Med.* 61:303–306, 1990.

36. Frey, M. A. B., K. L. Mathes, and G. W. Hoffler. Aerobic fitness in women and responses to lower body negative pressure. *Aviat. Space Environ. Med.* 58:1149–1152, 1987.

37. Frick, M. H., R. O. Elovainio, and T. Somer. The mechanism of bradycardia evoked by physical training. *Cardiologia* 51:46–54, 1967.

38. Geyssant, A., G. Geelen, Ch. Denis, A. M. Allevard, M. Vincent, E. Jarsaillon, C. A. Bizollan, J. R. Lacour, and Cl. Gharib. Plasma vasopressin, renin activity, and aldosterone: effect of exercise and training. *Eur. J. Appl. Physiol.* 46:21–30, 1981.

39. Gilbert, C. A., and P. M. Stevens. Forearm vascular responses to lower body negative pressure and orthostasis. *J. Appl. Physiol.* 21:1265–1272, 1966.

40. Goldsmith, S. R., G. S. Francis, and J. N. Cohn. Effect of head-down tilt on basal plasma norepinepherine and renin activity in humans. *J. Appl. Physiol.* 59:1068–1071, 1985.

41. Goldsmith, S. R., G. S. Francis, A. W. Cowley, and J. N. Cohn. Response of vasopressin and norepinephrine to lower body negative pressure in humans. *Am. J. Physiol.* 243:H970–H973, 1982.

42. Goldwater, D. J., M. DeLada, A. Polese, L. Keil, and J. A. Luetscher. Effect of athletic conditioning on orthostatic tolerance after prolonged bedrest. *Circulation* 62:287, 1980.

43. Gove, P. B. (ed). *Webster's Third New International Dictionary of the English Language Unabridged.* Springfield, MA: Merriam-Webster, 1986, p. 1837.

44. Greenleaf, J. E., P. J. Brock, and D. Sciaraffa. Effect of physical training in cool and hot environments on +Gz acceleration tolerance in women. *Aviat. Space Environ. Med.* 56:9–14, 1985.

45. Greenleaf, J. E., P. J. Brock, D. Sciaraffa, A. Polese, and R. Elizondo. Effects of exercise-heat acclimation on fluid, electrolyte, and endocrine responses during tilting and +Gz acceleration in women and men. *Aviat. Space Environ. Med.* 56:683–689, 1985.

46. Greenleaf, J. E., E. R. Dunn, C. Nesvig, L. C. Keil, M. H. Harrison, G. Geelen, and S. E. Kravik. Effect of longitudinal physical training and water immersion on orthostatic tolerance in men. *Aviat. Space Environ. Med.* 59:152–159, 1988.

47. Greenleaf, J. E., R. F. Haines, E. M. Bernauer, J. T. Morse, H. Sandler, R. Armbruster, L. Sagan, and W. Van Beaumont. +Gz tolerance in man after 14-day bedrest periods with isometric and isotonic exercise conditioning. *Aviat. Space Environ. Med.* 46:671–678, 1975.

48. Harrison, M. H. Athletes, astronauts, and orthostatic tolerance. *Sports Med.* 3:428–435, 1986.

49. Harrison, M. H., S. E. Kravik, G. Geelen, L. Keil, and J. E. Greenleaf. Blood pressure and plasma renin activity as predictors of orthostatic intolerance. *Aviat. Space Environ. Med.* 56:1059–1064, 1985.

50. Holmgren, A., F. Mossfeldt, T. Sjöstrand, and G. Ström. Effect of training on work capacity, total hemoglobin, blood volume, heart volume, and pulse rate in recumbent and upright positions. *Acta Physiol. Scand.* 50:72–83, 1960.

51. Hudson, D. L., M. L. Smith, H. Graitzer, and P. B. Raven. Fitness-related differences in response to LBNP during sympathetic blockade with metoprolol. *Fed. Proc.* 45:643, 1986.

52. Hudson, D. L., M. L. Smith, and P. B. Raven. Physical fitness and hemodynamic response of women to lower body negative pressure. *Med. Sci. Sports Exerc.* 19:375–381, 1987.

53. Hyman, A. S. The postural mean blood pressure index. A simple test of general physical fitness. *J. Sports Med. Phys. Fitness* 2:218–220, 1960.

54. Jingu, S., A. Takeshita, T. Imaizumi, M. Nakamura, M. Shindo, and H. Tanaka. Exercise training augments cardiopulmonary baroreflex control of forearm vascular resistance in middle-aged subjects. *Jpn. Circ. J.* 52:162–168, 1988.

55. Johnson, R. L., G. W. Hoffler, A. E. Nicogossian, S. A. Bergman, Jr., and M. M. Jackson. Lower body negative pressure: Third manned Skylab mission. R. S. Johnston, and L. F. Dietlein (eds). *Biomedical Results from Skylab.* Washington, D.C.: National Aeronautics and Space Administration, 1977, p. 284–312 (NASA SP-377).

56. Kilbom, A. Physical training with submaximal intensities in women. I. Reaction to exercise and orthostasis. *Scand. J. Clin. Lab. Invest.* 28:141–161, 1971.

57. Kilbom, A., L. H. Hartley, B. Saltin, J. Bjure, G. Grimby, and I. Astrand. Physical training in sedentary middle-aged and older men. I. Medical evaluation. *Scand. J. Clin. Lab. Invest.* 24:315–322, 1969.

58. Kingwell, B. A., A. M. Dart, G. L. Jennings, and P. I. Korner. Exercise training reduces the sympathetic component of the blood pressure-heart rate baroreflex in man. *Clin. Sci.* 82:357–362, 1992.

59. Klein, K. E., F. Backhausen, H. Bruner, J. Eichhorn, D. Jovy, J. Schotte, L. Vogt, and H. W. Wegmann. Die Abhängigkeit der Orthostase-und Beschleunigungs-toleranz von Körperbau und Leistungsfähigkeit. *Arbeitsphysiologie* 26:205–226, 1968.

60. Klein, K. E., H. Brüner, D. Jovy, L. Vogt, and H. M. Wegmann. Influence of stature and physical fitness on tilt-table and acceleration tolerance. *Aerospace Med.* 40:293–297, 1969.

61. Klein, K. E., H. M. Wegmann, H. Brüner, and L. Vogt. Physical fitness and tolerances to environmental extremes. *Aerosapce Med.* 40:998–1001, 1969.

62. Klein, K. E., H. M. Wegmann, and P. Kuklinski. Athletic endurance training—advantage for space flight?: The significance of physical fitness for selection and training of spacelab crews. *Aviat. Space Environ. Med.* 48:215–222, 1977.

63. Korobkov, A. V., L. A. Ioffe, M. A. Abrikosova, and Yu.M. Stoyda. Dynamics of orthostatic tolerance of athletes after forty-day hypokinesia. *Kosm. Biol. Med.* 2:33–40, 1968.

64. Länsimies, E. A., and E. Rauhala. Orthostatic tolerance and aerobic capacity. *Aviat. Space Environ. Med.* 57:1158–1164, 1986.

65. Levine, B. D., J. C. Buckey, J. M. Fritsch, C. W. Yancy, Jr., D. E. Watenpaugh, P. G. Snell, L. D. Lane, D. L. Eckberg, and C. G. Blomqvist. Physical fitness and cardiovascular regulation: mechanisms of orthostatic intolerance. *J. Appl. Physiol.* 70:112–122, 1991.

66. Levine, B. D., L. D. Lane, J. C. Buckey, D. B. Friedman, and C. G. Blomqvist. Left ventricular pressure-volume and Frank-Starling relations in endurance athletes. Implications for orthostatic tolerance and exercise performance. *Circulation* 84:1016–1023, 1991.

67. Lightfoot, J. T., R. P. Claytor, D. J. Torok, T. W. Journell, and S. M. Fortney. Ten weeks of aerobic training do not affect lower body negative pressure responses. *J. Appl. Physiol.* 67:894–901, 1989.

68. Lijnen, P., P. Hespel, S. Van Oppens, R. Fiocchi, W. Goossens, E. Vanden Eynde, and A. Amery. Erythrocyte 2, 3-diphosphoglycerate and serum enzyme concentrations in trained and sedentary men. *Med. Sci. Sports Exerc.* 18:174–179, 1986.

69. Luft, U. C., J. A. Loeppky, M. D. Venters, E. R. Greene, M. W. Eldridge, D. E. Hoekenga, and K. L. Richards. Tolerance of lower body negative pressure (LBNP) in endurance runners, weightlifters, swimmers and nonathletes. Albuquerque: Lovelace Foundation, *NASA Report NAS 9–15483*, 1980, p. 1–35.

70. Luft, U. C., J. A. Loeppky, M. D. Venters, and Y. Kobayashi. The effects of acute diuresis with Lasix on the volume and composition of body fluids and the responses to lower body negative pressure. Albuquerque: Lovelace Foundation, *NASA Report NAS 9–15483*, 1978, p. 1–99.

71. Luft, U.C., L. G. Myhre, J. A. Loeppky, and M. D. Venters. A study of factors affecting tolerance to gravitational stress simulated by lower body negative pressure. Albuquerque: Lovelace Foundation, *NASA Report NAS 9–14472*, 1976, p. 1–60.

72. Mack, G. W., X. Shi, H. Nose, A. Tripathi, and E. R. Nadel. Diminished baroreflex control of forearm vascular resistance in physically fit humans. *J. Appl. Physiol.* 63:105–110, 1987.

73. Mack, G. W., C. A. Thompson, D. F. Doerr, E. R. Nadel, and V. A. Convertino. Diminished baroreflex control of forearm vascular resistance following training. *Med. Sci. Sports Exerc.* 23:1367–1374, 1991.

74. Mancia, G., and A. L. Mark. *Handbook of Physiology*. Section 2: The cardiovascular system, Vol. III, Part 2. Arterial baroreflexes in humans. Bethesda, MD: American Physiological Society, 1983, p. 755–793.

75. Mangseth, G. R., and E. M. Bernauer. Cardiovascular response to tilt in endurance trained subjects exhibiting syncopal reactions. *Med. Sci. Sports Exerc.* 12:140, 1980.

76. Mann, G. V., H. L. Garrett, A. Farhi, H. Murray, T. Billings, E. Shute, and S. E. Schwarten. Exercise to prevent coronary heart disease. *Am. J. Med.* 46:12–27, 1969.

77. Mark, A. L., F. M. Abboud, and A. E. Fitz. Influence of low- and high-pressure baroreceptors on plasma renin activity in humans. *Am. J. Physiol.* 235:H29–H33, 1978.

78. Michel, E. L., J. A. Rummel, C. F. Sawin, M. C. Buderer, and J. D. Lem. Results of Skylab medical experiment M171—metabolic activity. R. S. Johnston, and L. F. Dietlein (eds). *Biomedical Results from Skylab*. Washington, D.C.: National Aeronautics and Space Administration, 1977, p. 372–387 (NASA SP-377).

79. Molzahn, M., Th. Dissmann, S. Halim, F. W. Lohmann, and W. Oelkers. Orthostatic changes in haemodynamics, renal function, plasma catecholamines and plasma renin concentration in normal and hypertensive man. *Clin. Sci.* 42:209–222, 1972.

80. Oparil, S., C. Vassaux, C. A. Sanders, and E. Haber. Role of renin in acute postural homeostasis. *Circulation* 41:89–95, 1970.

81. Oscai, L. B., B. T. Williams, and B. A. Hertig. Effect of exercise on blood volume. *J. Appl. Physiol.* 24:622–624, 1968.

82. Pawelczyk, J. A., W. L. Kenney, and P. Kenney. Cardiovascular responses to head-up tilt after an endurance exercise program. *Aviat. Space Environ. Med.* 59:107–112, 1988.

83. Pawelczyk, J. A., S. Stern, and P. B. Raven. Baroreflexes are less effective in endurance athletes. *Med. Sci. Sports Exerc.* 21:S42, 1989.

84. Raven, P. B., D. Rohm-Young, and C. G. Blomqvist. Physical fitness and cardiovascular response to lower body negative pressure. *J. Appl. Physiol.* 56:138–144, 1984.

85. Raven, P. B., and M. L. Smith. Physical fitness and its effect on factors affecting orthostatic tolerance. *Physiologist* 27:S59–S60, 1984.

86. Raven, P. B., and G. H. Stevens. Endurance exercise training reduces orthostatic tolerance in humans! *Physiologist* 33:S56–S58, 1990.

87. Rogge, J. D., and W. W. Moore. Influence of lower body negative pressure on peripheral venous ADH levels in man. *J. Appl. Physiol.* 25:134–138, 1968.

88. Sassard, J., M. Vincent, G. Annat, and C. A. Bizollon. A kinetic study of plasma renin and aldosterone during changes of posture in man. *J. Clin. Endocrinol. Metab.* 42:20–27, 1976.

89. Sather, T. M., V. A. Convertino, D. J. Goldwater, L. C. Keil, R. Kates, and L. D. Montgomery. Vasoactive neuroendocrine responses associated with orthostatic tolerance in man. *Fed. Proc.* 44:817, 1985.

90. Sather, T. M., D. J. Goldwater, L. D. Montgomery, and V. A. Convertino. Cardiovascular dynamics associated with tolerance to lower body negative pressure. *Aviat. Space Environ. Med.* 57:413–419, 1986.

91. Scheuer, J., and C. M. Tipton. Cardiovascular adaptations to physical training. *Annu. Rev. Physiol.* 39:221–251, 1977.

92. Seals, D. R., and P. B. Chase. Influence of physical training on heart rate variability and baroreflex circulatory control. *J. Appl. Physiol.* 66:1886–1895, 1989.

93. Seals, D. R., and R. G. Victor. Regulation of muscle sympathetic nerve activity during exercise in humans. *Exerc. Sport Sci. Rev.* 19:313–349, 1991.

94. Segar, W. E., and W. W. Moore. The regulation of antidiuretic hormone release in man: I. Effects of change in position and ambient temperature on blood ADH levels. *J. Clin. Invest.* 47:2143–2151, 1968.

95. Sheldahl, L. M., F. E. Tristani, J. A. Barney, L. Groban, S. Levandoski, J. Christie, and J. J. Smith. Effect of endurance exercise training on hemodynamic response to postural stress. *Fed. Proc.* 45:282, 1986.

96. Shvartz, E. Relationship between endurance and orthostatic tolerance. *J. Sports Med.* 8:75–80, 1968.

97. Shvartz, E. Effect of gymnastic training on orthostatic efficiency. *Res. Q.* 39:351–354, 1968.

98. Shvartz, E. Effect of two different training programs on cardiovascular adjustments to gravity. *Res. Q.* 40:575–581, 1969.

99. Shvartz, E., V. A. Convertino, L. C. Keil, and R. F. Haines. Orthostatic fluid-electrolyte and endocrine responses in fainters and nonfainters. *J. Appl. Physiol.* 51:1404–1410, 1981.

100. Shvartz, E., A. Meroz, A. Magazanik, Y. Shoenfeld, and Y. Shapiro. Exercise and heat orthostatism and the effect of heat acclimation and physical fitness. *Aviat. Space Environ. Med.* 48:836–842, 1977.

101. Shvartz, E., and N. Meyerstein. Effect of heat and natural acclimatization to heat on tilt tolerance of men and women. *J. Appl. Physiol.* 28:428–432, 1970.

102. Shvartz, E., and N. Meyerstein. Relation of tilt tolerance to aerobic capacity and physical characteristics. *Aerospace Med.* 43:278–280, 1972.

103. Shvartz, E., N. B. Strydom, and H. Kotze. Orthostatism and heat acclimation. *J. Appl. Physiol.* 39:590–595, 1975.

104. Smith, J. J., and T. J. Ebert. General response to orthostatic stress. J. J. Smith (ed). *Circulatory Response to the Upright Posture.* Boca Raton, FL: CRC Press, 1990, p. 1–46.

105. Smith, M. L., H. M. Graitzer, D. L. Hudson, and P. B. Raven. Baroreflex function in endurance- and static exercise-trained men. *J. Appl. Physiol.* 64:585–591, 1988.

106. Smith, M. L., and P. B. Raven. Cardiovascular responses to lower body negative pressure in endurance and static exercise-trained men. *Med. Sci. Sports Exerc.* 18:545–550, 1986.

107. Stegemann, J. Beziehungen zwischen Trainingszustand und Orthostasetoleranz. *Cardiology* 61:(Suppl. 1):255–266, 1976.

108. Stegemann, J., A. Busert, and D. Brock. Influence of fitness on the blood pressure control system in man. *Aerospace Med.* 45:45–48, 1974.

109. Stegemann, J., H.-D. Framing, and M. Schiefeling. Der Einfluss einer 6 stündigen Immersion in thermoindifferentem Wasser auf die Regulation des Kreislaufs und die Leistungsfähigkeit bei Trainierten und Untrainierten. *Pflügers Arch.* 312:129–138, 1969.

110. Stegemann, J., U. Meier, W. Skipka, W. Hartlieb, B. Hemmer, and U. Tibes. Effects of a multi-hour immerson with intermittent exercise on urinary excretion and tilt table tolerance in athletes and nonathletes. *Aviat. Space Environ. Med.* 46:26–29, 1975.

111. Tabakin, B. S., J. S. Hanson, and A. M. Levy. Effects of physical training on the cardiovascular and respiratory response to graded upright exercise in distance runners. *Br. Heart J.* 27:205–210, 1965.

112. Takeshita, A., S. Jingu, T. Imaizumi, Y. Kunihiko, S. Koyanagi, and M. Nakamura. Augmented cardiopulmonary baroreflex control of forearm vascular resistance in young athletes. *Circ. Res.* 59:43–48, 1986.

113. Terjung, R. L., K. M. Baldwin, J. Cooksey, B. Samson, and R. A. Sutter. Cardiovascular adaptation to twelve minutes of mild daily exercise in middle-aged sedentary men. *J. Am. Geriat. Soc.* 21:164–168, 1973.

114. Tesch, P. A., H. Hjort, and U. I. Balldin. Effects of strength training on G tolerance. *Aviat. Space Environ. Med.* 54:691–695, 1983.

115. Thornton, W. E., and G. W. Hoffler. Hemodynamic studies of the legs under weightlessness. R. S. Johnston, and L. F. Dietlein (eds). *Biomedical Results from Skylab.* Washington, D.C.: National Aeronautics and Space Administration, 1977, p. 324–329 (NASA SP-377).

116. Tipton, C. M. Exercise, training and hypertension: an update. *Exerc. Sports Sci. Rev.* 19:447–505, 1991.

117. Turner, A. H. The circulatory minute volumes of healthy young women in reclining, sitting and standing position. *Am. J. Physiol.* 80:601–630, 1927.

118. Van Lieshout, E. J., J. J. Van Lieshout, J. Krol, M. Simons, and J. M. Karemaker. Assessment of cardiovascular reflexes is of limited value in predicting maximal $+Gz$ tolerance. *Aviat. Space Environ. Med.* 63:21–26, 1992.

119. Vroman, N. B., J. A. Healy, and R. Kertzer. Cardiovascular response to lower body negative pressure (LBNP) following endurance training. *Aviat. Space Environ. Med.* 59:330–334, 1988.

120. Wessel, J. A. An investigation of the relation between man's fitness for strenuous work and his ability to withstand high headward acceleration. Doctoral dissertation, University of Southern California, Los Angeles, CA, 1950. 109p.

121. Whinnery, J. E., and M. J. Parnell. The effects of long-term aerobic conditioning on $+Gz$ tolerance. *Aviat. Space Environ. Med.* 58:199–204, 1987.

122. White, W. J., J. W. Nyberg, P. D. White, R. H. Grimes, and L. M. Finney. Biomedical potential of a centrifuge in an orbiting laboratory. Air Force Systems Command, Los Angeles Air Force Station, CA. *Report No. SSD-TDR-64–209-supplement*, 1965, 120p. (Douglas Aircraft Company Report SM-48703).

123. Winder, W. W., J. M. Hagberg, R. C. Hickson, A. A. Ehsani, and J. A. McLane. Time course of sympathoadrenal adaptation to endurance exercise training in man. *J. Appl. Physiol.* 45:370–374, 1978.

124. Winder, W. W., R. C. Hickson, J. M. Hagberg, A. A. Ehsani, and J. A. McLane. Training-induced changes in hormonal and metabolic responses to submaximal exercise. *J. Appl. Physiol.* 46:766–771, 1979.

8
Thermoregulation in Women
LOU A. STEPHENSON, Ph.D., MARGARET A. KOLKA, Ph.D.

INTRODUCTION

Early investigations concerning thermoregulation in women emphasized direct comparisons to men; eventually the importance of controlling for physical fitness, heat acclimation, body fat, and size before comparing men and women was recognized [2, 29, 39, 93]. More recent studies have emphasized the importance of controlling for menstrual cycle phase in thermoregulatory studies [19, 23, 55, 58, 59, 68]. Since it has become obvious that the reproductive cycle has profound thermoregulatory effects, the interactions between endocrine and thermoregulatory systems must be clarified. Future study of thermoregulation in women should focus on the complex integration of these and other regulatory systems to understand the unique thermoregulatory responses of women.

Neuroendocrine variations during the menstrual cycle modulate brain function via numerous mechanisms including changes in receptor number and sensitivity, changes in pulse frequency and amplitude, as well as by other factors [32, 60, 86, 97]. The importance of reproductive neuroendocrine variations on thermoregulation, cardiovascular regulation, metabolic regulation, and fluid volume regulation is now being appreciated through both systemic [5, 27, 38, 50, 58, 59, 94, 111, 113–116] and in vitro preparation studies [10, 12, 109, 110]. In neuronal single unit activity studies, steroidal reproductive hormones have been implicated as potential modulators of integrative neurons involved in temperature regulation. Specifically, neurons isolated from the preoptic region are responsive to more than one input; a temperature-sensitive neuron may also be estrogen sensitive [10, 110]. In fact, the degree of overlap in neuronal responses to multiple factors [10, 12] indicates that neurons are not, for the most part, functionally specific [11]. Still, a small percentage of neurons are responsive to nonthermal stimuli, but not temperature, and some neurons, when tested for many different stimuli, are sensitive only to temperature [9]. Multiple sensitivity of hypothalamic neurons may be one way to integrate function among several regulatory systems [10, 12, 109, 110]. These studies are particularly useful in interpreting interactions between the reproductive system and thermoregulation and should stimulate more in vivo studies.

It is difficult to separate thermoregulation from fluid volume or cardiovascular regulation when gauging systemic responses to a stressor, such as exercise, heat exposure, or cold exposure. The usual experimental approach when studying thermoregulation in humans is to assume that fluid volume or cardiovascular regulation is static during the experiment. Such untenable assumptions are made because it is so difficult to control more than one regulatory system during experiments in humans. In women, one solution to dealing with the complex interactions among several regulatory systems is to study thermoregulation or fluid volume regulation in a defined phase of the menstrual cycle. Thus, if menstrual cycle phase is consistent, it is assumed that the interaction of multiple regulatory systems is consistent, even though all those regulatory systems are not monitored simultaneously. It would be ideal to study whole-body responses of several regulatory systems simultaneously, especially when those regulatory systems interact with each other as do thermoregulation and cardiovascular and fluid volume regulation. That is nearly an impossible task, due to the enormous resources needed to accomplish such research. In effect, studies of whole-body responses to exercise of interdependent regulatory systems are done in a way in which the regulatory system that is not actively being studied is held as constant as possible. Because research is conducted in this genre, we will review the responses of women to exercise and thermal stresses with the focus being on each regulatory system. Perhaps, preliminary conclusions might be drawn about the interaction of the regulatory systems across the menstrual cycle, especially in regard to the impact of reproductive status on each.

To begin, a model of thermoregulation will be presented, followed by a brief description of reproductive physiology of women. The major focus of the review will be thermoregulation in women who have normal menstrual function. Imbedded in the discussion will be the impact of the menstrual cycle on fluid volume regulation during exercise, heat stress, or cold stress. Special aspects of thermoregulation in women will also be considered that may help us understand the factors that affect the integrative function of thermoregulation. In addition, the impact of menstrual dysfunction, pregnancy, and menopause on thermoregulation will be reviewed. Finally, suggestions for future research and essential considerations for research design in thermoregulatory studies of women are stated.

TEMPERATURE REGULATION

Autonomic control of thermoregulation has been reported in many regions of the central nervous system (CNS) and summarized recently by Boulant et al. [9]. The most thermosensitive of these regions are the preoptic area, anterior hypothalamus, and septum (PO/AH [7]). Lesion, thermal, or electrical stimulation and neuronal preparation studies indicate the PO/AH senses changes in peripheral temperature and in its own temperature, and integrates both to modulate heat loss, heat conservation, and heat production responses as appropriate [7]. Whole-body thermoregulatory responses in humans are often interpreted in terms of a proportional control model of thermoregulation. Hammel's model [52] may also describe human thermoregulatory responses because it contains the necessary components to explain observed whole-body thermoregulatory responses. The following equation describes Hammel's model of thermoregulation [52]:

$$R - R_o = \alpha_R (T_h - T_{set})$$

R is the response of the thermoregulatory effector, R_o is the initial thermoregulatory effector response prior to the pertubation, T_h is the hypothalamic temperature, while T_{set} is the set-point temperature for initiation of thermoregulatory effector neuronal activity; α_R is a proportionality constant that is equal to the change in response per unit change in temperature and an index of hypothalamic thermosensitivity. α_R is positive for heat dissipation responses and negative for heat conservation and heat production. Factors modulating thermoregulation act by affecting T_{set} or α_R. To include the modifications of thermoregulatory effector responses due to changes in skin temperature, an additional term can be added to the right side of the equation [52]. For a detailed discussion of the impact of skin temperature on thermoregulatory effector function in humans, please see reviews by Boulant [7], Brenglemann [13], and Johnson [63].

The *top part* of Figure 8.1 shows a neuronal scheme adapted from Boulant [8] to represent a proportional control system as proposed by Hammel [51]. It shows that skin thermoreceptors stimulate warm-sensitive (W) and temperature-insensitive (I) neurons in the PO/AH. The input from these temperature-sensitive and temperature-insensitive neurons are integrated by thermoregulatory effector neurons in the PO/AH to modulate heat loss, heat conservation, and heat production, depending on the summation of the inputs. For example, if warm thermoreceptors from the skin stimulate W neurons to increase firing frequency, excitatory input from W neurons to the heat-loss effector neurons is enhanced while the inhibitory input from I neurons will remain constant. The integrated effect would be to ↓ T_{set} of the heat-loss effector neurons so that heat loss would occur at a lower hypothalamic temperature when the skin was warm. Also, W neurons would inhibit cold-sensitive (C) neurons so that the integration of I input (excitatory) and W neuron input (inhibitory) would decrease the firing

FIGURE 8.1
Schematic representation of central thermoregulation in humans. Input from peripheral and central thermoreceptors is integrated and the appropriate thermoregulatory effector response (**R**) *is initiated. This simplified diagram was adapted from Boulant, J. A. [Thermoregulation. P. Mackowiak (ed).* Fever. Basic Mechanisms and Managements. New York: Raven Press, 1991] *and Hammel* [H. T. Neurons and temperature regulation. W. S. Yamamoto, and J. R. Brobek (eds). Physiological Controls and Regulations. *Philadelphia: W. B. Saunders, 1965.*], *and represents warm-sensitive* (**W**), *cold-sensitive* (**C**), *and temperature-insensitive* (**I**) *neurons in the PO/AH.*

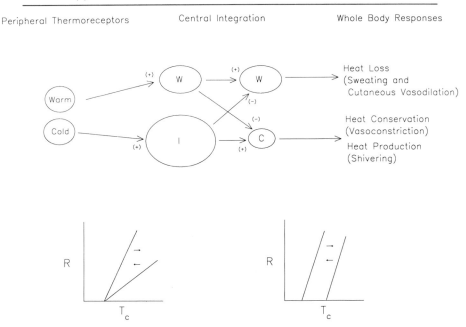

rate of C neurons. This would decrease the T_{set} of neuronal effectors for heat conservation and heat production. In other words, a lower hypothalamic temperature is needed to activate heat conservation and heat production mechanisms when skin temperature is warm.

Cold thermoreceptors in the skin provide excitatory input to I neurons. The increased firing rate of I neurons provides excitatory input C neurons to increase firing rate, thereby decreasing the T_{set} of the thermoregulatory effector neurons controlling heat conservation and heat production mechanisms. Therefore, the effect of a cold skin is to increase the hypothalamic temperature at which heat conservation, as well as heat loss, mechanisms are activated. Also, the increased firing rate of I neurons inhibits the firing rate of heat-loss effector neurons.

If the inputs of the temperature-sensitive and I neurons are equal and opposite to each other, the PO/AH is at the set-point temperature and whole-body thermoregulatory effectors are in equilibrium [7]. When the PO/AH temperature is greater than T_{set}, there is an increased firing rate of the W neurons and the effector neurons driving heat-loss responses are activated. This activation results in a proportional increase in cutaneous vasodilation and sweating as a function of the magnitude of the difference between T_h and T_{set} [51, 52]. When the PO/AH temperature is less than T_{set}, the firing rate of C neurons increases, and the effector neurons driving heat conservation and heat production mechanisms are activated in proportion to the magnitude of the difference between T_h and T_{set}.

The *bottom* of Figure 8.1 shows a simplistic scheme for whole-body thermoregulatory responses in humans. The same parameters are used in these diagrams, the only difference being that PO/AH temperature in humans is not measured, so the best approximation of the regulated temperature is used. In humans, esophageal temperature (T_{es}) has been advanced as the best index of brain temperature [14].

The *bottom* of Figure 8.1 illustrates several concepts used to explain how human thermoregulation may be adapted or modified. Whole-body effector responses (R), which are measured during exercise or during exposure to a hot environment, are plotted as a function of core temperature. If R is a heat dissipatory response as depicted here, R increases in proportion to the increase in core temperature as predicted by a proportional control model of thermoregulation. The *left bottom panel* shows a change in the slope of the $R:T_c$ relationship caused by some factor that affects thermoregulation. In Hammel's model [52], this slope is the term α_R. For a given change in core temperature, the change in the thermoregulatory effector response is less when the slope is reduced. In human thermoregulatory experiments, this change in slope is interpreted as a change in central thermosensitivity. That is, central integration or peripheral thermoregulatory effector response is modified so that the same change in core temperature causes less change in effector response. An example of altered central thermosensitivity is sleep deprivation, which decreases the central thermosensitivity of the sweating response during exercise [71, 103].

In human thermoregulation, any changes in PO/AH activity of thermoregulatory effector neurons indicative of set-point changes have to be interpreted from whole-body responses. Modulation of the core temperature threshold for onset of thermoregulatory effector response is determined as shown in the *bottom right panel* of Figure 8.1. The core temperature threshold for a thermoregulatory response during exercise or heat exposure is that temperature above which the effector response is greater than the control response in an individual resting in a thermoneutral environment. A decrease in the core temperature threshold for onset of a thermoregulatory effector response is interpreted as a decrease in the set-point temperature for neuronal activation of that thermoregulatory effector response. Both heat acclimation and physical training decrease the core temperature threshold for onset of cutaneous vasodilation and sweating [91, 96], while dehydration causes an increase in the core temperature threshold for onset of thermoregulatory effectors acting to dissipate heat [90]. Depending on the time of day used as the reference, the core temperature thresholds for onset of cutaneous vasodilation and sweating are either increased or decreased [117]. These threshold modifications may be the most useful indicator in human thermoregulation that there has been a change in the set-point temperature.

MENSTRUAL CYCLE

The reproductive system has an important role in modulating thermoregulation in women, at least in that core temperature is regulated at a higher temperature during the luteal phase compared with the follicular phase of the menstrual cycle. This regulated elevation in basal body temperature during the luteal phase may be necessary to provide the proper environment for implantation of the zygote in the uterus or it may be a vestigial event resulting from cyclic neuroendocrine changes in the brain. No matter how the luteal phase elevation in basal body temperature evolved, it is an interesting feature of thermoregulation in humans. Before reviewing how the menstrual cycle affects thermoregulation, a brief and simplified description of female reproductive physiology is presented. The detailed diagram of the reproductive system of women, modified from Fink [32], depicts the complex neuroendocrine interactions that occur throughout the reproductive cycle in the brain, including the hypothalamus, the anterior pituitary gland, and in the ovary and uterus (Fig. 8.2). Other factors that influence reproductive integration, such as light and circadian pacemakers, are also indicated. Figure 8.3 (modified from Fink [32] and McLachlan et al. [86]) shows the variation in circulating hormones from the pituitary and ovary, and core temperature changes.

The term "menstrual cycle" describes the approximately monthly rhythm in the function of the uterine endometrium, while the term "ovarian cycle" describes the cyclic change in ovarian function over the same time. The terminology of the ovarian and menstrual cycles is often interchanged so that the terms "follicular" and "luteal" phases of the menstrual cycle connote changes in ovarian hormone status. Because the ovarian and uterine cycles are the same length, the generic term "menstrual cycle" is used to include both of these cycles, as well as the neuroendocrine cycle of the brain. The reproductive cycle varies in

FIGURE 8.2

Schematic diagram of the female reproductive system including the hormonal interactions among the **brain, hypothalamus, pituitary, ovary** *and* **uterus** *during a 30-day menstrual cycle. This figure was modified from Fink, G. Gonadotropin secretion and its control. E. Knobil and J. D. O'Neill (eds).* The Physiology of Reproduction. *Vol. 1. New York: Raven Press, 1988.*

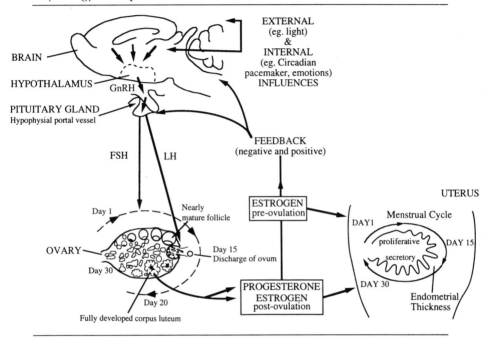

women from 27–35 days [122], but for this review, a reproductive cycle length of 30 days will be used.

The onset of menses is designated as the first day of the menstrual cycle in Figures 8.2 and 8.3. This presentation of time of the menstrual cycle is fine for a review, but it is more useful to depict changes in ovarian and pituitary hormones during the reproductive cycle as a function of time from the luteinizing hormone (LH) surge. The LH surge can then be used as a biological marker for each individual to standardize menstrual cycles of varying length. The time during which the follicle grows and matures is called the follicular phase of the ovarian cycle (days 1–14). Menses occurs from day 1 through approximately day 7, during which time the process of follicle recruitment occurs in the ovary [49, 60]. Several follicles (cohort) grow when follicle-stimulating hormone (FSH) is at a fairly high concentration from days 2–5 [86]. By approximately day 7, a dominant follicle is evident (Fig. 8.2), FSH decreases, and the rest of the cohort become atretic. As the dominant

FIGURE 8.3
*Schemactic representation of pituitary (**LH** and **FSH**) and ovarian (**estradiol, progesterone,** and **inhibin**) hormonal and daily core temperature (**T**$_C$) fluctuations during a 30-day menstrual cycle. This figure was modified from Fink, G., Gonadotropin secretion and its control. E. Knobil and J. D. O'Neill (eds).* The Physiology of Reproduction. *Vol. 1. New York: Raven Press, 1988, and McLachlan, R. I., D. M. Robertson, D. L. Healey, H. G. Burger, and D. M. deKrester. Circulating immunoreactive inhibin levels during the normal menstrual cycle.* J. Clin. Endocrinol. Method. *65:954–961, 1987.*

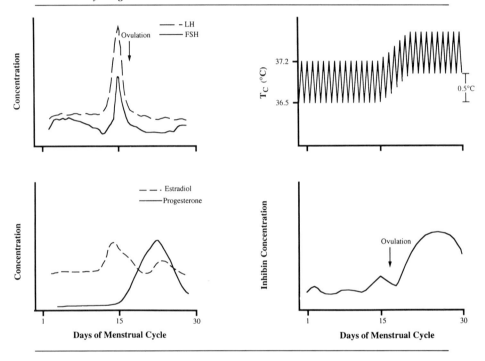

follicle increases in size (days 7–14), it produces greater quantities of estradiol and some progesterone (Fig. 8.3 [43]). The theca cells of the follicle become more vascularized [82]. Circulating estradiol secreted from the dominant follicle is necessary for the proper pulsatile frequency and amplitude in the secretion of gonadotropin-releasing hormone (GnRH) by the anterior hypothalamus [32, 60] in response to a neural pulse-generating signal [32, 134]. The combination of estradiol and GnRH increases the sensitivity of the gonadotropes in the anterior pituitary gland so that both FSH and LH secretion are increased [32]. In addition, increased circulating estradiol stimulates the endometrium of the uterus [21] during the proliferative phase of the menstrual cycle (days 7–14). By day 13–14, estradiol secretion from the dominant follicle is at its peak [43, 60, 86], and progesterone is slightly elevated.

In response to a neural signal [32], a GnRH surge is generated approximately 12 hr after the estradiol peak [60] causing both the FSH and LH surge on day 14–15 (Fig. 8.3). LH stimulation of the dominant follicle causes increased follicular blood flow and edema as well as increased prostaglandin synthesis. About 9 hr after the LH surge [60], ovulation occurs (Fig. 8.2) by follicle rupture [82].

After the LH surge and ovulation, the follicle involutes to become the corpus luteum. The gonadotropin surges and prolactin (PRL) secretion trigger changes in the enzymes of the granulosa (FSH, LH, PRL) and theca (LH, PRL) cells of the follicle so that they change from producing mainly estrogen to secretion of large amounts of progesterone [43]. The luteal phase of the ovarian cycle lasts 14 days, and the ovarian and pituitary hormones fluctuate during that time (Fig. 8.3). LH maintains the corpus luteum and enables progesterone secretion to become maximal during the midluteal phase [43]. During the luteal phase, estrogen and progesterone stimulate secretory activity in the uterine endometrium to support implantation (Fig. 8.2). Inhibin, another hormone secreted by the corpus luteum (Fig. 8.3 [112]), has approximately the same pattern of release during the luteal phase as does progesterone [86]. McLachlan et al. [86] have proposed that inhibin acts to decrease FSH release from the anterior pituitary during the luteal phase to arrest follicle stimulation. The LH pulse interval is greatly increased in the late luteal phase [49], probably because of changes in the GnRH pulse generator [97, 121]. When inhibin decreases in late luteal phase, FSH secretion increases, which begins the process of recruitment of the next cohort of follicles [49, 86, 112]. Progesterone and estradiol secretion also decrease dramatically in the late luteal phase, which is associated with curtailment of endometrial secretion and triggers endometrial necrosis and sloughing. Initiation of menses occurs and the reproductive cycle is repeated.

Considerations for Timing of Experiments

Core temperature exhibits a rhythm during the menstrual cycle in which body temperature is approximately 0.4°C higher in the luteal phase (after ovulation) than during the follicular phase [69, 98]. In addition, there is also a circadian rhythm in body temperature as shown in Figures 8.3 and 8.4 [113]. The impact of these distinct rhythms on resting esophageal (core) temperature for four women at two different times of day during the follicular and luteal phases of the menstrual cycle is shown on the *left side* of Figure 8.4. These resting body temperatures range from 36.76°C during early morning in the follicular phase to 37.48°C during the afternoon of the luteal phase, a 0.72°C (1.30°F)

FIGURE 8.4
Mean ± SD equilibrated esophageal temperatures measured at rest and during exercise (60% peak V̇O₂) for experiments conducted in the early mornings and midafternoons during the follicular and luteal phases of the menstrual cycle. Environmental conditions were 35°C, 30% relative humidity (rh). Adapted from Stephenson, L. A., and M. A. Kolka. Menstrual cycle phase and time of day after reference signal controlling arm blood flow and sweating. Am. J. Physiol. 249:R186–R191, 1985.

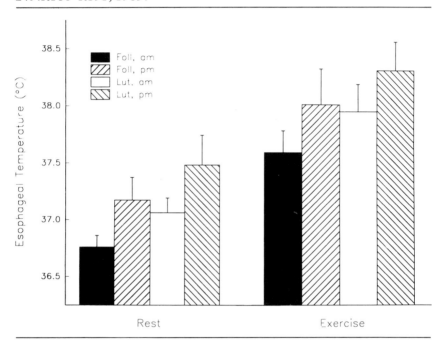

difference in resting core temperature! Statistical analysis of the individual data on the *left side* (resting) of Figure 8.4 indicates that core temperature is significantly different at all measured times (P<0.01).

Furthermore, the exercise data presented on the *right side* of Figure 8.4 indicate that resting core temperature recorded in the afternoon of the luteal phase is very similar to the core temperature measured during 30 minutes of moderate exercise in the early morning of the follicular phase experiments. If either the time of day, or menstrual cycle phase are mixed in the individual data that comprise the mean data shown in Figure 8.4 (for example, two subjects in each of morning, afternoon, follicular phase, or luteal phase), statistical differences in core temperature disappear (P=0.48). This example shows the effect about which Cunningham et al. [24] warned when they stated: "Such an experimental design tends to maximize variability within each phase, and to minimize the difference between the follicular and luteal phases."

Both experimental design and timing of experiments can influence the findings of a particular investigation. Many published papers indicate no clear difference in measured thermoregulatory parameters between menstrual cycle phases or between genders [2, 36, 129]. Generally, a closer examination indicates that the starting point in core temperature for the women used in those studies was mixed by time of day or menstrual cycle phase, thus there was an a priori bias toward finding insignificant differences. Not only can the timing of steady-state exercise or equilibrated resting temperatures affect statistical comparisons and the significance of research findings, but in addition, the core temperature thresholds for thermoregulatory effectors (sudomotor, vasomotor, shivering) are affected by time of day and menstrual cycle phase. This point is illustrated (Fig. 8.5) for the same core temperature data shown in Figure 8.4. In this example, the pattern of variability in resting core temperature is similar to that of both sudomotor and

FIGURE 8.5

Mean ± SD esophageal temperatures at rest during the morning and afternoons of both follicular and luteal phase experiments (**closed circles**). *The core temperature for the onset of sweating* (**squares**) *and skin blood flow* (**triangles**) *during exercise are superimposed on the resting core temperature data for circadian and menstrual cycle variability.*

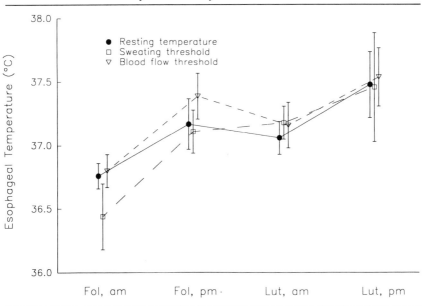

vasomotor core temperature thresholds. Clearly, menstrual cycle phase, as well as time of day, must be controlled when evaluating thermoregulatory function in women [113].

PHYSIOLOGICAL RESPONSES

The tolerated core temperature in humans is relatively narrow, ranging from 36–40°C [131]. Outside of this temperature range, thermoregulation is impaired or even lost. Humans routinely change their behavior to offset possible changes in body temperature, and have exquisite physiological mechanisms to regulate body temperature closely.

Cold Stress
At rest in a neutral environment, blood flow to the skin can be 0.2–0.3 liters·min^{-1} and, under severe cold stress, skin blood flow approaches zero [64]. During mild cooling of the skin and core, venoconstriction of cutaneous vessels increases the volume of the deeper veins. If cooling of the skin and core is more severe, additional heat-conserving vasoconstriction of surface vessels occurs, further increasing the volume of deeper veins [99]. Increased central venous blood volume inhibits antidiuretic hormone (ADH) release, which then causes diuresis and water loss. Elevated cardiac output, cardiac stroke volume, arterial pressure, and total peripheral resistance can accompany severe cold stress [99]. At rest in the cold, heat production increases secondarily to the initial venoconstriction and vasoconstriction [80] by increased metabolic rate and shivering. Since heat is lost from the body proportionally to surface area/mass, and smaller individuals have a smaller thermal mass and larger surface area to mass, smaller individuals (i.e., women) are less resistant to cold stress than larger individuals.

Exercise is associated with cutaneous vasoconstriction [64], which when combined with cold stress increases vasoconstrictor outflow to cutaneous arterioles to increase insulation and decrease heat loss from the body surface. During exercise in moderately cold environments, heat production dramatically increases and heat retention can be controlled behaviorally by varying the layers of clothing worn [41].

Differences in thermal mass, body surface area, surface area to mass, limb proportions, and distribution and amount of body fat all influence heat exchange in a cold environment by affecting heat production (lower muscle mass = lower heat production), insulation, or effective area for heat loss. Over 50 years ago, it was recognized that little was known about responses of women upon exposure to environmental cold stress [53]. Since that time, many descriptive studies comparing gender responses to cold stress have been done, but little effort has been spent to examine possible physiological mechanisms for differences between the genders, or the possible influence of menstrual cycle phase [44]. Nunneley [93] and, more recently, Graham [45], have summarized gender differences in the responses to cold stress (in both air and water) at rest and during exercise. In general, women resting in a cold environment have lower skin temperatures and, therefore, lower core to skin thermal conductance than men [24, 30, 45, 53, 133]. In cold-water immersion, women cool at faster rates than men [56, 76, 84].

In the mid-1980s, Hessemer and Brück characterized the effect of varying menstrual cycle phase on thermoregulation in women exposed to cold air [58, 59]. Heat production (metabolic rate) and electrical muscular activity were measured during cold exposure to ascertain the onset of shivering in the midfollicular and midluteal phases of the menstrual cycle. As earlier noted, body temperature is regulated at a higher level in the luteal phase in women with normal ovulatory menstrual cycles. This higher body temperature at rest, 0.6°C in this study, was associated with a higher core temperature threshold for heat production, measured by both increased muscular activity and increased oxygen consumption. These core temperature thresholds averaged 0.47°C higher in luteal phase experiments than in follicular phase experiments (see Fig. 8.6). So, the core temperature thresholds for the onset of thermoregulatory effectors to prevent body cooling occurred at higher core temperatures in the luteal phase compared with the follicular phase. Over 20 yr ago, two different laboratories demonstrated behavioral thermoregulatory changes to cooling [23, 68]. These behavioral changes were: *(a)* women sensed skin cooling more quickly in the luteal phase [68], and *(b)* women had a higher skin temperature preference in the luteal phase [23]. Both behavioral [23, 68] and autonomic thermoregulatory function [58, 59] were altered during the luteal phase so that the higher core temperature was maintained. Both of these modifications are consistent with an ↑ T_{set} in the luteal phase of the menstrual cycle.

During exposure to cold water, skin temperature is held constant or "clamped" so gender differences observed in skin temperature during cold air stress disappear. In general, women cool faster in cold water than men do [56, 76, 84]. In fact, in men and women matched for body fat percentage, McArdle et al. [84] observed faster cooling rates in both 20°C and 24°C water in women. Kollias et al. observed that women (22% fat) cooled at the same rate as men (15% fat) in 20°C water [76]. Increased body fat in women does provide insulation during water immersion [45], but the larger surface area to mass ratio and lower mass contributing to heat production in women certainly contribute to faster cooling during water immersion in women compared with men. At warmer water temperatures, Rennie et al. reported that women required a warmer water temperature than men did during water immersion that could be tolerated for 3 hr [95]. Women have a similar heat production effector response (increased metabolism to decreased core temperature)

FIGURE 8.6

Summary of changes in thermoregulatory effector (**R**) *function, during* **follicular** *and* **luteal** *phase experiments, showing the higher core temperature thresholds for both heat loss and heat production mechanisms.* **SkBF**, *skin blood flow [113];* **m$_s$**, *local sweating [73, 113];* **EMA**, *electrical muscular activity [58];* **ABF**, *arm blood flow [58, 59];* **ThBF**, *thumb blood flow [58];* **M**, *metabolic rate [58].*

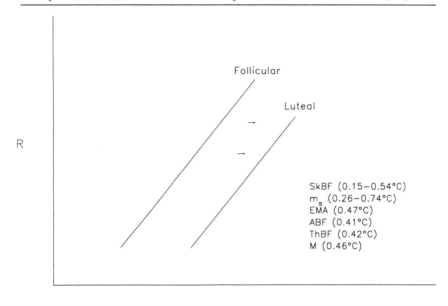

as men have during cold water exposure even though women cool at a faster rate than men do [56, 84].

In studies combining cold-water immersion with exercise, there are no differences in cooling if men and women exercise at the same absolute work intensity [76, 85]. However, the women are exercising at a higher percentage of their maximal aerobic power, which directly relates to the rate and amount of heat storage [101]. Yet, if men and women exercise at the same percentage of their maximal aerobic power, women cool faster than men do [44], illustrating the imbalance between heat loss and heat production.

Women have lower skin temperatures than men during cold air exposure [24, 53, 118, 124, 133], perhaps because of their greater body fat. The lower temperature of the general body surface reduces the gradient for sensible heat flux between the skin and the environment and helps prevent a decrease in core temperature during cold exposure [53]. Hardy et al. [53] and Wyndham and colleagues [133] reported similar core temperatures in men and women exposed to cold air at rest, while Cunningham et al. [24] and Wagner and Horvath [125] reported slightly higher core temperatures in women than men resting in the cold. There were no differences between genders in the skin temperature of acral areas, so women are probably not at a greater risk for peripheral cold injuries than men [124, 133].

The lower skin temperature seen in women at rest in cold environments is also observed during exercise [44, 46, 118, 126]. At similar absolute exercise intensities [46], men increase heat production whereas women decrease skin temperature (lower thermal conductance from core to skin) to maintain core temperature. However, during exercise at similar relative exercise intensities, core temperature in women decreases after 2 hr while men maintain their core temperature during that time [44]. This is another indication that heat loss exceeds heat production and heat conservation faster during exercise in a cold environment in women than in men.

Although $\uparrow$ T_{set} was described by the higher core temperature threshold for the onset of heat production during the luteal phase of the menstrual cycle [58, 59], additional studies of thermoregulatory effector function during cold exposure throughout the menstrual cycle are necessary. Graham [44] was unable to detect differences in rectal and skin temperature responses during exercise in cold air between the follicular and luteal phases. Mittleman and Mekjavic [88] have recently described a method for characterizing heat production effector responses as a function of decreasing esophageal temperature during cold-water immersion. Using their techniques, effector changes in heat conservatory and heat-producing thermoregulatory function associated with reproductive status may be characterized during water immersion.

Heat Stress
Exposure to the heat, even in a resting individual, requires active thermoregulatory effector mechanisms to maintain core temperature. During exercise, muscular contraction results in increased heat production, whereas at rest, when the ambient temperature is higher than the skin surface temperature, heat will be transferred from the environment to the body. Skin temperature is set by the environmental temperature and will reach a level imposed by the ambient conditions [42]. The same conductive and convective heat exchange avenues that remove heat from the body core to the skin surface transport heat from the body surface to the core. When core or skin temperatures are elevated, heat loss mechanisms are activated (via proportional control, Fig. 8.1), and sweat secretion and blood flow to the skin surface increase. Heat can then be eliminated by evaporative heat loss and by dry heat loss (if skin temperature exceeds ambient temperature). Evaporative heat loss is determined by the water vapor pressure gradient between the skin and

the environment. High sweating rates increase body water loss, initially from extracellular compartments. In addition, a greater proportion of the blood volume is directed to the skin vascular beds for heat dissipation from the core to the skin and from skin to the environment. In fact, skin blood flow can reach 8 liters $\cdot$min^{-1} or up to 60% of the cardiac output during heat stress [64], which will increase cardiovascular strain.

During exercise, if the heat of muscular contraction is not dissipated, core temperature would increase to an intolerable level within minutes. However, after a short time lag, increasing core temperature is sensed by the PO/AH, and neurons activating sweat secretion are stimulated. Subsequently, heat loss occurs by evaporation at the skin surface. If the water vapor pressure in the ambient air is high, evaporation of secreted sweat will not occur, and heat will not be dissipated. In the same way, increasing core temperature results in increased blood flow to the skin surface. At the skin, heat can be transferred to the environment by radiative and convective (R+C, dry) heat flux when the skin temperature is higher than the ambient temperature. If the ambient temperature is warmer than the skin surface temperature, heat is gained by the body.

Haslag and Hertzman [55] demonstrated that the onset of thermoregulatory sweating during whole body heating occurred at a higher core temperature in women during their luteal phase compared with their follicular phase. In addition, as mentioned earlier, women preferred a higher skin temperature in the luteal phase than during the follicular phase [23]. These observations suggested that the higher core temperature observed in the luteal phase was regulated. Changes in both behavioral and physiological thermoregulation [23, 55] were attributed to an elevation in the thermoregulatory set-point during the luteal phase of the human menstrual cycle. Thus, in a warm environment, the threshold for onset of sweating is at a higher temperature during the luteal phase in resting women, which serves to regulate core temperature at the higher temperature [55]. Central thermosensitivity is apparently not affected by the menstrual cycle, at least in the follicular and ovulatory phases, as indicated by thermal latency and sensitivity of sweat glands to acetyl-β-methylcholine stimulation [102].

The higher core temperature for sweating onset in women resting in a hot environment in their luteal phase compared with their follicular phase was confirmed by Bittel and Henane [6]. More recently, the effect of the menstrual cycle on effector function in women was investigated at rest and during exercise by two laboratories (Fig. 8.6 [58, 59, 73, 113]). Stephenson and Kolka reported higher core temperature thresholds for onset of both thermoregulatory sweating [73, 113] and cutaneous vasodilation [113] during exercise in a hot environment for women in the luteal phase of the menstrual cycle when compared with the follicular phase. Threshold changes in the onset of sweating and skin blood flow demonstrate that the thermoregulatory set-point was increased in the luteal phase, and fulfill the criterion [40] that a change in the thermoregulatory set-point must be observed by parallel changes in all involved thermoregulatory effectors (see Fig. 8.6).

Gender differences in autonomic thermoregulatory effector function during exercise have been reported [24, 92, 96]. The core temperature thresholds for both sweating and vasodilation were higher in women than in men. Menstrual cycle phase was not standardized in these studies [24, 92, 96], although it had been previously reported that preovulatory women respond to body heating similarly to men, but different than their own postovulatory responses [55]. The observations of these investigators [24, 92, 96] are similar to those reported by Fox et al. [34] and Morimoto et al. [89] and suggest that at a given core temperature, sweating and skin blood flow are lower in women compared with men. Men and women were compared while working at the same absolute exercise intensity, which required women to exercise closer to their maximal aerobic power than did the men [92, 96].

If the data of untrained men and trained women are compared [92], the differences between the men and the women narrow, even when the menstrual cycle phase of the women is not standardized. Also, if there was a disparity in training history between the men and the women, autonomic effector function may not be all that different between women in the follicular phase and men. In support of this, training appears to ↓ T_{set} as indicated by a lower core temperature threshold for the onset of cutaneous vasodilation and sweating during exercise [96]. In fact, the thermoregulatory responses of men and women were shown to be similar during exercise and moderate heat stress [74, 75] when the women were studied in only the follicular phase of the menstrual cycle, and the women had trained as many years as the men did. There were no differences in either the core temperature thresholds or the slopes of skin blood flow and sweating to core temperature between men and women (follicular phase) during the same environmental and exercise stress [74, 75]. If thermoregulatory effector responses are to be compared between genders, or if both men and women comprise the study population, it is essential that women be studied in the early follicular phase.

There were a number of other investigations between 1940 and 1978 that described how women respond to heat exposure [15, 30, 34, 40, 53, 55, 68, 89, 102, 127, 132]. Nunneley [93], in her review of 1978, interpreted these data as being qualitatively similar between men and women. Yet, for the most part, women had higher core and skin temperatures, higher heart rates, lower sweating rates, and later onset of sweating (determined by time and core temperature) than men had when both groups were exposed to the same environment. In 1969 Fox et al. [34] and in 1975 Bittel and Henane [6] reported that women began to sweat at higher core temperatures than did men, suggesting a delay in thermoregulatory heat loss that could lead to decreased heat tolerance. Wyndham et al. [132] and Morimoto et al. [89] reported lower sweating rates during heat exposure in women compared to men. However, Haslag and Hertzman [55] reported that the women studied before ovulation had similar sweating onset during passive heating to men. In these early studies, the men were more fit than were the women. Since tolerance to heat is related to aerobic fitness [16, 29, 39], some of the reported differences in heat tolerance between men and women might be, again, accounted for by differences in aerobic fitness. Anthropometric differences between genders can also affect heat loss to the environment, since women generally have a larger surface area to mass, heat gain is greater in severely hot environments [93]. Therefore, women may be at a disadvantage in severely hot environments.

Many studies were done comparing the responses of men and women to heat stress in the late 1970s and early 1980s [2, 3, 22, 25, 29, 31, 33, 35–37, 61, 62, 106–108, 128–130]. These papers compared men and women exercising at low intensities in a wide range of hot and humid environments. Some studies considered individual characteristics such as maximal aerobic power, body fat, or body surface area in an attempt to eliminate differences between men and women associated with any of these factors [2, 29, 35, 36, 107, 128]. In all cases, men had higher sweating rates than women did during light exercise in hot, dry conditions. Otherwise, the responses of men and women were similar during light exercise in warm to hot environments. Unfortunately, few of these investigators controlled experiments for menstrual cycle phase [2, 36, 62, 130], and only Horvath and Drinkwater [62] showed differences in resting core temperature between menstrual cycle phase. The general findings suggest that during light to moderate exercise in dry heat, women sweat less and have higher heart rates and core temperatures than do men [2, 35–37, 107]. If men and women exercise at the same percentage of their maximal aerobic power, and are matched for cardiovascular fitness, these differences narrow, especially during light exercise [2, 35–37, 107, 128]. Men still have higher sweating rates in dry environments. However, it was also reported that women may be more efficient "sweaters" during exercise in humid environments, as more of their secreted sweat was evaporated and less sweat drippage occurred [2, 35].

It has been suggested that during long duration exercise or heat exposure, differences observed in resting core temperature during the follicular and luteal phases of the menstrual cycle will be eliminated, and may be one reason for the lack of significant findings in some studies [58, 59]. Esophageal temperature data for a single exercising subject (80% peak $\dot{V}O_2$, 35°C) are shown in Figure 8.7 for both the follicular and luteal phases (Stephenson and Kolka, unpublished observations). At no time during the first 30 minutes of heavy exercise was the difference in core

FIGURE 8.7

Esophageal temperature *during exercise (80% peak* V̇o₂*) in both the* **follicular** *and* **luteal** *phases of the subject's menstrual cycle. Environmental conditions of the experiments were 35°C, 20% rh (Stephenson and Kolka, unpublished observations).*

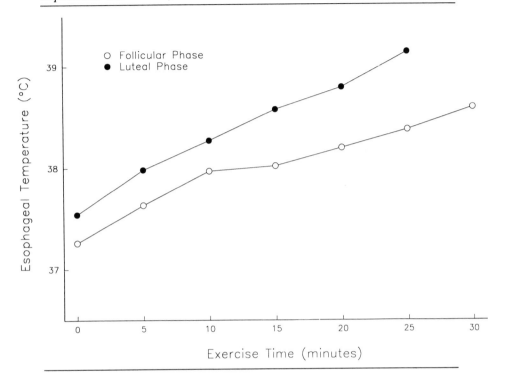

temperature less than that observed at rest between menstrual cycle phases. In fact, it appears that the difference in core temperature may be increasing. During 2 hr of low-intensity exercise in a hot environment, core temperature differences observed at rest among the follicular, ovulatory, and luteal phases were increased by approximately the same magnitude [19]. Further, it was recently reported by Pivarnik and colleagues [94] that, during exercise (65% peak V̇o₂) in a cool environment (22°C), rectal temperature continued to increase throughout a 1-hr experiment during the luteal phase, whereas during the follicular phase, rectal temperature reached a steady-state after approximately 30 min. Also, the heart rate was significantly increased during exercise in the luteal phase when compared with the follicular phase. It was suggested that the inability of women to reach thermal equilibrium during exercise in the luteal phase was mediated by progesterone [94].

Skin blood flow responses are different during the follicular and luteal phases of the menstrual cycle [1, 58, 59, 67, 68, 113, 116]. In general, limb blood flow is higher during the luteal phase compared with the follicular phase [4, 58, 59, 67, 68], which indicates that vascular responses vary with the changes in hormonal status during the menstrual cycle. Stephenson and Kolka have shown that the onset of vasoconstrictor activity during sustained heavy exercise is at both a higher skin blood flow and core temperature during the luteal phase than the follicular phase [116]. These observations suggest that heat transfer to and from the skin surface can be modified by menstrual cycle phase.

Postmenopausal women have similar thermoregulatory responses to 2 hr of heat exposure as do younger women [28]. The time and core temperature at which sweating was initiated, heat storage, skin blood flow, evaporative heat loss, and plasma volume changes were not different between the two groups of women, although phase of the menstrual cycle was not controlled in the premenopausal group. Drinkwater et al. [28] concluded that the function of the sweating mechanism of active postmenopausal women was not different from premenopausal women.

Fluid Volume Issues
Changes in vascular and extravascular fluid volumes impact significantly on thermoregulatory function, as sweating and skin blood flow responses to heating or exercise are attenuated when these fluid volumes are decreased (see [54] for review). Plasma volume decreases in euhydrated women at rest in hot environments [105, 114]. However, Wells and Horvath reported higher plasma volumes in women resting in a hot environment [129]. In most cases, during treadmill [29] and cycle exercise [33, 38, 72, 114, 115] in hot environments, plasma volume decreases. An expansion of the plasma volume after treadmill exercise was reported [130]; however, these data were complicated by positional changes in the subjects between blood samples [54]. Also, in one study [104], hemodilution occurred in both men and women during light exercise on a treadmill in a hot environment, but the resting blood sample was drawn in a cool environment. Increased skin temperature upon moving from a cool to a hot environment would be expected to cause a hemodilution [54].

Differences in plasma volume during the follicular and luteal phases of the menstrual cycle at rest or during exercise have been reported [38, 72, 114, 115]. Other investigators [33, 129, 130] indicated equivocal results. Those studies reporting differences show that resting plasma volume is lower during the luteal phase than the follicular phase [72, 114, 115], and a greater volume of vascular fluid is shifted during exercise and/or heat stress during the follicular phase than the luteal phase [38, 72, 114, 115]. There is some evidence [114] that a lower limit for plasma volume reduction during exercise or heat stress exists during the luteal phase. The variations in plasma volume at rest and during exercise that are observed during different menstrual cycle phases are similar in magnitude to the reported effects of posture, skin temperature, or perhaps even exercise intensity [54].

Aldosterone [27, 48, 66], plasma renin activity (PRA) [115], renin [66], and angiotensin [66] are higher in the luteal phase compared with the follicular phase of the menstrual cycle. The higher concentrations of these fluid regulatory hormones persist during both moderate [115] and heavy exercise [27] as aldosterone [115], PRA [27, 115], and vasopressin PVP [27] are higher during, and following, exercise in the luteal phase than the follicular phase. The increased aldosterone, PRA, and PVP during the luteal phase are consistent responses to the stimulus of decreased plasma volume. Each of these hormones will act to maintain fluid intravascularly and each participates in blood pressure regulation.

MENOPAUSE, PREGNANCY AND MENSTRUAL DYSFUNCTION

It is sometimes discouraging to study the physiology of women because our understanding of how the reproductive cycle impacts on other regulatory systems is far from complete. However, changes in reproductive status such as menopause, pregnancy, or menstrual dysfunction might provide an excellent opportunity to study how the reproductive system interacts with other regulatory systems, in particular, thermoregulation.

Amenorrhea/Menstrual Dysfunction
Amenorrhea is the term used to describe the absence of menses and is associated with infertility. Reduced follicular phase length and luteal phase insufficiency are other types of menstrual dysfunction associated with abnormal menstrual cycle length and anovulation [123]. In 1940, Hardy and DuBois observed that an amenorrheic female did not increase her metabolism during exposure to cold air like eumenorrheic women did [53]. These authors were not convinced that this observation was significant. It was shown 50 years later that amenorrheic women have lower core temperatures than eumenorrheic women when both groups rested in a cool (22°C) environment [47]. Core and skin temperature responses to cooling (22°C and 5°C) at rest and during exercise were similar between amenorrheic and eumenorrheic women. However, the amenorrheic women had lower finger temperatures than the eumenorrheic women while resting at 22°C [47]. In addition, increased heat production in response to body cooling was delayed in amenorrheic compared with eumenorrheic women. Conversely, there were no reported differences in core temperature, skin temperature, or sweating rate between amenorrheic and eumenorrheic women during light treadmill exercise in a hot environment [37].

In another report [94], a woman was studied during an hour of moderate exercise during both the follicular and luteal phases of her menstrual cycle. Low progesterone concentration measured during the luteal phase indicated luteal insufficiency and it was presumed that she did not ovulate. The resting core temperature of this woman was lower in the luteal than in the follicular phase, which likely indicates that T_{set} was not increased in her "luteal" phase. This woman also did not exhibit the uncompensated increase in rectal temperature during the last 20 min of exercise as the other women did [94]. One reason that her core temperature was maintained during prolonged exercise in the luteal phase was that her skin temperature was about 1°C higher than the mean skin temperature of the normally ovulating women. Increased skin temperature would increase dry heat loss, thereby decreasing heat storage. Also, the anovulatory woman did not have an increased heart rate during exercise in the luteal phase as the normally ovulating women did, which reflects her lower cardiovascular strain in conjunction with lower heat storage. Pivarnik et al. [94] attributed the better thermoregulatory capability of the anovulatory woman to her low progesterone concentration in the luteal phase.

Pregnancy
Physiological changes associated with pregnancy can impact on thermoregulatory function in women. McMurray and Katz [87] have recently reviewed critical issues associated with thermoregulation during pregnancy. Possible teratogenic effects of increased body temperature during exercise and/or heat stress early in pregnancy, and the maintenance of uterine blood flow as pregnancy continues, are of primary concern. Two studies reported thermoregulatory function during aerobic exercise through 32 weeks of gestation [20, 65]. The intensity of the exercise decreased with time of pregnancy. However, these women were able to regulate core temperature effectively in temperate environments into the third trimester [20, 65, 87]. In general, exercise at either high intensity or long duration is probably not appropriate during pregnancy due to the risks of hyperthermia and dehydration [87]. There is no evidence that temperature regulation is impaired, but blood pressure regulation can be adversely affected by pregnancy. Therefore, thermoregulation might also be influenced because the two systems closely interact [99].

Menopause
The process of menopause begins when normal cyclic ovarian function is intermittently disrupted, and is manifested by either reduced follicular phase length or luteal phase dysfunction [123]. Both conditions are associated with anovulatory cycles. Steroidogenesis by the follicle and the corpus luteum are impaired so that the neuroendocrine balance of the

menstrual cycle is upset [123], which causes further disruption of follicle growth (Fig. 8.2). The process of menopause is complete when the follicles within the ovary are depleted. Estrogen, progesterone, and probably inhibin concentrations are markedly reduced while FSH and LH concentrations are greatly increased [123]. It is thought that GnRH is secreted in high concentration during the process of menopause and is the stimulus for the elevated LH concentrations. Hot flashes are experienced by 75% of women undergoing menopause [77]. Estrogen and progesterone replacement therapy is effective in reducing hot flashes.

The changes in thermoregulatory effector function that occur during menopause present an interesting topic for students of temperature regulation [79]. The hot flush or hot flash is associated with physical and emotional discomfort [77, 78]. During a hot flash, a woman will have increased blood flow (higher skin temperature) and sweating at various areas of the skin surface [123]. These events occur more often when the skin is hot (high environmental temperature) than when the skin is cool [78]. Lomax et al. [83] have suggested that the hot flash is triggered by a downward setting of the regulated core temperature or $\downarrow T_{set}$, which immediately gives rise to a "feeling of hotness." A $\downarrow T_{set}$ is then followed by $\uparrow$ thermoregulatory heat dissipation effector activity, that is, sweating and increased blood flow to the skin surface to dissipate body heat so that core temperature decreases to the transiently $\downarrow T_{set}$. It has been suggested that vasomotor changes associated with a hot flash are related to the pulsatile LH release, or perhaps to GnRH activity in the PO/AH [120].

Menopausal hot flashes are of short duration [78] and may be initiated by a transient decrease in T_{set}. Such a short duration shift in T_{set} is a somewhat unique observation in thermoregulatory integrative function. In contrast, the circadian alteration in T_{set} develops over several hours. Another quickly developing modulation in T_{set} may be associated with transitions between arousal states [57, 81, 100]. The postulated $\downarrow T_{set}$ of the hot flash is temporally consistent with changes in GnRH, FSH, and/or LH pulses, but could just as easily be associated with neurotransmitter oscillator(s) or pulse generators because the hot flash appears to precede increased LH [120, 123]. Withdrawal of the cyclic feedback action of estrogen and progesterone during menopause would be expected to alter the pulse frequency and/or pulse amplitude of neuromodulators controlling hypothalamic release of GnRH because that normally happens during the menstrual cycle [97, 134]. Studies that show that individual temperature-sensitive and I neurons are multisensory [10, 12] suggest that menopausal neuroendocrine modulations could impact on either or both of these PO/AH neuronal populations to $\downarrow T_{set}$. For example, a transient change in neuroendocrine pulse frequency or amplitude might increase the firing rate of W neurons. The equilibrium with input from I neurons is upset, which increases the firing rate of those neurons driving heat-loss effectors (Fig. 8.1). The same effect could occur by neuroendocrine modulation, which reduces inhibitory input of I neurons. The summation of inputs would increase the firing rate of those neurons initiating sweating and cutaneous vasodilation. The observation that warm skin is associated with more frequent hot flashes [78] is consistent with the proportional control of thermoregulation. In a warm environment, afferent input from warm skin would increase the firing rate of W neurons such that the inhibitory input to the neurons affecting heat loss mechanisms is exceeded. This also would have the effect of ↓ T_{set} and would initiate sweating and cutaneous vasodilation.

Estrogen Replacement Therapy
Estrogen replacement therapy (ERT) is commonly prescribed at or around menopause to decrease physiological symptoms of estrogen withdrawal, such as the occurrence of hot flashes [77]. Kronenberg et al. [77] and Lomax [83] have suggested the estrogen withdrawal at menopause ↓ T_{set}. However, estradiol increases the firing of W neurons and decreases core temperature [10, 11, 110]. Menopause is a condition of very low estrogen concentration and it does not seem likely that there would be episodic pulses of estrogen reaching the PO/AH. Apparently, the effect of estrogen withdrawal is to change other neuroendocrine factors, perhaps the neurotransmitter mediating GnRH pulse generation, which, in turn, has an effect on the thermoregulatory neurons. Estrogen replacement therapy (Premarin or Estraderm) in postmenopausal women decreased core temperature at rest and during exercise, decreased heart rate and arm blood flow during exercise, and decreased the esophageal temperature for the onset of arm blood flow and sweating [119]. These observations [119], combined with the observations of increased firing rate for W PO/AH neurons by Silva and Boulant [110], suggest that estrogens may ↓ T_{set}.

SUMMARY AND FUTURE CONSIDERATIONS

Reproductive physiology is an important modulator of thermoregulatory function in women. The mechanism causing the increase in the thermoregulatory set-point in the luteal phase of the ovarian cycle is not known, but integration among higher brain centers and the hypothalamic-hypophyseal-ovarian axis are involved. One of these integrative events, or a combination of events, apparently causes heat-loss effector neurons to be activated at a higher core temperature compared with the follicular phase. Heat retention and production effectors are also activated at a higher temperature during the luteal phase than in the follicular phase as evidenced by whole-body thermoregulatory responses of women.

To stimulate future research on thermoregulatory function in women and to provoke modification of current neuronal models of thermoregulation, a few speculative thoughts about how T_{set} is increased during the luteal phase are presented. If Hammel's model of thermoregulation [51, 52] is used, the luteal T_{set} elevation could be modified through a mechanism similar to the elevation in T_{set}, which occurs during fever. Boulant [8] has reviewed how a pyrogen caused an elevation in T_{set} and has presented evidence that this response was consistent with Hammel's model of thermoregulation. In short, the pyrogen decreases the firing rate of W neurons. This causes the equilibrium temperature, at which the excitatory input from W neurons is equal to the inhibitory input from I neurons, to increase, thereby effecting an increase in T_{set}. An elevated T_{set}, in turn, causes heat-loss effector neurons to be activated at a higher temperature, and causes activation of neurons effecting heat retention and heat production mechanisms. Therefore, the body temperature is increased to the new set-point temperature [8]. Thermoregulatory modifications may be as subtle as a behavioral change or vasoconstriction of cutaneous blood vessels when there is a small increase in T_{set} or as obvious as intense shivering to produce heat, which increases core temperature when T_{set} is elevated substantially.

In fever, several pyrogens have been identified [70], among them interleukin-1 (IL-1) and interleukin-6 (IL-6). In the luteal phase, basal body temperature is elevated for days and the 0.4°C-elevation in T_{set} is comparable with a low-grade fever. Cannon and Dinarello [17] have shown that there is increased IL-1 circulating during the luteal phase, which could explain this T_{set} elevation if the increased IL-1 identified is acting to decrease firing rate of W neurons in the hypothalamus. T_{set} may be elevated during the luteal phase by increased inhibitory input of I neurons to heat-loss effector neurons and/or by increased excitatory input to C neurons. This will increase the firing rate of heat retention effector neurons and will increase heat production. This possibility, without evidence from neuronal studies, is attractive because estradiol and progesterone feedback to the brain modulates hypothalamic GnRH release. Hypothalamic modulation of GnRH is just one of many complex neuroendocrine interactions that occur during the luteal phase. It is not hard to imagine that any one of many neuroendocrine events occurring during the time of ovulation and the luteal phase may be increasing the firing rate of I neurons to cause an increased T_{set}. Progesterone injected intramuscularly in amenorrheic or ovariectomized women caused body temperature to increase [26]. Also, when there is little or limited increase in progesterone concentration in the luteal phase, basal body temperature does not increase despite surges in LH and FSH [18]. Although increased progesterone is the most often proposed mechanism for mediating the ↑ T_{set} [23, 58, 59, 68, 113] and other thermoregulatory modifications in the luteal phase [94], there are many other possibilities. If an ovarian factor is responsible for ↑ T_{set} during the luteal phase, inhibin might be just as likely a candidate as progesterone is, because both fit the same temporal pattern of secretion (Fig. 8.3). Other potential stimuli for mediating the ↑ T_{set} in the luteal phase are interactions between fluid volume regulation and thermoregulation, including multisensory neurons [10 12, 109] and whole-body responses.

To summarize, thermoregulation in women of reproductive age is characterized by increased core temperature thresholds for onset of all thermoregulatory effectors during exercise, heat, and cold exposure during the luteal phase of the menstrual cycle [23, 55, 58, 59, 73, 113]. Higher core temperature thresholds for onset of thermoregulatory effector function are consistent with ↑ T_{set} in the luteal phase. Thermoregulation may be somewhat compromised during prolonged exercise or heat exposure in the luteal phase [94, 114], perhaps due to the smaller plasma volume [38, 114]. Postmenopausal women have the same thermoregulatory effector response (sweating) to increased core temperature during heat exposure as have premenopausal women [28]. Perimenopausal and postmenopausal women have a lower resting core temperature and lower core temperature thresholds for onset of sweating and cutaneous vasodilation during exercise (↓ T_{set}) after estrogen replacement therapy than they did before therapy [119].

ACKNOWLEDGMENTS

We thank S. Yazzi and S. Millett for bibliographic assistance and J. Gonzalez and L. Blanchard for drawing the illustrations. The editorial feedback from L. Blanchard, J. DeLuca, and L. Levine was greatly appreciated. We thank Drs. M. N. Sawka, R. R. Gonzalez, and K. B. Pandolf for reviewing the manuscript.

REFERENCES

1. Altura, B. M. Sex and estrogens and responsiveness of terminal arterioles to neurohypophyseal hormones and catecholamines. *J. Pharmacol. Exper. Ther.* 193:403–412, 1975.
2. Avellini, B. A., E. Kamon, and J. T. Krajewski. Physiological responses of physically fit men and women to acclimation to humid heat. *J. Appl. Physiol.* 49:254–261, 1980.
3. Avellini, B. A., Y. Shapiro, K. B. Pandolf, N. A. Pimental, and R. F. Goldman. Physiological responses of men and women to prolonged dry heat exposure. *Aviat. Space Environ. Med.* 51:1081–1085, 1980.
4. Bartelink, M. L., H. Wollersheim, A. Theeuwes, D. Van Duren, and T. Thien. Changes in skin blood flow during the menstrual cycle: the influence of the menstrual cycle on the peripheral circulation in healthy female volunteers. *Clin. Sci.* 78:527–532, 1990.

5. Baylis, P. H., B. A. Spruce, and J. Burd. Osmoregulation of vasopressin secretion during the menstrual cycle. R. W. Schrier (ed). *Vasopressin*. New York: Raven Press, 1985, pp. 241–247.
6. Bittel, J., and R. Henane. Comparison of thermal exchanges in men and women under neutral and hot conditions. *J. Physiol. (London)* 250:475–489, 1975.
7. Boulant, J. A. Hypothalamic control of thermoregulation. Neurophysiological basis. P. J. Morgane and J. Panksepp (eds). *Handbook of the Hypothalamus*. Vol. 3 part A, New York: Marcel Dekker, Inc., 1980, pp. 1–82.
8. Boulant, J. A. Thermoregulation. P. Mackowiak (ed.). *Fever: Basic Mechanisms and Managements*. New York: Raven Press, 1991, pp. 1–21.
9. Boulant, J. A., M. C. Curras, and J. B. Dean. Neurophysiological aspects of thermoregulation. L. C. H. Wang (ed). *Advances in Comparative and Environmental Physiology*. Vol. 4, Berlin: Springer-Verlag, 1989, pp. 118–155.
10. Boulant, J. A., and N. L. Silva. Interactions of reproductive steroids, osmotic pressure, and glucose on thermosensitive neurons in preoptic tissue slices. *Can. J. Physiol. Pharmacol.* 65:1267–1273, 1987.
11. Boulant, J. A., and N. L. Silva. Multisensory hypothalamic neurons may explain interactions among regulatory systems. *News Physiol. Sci.* 4:245–248, 1989.
12. Boulant, J. A., and N. L. Silva. Neuronal sensitivities in preoptic tissue slices: interactions among homeostatic systems. *Brain Res. Bull.* 20:871–878, 1988.
13. Brengelmann, G. L. Circulatory adjustments to exercise and heat stress. *Ann. Rev. Physiol.* 45:191–212, 1983.
14. Brengelmann, G. L. Dilemma of body temperature measurement. K. Shiraki and M. K. Yousef (eds). *Man in Stressful Environments. Thermal and Work Physiology*. Springfield, IL: Charles C Thomas, 1987, pp. 5–22.
15. Brouha, L., P. E. Smith, Jr., R. D. E. Lanne, and M. E. Maxfield. Physiological reactions of men and women during muscular activity and recovery in various environments. *J. Appl. Physiol.* 16:133–140, 1961.
16. Byrd, R., L. Stewart, C. Torranin, and O. M. Berringer. Sex differences in response to hypohydration. *J. Sports Med.* 17:65–68, 1977.
17. Cannon, J. G., and C. A. Dinarello. Increased plasma interleukin-1 activity in women after ovulation. *Science* 227:1247–1249, 1985.
18. Cargille, C. M., G. T. Ross, and T. Yoshimi. Daily variations in plasma follicle stimulating hormone, luteinizing hormone and progesterone in the normal menstrual cycle. *J. Clin. Endocrinol.* 29:12–19, 1969.
19. Carpenter, A. J., and S. A. Nunneley. Endogenous hormones subtly alter women's response to heat stress. *J. Appl. Physiol.* 65:2313–2317, 1988.
20. Clapp, J. F., III, M. Wesley, and R. H. Sleamaker. Thermoregulatory and metabolic responses to jogging prior to and during pregnancy. *Med. Sci. Sports Exerc.* 19:124–130, 1987.
21. Clark, J. H., and B. M. Markaverich. Actions of ovarian steroid hormones. E. Knobil and J. D. Neill (eds). *The Physiology of Reproduction*. Vol. 1, New York: Raven Press, 1988, pp. 675–724.
22. Cohen, J. S., and C. V. Gisolfi. Effects of interval training on work-heat tolerance of young women. *Med. Sci. Sports Exerc.* 14:46–52, 1982.
23. Cunningham, D. J., and M. Cabanac. Evidence from behavorial thermoregulatory responses of a shift in setpoint temperature related to the menstrual cycle. *J. Physiol. (Paris)* 63:236–238, 1971.
24. Cunningham, D. J., J. A. J. Stolwijk, and C. B. Wenger. Comparative thermoregulatory responses of resting men and women. *J. Appl. Physiol.* 45:908–915, 1978.
25. Davies, C. T. M. Thermoregulation during exercise in relation to sex and age. *Eur. J. Appl. Physiol.* 42:71–79, 1979.
26. Davis, M. E., and N. W. Fugo. The cause of physiologic basal temperature changes in women. *J. Clin. Endocrinol.* 8:550–563, 1948.

27. De Souza, M. J., C. M. Maresh, M. S. Maguire, W. J. Kraemer, G. Flora-Ginter, and K. L. Goetz. Menstrual status and plasma vasopressin, renin activity, and aldosterone exercise response. *J. Appl. Physiol.* 67:736–743, 1989.

28. Drinkwater, B. L., J. F. Bedi, A. B. Loucks, S. Roche, and S. M. Horvath. Sweating sensitivity and capacity in relation to age. *J. Appl. Physiol.* 53:671–675, 1982.

29. Drinkwater, B. L., J. E. Denton, I. C. Kupprat, T. S. Talag, and S. M. Horvath. Aerobic power as a factor in women's response to work in hot environments. *J. Appl. Physiol.* 41:815–821, 1976.

30. DuBois, E. F., F. G. Ebaugh, and J. D. Hardy. Basal heat production and elimination of thirteen normal women at temperatures from 22°C to 35°C. *J. Nutr.* 48:257–293, 1952.

31. Fein, J. T., E. M. Haymes, and E. R. Buskirk. Effects of daily and intermittent exposures on heat acclimation of women. *Int. J. Biometeor.* 19:41–52, 1975.

32. Fink, G. Gonadotropin secretion and its control. E. Knobil and J. D. Neill (eds). *The Physiology of Reproduction.* Vol. 1, New York: Raven Press, 1988, pp. 1349–1377.

33. Fortney, S. M., and L. C. Senay, Jr. Effects of training and heat acclimation on exercise responses of sedentary females. *J. Appl. Physiol.* 47:978–984, 1979.

34. Fox, R. H., B. E. Lofstedt, P. M. Woodward, E. Erickson, and B. Werkstrom. Comparison of thermoregulatory function in men and women. *J. Appl. Physiol.* 26:444–453, 1969.

35. Frye, A. J., and E. Kamon. Responses to dry heat of men and women with similar aerobic capacities. *J. Appl. Physiol.* 50:65–70, 1981.

36. Frye, A. J., and E. Kamon. Sweating efficiency in acclimated men and women exercising in humid and dry heat. *J. Appl. Physiol.* 54:927–977, 1983.

37. Frye, A. J., E. Kamon, and M. Webb. Responses of menstrual women, amenorrheal women, and men to exercise in a hot, dry environment. *Eur. J. Appl. Physiol.* 48:279–288, 1982.

38. Gaebelein, C. J., and L. C. Senay, Jr. Vascular volume dynamics during ergometer exercise at different menstrual phases. *Eur. J. Appl. Physiol.* 50:1–11, 1982.

39. Gisolfi, C. V., and J. S. Cohen. Relationships among training, heat acclimation, and heat tolerance in men and women: the controversy revisited. *Med. Sci. Sports* 11:56–59, 1979.

40. Gisolfi, C. V., and C. B. Wenger. Temperature regulation during exercise: old concepts, new ideas. R. L. Terjung (ed). *Exercise Sports Sciences Reviews.* Vol. 14, Lexington: Collamore, 1984, pp. 339–372.

41. Gonzalez, R. R. Biophysical and physiological integration of proper clothing for exercise. K. B. Pandolf (ed). *Exercise and Sports Sciences Reviews.* Vol. 15, New York: Macmillan, 1987, pp. 261–295.

42. Gonzalez, R. R., L. G. Berglund, and A. P. Gagge. Indices of thermoregulatory strain for moderate exercise in the heat. *J. Appl. Physiol.* 44:889–899, 1978.

43. Gore-Langton, R. E., and D. T. Armstrong. Follicular steroidogenesis and its control. E. Knobil and J. D. Neill (eds). *The Physiology of Reproduction.* Vol. 1, New York: Raven Press, 1988, pp. 331–385.

44. Graham, T. E. Alcohol ingestion and sex differences on the thermal responses to mild exercise in a cold environment. *Hum. Biol.* 55:463–476, 1983.

45. Graham, T. E. Thermal, metabolic and cardiovascular changes in men and women during cold stress. *Med. Sci. Sports Exerc.* 20:S185–S192, 1988.

46. Graham, T. E., and M. D. Lougheed. Thermal responses to exercise in the cold: influence of sex differences and alcohol. *Hum. Biol.* 57:687–698, 1985.

47. Graham, T. E., M. Viswanathan, J. P. Va Dijk, A. Bonen, and J. C. George. Thermal and metabolic resposes to cold by men and by eumenorrheic and amenorrheic women. *J. Appl. Physiol.* 67:282–290, 1989.

48. Gray, M., K. S. Strausfeld, M. Watanabe, E. A. H. Sims, and S. Solomon. Aldosterone secretory rates in the normal menstrual cycle. *J. Clin. Endocrinol.* 28:1269–1275, 1968.

49. Greenwald, G. S., and P. F. Terranova. Follicular selection and its control. E. Knobil and J.D. Neill (eds). *The Physiology of Reproduction.* Vol. 1, New York: Raven Press, 1988, Vol. 1, pp. 387–445.
50. Hackney, A. C. Effects of the menstrual cycle on resting muscle glycogen content. *Horm. Metabal. Res.* 22:644, 1990.
51. Hammel, H. T. Neurons and temperature regulation. W. S. Yamamoto and J. R. Brobek (eds). *Physiological Controls and Regulations.* Philadelphia: W. B. Saunders, 1965, pp. 71–97.
52. Hammel, H. T., D. C. Jackson, J. A. J. Stolwijk, J. D. Hardy, and S. B. Stromme. Temperature regulation by hypothalamic proportional control with an adjustibale set point. *J. Appl. Physiol.* 18:1146–1154, 1963.
53. Hardy, J. D., and E. F. DuBois. Differences between men and women in their response to heat and cold. *Proc. Nat. Acad. Sci.* 26:389–398, 1940.
54. Harrison, M. H. Effects of thermal stress and exercise on blood volume in humans. *Physiol. Rev.* 65:149–209, 1985.
55. Haslag, S. W. M., and A. B. Hertzman. Temperature regulation in young women. *J. Appl. Physiol.* 20:1283–1288, 1965.
56. Hayward, J.S., J. D. Eckerson, and M. L. Collins. Thermal balance and survival time prediction of man in cold water. *Can. J. Physiol. Pharmacol.* 53:21–32, 1975.
57. Heller, H. C., S. Glotzbach, D. Grahn, and C. Raedeke. Sleep-dependent changes in the thermoregulatory system. R. Lydic and J. F. Biebuyck (eds). *Clinical Physiology of Sleep.* Bethesda, MD: American Physiological Society, 1988, pp. 145–158.
58. Hessemer, V., and K. Brück. Influence of menstrual cycle on shivering, skin blood flow, and sweating responses measured at night. *J. Appl. Physiol.* 59:1902–1910, 1985.
59. Hessemer, V., and K. Brück. Influence of menstrual cycle on thermoregulatory, metabolic, and heart rate responses to exercise at night. *J. Appl. Physiol.* 59:1911–1917, 1985.
60. Hodgen. G. D. Neuroendocrinology of the normal menstrual cycle. *J. Reproduc. Med.* 34:68–75, 1989.
61. Horstman, D. H., and E. Christensen. Acclimation to dry heat: active men vs. active women. *J. Appl. Physiol.* 52:825–831, 1982.
62. Horvath, S. M., and B. L. Drinkwater. Thermoregulation and the menstrual cycle. *Aviat. Space Environ. Med.* 53:790–794, 1982.
63. Johnson, J. M. Exercise and the cutaneous circulation. J. O. Holozsy (ed). *Exercise and Sport Sciences Reviews.* Vol. 20, Baltimore: Williams & Wilkins, 1992, pp. 59–97.
64. Johnson, J. M., G. L. Brengelmann, J. R. S. Hales, P. M. Vanhoutte, and C. B. Wenger. Regulation of the cutaneous circulation. *Fed. Proc.* 45:2841–2850, 1986.
65. Jones, R. L., J. J. Botti, W. M. Anderson, and N. L. Bennett. Thermoregulation during aerobic exercise in pregnancy. *Obstet. Gynecol.* 65:340–345, 1985.
66. Kaulhausen, H., G. Leyendecker, G. Benker, and H. Breuer. The relationship of the renin-angiotensin-aldosterone system to plasma gonadotropin, prolactin, and ovarian steroid patterns during the menstrual cycle. *Arch. Gynak.* 225:179–200, 1978.
67. Keates, J. S., and D. E. Fitzgerald. Limb volume and blood flow changes during the menstrual cycle. *Angiol.* 20:624–627, 1969.
68. Kenshalo, D. R. Changes in the cool threshold associated with phases of the menstrual cycle. *J. Appl. Physiol.* 21:1031–1039, 1966.
69. Kleitman, N., and A. Ramsaroop. Periodicity in body temperature and heart rate. *Endocrinology* 43:1–20, 1948.
70. Kluger, M. J. Fever: Role of pyrogens and cryogens. *Physiol. Rev.* 71:93–127, 1991.
71. Kolka, M. A., and L. A. Stephenson. Exercise thermoregulation after prolonged wakefulness. *J. Appl. Physiol.* 64:1574–1579, 1988.
72. Kolka, M. A., and L. A. Stephenson. Plasma volume loss during maximal exercise in females. *The Physiologist* 33:A73, 1990.

73. Kolka, M.A., L. A. Stephenson, and R. R. Gonzalez. Control of sweating during the human menstrual cycle. *Eur. J. Appl. Physiol.* 58:890–895, 1989.

74. Kolka, M. A., L. A. Stephenson, and R. R. Gonzalez. Depressed sweating during exercise at altitude. *J. Thermal. Biol.* 14:167–170, 1989.

75. Kolka, M. A., L. A. Stephenson, P. B. Rock, and R. R. Gonzalez. Local sweating and cutaneous blood flow during exercise in hypoxic environments. *J. Appl. Physiol.* 62:2224–2229, 1987.

76. Kollias, J., L. Bartlett, B. Bergsteinova, J. S. Skinner, E. R. Buskirk, and W. L. Nicholas. Metabolic and thermal responses of women during cooling in cold water. *J. Appl. Physiol.* 36:577–580, 1974.

77. Kronenberg, F. Hot flashes: epidemiology and physiology. *Ann. N.Y. Acad. Sci.* 592:52–86, 1990.

78. Kronenberg, F., and R. M. Barnard. Modulation of menopausal hot flashes by ambient temperature. *J. Therm. Biol.* 17:43–49, 1992.

79. Kronenberg, F., and J. A. Downey. Thermoregulatory physiology of menopausal hot flashes: a review. *Can. J. Physiol. Pharmacol.* 65:1312–1324, 1987.

80. LeBlanc, J. *Man in the Cold.* Springfield, IL: Charles C Thomas, 1975.

81. Lindsley, J. G., L. Levine, M. A. Kolka, and L. A. Stephenson. Esophageal temperature decrease anticipates REM sleep onset. *Sleep Res.* 20A:546, 1991.

82. Lipner, H. Mechanism of mammalian ovulation. E. Knobil and J. D. Neill (eds). *The Physiology of Reproduction.* Vol. 1, New York: Raven Press, 1988, pp. 447–488.

83. Lomax, P., J. G. Bajorek, and I. V. Tataryn. Thermoregulatory changes following the menopause. Z. Szelényi and M. Székelv (eds). *Contributions to Thermal Physiology.* Vol. 32, Budapest: Akadémiai Kiadó, 1981, pp. 41–44.

84. McArdle, W. D., J. R. Magel, T. J. Gergley, R. J. Spina, and M. M. Toner. Thermal adjustment to cold-water exposure in resting men and women. *J. Appl. Physiol.*56: 1565–1571, 1984.

85. McArdle, W. D., J. R. Magel, R. J. Spina, T. J. Gergley, and M. M. Toner. Thermal adjustment to cold-water exposure in exercising men and women. *J. Appl. Physiol.* 56:1572–1577, 1984.

86. McLachlan, R. I., D. M. Robertson, D. L. Healy, H. G. Burger, and D. M. de Kretser. Circulating immunoreactive inhibin levels during the normal human menstrual cycle. *J. Clin. Endocrinol. Metabol.* 65:954–961, 1987.

87. McMurray, R. G., and V. L. Katz. Thermoregulation in pregnancy. *Sports Med.* 10:146–158, 1990.

88. Mittleman, K. D., and I. B. Mekjavic. Effect of occluded venous return on core temperature during cold water immersion. *J. Appl. Physiol.* 65:2709–2713, 1988.

89. Morimoto, T., Z. Slabachova, R. K. Naman, and F. Sargent, II. Sex differences in physiological reactions to thermal stress. *J. Appl. Physiol.* 22:526–532, 1967.

90. Nadel, E. R., S. M. Fortney, and C. B. Wenger. Effect of hydration state on circulatory and thermal regulations. *J. Appl. Physiol.* 49:715–721, 1980.

91. Nadel, E. R., K. B. Pandolf, M. F. Roberts, and J. A. J. Stolwijk, Mechanisms of thermal acclimation to exercise and heat. *J. Appl. Physiol.* 37:515–520, 1974.

92. Nadel, E. R., M. F. Roberts, and C. B. Wenger. Thermoregulatory adaptations to heat and exercise: comparative responses of men and women. L. Folinsbee (ed). *Environmental Stress: Individual Human Adaptations.* New York: Academic Press, 1978, pp. 29–37.

93. Nunneley, S. H. Physiological responses of women to thermal stress: a review. *Med. Sci. Sports* 10:250–255, 1978.

94. Pivarnik, J. M., C. J. Marichal, T. Spillman, and J. R. Morrow, Jr. Menstrual cycle phase affects temperature regulation during endurance exercise. *J. Appl. Physiol.* 72:543–548, 1992.

95. Rennie, D. W., B. G. Covino, B. J. Howell, S. H. Song, B. S. Kang, and S. K. Hong. Physical insulation of Korean diving women. *J. Appl. Physiol.* 17:961–966, 1962.

96. Roberts, M. F., C. B. Wenger, J. A. J. Stolwijk, and E. R. Nadel. Skin blood flow and sweating changes following exercise training and heat acclimation. *J. Appl. Physiol.* 43:133–137, 1977.

97. Rossmanith, W. G., and S. S. C. Yen. Sleep-associated decrease in luteinizing hormone pulse frequency during the early follicular phase of the menstrual cycle: evidence for an opioidergic mechanism. *J. Clin. Endocrinol. Metab.* 65:715–718, 1987.

98. Rothchild, I., and A. C. Barnes. Effects of dosage, and of estrogen, androgen or salicylate administration on degree of body temperature elevation induced by progesterone. *Endocrinology* 50:485–496, 1952.

99. Rowell, L. B. *Human Circulation. Regulation during Physical Stress.* New York: Oxford University Press, 1986.

100. Sagot, J. C., C. Amoros, V. Candas, and J. P. Libert. Sweating responses and body temperatures during nocturnal sleep in humans. *Am. J. Physiol.* 252:R462–R470, 1987.

101. Saltin. B., and L. Hermansen. Esophageal, rectal and muscle temperature during exercise. *J. Appl. Physiol.* 21:1757–1762, 1966.

102. Sargent, F., and K. P. Weinman. Eccrine sweat gland activity during the menstrual cycle. *J. Appl. Physiol.* 21:1685–1687, 1966.

103. Sawka, M. N., R. R. Gonzalez, and K. B. Pandolf. Effects of sleep deprivation on thermoregulation during exercise. *Am. J. Physiol.* 246:R72–R77, 1984.

104. Sawka, M. N., M. M. Toner, R. P. Francesconi, and K. B. Pandolf. Hydration and exercise: effects of heat acclimation, gender, and environment. *J. Appl. Physiol.* 55:1147–1153, 1983.

105. Senay, L. C. Body fluids and temperature responses of heat-exposed women before and after ovulation with and without rehydration. *J. Physiol. (London)* 232:209–219, 1973.

106. Shapiro, Y., K. B. Pandolf, B. A. Avellini, N. A. Pimental, and R. F. Goldman. Heat balance and transfer in men and women exercising in hot-dry and hot-wet conditions. *Ergonomics* 24:375–386, 1981.

107. Shapiro, Y., K. B. Pandolf, B. A. Avellini, N. A. Pimental, and R. F. Goldman. Physiological responses of men and women to humid and dry heat. *J. Appl. Physiol.* 49:1–8, 1980.

108. Shapiro, Y., K. B. Pandolf, and R. F. Goldman. Sex differences in acclimation to a hot-dry environment. *Ergonomics* 23:635–642, 1980.

109. Silva, N. L., and J. A. Boulant. Effects of osmotic pressure, glucose, and temperature on neurons in preoptic tissue. *Am. J. Physiol.* 247:R335–R345, 1984.

110. Silva, N. L., and J. A. Boulant. Effects of testosterone, estradiol, and temperature on neurons in preoptic tissue slices. *Am. J. Physiol.* 250:R625–R632, 1986.

111. Spruce, B. A., P. H. Baylis, J. Burd, and M. J. Watson. Variation in osmoregulation of arginine vasopressin during the human menstrual cycle. *J. Clin. Endocrinol.* 22:37–42, 1985.

112. Steinberger, A., and D. N. Ward. Inhibin. E. Knobil and J. D. Neill (eds). *The Physiology of Reproduction.* Vol. 1, New York: Raven Press, Ltd., 1988, pp. 567–583.

113. Stephenson, L. A., and M. A. Kolka. Menstrual cycle phase and time of day alter reference signal controlling arm blood flow and sweating. *Am. J. Physiol.* 249:R186–R191, 1985.

114. Stephenson, L. A., and M. A. Kolka. Plasma volume during heat stress and exercise in women. *Eur. J. Appl. Physiol.* 57:573–581, 1988.

115. Stephenson, L. A., M. A. Kolka, R. Francesconi, and R. R. Gonzalez. Circadian variations in plasma renin activity, catecholamines and aldosterone during exercise in women. *Eur. J. Appl. Physiol.* 58:756–764, 1989.

116. Stephenson, L. A., M. A. Kolka, and R. R. Gonzalez. Effect of the menstrual cycle on the control of skin blood flow during exercise (abstract). *Fed. Proc.* 45:407, 1986.

117. Stephenson, L. A., C. B. Wenger, B. H. O'Donovan, and E. R. Nadel. Circadian rhythm in sweating and cutaneous blood flow. *Am. J. Physiol.* 246:R321–R324, 1984.
118. Stevens, G. H., T. E. Graham, and B. A. Wilson. Gender differences in cardiovascular and metabolic responses to cold and exercise. *Can. J. Physiol. Pharmacol.* 65:165–171, 1987.
119. Tankersley, C. G., W. C. Nicholas, D. R. Deaver, D. Mikita, and W. L. Kenney. Estrogen replacement in middle-aged women: thermoregulatory responses to exercise in the heat. *J. Appl. Physiol.* 73:1238–1245, 1992.
120. Tataryn, I. V., D. R. Meldrum, A. M. Frumar, and H. L. Judd. LH, FSH and skin temperature during the menopausal hot flash. *J. Clin. Endocrinol. Metabol.* 49:152–154, 1979.
121. Turek, F. W., and E. V. Cauter. Rhythms in reproduction. E. Knobil and J. D. Neill (eds). *The Physiology of Reproduction.* Vol. 2, New York: Raven Press, 1988, pp. 1789–1830.
122. Vollman, R. F. The menstrual cycle E. A. Friedman (ed). *Major Problems in Obstetrics and Gynaecology.* Vol. 7, Philadelphia: W. B. Saunders, 1977.
123. Vom Saal, F. S., and C. E. Finch. Reproductive senescence: phenomena and mechanisms in mammals and selected vertebrates. E. Knobil and J. D. Neill (eds). *The Physiology of Reproduction.* Vol. 2, New York: Raven Press, 1988, pp. 2351–2413.
124. Wagner, J. A., and S. M. Horvath. Cardiovascular reactions to cold exposures differ with age and gender. *J. Appl. Physiol.* 58:187–192, 1985.
125. Wagner, J. A., and S. M. Horvath. Influences of age and gender on human thermoregulatory responses to cold exposures. *J. Appl. Physiol.* 58:180–186, 1985.
126. Walsh, C. A., and T. E. Graham. Male-female responses in various body temperatures during and following exercise in cold air. *Aviat. Space Environ. Med.* 57:966–973, 1986.
127. Weinman, K. P., Z. Slabochova, E. M. Bernauer, T. Morimoto, and F. Sargent, II. Reactions of men and women to repeated exposure to humid heat. *J. Appl. Physiol.* 22:533–538, 1967.
128. Wells, C. L. Responses of physically active and acclimated men and women to exercise in a desert environment. *Med. Sci. Sports Exerc.* 12:9–13, 1980.
129. Wells, C. L., and S. M. Horvath. Heat stress responses related to the menstrual cycle. *J. Appl. Physiol.* 35:1–5, 1973.
130. Wells, C. L., and S. M. Horvath. Responses to exercise in a hot environment as related to the menstrual cycle. *J. Appl. Physiol.* 36:299–302, 1974.
131. Wenger, C. B., and J. D. Hardy. Temperature regulation and exposure to heat and cold. J. F. Lehmann (ed). *Therapeutic Heat and Cold.* 4th Ed., Baltimore: Williams & Wilkins, 1990, pp. 150–178.
132. Wyndham, C. A., J. F. Morrison, and C. G. Williams. Heat reactions of male and female caucasians. *J. Appl. Physiol.* 20:357–364, 1965.
133. Wyndham, C. A., J. F. Morrison, C. G. Williams, G. A. G. Bredell, J. Peter, M. J. Von Rahden, A. J. Van Rensberg, and A. Monro. Physiological reactions to cold of caucasian females. *J. Appl. Physiol.* 19:877–880, 1964.
134. Yen, S. S. C., M. E. Quigley, R. L. Reid, J. F. Ropert, and N. S. Cetal. Neuroendocrinology of opioid peptides and their role in the control of gonadotropin and prolactin secretion. *J. Obstet. Gynecol.* 152:485–493, 1985.

9
Skeletal Muscle Regeneration and Plasticity of Grafts

TIMOTHY P. WHITE, Ph.D.
STEVEN T. DEVOR, M.S.

INTRODUCTION

Skeletal muscle fiber degeneration and subsequent regeneration follows from widespread damage to the fiber induced by a variety of insults including free grafting operations, other mechanical and chemical trauma, ischemia, exposure to extreme heat and cold, and some diseases [25, 30, 68, 112, 141]. Moreover, subtle and focal areas of degeneration-regeneration in skeletal muscle can result from excessive stretch, specific types and durations of exercise (particularly those with a bias toward lengthening contractions), and denervation or mild compression. An ongoing presence of a population of regenerating skeletal muscle fibers may be an inevitable and normal consequence of an active life-style.

To explore facets of muscle fiber degeneration and regeneration, a graft-ischemia model has been employed in many laboratories. Results from this model provide the primary basis of this review. Experiments that initiated the characterization of the structural and functional correlates of fiber degeneration and regeneration were done primarily with the extensor digitorum longus (EDL) muscle of rats and cats. Investigations into postgrafting procedures employed to alter graft structure and function have studied primarily the soleus, EDL, and gastrocnemius muscles of the rat. The soleus muscle is most often chosen in postgrafting improvement studies because it is a muscle recruited frequently during standing and locomotion [133, 144].

In this review, we aspire to clarify that the study of skeletal muscle regeneration is a fertile and promising area of research in myogenesis. As discussed recently by Gunning and Hardeman [71], among others, "the generation of adult skeletal muscle is increasingly proving to be an attractive system for studying the mechanisms that govern tissue differentiation and maturation." We submit that the grafting of skeletal muscle and the ensuing degeneration-regeneration of muscle fibers is a useful model for the study of many regulatory aspects of skeletal muscle development and maturation. Unlike ontogenetic development studied in utero or in ovo, a host animal of sufficient size and age is employed in the graft model that allows one to manipulate variables experimentally such as the degree of reinnervation, the components of physical activity, and the level of circulating endocrines. With some liberties of literal interpretation, one may consider the skeletal muscle graft model to be one of tissue culture in vivo.

This line of research also has applied clinical significance in the postgrafting management of patients who have undergone free graft operations of skeletal muscles for repair in sites of muscle impairment. Skeletal muscle graft operations are a useful procedure for reconstruction in sites of muscle dysfunction, such as partial facial paralysis, anal or urinary incontinence, and forelimb muscle ablation, [61, 62, 84, 86, 87, 100]. When these surgical procedures are done with large muscle masses, it is most common today to repair the vasculature, thereby allowing for the majority of muscle cells to survive the graft operation. However, muscle fibers will degenerate and regenerate in cases where vascular repair of small or large muscle grafts is not possible or fully successful, or if the clinical decision is made to not repair the vasculature [61, 62, 73, 82]. Individuals with populations of regenerating muscle fibers caused by disease, exposure to myotoxic anesthetics or snake venom, direct physical trauma, or excessive exercise (particularly if lengthening contractions predominate) are also potential benefactors of research in skeletal muscle regeneration and plasticity.

This review is divided into five major sections. The second section summarizes the major operative procedures and the sequence of early degenerative and regenerative events. The third section reviews the biochemical, molecular, morphological, and physiological characteristics of muscle grafts that develop and stabilize with time. The fourth section focuses on studies of selected postgrafting interventions that alter the gross components of physical activity and induce adaptations in muscle grafts. The fifth section provides a brief summary.

The content is not exhaustive of the entire field of skeletal muscle regeneration and the plasticity of grafts because of space limitations. The interested reader is directed to other salient reviews [2, 17, 20, 22, 23, 25, 30, 68, 112].

SKELETAL MUSCLE REGENERATION

Skeletal muscle development and maturation, both ontogeny and regeneration, is characterized by a well-defined sequence of molecular and cellular events that result in myoblasts proliferating, fusing, and differentiating into muscle cells [9, 30, 63, 68, 75, 112, 125, 126, 127]. With ontogeny, there is a family of myoblasts (embryonic, fetal, and adult-satellite) that give rise to a diversity of fiber types [94, 125]. There are important distinctions between the members of the family of myoblasts. For example, embryonic myoblasts have a predetermined commitment to a specific fiber-type lineage [125, 127], whereas adult-satellite myoblasts of young rodents are not restricted to fusing with specific postnatal fiber type [78]. However, with muscle regeneration it is the adult myoblast, commonly referred to as the satellite cell, that is the primary if not exclusive muscle precursor cell.

The ultimate expression of a definitive adult phenotype of skeletal muscle is a complex process of commitment and modulation. Fiber diversity is rooted in, but not exclusively determined by, the myoblast of origin. Myogenesis is regulated by factors intrinsic and extrinsic to the muscle cell, including those associated with the family of myoblasts, innervation, the extracellular matrix, hormones, growth factors, and sufficient recruitment and biomechanical loading of the muscle or graft [3, 7, 46, 48, 59, 68, 71, 85, 94, 99, 104, 111, 114, 116, 117, 125, 129, 145].

Operative Procedures

In a free muscle graft [29], the muscle is freed completely from its original anatomical site and replaced (i.e., orthotopic graft) or moved to an alternative site (i.e., heterotopic graft). Once the muscle is freed, the proximal and distal tendon stumps of the graft are sutured to the corresponding tendon stumps in the recipient site. There are no apparent differences in structural and functional attributes of EDL muscles that are grafted orthotopically or heterotopically into the contralateral EDL site [58, 92]. However, if the muscle is placed in an atypical site with different innervation and loading characteristics, the graft will assume site-specific characteristics [45, 61, 84, 86, 142].

In free muscle grafts of rats, no attempt is made to re-establish blood perfusion by vascular anastomoses as grafts revascularize spontaneously [76]. With larger grafts in large host animals, the vasculature is typically repaired and this results in fiber survival rather than initiation of degeneration and regeneration [14, 15, 69, 84, 88].

If skeletal muscle is denervated for a short time before the grafting operation, there are no permanent changes on the degree of regeneration [28, 58, 90]. If the period of denervation is prolonged before the grafting operation, there is a subsequent impairment in the structure and function of the muscle grafts [26, 70].

Although skeletal muscle can regenerate in the absence of functional innervation, final differentiation requires re-establishment of neural connections with the host animal [25, 26, 32, 33, 69, 70, 74]. The different models of reinnervation will impact the rate and magnitude of regeneration, as detailed later in this review. One of four procedures is typically used to re-establish neural connections in the recipient site:

1. Allow the nerve to reinnervate spontaneously from the cut ends of the motor nerves lying in the vicinity of the graft (i.e., standard graft);

2. Implant the nerve stump(s) of the recipient site into the graft muscle at the time of the graft operation (i.e., nerve-implant graft);
3. During the graft operation, the motor nerve branches leading into a muscle are not cut, although the tendon and blood supply are severed (i.e., nerve-intact graft); with this technique it is important to recognize that neuromuscular transmission is not functional for 1–2 weeks even though the nerve is left structurally intact [32]; or
4. Repair the nerve stumps with a neuroanastomosis (i.e., nerve-repaired graft); Because of size limitations with the nerve, this procedure is currently not technically possible with small nerves in rats, such as with branches of the tibial or peroneal nerves that innervate the soleus or EDL muscles, respectively; It is possible, however, to anastomose large nerves in the rat and other species; For example, branches of the tibial nerve are anastomosed during grafting of the medial gastrocnemius muscle in rats [54].

Unlike with the EDL muscle, the soleus muscle in rats will not properly reinnervate de novo unless the nerve is left intact or the severed nerve is reimplanted during the graft operation [37, 39, 118, 145]. This phenomenon likely results from when the motor nerve is severed during a graft operation, it retracts significantly further away from the soleus muscle compared with the same circumstance in the EDL muscle. Although this has not been rigorously tested, the degree or angle of nerve retraction in the soleus muscle model appears to preclude the possibility for spontaneous reinnervation [139]. The fact remains, however, that interpretation of results is limited in experiments involving soleus muscle grafts unless there has been some facilitation of functional reinnervation.

There are no intrinsic differences in the regenerative capacity of EDL and soleus muscle grafts when the operation is performed with the nerve intact [37]. This interpretation is based only on the morphological variables of mass, length, fiber-type distribution, and fiber cross-sectional area, but is likely true for other attributes as well. The similar regenerative capacity observed in muscles of essentially diametrically opposite myosin isoforms in young adult animals is fortunate for it allows a degree of generalization regarding experimental results that have used different muscles.

Early Molecular and Cellular Sequelae
Successful skeletal muscle regeneration requires revascularization, cellular infiltration and phagocytosis of necrotic muscle fibers, proliferation and fusion of muscle precursor cells, reinnervation, and recruitment and loading. The early regenerative development and maturation of free muscle grafts is similar regardless of the operative treatment of the nerve

at the time of grafting [24, 30, 68]. During the first few hours after grafting, over 95% of the muscle cells become ischemic and necrose. The necrotic muscle cells are located almost exclusively in the ischemic center of a graft, while approximately 2–5% of the peripherally located cells survive. Survival of these muscle cells presumably results from the diffusion of oxygen and nutrients from extramuscular space. The percentage of ischemic degenerating muscle cells can be increased to 100% if grafts are treated with a myotoxic anesthetic, such as bupivacaine or other anesthetics, at the time of grafting [8, 21, 29, 60, 80].

In skeletal muscle regeneration induced by muscle contractions and other trauma, the elevation of intracellular calcium appears to be a common mediator [4, 68]. Lengthening contractions are common and are particularly known to induce injury to muscle fibers [93]. Polyethylene glycol-superoxide dismutase (PEG-SOD) administered before lengthening contractions reduced the subsequent degree of degeneration and regeneration [148]. PEG-SOD is a free radical scavenger that likely interrupts the free radical-induced calcium-mediated phospholipase breakdown of membranes. Similarly, the administration of bromelain attenuates the development of contraction-induced injury in hamster EDL muscle [136]. Although the mechanism by which this proteolytic enzyme provides its effect is unclear, it may work through a generalized reversal of the negative consequences of the inflammatory process and/or attenuation of the production or action of oxygen-free radicals [136].

REVASCULARIZATION. Revascularization is the first critical process that occurs in muscle regeneration [21, 25, 73, 76, 143]. It is not currently understood how functional vascular connections are made between a whole-muscle free graft and the vasculature of the site to which the graft has been placed. Following standard whole skeletal muscle grafting procedures, the peripheral vascular elements associated with the thin rim of surviving muscle cells in the periphery will likely survive [12, 19, 73, 76]. However, the vast majority of the vascular endothelium and other foundations of the vasculature will degenerate. To replace the lost vasculature, capillary sprouts grow inward from host vessels to the graft, or outward from the surviving vascular fragments within the periphery of the graft to the host site, or a combination of these two processes [12]. It is recognized that the extent and success of spontaneous revascularization of standard free-muscle grafts is contingent upon the vascularity of the recipient size in concert with the mass of the ischemic graft that needs to be revascularized. Low vascularity in the recipient site or grafting of large masses leads to a poor degree of success.

The extent to which a free graft regains structure and function initially depends largely on the degree and timing of the revascularization [25]. Blood vessels begin to grow into many sites along the surface of muscle grafts in rats starting about 2 days after grafting, and thereafter, the vessels spread throughout the graft [76]. In freely grafted EDL muscle of rats, most large vessels are ischemic and capillaries have degenerated at *day 1* postgrafting. From *days 3–10,* new vessels grow centripetally into the graft; 5–7 days are required for the spontaneously generated blood vessels to contact the most central region of 100- to 150-mg EDL grafts in the rat. New vessels seem to grow along a path of least resistance, as some enter into lumens of degenerated vessels, use original vessels as vascular channels, grow in interstitial spaces, or grow within the basal laminae of degenerating muscle fibers or nerves [30, 76]. Mechanisms regulating angiogenesis have been reviewed recently by Hudlicka et al. [77].

CELLULAR INFILTRATION. Distinct zones of degeneration and regeneration pass through the muscle in a centripetal pattern following the onset of revascularization [24, 30]. Vascular sprouts that appear in muscle grafts are characterized by inward growth and are typically intimately associated with dense accumulations of blood-borne phagocytes that facilitate cell-mediated degeneration.

MUSCLE PRECURSOR CELLS. After phagocytosis of the necrotic tissue, regeneration of new muscle fibers begins: they arise primarily if not exclusively from the satellite cell population that survives the ischemic episode [3, 83, 89, 122, 124]. Miranda Grounds [68] cautions that since muscle precursor cells cannot be definitively identified during the early stages of proliferation, one cannot totally exclude the possibility that other types of muscle precursor cells might be a source in vivo. Myogenic cells do not survive in the ischemic core of muscle grafts, and either migrate to areas of the graft as needed [105], or migrate toward the periphery and then return to the central core [122]. After closed contusion injury to skeletal muscle, the vast majority of myoblasts arise from local precursor cells whereas satellite cells recruited from surviving tissue do not contribute much to the regeneration [79].

Alexander Mauro's classic publication [89] first identified the satellite cell in skeletal muscle, a term derived from its peripheral location in the cell between the basal lamina (also termed the basement membrane or external lamina) and the plasma membrane (also termed the sarcolemma or plasmalemma). This cell is currently referred to by some as an adult myoblast or adult-satellite myoblast, reflecting its physiological importance rather than anatomical location [125]. The process of myogenesis gives rise not only to myoblasts, myotubes and myofibers, but also to mononuclear "satellite" cells that are presumably derived from a population of myoblasts that do not align or fuse with the developing myotube, but rather may simply be carried forward near the surface of the myofibers under the basal lamina [141]. Satellite cells constitute between 2% and 10% of the total fiber-associated myonuclei in young and adult vertebrates. There are differences in the number of satellite cells in different types of muscle and in muscles of animals at different ages [64, 120, 121]. A relatively high population of satellite cells exists in the immediate postnatal period (approximately 30% of all myonuclei), followed by a precipitous drop early in life [17, 121]. This, in turn, is followed by a slow decline to even lower populations with advanced age [64, 124]. There is a pronounced increase in the number of true myonuclei within a myofiber during ontogenetic growth, yet soon after birth, true myonuclei are not themselves capable of mitosis.

Moss and LeBlond [97] first demonstrated that the increase in the number of true myonuclei and the associated increase in fiber cross-sectional area resulted from the division of satellite cells and the subsequent fusion of one or both daughter cells in the developing syncytium. In skeletal muscle of adult animals, satellite cells are normally mitotically quiescent and function essentially as a reserve stem cell population. Satellite cells are capable of migration, proliferation, and differentiation under a variety of conditions in myofibers, such as following free graft operations [83, 118, 119]. It is interesting to note that the number of satellite cells in a stable free-muscle graft does not differ from that in a nongrafted muscle [120].

Regenerating muscle cells evolve through the mononuclear myoblast phase and then fuse to form multinucleated myotubes [30, 68]. Although its presence is not obligatory, the basal lamina survives grafting procedures, and provides a scaffold for new myotube formation [16, 75, 132]. Myotubes and then myofibers undergo maturation following essentially the same steps as during normal ontogeny, as long as proper revascularization, reinnervation, and recruitment-loading occurs. Although there are some distinctions, the pattern of expression of myosin heavy chain (MHC) in grafted skeletal muscle in which fibers degenerate and regenerate clearly parallels the embryonic-neonatal-adult pattern observed in the ontogeny of skeletal muscle [30, 34, 85, 114, 137, 138]. Regenerating rat skeletal muscle fibers begin to contract in a rudimentary fashion within a week postgrafting [24, 29, 32]. Ultimately, an essentially normal-appearing cross-striated muscle fiber results.

REINNERVATION AND RECRUITMENT. Functional innervation is crucial for the maturation of regenerating muscle [20, 32, 33, 70, 145]. The seminal experiments by Bruce Carlson on graft reinnervation have employed the free standard EDL muscle graft in the rat. Regenerating nerve fibers begin to enter grafts at 1–2 weeks postgrafting, and functional neuromuscular junctions appear during the third week [30, 32, 147]. Innervation stabilizes at about 60% of control muscle value [30, 32], and Womble [147] determined the number of neuromuscular junctions in standard free grafts of the EDL muscle to be 10–45% of control muscle value. In grafts, the motor end-plates (MEPs) are often not normal morphologically [74].

There have been few experiments on the sensory nervous system of grafts. The frequency of observing muscle spindles is about one-half that of control muscle values [28, 110]. Spindle structure is also not normal, as there appears to be incomplete innervation or regeneration of spindles, and incomplete differentiation of intrafusal fibers. Nuclear bag fibers were not present, although occasional nuclear chain fibers were [109].

Careful experiments of reinnervation have not been conducted with soleus muscle grafts. It is known, however, that the grafts become functionally reinnervated with time. Choline acetyltransferase activity returned to control soleus values by *week 8* after grafting and pro-nounced depletion of glycogen occurred in 8-week grafts during an exhaustive run [145]. At *week 8* postgrafting, electromyographic activity in soleus muscle grafts in rats was not different from control muscle value [144].

When reinnervation is facilitated at the time of grafting, improve-ments are noted in the degree of innervation and regeneration. In nerve-intact grafts, the rate at which reinnervation became functional was more rapid, and choline acetyltransferase activity and morphologi-cal evidence of reinnervation was more pronounced [32] compared with standard EDL grafts of rats. When the grafting operation includes nerve anastomosis, one would expect some impairment in reinnervation compared with control muscle or experimental nerve-intact procedures. In vascularized, nerve-repaired grafts of medial gastrocnemius muscle in rats, the number and size of motor units are impaired by approximate-ly 20% compared with control muscle [54].

Structural and functional attributes of grafts were improved by treatment with subsequent nerve-crush 7 days postgrafting, and by forskolin administration [18]. Secondary nerve crush is known to facilitate the rate and number of nerve fibers that regenerate. Forskolin stimulates the production of cyclic adenosine monophosphate (cAMP) in both regenerating nerves and muscle, which, in turn, can enhance nerve regeneration and modulate muscle differentiation, protein synthesis, and capillary growth [18].

The impact of enhanced reinnervation on the success of regeneration is evidenced in structural and functional variables. Unlike with standard grafts of rats, nerve-intact grafts do not have a persistent deficit in mass, and the deficits in maximum isometric force and power are less [32, 37, 52, 53]. The fiber type distribution of nerve-intact grafts does not differ from control muscle value, whereas the average fiber cross-sectional area was 60–70% of control muscle value [37]. There is a slight deficiency of the subsequent impact of surgical nerve repair compared with the nerve-intact experimental procedure. In rats, for example, vascularized and nerve-anastomosed grafts of the medial gastrocnemius muscle have a mass, fiber cross-sectional area, maximum force capacity, and estimat-ed fiber number that are 25–40% less than control muscle value.

However, of these same variables in nerve-intact EDL grafts, only maximum force demonstrates an impairment and its magnitude is only 15–20% [53]. In large muscle models, there is variability in the response of fiber cross-sectional area to the facilitation of reinnervation [55, 90]. However, there is significant improvement in mass, number of fibers, and function with nerve repair or with use of the nerve-intact procedure at the time of grafting. These observations are consistent with the notion that the success of reinnervation is an important factor that affects graft development and maturation.

CHARACTERISTICS OF MUSCLE GRAFTS

The morphological and physiological characteristics of skeletal muscle undergo pronounced changes after grafting. After a period of degeneration, the changes reflect the regenerative development and maturation of grafts. Structural and functional characteristics of grafts reach a plateau with time, the duration of which depends upon many biological factors. The achievement of near-stable or stable values for structural and functional variables will occur typically from 8–16 weeks postgrafting in rat models [32, 37, 145]. In larger species, including human beings, it takes several months for variables to stabilize [56, 58, 61, 98, 142].

In stable grafts, several structural and functional variables do not achieve values of control muscle [25, 52–54, 88, 123, 129, 145]. In the absence of postgrafting interventions, the nature and magnitude of the structural and functional deficits depend on the mass of muscle grafted, the degree of surgical facilitation of reinnervation and revascularization at the time of grafting, and characteristics of the anatomical site to which the muscle is grafted. Functional deficits in grafts will presumably limit the usefulness of the graft to the host organism during physical activities that require endurance or high power. This observation, from a practical perspective, has been one impetus for the design of experiments that evaluate the efficacy of postgrafting interventions that are designed to improve graft structure and function.

Regenerating muscle is significantly more active in the incorporation of ^{35}S-methionine into protein than is control muscle [80]. The hormonal sensitivity of grafts is evident, as treatment with testosterone proprionate increased graft mass, fiber cross-sectional area, and function [31].

Many characteristics of skeletal muscle grafts are greatly influenced by the amount of muscle mass grafted and the operative procedures. As detailed earlier in this review, techniques to enhance reinnervation or essentially to maintain the vascular supply during grafting have particular impact on the outcome. As a consequence, the ensuing presentation of graft characteristics must take these considerations into account. For each variable, we first discuss results from the smaller rat models before those from larger cat and rabbit models. In all cases where known, we clarify the impact of operative procedure on the variable of interest.

Morphological Attributes

In rat models, the mass and fiber cross-sectional area of standard grafts range from 35–65% of control muscle values as late as *week 16* [32, 35, 36, 53, 145]. The fiber-type distribution in different experiments either does not differ from, or closely approximates, control muscle values for grafts of both soleus and EDL muscle [35–37]. There is evidence of increased fiber branching in EDL grafts in mice [102] and in rats [10]. Compared with nongrafted control muscle, in free standard EDL muscle grafts of mice, the number of fibers in a mature graft is about 30% less than the value of control muscle [102], whereas in the rat EDL graft the number of fibers is estimated not to differ from control muscle value [29, 32, 35, 52, 53]. There is no reason to expect these group comparisons to be invalid, but the fiber numbers were obtained from histological cross-sections and the values are about 75% of the value obtained directly via nitric acid digestion [43, 65].

Compared with values for nongrafted control muscle, the inulin space was 135% and the connective tissue protein was 177% for soleus muscle grafts [123]. For soleus muscle grafts, total muscle length and fiber length were 91% and 123% of respective control muscle values. When capillarity is expressed as capillaries/mm^2 of muscle or graft, the value of grafts was 40% greater than that of control muscle [35]. However, this apparent increase is the result primarily of the smaller fiber cross-sectional area, as capillarity expressed as a capillary/fiber ratio did not differ between graft and control muscle. For soleus grafts in rats, the reduced total protein was associated with a concomitant increase in the percentage of connective tissue protein [123]. This may reflect an increase of endomysial connective tissue protein relative to the intercellular scaffold normally observed in the degeneration-regeneration of skeletal muscle.

In rats, the distribution of fiber areas for single motor units was broader in EDL grafts than in control muscle, whereas the average innervation ratios did not differ [41, 42]. In approximately 20% of the motor units studied in grafts, fibers were tightly clustered in a localized region, suggesting an increased presence of axonal sprouting during regeneration.

In models where larger muscles are freely grafted under standard conditions, one major difference compared with models of smaller muscles is the persistence of a necrotic core and significant elevation in connective tissue in the graft [55, 56, 58, 87, 88, 90–92]. This may reflect the distance that revascularization must proceed, for in large vascular repaired grafts, the necrotic core is not present and, although connective tissue concentration is elevated, it remains as a small fraction of the total muscle mass [14, 15]. Reinnervation of relatively large standard grafts is also slow and incomplete [55].

In free EDL muscle grafts in cats, the mass at 26 weeks postgrafting was 60–70% of control muscle value, whereas the average fiber cross-sectional area exceeded control value [55, 91, 92, 98]. In this model with relatively large amounts of noncontractile tissue, the regenerated muscle fibers hypertrophied apparently in response to the high loads placed upon them when recruited. The distribution of fiber types in cat EDL grafts is different than control muscle, with fewer Type I fibers and more Type IIb [92]. In the cat, the number of fibers is estimated at 39,000 for control EDL muscle, 9000 for standard grafts, 15,000 for nerve-anastomosed grafts, and 20,000 for nerve-intact grafts [55]. Measures of capillarity were approximately 50% of normal values in cat EDL muscle grafts [55, 91, 143]. Selected cellular and matrix components of large gracilis muscle grafts in the dog (about 75 at time of operation) were studied 9–12 months after orthotopic grafting with neurovascular repair [88]. Reductions compared with control muscle were observed for wet mass (29% reduction) and concentrations of noncollagenous protein (13%), DNA (28%), and RNA (34%). Collagen concentration increased 41% in grafts, myofibrillar ATPase (34%), and α-glycerophosphate dehydrogenase (25%) were reduced, while citrate synthase did not differ.

Contractile Attributes
When one studies the functional attributes of whole grafts or their motor units, some functional properties return to control value while others remain impaired [51, 52, 54, 55, 58, 88, 123, 143]. There is a substantial improvement in the degree of functional recovery achieved by the nerve-intact compared with standard grafts. This is because of a larger functional mass in the former model that results primarily from the facilitated reinnervation, and not because of any significant difference in the degree of revascularization.

Contractile properties of standard and nerve-intact grafts of the EDL muscle of rats were studied in vitro from 2–8 weeks after graft operations [51]. At 2–3 weeks postgrafting, the time-to-peak tension of both graft types was approximately 2-fold longer than values of control muscle. By *week 8*, values for both graft types reached control value. The response of one-half relaxation time qualitatively followed the same pattern as for time-to-peak tension. During the early postgrafting period, the maximum capacity to develop isometric force (P_o) in grafts was depressed to about 20% of control muscle value. The ability to generate force increased with time, and the rate of improvement was greater in nerve-intact grafts than in standard grafts. At *week 8*, the P_o of standard and nerve-intact grafts was 57% and 91% of control muscle values, respectively. When P_o is normalized to muscle fiber cross-sectional area (i.e., specific force), values were depressed early following grafting and were greater in nerve-intact vs. standard grafts. By *week 8*, the nerve-intact values did not differ from control muscle, whereas the value for standard grafts was 67% of control value. Although subtle differences exist between the recovery of functional attributes of soleus and EDL grafts, the attributes are qualitatively similar [123]. For example, the time-to-peak tension and half-relaxation times recovered fully by *week 8* in EDL grafts but were 6% slower in soleus grafts, and P_o was 40% of control value in soleus grafts compared with 57% in EDL grafts. Specific force in soleus grafts was 76% of control value.

Physiological properties of motor units were studied in standard and nerve-intact grafts of the EDL muscle in rats [40, 41]. Motor units from both types of grafts evidenced a mean and range of time-to-peak twitch tensions that did not differ from control muscle. Evidence was presented indicating no loss of motor units in nerve-intact grafts, although their size was approximately 20% less than in control muscle. However, in standard grafts, there was a 45% decrease in the number of motor units and a 20% decrease in the size of each motor unit compared with control muscle values. The motor unit data also reflect the more complete reinnervation of grafts with the experimental nerve-intact procedure.

In cats, the first comprehensive study of free standard EDL grafts studied the time course of contractile properties from 6–63 weeks postgrafting [58]. At the time of the graft operation, the muscle mass ranged from 2–6 g. The absolute maximum isometric force (P_o) increased from 2% of control muscle value at *week 6* to 26% by *week 63*. One major cause of the sustained deficit in P_o in the relatively large grafts, compared with grafts in rats, is likely because the center of the large graft is not completely revascularized and, thus, a core of necrotic tissue remained [25, 143]. When P_o is normalized to estimated viable muscle fiber cross-sectional area, the value was not different between long-term free standard grafts and control muscle values. Furthermore, when grafts in the 2- to 6-g range are grafted in cats with vascular repair, there is a 70% improvement in P_o [53]. With regard to isometric contraction times, grafts in cats had longer times to reach peak tension and for half-relaxation, and slower maximum velocity of shortening during the first 25 weeks postgrafting [58]. From *weeks 25–63*, these values approximated control muscle values. Grafts of this size were significantly more fatigable then control muscles [58, 143]. With respect to motor units in large, nerve-intact EDL grafts in cats, there is essentially full recovery to control muscle values for size, number, and contractile properties from 21–39 weeks postgrafting [115].

In 9-g rectus femoris muscle grafts in rabbits, when the vasculature is left intact during grafting, the capacity to generate isometric force was 50% and 65%, respectively, for absolute values and for values normalized to muscle cross-sectional area [15]. The wet mass of vascularized grafts was 75% of control muscle value, and the grafts maintained the bipinnate architecture and normal fiber length of control rectus femoris muscle. The muscle fiber cross-sectional area was 77% of control muscle value. The concentration of connective tissue of grafts was almost 4-fold greater in grafts than in control muscle, and there were no differences in interstitial space. The difference in connective tissue can explain approximately 5% of the 35% deficit in specific P_o, and the remaining 30% remains unexplained. In vascularized grafts of the rectus femoris muscle in rabbits, the nerve and vascular repair do not contribute to the impaired function [69]. It seems that factors associated with tendon repair bear responsibility for the functional impairments.

Metabolic Attributes
Two weeks after grafting, the oxidative capacity of whole muscle homogenates of soleus muscle grafts in rats was 20% of the control muscle value [145]. Oxidative capacity increased to 50% of control value by *week 6*, and did not change thereafter. Cytochrome *c* is depressed in EDL grafts compared with control muscle [35]. The loss of oxidative capacity in marcaine-treated grafts was paralleled by a drop in activity of monamine oxidase, suggesting diminished mitochondrial protein [107]. In minced gastrocnemius grafts, there was a return to pyruvate-malate oxidative capacity to 85% of control muscle value by 6.5 weeks postgrafting [130]. The reason for the disparate response between free and minced models is not known.

Selected aspects of glycogen metabolism have been studied in muscle grafts of rats [134, 135]. There appears a transient elevation in hexose monophosphate shunt activity early following grafting [107]. At 10 weeks after grafting the EDL muscle, three patterns were evident for glycolytic enzymes:

1. An early and sustained increase in activities of hexokinase and glucose-6-phosphate dehydrogenase;
2. An early decline and continued deficit in phosphorylase activity; expression of the muscle glycogen phosphorylase gene is depressed in free grafts of EDL muscle in rats compared with control muscle [66]; also, an early and sustained deficit was noted in activities of phosphofructokinase, and cytoplasmic α-glycerophosphate dehydrogenase; and
3. An early decrease and return to control muscle value for lactate dehydrogenase, pyruvate kinase, creatine kinase, and adenylate kinase.

Studies in vivo and in vitro reflect a modest impairment in glycogen metabolism. Resting concentration of glycogen in nerve-implant soleus grafts were 70% of the control muscle value at *week 1* after grafting, and increased to 85% by *week 4* [145]. In response to an acute bout of exhaustive running exercise (45 min), glycogen concentration decreased to 75% and 45% of resting values at 1 and 4 weeks after grafting, respectively. A similar acute bout of running decreased glycogen concentration of nongrafted soleus muscle to 40% of the resting value. Exercise-induced and fasting-induced decreases in glycogen concentration have also been noted in EDL and soleus grafts in the rat [96]. Cage rest and refeeding allowed glycogen concentrations to replete. EDL muscle grafts stimulated in an anaerobic environment in vitro demonstrate a reduction in capacity for glycolytic metabolism [146]. At 11 weeks postgrafting, grafts produced approximately 60% of the lactate generated by control EDL muscles with similar stimulation parameters, and developed 50% of the estimated increase in H^+. During repeated contractions, grafts maintained concentrations of ATP while decreasing phosphocreatine.

Few experiments have been done on the metabolic attributes of large grafts in cats or other species. It is known that in EDL grafts of cats, the oxidative capacity was depressed and reached 55% of control muscle value at *week 26* [55, 91].

Muscle Blood Flow

It has been documented that the ability of standard EDL muscle grafts in the cat to regulate blood flow in response to twitch contractions is impaired [143]. When maximum flow is expressed relative to total muscle mass, the maximum value is approximately 25% of control value [143]. When these data are corrected for an estimate of viable muscle mass, the maximum values are 25% greater than in control muscle [52]. In either case, maximum value is reached in grafts at 1 twitch/sec rather than 4 twitches/sec for control EDL muscle, suggesting an impairment in regulatory mechanisms. The ability of newly formed vasculature to respond to topical treatments of adenosine and norepinephrine is also diminished [12, 13]. Taken in aggregate, these results suggest that arterioles in grafted muscle may have a diminished capacity to regulate blood flow when work demands dictate a need, and this undoubtedly relates to the increased fatigability of these types of grafts.

In contrast, when graft operations are done with neurovascular repair or with leaving the nerve and vasculature intact, there is minimal change compared with control muscle in the total or regional blood flow at rest and during contractions [14]. An adequate blood flow does not appear to contribute to the deficits in force production in the vascularized graft model.

Fatigability

Fatigability measured in vitro for EDL grafts in rats demonstrated a complex pattern. At 2 weeks postgrafting and when grafted with standard procedures, grafts were more resistant to fatigue than control EDL muscles, whereas the fatigability of grafts was not different from control value with the nerve-intact procedure [51]. By *week 8,* both graft types were more resistant to fatigue than control muscle, and this was confirmed in a second study conducted in situ [35].

To study the relationships among oxidative capacity, substrate depletion and fatigability of muscle grafts in situ, soleus muscles were grafted with nerve-implant in female rats [42]. Fatigability was measured in grafts and in control muscles from age-matched rats 10 weeks postgrafting. Intramuscular glycogen and triglyceride concentrations were also measured before and after the fatigue protocol. Even though stabilized soleus grafts have a reduced oxidative capacity compared to control soleus muscles [145], no difference was observed between groups for either the rate of decline in tension during the in situ fatigue test nor in the relative tension developed at the end of the protocol. Glycogen concentration did not decrease significantly during the fatigue protocol in either group. Compared with control soleus muscle, the triglyceride concentration in soleus grafts was significantly higher before the fatigue protocol. The fatigue protocol induced a greater decline in triglyceride concentration in the grafts compared with control muscle. It is apparent that the reduced oxidative capacity of soleus grafts is not associated with a change in fatigability in situ, and that the pattern of substrate utilization is qualitatively similar in grafts and control muscles.

Large free-muscle grafts of the EDL muscle are less resistant to fatigue than control muscles in the cat [55, 143]. However, when large muscles are grafted with vascular repair, the resistance to fatigue is either not altered from control muscle value [14, 88] or increases [69].

Aging
The age of the rat that serves as a host for a muscle graft is an important determinant of the success of skeletal muscle regeneration. An early study by Gutmann and Carlson [72] demonstrated that freely grafted muscle in old rats regenerates poorly compared with young rats. In a qualitative histological study, Sadeh [113] found that degeneration-regeneration induced by bupivacaine was depressed 3-fold in 24-month rats compared with 3-month rats. Carlson and Faulkner [27] demonstrated that muscle harvested from young or old rats and grafted into young rats regenerated better than muscle from hosts of either age grafted into old rats. This was evidenced by an approximate 2- to 3-fold difference in mass and maximum isometric force by 8 weeks postgrafting. This study led to the conclusion that the poor regeneration of muscles in old animals is a function of the environment for regeneration provided by the host organism and not necessarily due to an intrinsic limitation of the grafted muscle itself.

With muscle in aging animals, there is a diminished response of axons to regenerate or reinnervate MEPs after perturbation [103]. One obvious consequence of impaired reinnervation concomitant with grafting in an old host is a reduced nerve-muscle fiber interaction and impaired ability to generate and maintain power. In adult and old rats, Clark and White studied the adaptive response of MEPs and muscle fibers to reinnervation of nongrafted EDL muscle by branches of the peroneal nerve (self-reinnervation) or the tibial nerve (i.e., cross-reinnervation) [38]. There was an age-associated decrease in the reinnervation of muscle following nerve section, as evidenced by an increased number of noninnervated MEPs and decreased neuronal contact with innervated MEPs. The conversion of fiber type after cross-reinnervation correlated closely with the number of innervated MEPs, suggesting that innervated fibers in old rats are capable of adapting to a new stimulus. Thus, we hypothesize a major reason for impaired muscle development and maturation in old animals is because of deficient reinnervation.

Disparity Between Shortening Velocity and Myofibrillar ATPase Activity
The major structural and functional proteins in skeletal muscle are the myofibrillar proteins, which include contractile proteins (MHC; myosin light chain, MLC; and actin) and regulatory proteins (troponin and tropomyosin). MHC is the largest and most predominant myofibrillar protein that functions to provide structural integrity, enzymatic activity (myosin ATPase), and regulation of the power developed by fibers. At least five distinct isoenzymes of MHC have been detected in mammalian limb skeletal muscle: two developmental forms (embryonic and neonatal) and three adult forms (two with high ATPase activity termed "fast," and one with low ATPase activity termed "slow") [6, 71]. The isoforms of the contractile and regulatory proteins of control limb muscle dictate, in large part, the functional parameters [67, 106].

In soleus muscle grafts of rats, the extrapolated shortening velocity at zero load did not differ from control muscle value 8 weeks postgrafting [123]. This is in contrast to the myofibrillar ATPase activity in grafts that was depressed to 70% of control muscle values [50]. The observation is similar to the altered relationship in grafted gracilis muscle in the dog [88]. There was a 34% reduction in ATPase activity in gracilis muscle grafts, and in three of the five grafts studied, the maximum velocity of shortening (V_{max}) did not differ from values of three of five control muscles studied. However, there were two grafts and two control muscles that had relatively low and high V_{max}, respectively. In the soleus grafts, the ATPase activity was measured on a suspension of myofibrillar proteins, and values reported are relative to a standard protein concentration of the suspension [50]. Thus, the ATPase activity reflects both the activity of the specific myosin isoforms and the stoichiometric relationship of myofibrillar proteins within the suspension.

To gain further insight into the depression of ATPase activity in light of a normal maximum velocity of shortening, the relative amount of proteins within the myofibrillar suspension were characterized and quantified [50]. Eight weeks after bilateral nerve-implant soleus graft surgery, muscles were excised, blotted, and weighed. Ten control soleus muscles were also removed from age-matched rats. Aliquots from the myofibrillar suspension were prepared for SDS polyacrylamide gel electrophoresis [47]. Samples containing 10–20 μg of protein, were separated on a gradient gel (5–15% T) that was subsequently scanned by laser densitometry to assess the proteins quantitatively. It was found that stable soleus muscle grafts expressed a stoichiometric relationship between the myofibrillar proteins that does not differ from control soleus muscle. MHC was the predominant protein in the suspension, and values ranged from 37 ± 1% to 41 ± 1% of the total protein for control muscle and grafts, respectively. Actin content in each sample was 33 ± 2% and 29 ± 1% for control and grafted muscle, respectively. Thus, the basis of the different relationship between maximum velocity of shortening and ATPase activity in grafts compared with control muscles remains to be determined. It would seem fruitful to pursue differences in actin isoforms, the regulatory proteins, and the calcium handling ability of the plasma membrane and sarcoplasmic reticulum.

PLASTICITY OF MUSCLE GRAFTS

Nongrafted skeletal muscle is recognized to be a highly plastic tissue. Skeletal muscle adaptation to chronic increases and decreases in the components of physical activity are evidenced by changes of molecular and cellular attributes that alter the functional capacity of muscle fibers (reviewed in [11, 57, 104, 111]). A stimulus for muscle adaptation occurs when a change in the habitual level of activity is sufficiently different from that which the muscle fibers are accustomed, and the atypical (increased or decreased) level is sustained for a sufficient duration to allow for the alteration in the expression of affected proteins (contractile, regulatory, structural, and/or metabolic).

Depending upon the gross nature of the stimulus, adaptations in nongrafted skeletal muscle include: (*a*) an impaired capacity to generate or maintain power in response to a chronic reduction in the components of physical activity; (*b*) an enhanced capacity to develop power with training that emphasizes increased biomechanical afterload; and (*c*) an enhanced capacity to sustain power with training that emphasizes elevated frequency of recruitment. Adaptations to increased components of physical activity can occur independently or, if the stimulus is appropriate, concurrently. Moreover, skeletal muscle adaptations are readily reversible when the stimuli for adaptation are removed.

Significant progress has been made in documenting that changes in the habitual level of the components of physical activity will alter the molecular, cellular, biochemical, morphological, and physiological characteristics of muscle grafts. In particular, this section will focus on studies that have experimentally manipulated the gross components of physical activity with interventions that have a bias to a relatively high or low frequency of recruitment and/or biomechanical load. Repetitive contractions associated with treadmill running and chronic electrical stimulation have been used primarily to affect the frequency of recruitment. Myectomy of muscles synergistic to the graft has been used to increase biomechanical load, and exposure of grafts to microgravity with hindlimb suspension has been used to decrease load. Some experiments have combined these interventions in an attempt to understand their interaction in the regulation of skeletal muscle regeneration. Although there are limited exceptions, the consensus of published work indicates that grafts adapt to postgrafting programs of endurance training, increased functional load by removal of synergistic muscles, chronic low frequency stimulation, and microgravity induced by hindlimb suspension.

Adaptations to Chronic Running
Using female Wistar rats, White et al. [145] grafted the soleus muscle with the nerve-implant technique and the impact of subsequent chronic running on muscle regeneration was studied through 16 weeks postgrafting. At the time that this descriptive study was initiated, there were unresolved experimental questions:

1. As the grafts were initially void of functional innervation, what time following the graft operation would be effective or optimal to begin training?
2. Would there be a differential impact of running intensity?
3. What duration of training would lead to a plateau in the adaptive responses?

It was known that stable grafts in untrained rats were smaller in cross-sectional area than control muscle, and less capable of generating force. Since training adaptations result from a sufficiently intense stimulus relative to the capacity of a muscle, it was hypothesized that running would induce adaptive responses in mass and metabolic parameters of grafts because of the aforementioned deficits. We recognized that nongrafted muscle mass would not be expected to adapt to running, although the metabolic adaptations (oxidative capacity, and others) were expected and well documented.

Running exercise was done on a motor-driven treadmill 5 days/week

[145]. The nature of the whole-body exercise stimulus determined the rate, magnitude, and type of adaptations of muscle grafts. Easy running (15 m/min; 15% grade; 1 hr/day) had no effect on graft mass and total protein content, even when the duration of conditioning was extended for 12 weeks. Conversely, sprint (50 m/min; 15% grade; 10 min/day) and endurance (30 m/min; 15% grade; 1 hr/day) running for 4 weeks initiated at 4 or 8 weeks after grafting increased the graft mass and total protein content by 30% compared with age-matched grafts from untrained rats. There is variability in the magnitude of exercise-induced growth of soleus grafts induced by running. In some cohorts of animals, run-training did not improve mass [123]. The reason for a lack of a training adaptation in the study by Segal et al. was largely because the mass of nontrained grafts was significantly larger than values of similar untrained groups in other studies. There may have been subtle differences in the operative procedure, perhaps enhanced resting tension at the time of grafting, that led to this anomalous result.

The effect of endurance training on the distribution of fiber size and fiber type of soleus muscle grafts was addressed by Clark et al. [36]. Orthotopic graft operations were performed with nerve-implant on 6-week-old rats. A cohort of animals began running 4 weeks later. Run-training increased graft mass 34% over the nonrun graft value of 82 ± 7 mg at 8 weeks postgrafting. Mass continued to increase through *week 16*, but the magnitude of change was smaller. Running had no effect on fiber cross-sectional area of grafts through *week 8*. Continued running through *week 16* increased fiber area by 21% over nonrun graft values (1193 ± 115 μm²), and had the greatest effect on the cross-sectional area of Type I fibers, a transient effect on Type IIb fibers and no effect on Type IIa fibers. By *week 16*, muscle fiber-type distribution was not different among nongrafted muscles or grafts from untrained and run-trained animals. It is apparent that the effect of run-training on muscle mass and fiber cross-sectional area differs with respect to the time course and magnitude of the increase. When recruitment frequency of grafts is increased by daily swimming, there is a small and transient increase in fiber diameter [101].

Several explanations are possible for the dissociation in the adaptive response between mass and fiber cross-sectional area [36]. It remains for experimental evidence to determine if exercise-induced changes in fiber architecture, fiber number, degree of fiber branching, or other attributes provide explanations for the aforementioned dissociation.

Grafting procedures in which the muscle is excised, minced into 1-mm³ pieces, and repacked into a limb muscle site have been used to evaluate myogenic potential [19, 22, 124]. Compared with control muscle and free grafts, minced muscle grafts have a high content of connective tissue, numerous cellular adhesions, and poor ultrastructural organization and functional properties. Van Handel et al. [130] investigated the adaptive response to running of minced gastrocnemius muscle grafted to the vacated site of the triceps surae muscle group in rats. A running group engaged in easy treadmill exercise (final level: 21.5 m/min, 15% grade, 1 hr/day, 5 days/week) for 6.5 weeks after grafting. The mass of grafts from untrained rats was 760 ± 58 mg compared with 1063 ± 56 mg from the trained rats. Despite the limitations of minced grafts, running exercise increased the tissue wet mass by 40%.

In mice, the effect of run-training before and after the grafting of EDL muscle was studied [108]. Satellite cells in grafts of trained mice were synthesizing DNA and grafts appeared vascularized substantially earlier than in other studies from this laboratory without run-training. Morphometric analysis indicated cellular hypertrophy and increased capillarity in grafts with run-training.

The oxidative capacity of muscle grafts is also improved with run-training. In soleus muscles grafted with the nerve-implant, the adaptive increase in oxidative capacity was less than that observed in mass, and became statistically significant only after long durations of running [145]. For example, endurance conditioning initiated 4 weeks after grafting increased pyruvate-malate oxidative capacity of whole-muscle homogenates 55%. However, the increase was observed only after 12 weeks of training and values were still only 70% of the value for control soleus muscle. In minced gastrocnemius muscle grafts, moderate run conditioning had no effect on phosphorylase, led to an 8% decrease in lactate dehydrogenase, and increased the oxidative capacity to values not different from those of control gastrocnemius muscle [130]. The reason for the different adaptive response of oxidative capacity to conditioning between free soleus grafts and minced gastrocnemius grafts is not known, but may reflect differences in initial control muscle values, degree of reinnervation, and the recruitment and loading patterns during standing and locomotion.

Mong et al. reported on the training-related adaptation of glycogen concentration of grafts [95]. Eight weeks after grafting of the soleus muscle with the nerve-intact procedure, comparisons were made between untrained and endurance-trained rats. Training was initiated 10 days postgrafting, and consisted of level treadmill running at 27 m/min for two 30-min periods per day. There was a 60% increase in the resting concentration of glycogen in grafts.

Adaptations to Chronic Electrical Stimulation
Chronic low-frequency stimulation is a powerful tool to alter phenotypic expression of several proteins in skeletal muscle. In nerve-intact EDL grafts, Ciske and Faulkner [35] evaluated the effects of approximately 4 weeks (8 hr/day) of 10-Hz stimulation that commenced 2 weeks after the graft operation. Compared with nonstimulated grafts, stimulated grafts demonstrated a 72% increase in the resistance to fatigue, a 65%

enhancement of oxidative capacity, a 30% increase in the number of capillaries per fiber, and a 45% greater number of capillaries/mm^2. In contrast, muscle wet mass, capacity to develop maximum isometric force, and fiber cross-sectional area were 20–30% less in the stimulated grafts compared with age-matched nonstimulated grafts. These results indicate that a period of low-frequency stimulation, during which grafts were chronically activated but not contracting against an appreciable increase in afterload, enhanced metabolic, and endurance characteristics. These improvements appear to be at the expense of variables associated with the capacity to generate force.

Adaptations to Microgravity
Soleus muscles and grafts are composed primarily of Type I motor units [37]. As a consequence, the change in soleus recruitment and loading patterns with running is small even if relatively large changes in overall running velocity are imposed on the animal [133, 144]. One experimental approach to increase the amount of change in recruitment and loading of soleus grafts is by exposing the grafts to microgravity by the ground-based technique of hindlimb suspension [81, 128]. With this technique, the plantarflexor muscles in the hindlimb are actively recruited [1], although the load on the muscle is minimized.

To decrease the biomechancial load on nerve-implant soleus grafts, the hindlimbs of rats were suspended from the cage floor [140]. Suspension was initiated 4 weeks after the graft operation, and continued through *week 8*, at which time the mass of grafts of suspended rats was 40 ± 4 mg, a value 50% of age-matched grafts from weight-bearing rats. Suspending the animals also decreased body mass to 65% of control muscle values. To account for differences in body mass, the graft mass was expressed as a ratio with body mass. The mass ratios for grafts in suspended animals was 75% of the value from weight-bearing rats. The cross-sectional area of muscle fibers of grafts from suspended rats was 30% of that from grafts in weight-bearing rats. In addition, there were notable differences in the histochemical demonstration of fiber types between grafts of weight-bearing and suspended rats. The grafts of suspended rats were composed of only 16% Type I fibers, 43% Type IIa, 14% Type IIb, and 27% Type IIc. This is in contrast to the grafts of weight-bearing rats that were 85% Type I, 11% Type IIa, and 4% Type IIb.

In another experiment, the hypothesis was tested that compared with grafts in cage-sedentary animals, decreased loading of grafts would reduce the rate of growth and differentiation of MHC isoforms [48]. Soleus muscles were grafted with the nerve-intact in female Wistar rats. Rats were then assigned to a cage-sedentary group (normal load) or a hindlimb suspension group (decreased load). Grafts were studied 0.5–5.0 weeks after the graft operation and initiation of load treatment.

With normal load, the mass and protein content of grafts declined through 1 week; thereafter, values increased at 1.83 mg mass/day and 0.49 mg protein/day. The rate of change for mass and protein content in grafts was less with decreased load (− 1.01 mg mass/day and − 0.05 mg protein/day, respectively) than with normal load. In grafts, the neonatal MHC peaked at 11 ± 1.6% of total MHC at 1 week in cage-sedentary rats, and was not evident at 3 weeks. Neonatal MHC in grafts of the suspended animals peaked at 11 ± 2.4% of total MHC at 2 weeks and was still present at 3 weeks (1.6 ± 1.1%). The proportion of fast MHC did not differ from 0.5 to 2.0 weeks between groups, and from 3–5 weeks, the grafts of the suspended animals were higher (55 ± 2.4%) compared with grafts of the cage-sedentary group (5 ± 0.7%). Biomechanical loading appears to be a significant factor that influences the rate of growth and differentiation of MHC in soleus muscle grafts of young adult rats.

Adaptations to Myectomy of Synergistic Muscles
When graft operations are done with the nerve-intact procedure, the muscle wet mass is not different from that of control muscle at *week 8* [37]. Four weeks after a nerve-intact soleus muscle graft procedure, Donovan and Faulkner removed the synergistic gastrocnemius muscle to increase the functional load [44]. Comparisons were made between grafts exposed to increased functional load and normal load through *week 16.* At *week 8,* the wet mass of grafts with increased functional load treatment was 139% of normally loaded grafts, and this difference persisted through 16 weeks. Muscle cross-sectional area demonstrated differences of similar magnitude at these times. The dry muscle mass at *week 8* for grafts exposed to increased functional load was 24% greater than grafts exposed to a normal load (P <0.05). At *week 16,* the difference due to load was 46%. Similar differences due to load condition were noted for the absolute capacity to develop maximum isometric force. These results are consistent with Turk et al. [129] who emphasized the importance of allowing a muscle graft to be loaded during contractions to enhance regeneration.

Three experiments were conducted to determine if types of grafts that normally have deficits in mass, compared with nongrafted muscle, would also adapt positively to myectomy of synergistic muscles. The early time course (0.5–5.0 weeks after grafting) of the adaptive response of soleus grafts to myectomy was investigated [48]. There was an acceleration in the daily rate of wet mass (112% increase) and protein (82% increase) accretion with myectomy of synergistic muscle compared with normal load conditions. There was no major impact of myectomy on the developmental sequence in regeneration of MHCs. In another experiment, the soleus muscle was grafted with the nerve-implant technique and 80% of the lateral gastrocnemius muscle was simultaneously removed. The wet mass of 8-week grafts was 92 ± 8 mg ($X \pm$ SEM; n = 8), which was 65% of control soleus muscle values. With myectomy of the lateral gastrocnemius muscle, the mass was 131 ± 11 mg (n = 8), a 45% increase [139]. The third experiment used the same graft model, and the synergistic muscle was excised at either 4 or 8 weeks postgrafting [49]. This resulted in a 34% increase in total protein content by 12 weeks postgrafting. Increases of similar magnitude were noted in the cross-sectional area of Type I and IIb fibers in the soleus grafts.

As elucidated earlier in this review, run-training can significantly increase the mass of soleus muscle grafts, yet values often remain lower than nongrafted muscle even with continued training. This observation raised the possibility that nerve-implant soleus grafts become resistant to a growth stimulus after a period of run-training. The hypothesis was thus tested that nerve-implant soleus grafts of rats previously run-trained would be refractory to the hypertrophic stimulus from myectomy of synergistic muscle [49]. Eight groups were studied that differed relative to the combination and order of treatments (running and myectomy of synergistic muscle), and the graft age at the time of the myectomy operation and analysis of tissues. The run-training before the myectomy operation did impair the magnitude of the adaptive response of total protein content to myectomy. When contrasting the change in total protein content from 8–12 weeks, the increase in grafts after myectomy was 33% for cage-sedentary rats and 15% for rats that had been previously running. The running-induced attenuation of the adaptive response of muscle grafts to the myectomy of synergistic muscles may reflect alterations in the pattern of motor unit recruitment and/or a limitation on the activation and proliferation of satellite cells in the muscle grafts.

Coan and Tomanek grafted the soleus muscle in male rats with no surgical reattachment of the nerve [39]. One week thereafter, the synergistic gastrocnemius muscle was excised. The myectomy of the synergist muscle resulted in a significant increase in the wet mass of grafts 2 days hence, but a large fraction of the increased mass was fluid, presumably resulting from an acute inflammatory response to the surgical trauma [5]. By 60 days, only 38% of the normally loaded and 21% of the grafts exposed to increased functional load persisted; the majority were resorbed likely as a result of inadequate reinnervation attributable to the standard operative procedure. At 11, 20, 40, and 60 days following grafting, the wet mass of the grafts that persisted in the legs with myectomy was 229, 205, 150, and 107% of normally loaded grafts, respectively. Similar negative results regarding changes due to increased functional load have been obtained by others [95].

Relative Plasticity of Grafted and Non-grafted Muscle
Chronic running increased wet mass and protein content of soleus muscle grafts, whereas nongrafted muscle will not typically adapt in this

fashion to this type of training. This raised the possibility that grafts are more adaptable to exercise conditioning that control muscle [145]. It was not possible to determine if increased plasticity in grafts compared with control muscles was a valid interpretation, however, as the relative exercise stimulus to grafts was unknown and likely differed from that in control soleus muscle. During locomotion, the EMG activity of soleus muscle grafts does not differ from control soleus muscle [144]. Furthermore, the capacity to develop maximum force is 55% less than for control muscle [123]. It seems clear, therefore, that the power developed by soleus grafts during running is a substantially higher percent of maximum than in control soleus muscle. High power activities have a bias to induce hypertrophy [57], so the running-induced growth of grafts compared to control muscle may merely reflect relatively different stimuli.

Markley et al. [86] compared free transplanted muscle and vascular-intact transposed muscle, both placed into the site of zygomaticus muscle in monkeys. The difference between operative techniques is of key importance as the fibers degenerate and regenerate in the transplantation, but survive in the transposition. It is interesting to note that when muscle fibers regenerate rather than survive, there is enhanced adapatability to the atypical site and its innervation, and a better approximation of the structure and function of zygomaticus muscle originally in the site. For example, the maximum capacity to develop P_o in nongrafted zygomaticus muscle is 10 ± 1 N/cm^2. Thirteen weeks after transplantation or transposition, P_o was 8 ± 2 (n.s.) and 4 ± 2 N/cm^2 (P<0.05), respectively. Fiber cross-sectional area was 2110 ± 140 μm^2 for control zygomaticus muscle, and 2300 ± 160 (n.s.) and 2890 ± 140 μm^2 (P<0.05) for transplanted and transposed muscle, respectively.

Donovan and Faulkner [45] compared skeletal muscle composed of surviving fibers (i.e., following transposition) with muscle grafts composed of regenerating fibers. They tested the hypothesis that compared with surviving fibers, regenerating fibers would adapt their structure and function more rapidly to an atypical site and innervation. The experiment involved either transposing or transplanting EDL muscles to soleus muscle sites, and vice versa. Eight weeks thereafter, selected isometric and isotonic contractile properties, and percentage distribution of Type II fibers, was measured. Regenerating fibers adapted more rapidly and almost completely in some cases than did the surviving fibers.

Mechanisms of Plasticity

Carraro [34] demonstrated that when a muscle comprised primarily of Type I fibers is grafted without the nerve, the fast isoform of MHC predominates in the stable graft. Moreover, the impaired regeneration of skeletal muscle in old host animals and in standard grafts compared with nerve-intact grafts in young hosts, is likely related to impaired reinnervation. Thus, overall, the result of studies in this area supports the interpretation that innervation, recruitment, and force (i.e., the biomechanical loading of a recruited muscle will result in force production) are critical variables in the regulation of regenerative muscle development and maturation.

Our working hypothesis at this point is that given proper reinnervation and revascularization, the lack of adequate force production by regenerating fibers is a primary extrinsic factor that impairs skeletal muscle regeneration. Much work remains to provide the definitive evidence for this hypothesis, as well as for elucidation of the molecular and cellular mechanisms by which force is transduced to the growth of muscle grafts. It should be noted that in another model of muscle development—tissue culture with embryonic chick muscle fibers—increased tension from externally applied stretching leads to fiber differentiation through many of the same mechanisms thought to be associated with fiber growth in vivo [131].

SUMMARY

The sequence of molecular and cellular events of muscle ontogeny leads to the proliferation, fusion, and differentiation of myoblasts to muscle cells. This sequence is closely paralleled in the grafting-ischemia model in which adult myoblast-satellite cells function as the muscle precursor cells. The study of skeletal muscle regeneration is a fertile and promising area of research in myogenesis. The early regenerative development and maturation of muscle is similar regardless of the perturbation that induced the degeneration-regeneration sequelae. In light of this, we maintain that the skeletal muscle graft model is useful to rigorously evaluate many regulatory aspects of skeletal muscle development and maturation in an adult animal host. One advantage of the graft model is that manipulation of the adult host, such as with exercise or hormone treatment, allows insight into their regulatory roles in muscle development and maturation. These approaches are often not possible for developing skeletal muscle in utero or in ovo.

After skeletal muscle grafting, many structural and functional characteristics change with time until they reach a stable value. Successful regeneration requires revascularization, cellular infiltration, phagocytosis of necrotic muscle fibers, proliferation and fusion of muscle precursor cells, reinnervation, and recruitment and loading. The time taken to reach stable values varies among different structural and functional variables, and many reach stable values that are less than those of control skeletal muscle. There are differences in the degree of regenerative success because of the size of muscle mass grafted. In small and large grafts, regeneration is enhanced by facilitation of the reinnervation. Regeneration is evident without vascular repair in grafts of up to approximately 6 g, although in all but the 100 to 150-mg grafts in rats, a significant necrotic core is present. Regeneration is typically unsuccessful when muscle masses greater than 6 g are grafted without vascular repair. Large muscles can be grafted with vascular repair, and in this case, the cellular response is quite different, as the majority of fibers survive rather than degenerate and regenerate.

Changing the components of physical activity during skeletal muscle regeneration can alter several attributes of the graft phenotype. The consensus of several experiments supports the interpretation that proper recruitment and force development by grafts are essential variables in the regulation of the development and maturation of muscle grafts. Morphological and physiological attributes of grafts adapt to changes in the habitual level of physical activity in a qualitatively similar fashion to control muscle. Further investigation into the mechanisms underlying the documented effects is necessary to advance our understanding of the molecular and cellular events underlying skeletal muscle regeneration and subsequent plasticity.

ACKNOWLEDGMENTS

The authors thank the valued colleagues and students who have informed or collaborated with the studies of skeletal muscle regeneration and plasticity. Sandra Ruland is thanked for her editorial comments during the development of this review. This review and several of the studies cited herein were supported by grants DE-07687 and AR-34298 of the National Institutes of Health.

REFERENCES

1. Alford, E., R.R. Roy, J.A. Hodgson, and V.R. Edgerton. Electromyography of rat soleus, gastrocnemius and tibialis anterior during hindlimb suspension. *Exp. Neurol.* 96: 635–649, 1987.
2. Allbrook, D. Skeletal muscle regeneration. *Muscle Nerve* 4:234–245, 1981.
3. Allen, R.E., and L.L. Rankin. Regulation of satellite cells during skeletal muscle growth and development. *Proc. Soc. Exp. Biol. Med.* 194:81–86, 1990.
4. Armstrong, R.B. Initial events in exercise-induced muscular injury. *Med. Sci. Sports Exerc.* 22:429–435, 1990.
5. Armstrong, R.B., P. Marum, P. Tullson, and C.W. Saubert, IV. Acute hypertrophic response of skeletal muscle to removal of synergists. *J. Appl. Physiol. Respir. Environ. Exercise Physiol.* 460:835–842, 1979.
6. Baldwin, K.M. Muscle development: neonatal to adult. R.L. Terjung (ed). *Exercise and Sports Science Reviews*, Vol. 12, 1984, pp. 1–19.
7. Bandman, E. Myosin isoenzyme transitions in muscle development, maturation and disease. *Int. Rev. Cytol.* 97:97–131, 1988.

8. Basson, M.D., and B.M. Carlson. Myotoxicity of single and repeated injections of mepivacaine (Carbocaine) in the rat. *Anesth. Analg.* 59:275–282, 1980.

9. Bischoff, R. Analysis of muscle regeneration using single myofibers in culture. *Med. Sci. Sports Exercise* 21:164–172, 1989.

10. Blaivas, M., and B.M. Carlson. Muscle fiber branching - differentiating between grafts in old and young rats. *Mech. Ageing Dev.* 60:43–53, 1991.

11. Booth, F.W., and D.B. Thomason. Molecular and cellular adaptation of muscle in response to exercise: perspectives of various models. *Physiol. Rev.* 71:541–585, 1991.

12. Burton, H.W., B.M. Carlson, and J.A. Faulkner. Microcirculatory adaptation to skeletal muscle transplantation. *Ann. Rev Physiol.* 49:439–451, 1987.

13. Burton, H.W., and J.A. Faulkner. The response of arterioles in skeletal muscle grafts to vasoactive agents. *Microvasc. Res.* 34:59–68, 1987.

14. Burton, H.W., T.R. Stevenson, R.C. Dysko, K.P. Gallagher, and J.A. Faulkner. Total and regional blood flows in vascularized skeletal muscle grafts in rabbits. *Am. J. Physiol.* 255 (*Heart Circ. Physiol.* 24): H1043–H1049, 1988.

15. Burton, H.W., T.R. Stevenson, T.P. White, J. Hartman, and J.A. Faulkner. Force deficit of vascularized skeletal muscle grafts in rabbits. *J. Appl. Physiol.* 66: 675–679, 1989.

16. Caldwell, C.J., D.L. Mattey, and R.O. Weller. Role of the basement membrane in the regeneration of skeletal muscle. *Neuropathol. Appl. Neurobiol.* 16:225–238, 1990.

17. Campion, D.R. The muscle satellite cell: a review. *Int. J. Cytol.* 87:225–251, 1984.

18. Carlsen, R.C., H.W. Klein, C.C. Matthews, and I.M. Gourley. Recovery of free muscle grafts in the rat: improvement is associated with an increase in cyclic adenosine monophosphate concentration or use of the condition/test paradigm. *Exp. Neurol.* 98:616–632, 1987.

19. Carlson, B.M. *The Regeneration of Minced Muscles.* Basel: Karger, 1972, pp. 1–128.

20. Carlson, B.M. The regeneration of skeletal muscle–a review. *Am J. Anat.* 137:119–149, 1973.

21. Carlson, B.M. A quantitative study of muscle fiber survival and regeneration in normal, predenervated and Marcaine-treated free muscle grafts in the rat. *Exp. Neurol.* 52:421–432, 1976.

22. Carlson, B.M. A review of muscle transplantation in mammals. *Physiologia Bohemoslovaca* 27:387–400, 1978.

23. Carlson, B.M. The regeneration of mammalian limbs and limb tissue. J.C. Daniels (ed). *Methods in Mammalian Reproduction.* New York: Academic, 1978, pp. 377–401.

24. Carlson, B.M. Regeneration of entire skeletal muscles. *Fed. Proc.* 45:1456–1480, 1986.

25. Carlson, B.M., and J.A. Faulkner. The regeneration of skeletal muscle fibers following injury: a review. *Med. Sci. Sports Exercise* 15:187–198; 1983.

26. Carlson, B.M., and J.A. Faulkner. Reinnervation of long-term denervated rat muscle freely grafted into an innervated limb. *Exper. Neurol.* 102:50–56, 1988.

27. Carlson, B.M., and J.A. Faulkner. Muscle transplantation between young and old rats: age of host determines recovery. *Am. J. Physiol.* 256 (*Cell Physiol.* 25): C1262–C1266, 1989.

28. Carlson, B.M., and E. Gutmann. Regeneration in free grafts of normal and denervated muscles in the rat: morphology and histochemistry. *Anat. Rec.* 183:47–62, 1975.

29. Carlson, B.M., and E. Gutmann. Free grafting of the extensor digitorum longus muscle in the rat after marcaine pretreatment. *Exp. Neurol.* 53:82–93, 1976.

30. Carlson, B.M., F.M. Hansen-Smith, and D.K. Magon. The life history of a free muscle graft. A. Mauro (ed). *Muscle Regeneration.* New York: Raven Press, 1979, pp. 493–507.

31. Carlson, B.M., A. Herbrychova, and E. Gutmann. Retention of hormonal sensitivity in free grafts of the levator ani muscle. *Exp. Neurol.* 63:94–107, 1979.

32. Carlson, B.M., P. Hnik, S. Tucek, R. Vejsasa, D. Bader, and J.A. Faulkner. Comparison between grafts with intact nerves and standard free grafts of rat extensor digitorum longus muscle. *Physiol. Bohemoslov.* 30:505–514, 1981.

33. Carlson, B.M., K.R. Wagner, and S.R. Max. Reinnervation of rat extensor digitorum longus muscles after free grafting. *Muscle Nerve* 2:304–307, 1979.

34. Carraro, U., L. Dalla Libera, and C. Catani. Myosin light and heavy chains in muscle regenerating in absence of the nerve: transient appearance of the embryonic light chain. *Exp. Neurol.* 79:106–117, 1983.

35. Ciske, P.E., and J.A. Faulkner. Chronic electrical stimulation of nongrafted and grafted skeletal muscles in rats. *J. Appl. Physiol.* 59:1434–1439; 1985.

36. Clark, K.I., P.G. Morales, and T.P. White. Mass and fiber cross-sectional area of soleus muscle grafts following training. *Med. Sci. Sports Exerc.* 21:432–436, 1989.

37. Clark, K.I., and T.P. White. Morphology of stable muscle grafts of rats: effects of gender and muscle type. *Muscle Nerve* 8:99–104, 1985.

38. Clark, K.I., and T.P. White. Neuromuscular adaptations to cross-reinnervation in 12- and 29-month Fischer 344 rats. *Am. J. Physiol.* 260 (*Cell Physiol.* 29):C96–C103, 1991.

39. Coan M.R., and R.J. Tomanek. The growth of regenerating soleus muscle transplants after ablation of the gastrocnemius muscle. *Exp. Neurol.* 71:278–294; 1981.

40. Coté, C., and J.A. Faulkner. Motor unit function in skeletal muscle autografts of rats. *Exp. Neurol.* 84:292–305, 1984.

41. Coté, C., and J.A. Faulkner. Characteristics of motor units in muscles of rats grafted with nerve intact. *Am. J. Physiol.* 250 (*Cell Physiol.* 19):C828–C833, 1986.

42. Coté, C., T.P. White, and J.A. Faulkner. Intramuscular substrate depletion and fatigability of soleus grafts in rats. *Can. J. Physiol. Pharmacol.* 66:829–832, 1988.

43. Daw, C.K., J.W. Starnes, and T.P. White. Muscle atrophy and hypoplasia with aging: impact of training and food restriction. *J. Appl. Physiol.* 64:2428–2432, 1988.

44. Donovan, C.M., and J.A. Faulkner. Muscle grafts overloaded by ablation of synergistic muscles. *J. Appl. Physiol.* 61:288–292, 1986.

45. Donovan, C.M., and J.A. Faulkner. Plasticity of skeletal muscle: regenerating fibers adapt more rapidly than surviving fibers. *J. Appl. Physiol.* 62:2507–2511, 1987.

46. Elmubarak, M.H., and K.W. Ranatunga. Differentiation of fast and slow muscles in the rat after neonatal denervation: a physiological study. *J. Muscle Res. Cell Motil.* 9:219–232, 1988.

47. Esser, K.A., M.O. Boluyt, and T.P. White. Separation of cardiac myosin heavy chains by gradient SDS-PAGE. *Am. J. Physiol.* 255 (*Heart Circ. Physiol.* 24):H659–H663, 1988.

48. Esser, K.A., and T.P. White. Biomechanical loading affects growth and differentiation of skeletal muscle grafts. *Med. Sci. Sports Exerc.* 22:S137, 1990.

49. Esser, K.A., and T.P. White. Prior running reduces hypertrophic growth of skeletal muscle grafts. *J. Appl. Physiol.* 69:451–455, 1990.

50. Esser, K.A., T.P. White, and S.S. Segal. Actin and myosin content in myofibrillar preparations from control and grafted soleus muscles. *Can. J. Sport Sci.* 13:11P, 1988.

51. Faulkner, J.A., and B.M. Carlson. Contractile properties of standard and nerve-intact muscle grafts in the rat. *Muscle Nerve* 8:413–418, 1985.

52. Faulkner, J.A., and C. Coté. Functional deficits in skeletal muscle grafts. *Fed. Proc.* 45:1466–1469, 1986.

53. Faulkner, J.A., P.J. Guelinckx, K.K. McCully, and T.P. White. Functional deficits in free and vascularized grafts. M. Frey and G. Freilinger (eds). *Proceedings of 2nd Vienna Muscle Symposium.* Vienna: Universitatverlag, 1986, pp. 68–72.

54. Faulkner, J.A., V.A. Kadhiresan, E.G. Wilkins, and C.A. Hassett. Properties of motor units in free standard grafts and in nerve-repaired vascularized grafts in rats. G. Freilinger, and M. Deutinger (eds). *Third Vienna Muscle Symposium.* Wien: Blackwell-MZV, 1992, pp. 41–48.

55. Faulkner, J.A., J.M. Markley, K.K. McCully, C.R. Watters, and T.P. White. Characteristics of cat skeletal muscles grafted with intact nerves or with anastomosed nerves. *Exp. Neurol.* 80:682–696, 1983.

56. Faulkner, J.A., L.C. Maxwell, S.A. Mufti, and B.M. Carlson. Skeletal muscle fiber

regeneration following heterotopic autotransplantation in cats. *Life Sci.* 19:289–296, 1976.

57. Faulkner, J.A., and T.P. White. Adaptations of skeletal muscle to physical activity. C. Bouchard, et al. (eds). *Exercise, Fitness and Health: A Consensus of Current Knowledge.* Champaign, IL: Human Kinetics, 1990, pp. 265–279.

58. Faulkner, J.A., J.H. Niemeyer, L.C. Maxwell, and T.P. White. Contractile properties of transplanted extensor digitorum longus muscles of cats. *Am J. Physiol.* 238 (*Cell Physiol.* 7):C120–126, 1980.

59. Florini, J.R., and K.A. Magri. Effects of growth factors on myogenic differentiation. *Am J. Physiol.* 256 (*Cell Physiol.* 25):C701–C711, 1989.

60. Foster, A.H., and B.M. Carlson. Myotoxicity of local anesthetics and regeneration of the damaged muscle fibers. *Anesth. Analg.* 58:727–736, 1980.

61. Freilinger, G., and M. Deutinger (eds). *Third Vienna Muscle Symposium.* Wien: Blackwell-MZV, 1992, pp. 1–403.

62. Freilinger, G., J. Holle, and B.M. Carlson. *Muscle Transplantation.* New York: Springer-Verlag; 1981.

63. Gambke, B., G.E. Lyons, J. Haselgrove, A.M. Kelly, and N.A. Rubestein. Thyroidal and neural control of myosin transitions during development of rat fast and slow muscles. *FEBS Lett.* 156:335–339, 1983.

64. Gibson, M.C., and E. Schultz. Age-related differences in absolute numbers of skeletal muscle satellite cells. *Muscle Nerve* 6:574–580, 1983.

65. Gollnick, P.D., B.F. Timson, R.L. Moore, and M. Riedy. Muscular enlargement and number of fibers in skeletal muscles of rats. *J. Appl. Physiol.* 50:936–943, 1981.

66. Gorin, F., P. Ignacia, R. Gelinas, and R.C. Carlsen. Abnormal expression of glycogen phosphorylase genes in regenerated muscle. *Am. J. Physiol.* 257 (*Cell Physiol.* 26): C495–C503, 1989.

67. Greaser, M.L., R.L. Moss, and P.J. Reiser. Variations in contractile properties of rabbit single muscle fibres in relation to troponin T isoforms and myosin light chains. *J. Physiol.* 406:85–98, 1988.

68. Grounds, M.D. Towards understanding skeletal muscle regeneration. *Path. Res. Pract.* 187:1–22, 1991.

69. Guelinckx, P.J., J.A. Faulkner, and D.A. Essig. Neurovascular-anastomosed muscle grafts in rabbits: functional deficits result from tendon repair. *Muscle Nerve* 11:745–751, 1988.

70. Gulati, A.K. Long-term retention of regenerative capability after denervation of skeletal muscle and dependency of late differentiation on innervation. *Anat. Rec.* 220:429–434, 1988.

71. Gunning, P., and E. Hardeman. Multiple mechanisms regulate muscle fiber diversity. *FASEB J.* 5:3064–3070, 1991.

72. Gutmann, E., and B.M. Carlson. Regeneration and transplantation of muscles in old rats and between young and old rats. *Life Sci.* 18:109–114, 1976.

73. Hakelius, L., and B. Nystrom. Blood vessels and connective tissue in autotransplanted free muscle grafts of the cat. *Scand. J. Plast. Reconstr. Surg.* 9:87–91, 1975.

74. Hansen-Smith, F.M. Development and innervation of soleplates in the freely grafted extensor digitorum longus (EDL) muscle in the rat. *Anat. Rec.* 207:55–67, 1983.

75. Hansen-Smith, F.M., and B.M. Carlson. Cellular responses to free grafting of the extensor digitorum longus muscle of the rat. *J. Neurol. Sci.* 41:149–173, 1979.

76. Hansen-Smith, F.M., B.M. Carlson, and K.L. Irwin. Revascularization of the freely grafted extensor digitorum longus muscle in the rat. *Am. J. Anat.* 158:65–82, 1980.

77. Hudlicka, O., M. Brown, and S. Egginton. Angiogenesis in skeletal and cardiac muscle. *Physiol. Rev.* 72:369–418, 1992.

78. Hughes, S., and H.M. Blau. Muscle fiber pattern is independent of cell lineage in postnatal rodent development. *Cell* 68:659–671, 1992.

79. Hurme, T., and H. Kalimo. Activation of myogenic precursor cells after muscle injury. *Med. Sci. Sports Exercise* 24:197–205, 1992.

80. Jones, G.H. Protein synthesis in bupivacaine (Marcaine)-treated, regenerating skeletal muscle. *Muscle Nerve* 5:281–290, 1982.

81. Kasper, C.E., T.P. White, and L.C. Maxwell. Running during recovery from hindlimb suspension induces transient muscle injury. *J. Appl. Physiol.* 68: 533–539, 1990.

82. Koshima, I., and T. Endo. Experimental study of vascularized muscle: multifactorial analysis of muscle regeneration following denervation. *J. Reconstr. Microsurg.* 5:225–230, 1989.

83. Lipton, B.H., and E. Schultz. Developmental fate of skeletal muscle satellite cells. *Science* 205:1292–1294, 1979.

84. Manktelow, R.T., and R.M. Zuker. Extremity reconstruction with functioning muscle transplantation—factors affecting functional return. G. Freilinger and M. Deutinger (eds). *Third Vienna Muscle Symposium.* Wien: Blackwell-MZV, 1992, pp. 234–243.

85. Marechal, G., K. Schwartz, G. Beckers-Bleukx, and E. Ghins. Isozymes of myosin in growing and regenerating rat muscles. *Eur. J. Biochem.* 138:421–428, 1984.

86. Markley, J.M., J.A. Faulkner, and C. Coté. Transplantation and transposition of skeletal muscles into the faces of monkeys. *Plast. Reconstr. Surg.* 84:424–431, 1989.

87. Markley, J.M., J.A. Faulkner, J.H. Niemeyer, and T.P. White. Functional properties of palmaris longus muscles of rhesus monkeys transplanted as index finger flexors. *Plast. Reconstr. Surg.* 76:574–577, 1985.

88. Martin, T.P., L.A. Gundersen, A.C. Vailas, V.R. Edgerton, and S.K. Das. Incomplete normalization of dog gracilis muscle grafts with neurovascular repair despite long-term recovery. *J. Appl. Physiol.* 68:687–692, 1990.

89. Mauro, A. Satellite cell of skeletal muscle fibers. *J. Biophys. Biochem. Cytol.* 9: 493–495, 1961.

90. Maxwell, L.C., J.A. Faulkner, J.M. Markley, and D.R. Winborn. Neuroanastomosis of orthotopically transplanted palmaris longus muscles. *Muscle Nerve* 2:44–52, 1979.

91. Maxwell, L.C., J.A. Faulkner, S.A. Mufti, and A.M. Turowski. Free autografting of entire limb muscles in the cat: histochemistry and biochemistry. *J. Appl. Physiol.* 44:431–437, 1978.

92. Maxwell, L.C., J.A. Faulkner, T.P. White, and F.M. Hansen-Smith. Growth of regenerating skeletal muscle fibers in cats. *Anat. Rec.* 209:153–163, 1984.

93. McCully, K.K., and J.A. Faulkner. Characteristics of lengthening contractions associated with injury to skeletal muscle fibers. *J. Appl. Physiol.* 61:293–299, 1986.

94. Miller, J.B. Myoblast diversity in skeletal myogenesis: how much and to what end? *Cell* 69:1–3, 1992.

95. Mong, F.S.F., J.L. Poland, and T.J. Breen. Exercise or overloading: effect on skeletal muscle grafts of rats. *Arch. Phys. Med. Rehabil.* 66:439–442, 1985.

96. Mong, F.S.F., J.L. Poland, and J.W. Poland. Glycogen and histological changes in muscle grafts of rats during fasting or exercise. *Can. J. Physiol. Pharmacol.* 60:387–391, 1982.

97. Moss, F.P., and C.P. LeBlond. Satellite cells as the source of nuclei in muscles of growing rats. *Anat. Rec.* 170:421–436, 1971.

98. Mufti, S.A., B.M. Carlson, L.C. Maxwell, and J.A. Faulkner. The free autografting of entire limb muscles in the cat: morphology. *Anat. Rec.* 188:417–429, 1977.

99. Narusawa, M., R.B. Fitzimons, S. Izumo, B. Nadal-Ginard, N.A. Rubenstein, and A.M. Kelly. Slow myosin in developing rat skeletal muscle. *J. Cell Biol.* 104:447–459, 1987.

100. Nicolai, J.-P.A. *Irreversible Facial Paralysis and its Treatment.* Amsterdam: Aan De Rijksuniversiteit Groningen, 1983.

101. Noah, E.M., R. Winkel, U. Schramm, and W. Kuhnel. Regeneration of neovascularized muscle transplants. Effects of innervation, reinnervation and exercise. Analyzed

by morphological and morphometric methods. G. Freilinger and M. Deutinger (eds). *Third Vienna Muscle Symposium.* Wien: Blackwell-MZV, 1992, pp. 127–144.

102. Ontell, M. Morphological aspects of muscle fiber regeneration. *Fed. Proc.* 45:1461–1465, 1986.

103. Pestronk, A., D.B. Drachman, and J.W. Griffin. Effects of ageing on nerve sprouting and regeneration. *Exp. Neurol.* 70:65–82, 1980.

104. Pette, D., and R.S. Staron. Cellular and molecular diversities of mammalian skeletal muscle fibers. *Rev. Physiol. Biochem. Pharmacol.* 116:1–76, 1990.

105. Phillips, G.D., D. Lu, V.I. Mitshov, and B.M. Carlson. Survival of myogenic cells in freely grafted rat rectus femoris and extensor digitorum longus muscles. *Am. J. Anat.* 180:365–372, 1987.

106. Reiser, P.J., R.L. Moss, G.G. Giulian, and M.L. Greaser. Shortening velocity in single fibers from adult rabbit soleus muscles is correlated with myosin heavy chain composition. *J. Biol. Chem.* 260:9077–9080, 1985.

107. Rifenberick, D.H., C.L. Koski, and S.R. Max. Metabolic studies of skeletal muscle regeneration. *Exp. Neurol.* 45:527–540, 1974.

108. Roberts, P., and J.K. McGeachie. The effects of pre- and post-transplantation exercise on satellite cell activation and the regeneration of skeletal muscle transplants: a morphometric and autoradiographic study in mice. *J. Anat.* 180:67–74, 1992.

109. Rogers, S.L. Muscle spindle formation and differentiation in regenerating rat muscle grafts. *Dev. Biol.* 94:265–283, 1982.

110. Rogers, S.L., and B.M. Carlson. A quantitative assessment of muscle spindle formation in reinnervated and non-reinnervated grafts of the rat extensor digitorum longus muscle. *Neuroscience* 6:87–94, 1981.

111. Roy, R.R., K.M. Baldwin, and V.R. Edgerton. The plasticity of skeletal muscle: Effects of neuromuscular activity. J.O. Holloszy (ed). *Exercise and Sport Sciences Reviews,* Vol. 19, 1991, pp. 269–312.

112. Russell, B., D.J. Dix, D.L. Haller, and J. Jacobs-El. Repair of injured skeletal muscle: a molecular approach. *Med Sci. Sports Exerc.* 24:189–196, 1992.

113. Sadeh, M. Effects of aging on skeletal muscle regeneration. *J. Neurol. Sci.* 87:67–74, 1988.

114. Salviati, G., R. Betto, and D. Danieli Betto. Polymorphism of myofibrillar proteins of rabbit skeletal-muscle fibres. *Biochem. J.* 207:261–272, 1982.

115. Sandercock, T.G., C. Coté, and J.A. Faulkner. Properties of motor units in nerve-intact autografts of cat extensor digitorum longus muscles. *J. Neurophysiol.* 62:231–238, 1989.

116. Sanes J.R. The extracellular matrix. A.G. Engel and B.Q. Banker (eds). *Myology,* Vol. 1. New York: McGraw Hill, 1986, pp. 155–175.

117. Sanes, J.R. Extracellular matrix molecules that influence neural development. *Ann. Rev. Neurosci.* 12:491–516, 1989.

118. Schmalbruch, H. Regeneration of soleus muscles of rat autografted in toto as studied by electron microscopy. *Cell Tissue Res.* 177:159–180, 1977.

119. Schmalbruch, H. Muscle regeneration: fetal myogenesis in a new setting. *Bibl. Anat.* 29:126–153, 1986.

120. Schultz, E. A quantitative study of satellite cells in regenerated soleus and EDL muscles. *Anat. Rec.* 208:501–506, 1984.

121. Schultz, E. Satellite cell behavior during skeletal muscle growth and regeneration. *Med. Sci. Sports Exerc.* 21:S181–S187, 1989.

122. Schultz, E., D.J. Albright, D.L. Jaryszak, and T.L. David. Survival of satellite cells in whole muscle transplants. *Anat. Rec.* 222:12–17, 1988.

123. Segal, S.S., T.P. White, and J.A. Faulkner. Architecture, composition and contractile properties of rat soleus muscle grafts. *Am. J. Physiol.* 250 (*Cell Physiol.* 19): C474–C479, 1986.

124. Snow, M. H. Myogenic cell formation in regenerating rat skeletal muscle injured by mincing. II. *Anat. Rec.* 168:201–218, 1977.

125. Stockdale, F.E. Myogenic cell lineages. *Dev. Biol.* 154:284–298. 1992.

126. Stockdale, F.E., and J.B. Miller. The cellular basis of myosin heavy chain isoform expression during development of avian skeletal muscles. *Dev. Biol.* 123:1–9, 1987.

127. Stockdale, F.E., J.B. Miller, J.L. Feldman, G. Lamson, and J. Hager. Myogenic cell lineages: commitment and modulation during differentiation of avian muscle. L.H. Kedes and F.E. Stockdale (eds). *Cellular and Molecular Biology of Muscle Development.* New York: Alan R. Liss, 1989, pp. 3–13.

128. Thomason, D.B., R.E. Herrick, D. Surdyka, and K.M. Baldwin. Time course of soleus muscle myosin expression during hindlimb suspension and recovery. *J. Appl. Physiol.* 63:130–137, 1987.

129. Turk, A.E., K. Ishida, M. Kobayashi, J. Narloch, B.M. Kinney, M.A. Verity, R.R. Roy, V.R. Edgerton, and T.A. Miller. The effects of dynamic tension and reduced graft size on muscle regeneration in rabbit free muscle grafts. *J. Plast. Reconstr. Surg.* 88:299–309, 1991.

130. Van Handel, P.J., P. Watson, J. Troup, and M. Pyley. Effects of treadmill running on oxidative capacity of regenerated skeletal muscle. *Int. J. Sports Med.* 2:92–96, 1981.

131. Vandenburg, H.H., S. Swasdison, and P. Karlisch. Computer-aided mechanogenesis of skeletal muscle organs from single cells in vitro. *FASEB J.* 5:2860–2867, 1991.

132. Vracko, R.E., and E.P. Benditt. Basal lamina: the scaffold for orderly cell replacement. Observations on regeneration of injured skeletal muscle fibers and capillaries. *J. Cell Biol.* 55:406–409, 1972.

133. Walmsley, B.J., J.A. Hodgson, and R.E. Burke. Forces produced by medial gastrocnemius and soleus muscles during locomotion in freely moving cats. *J. Neurophysiol.* 41:1202–1216, 1978.

134. Wagner, K.R., B.M. Carlson, and S.R. Max. Developmental patterns of glycolytic enzymes in regenerating skeletal muscle after autogenous free grafting. *J. Neurol. Sci.* 34:373–390, 1977.

135. Wagner, K.R., S.R. Max, E.M. Grollman, and C.L. Koski. Glycolysis in skeletal muscle regeneration. *Exp. Neurol.* 52:40–48, 1976.

136. Walker, J.A., F.J. Cerny, J.R. Cotter, and H.W. Burton. Attenuation of contraction-induced skeletal muscle injury by bromelain. *Med. Sci. Sports Exerc.* 24:20–25, 1992.

137. Whalen, R.G., J.B. Harris, G.S. Butler-Browne, and S. Sesodia. Expression of myosin isoforms during notexin-induced regeneration of rat soleus muscles. *Dev. Biol.* 141:24–40, 1990.

138. Whalen, R.G., S.M. Sell, G.S. Butler-Browne, K. Schwartz, P. Bouveret, and I. Pinset-Harstrom. Three myosin heavy chain isozymes appear sequentially in rat muscle development. *Nature* (London) 292:805–809, 1981.

139. White, T.P. Adaptations of skeletal muscle grafts to chronic changes of physical activity. *Fed. Proc.* 45:1470–1473, 1986.

140. White, T.P., G.J. Alderink, K.A. Esser, and K.I. Clark. Postoperative physical activity alters growth of skeletal muscle grafts. G. Freilinger and M. Deutinger (eds). *Third Vienna Muscle Symposium.* Wien: Blackwell-MZV, 1992, pp. 53–60.

141. White, T.P., and K.A. Esser. Satellite cell and growth factor involvement in skeletal muscle growth. *Med. Sci. Sports Exerc.* 21:S158–S163, 1989.

142. White, T.P., J.A. Faulkner, J.M. Markley, Jr., and L.C. Maxwell. Translocation of the temporalis muscle for treatment of facial paralysis. *Muscle Nerve* 5:500–504, 1982.

143. White, T.P., L.C. Maxwell, D.M. Sosin, and J.A. Faulkner. Capillarity and blood flow of transplanted skeletal muscles of cats. *Am. J. Physiol.* 241 (*Heart Circ. Physiol.* 10): H630–H636, 1981.

144. White, T.P., J.F. Villanacci, C. Gans, and D.J. Nelson. Electromyographic (EMG) activity of regenerating muscle during locomotion: effect of training. *Med. Sci. Sports Exerc.* 15:130–131, 1983.

145. White, T.P., J.F. Villanacci, P.G. Morales, S.S. Segal, and D.A. Essig. Exercise-induced adaptations of rat soleus muscle grafts. *J. Appl. Physiol.* 56:1325–1334, 1984.

146. Wineinger, M.A., F. Gorin, R. Tait, B. Froman, and R.C. Carlsen. Reduced glycolytic metabolism in regenerated fast-twitch skeletal muscle. *Am. J. Physiol.* 261 (*Cell Physiol.* 30): C169–C176, 1991.

147. Womble, M.D. The clustering of acetylcholine receptors and formation of neuromuscular junctions in regenerating mammalian muscle grafts. *Am. J. Anat.* 176:191–205, 1986.

148. Zerba, E., T.E. Komorowski, and J.A. Faulkner. Free radical injury to skeletal muscles of young, adult, and old mice. *Am. J. Physiol.* 258 (*Cell Physiol.* 27): C429–C435, 1990.

10
Fluid Replacement During Exercise

TIMOTHY DAVID NOAKES, M.B. Ch.B., M.D., F.A.C.S.M.

HISTORICAL INTRODUCTION

Included among the "Don'ts" in a 1909 monograph titled "Marathon Running" [152] was the admonition: "Don't get in the habit of drinking and eating in a Marathon race; some prominent runners do, but it is not beneficial." The advice of Arthur Newton, a leading ultramarathon runner of the first half of this century, who held world records for running distances from 50–130 miles [117] was similar: "Even in the warmest English weather, a twenty-six mile run ought to be manageable with no more than a single drink, or at most two" [115].

In 1957, the then holder of the world's four fastest times for the 42-km marathon footrace wrote: "There is no need to take any solid food at all (during a marathon race) and every effort should be made to do without liquid, as the moment food or drink is taken, the body has to start dealing with its digestion and in so doing some discomfort will almost invariably be felt" [135]. Another famous ultra-distance runner who set world records at 30, 40, and 50 miles in 1954 confirmed that this advice was widely accepted: "In those days it was quite fashionable not to drink, until one absolutely had to. After a race runners would recount with pride 'I only had a drink after 30 or 40 kilometres.' To run a complete marathon without any fluid replacement was regarded as the ultimate aim of most runners, and a test of their fitness." (J. Mekler, 1991, personal communication). This athlete, who once competed in a 100-mile race in which he first drank only after 75 miles, confirmed that this approach was still popular when he had run his last competitive ultramarathon race in 1969.

That these ideas could *ever* have held credence, let alone so recently, may seem absurd to the modern exercise physiologist. But the fluid requirements of athletes has attracted scientific interest only since the early 1970s. Virtually all of the textbooks of exercise physiology and sports medicine published before 1970 contain little or no reference to this topic [2, 12, 44, 52, 57, 89, 164]; one of the first to include a section on fluid replacement during exercise was the monograph by Costill [31]. Yet many studies showing the importance of adequate fluid replacement especially during industrial and military activities in the heat had already been published.

The building of the Hoover Dam near Boulder City, Nevada in the 1930s stimulated the first systematic studies of fluid (and electrolyte) requirements during work in temperatures ranging between 90–120°F. One early study described the clinical and biochemical features of so-called "heat cramps" in seven workers on this project [157]. Another study measured fluid intake and urine output during both work and rest [156] and concluded that construction work could be undertaken without major health risks even in these severe environmental conditions provided subjects were accommodated in air-conditioned lodgings [46]. Yet another early study showed that sweat sodium concentration fell within days of exposure to extreme heat becoming so low that "10 litres per day may be secreted without the necessity of an abnormal salt intake" [46].

More detailed studies by Adolph and Dill [7] showed that the daily fluid intakes of construction workers averaged about 4 liters/day but rose as a linear function of increasing maximum daily temperature. Sweat rates increased from a resting value of 400 ml/hr when sitting in shade, to maximum rates of 1500–1700 ml/hr during 1–2 hr of exercise in the heat. Subjects showed relatively little desire to drink during exercise; fluid ingestion was greatest immediately after exercise and with meals. In the absence of food ingestion, drinking stopped when approximately one-half of the fluid loss had been corrected. The authors suggested that: ". . since some solute as well as water was lost, only enough water was required by the subject to render the concentration of the body fluids equal to their previous state." They also noted that all the water ingested an hour before exercise was lost in urine before the onset of exercise. But if the fluid contained sodium chloride "the water was retained for several hours before it was required for the formation of sweat." Subsequent studies suggested that 1 or more liters of fluid with a sodium chloride content of 0.5–0.9% (80–140 mmol/liter) ingested 2–3 hr before exercise would·increase body fluid content [5].

Despite the clear reluctance of dehydrated subjects to replace their fluid losses fully during and immediately after exercise, their daily fluctuations in weight were no greater than those measured in winter climates, indicating that fluid imbalances were corrected diurnally: "All the deviations from water balance were on the negative side; water was expended and a debt built up, which was later paid off." In contrast, Dill [46] found that within minutes of being given water, the dog and the donkey (burro) replaced exactly all the fluid they had lost during exercise. In one case, a burro drank 12 liters in 5 minutes [46]. Among the mammals studied by then, therefore, dehydrated humans were unique in this inability to replace all the fluid lost during exercise, as soon as water was provided.

The demands of desert warfare during the Second World War stimulated the next and, possibly, the truly classic early studies of fluid replacement during exercise [5]. These magnificent studies established for the first time, many of the concepts that continue to intrigue modern physiologists. Interestingly, at the time the studies commenced, it was believed that men, like marathon runners, should be "trained to do without water." Among the classic findings were the following:

1. Maximal sweat rates during exercise under the most severe environmental desert conditions were of the order of 1.7 liters/hr; much higher rates were reported during exercise in conditions of high humidity (jungle heat). Sweat rates during exercise in desert heat rose as a linear function of body weight and, hence, metabolic rate and environmental temperature.

2. Sweat rates during exercise were not influenced by the level of dehydration. Thus, the capacity for evaporative heat loss during low-intensity exercise was not impaired by progressive dehydration. Despite this, the rectal temperature rose during exercise as a linear function of the level of dehydration.

3. Urine flow was reduced when levels of dehydration exceeded 3% but did not increase dehydration levels of 7%. Thus, progressive dehydration did not induce fluid conservation by decreasing urine output. Anuria was not detected in any subject under any conditions. The constant urine output was needed to excrete the solutes contained in urine.

4. Chloride was present in virtually all urine samples measured. Thus, "salt deficiency in the desert was not common."

5. Even when given free access to adequate fluids during exercise, subjects developed a progressive weight loss, termed "voluntary" dehydration. Food ingestion greatly increased fluid intake; at least one-half of the fluid ingested daily was taken with meals. Conversely, without an adequate fluid intake, food intake during meals was also reduced. But body weight was usually restored after the evening meal.

6. Unless corrected, the progressive dehydration that developed during exercise in the heat impaired physical performance. At low levels of dehydration, physical performance was impaired only during high-intensity exercise. Subjects became syncopal, however, and were unable to exercise even at low exercise intensities when their levels of dehydration exceeded 7%. Feelings of well-being and the ability to walk returned within minutes of the resumption of drinking. Maximal levels of dehydration compatible with life were of the order of 20%.

7. The fluid lost in sweat did not originate equally from the different fluid compartments but came predominantly from the extracellular compartment. This would impair cardiovascular function.

8. Heart rate and rectal temperature increased and stroke volume fell as

a linear function of increasing levels of dehydration. Rectal temperature rose 0.3°C for each 1% increase in the level of dehydration.

9. The level of dehydration correlated most accurately with the rise in rectal temperature, the standing heart rate, and the reduction in salivary flow. Salivary flow ceased at dehydration levels greater than 8%.

10. Sodium ingestion during exercise tended to increase the amount of fluid ingested and reduced the urine output.

These studies, which clearly established the value of fluid ingestion during exercise, made little immediate impact on the athletic community. The studies of Pugh et al. [138] and Wyndham and Strydom [169] finally drew attention to the need for fluid ingestion also by *athletes* during prolonged exercise.

Pugh et al. [138] showed that competitors drank only 400 ml during a marathon race (0.12 liters/hr) and developed a mean weight loss of 2.9 kg (5.9% of initial body weight). As fluid loss, sweat rate, and postrace rectal temperature were highest in the race winner, Pugh et al. [138] concluded that "a high tolerance to fluid loss" seemed to be an important requirement for success in distance running. But they did not propose any role for fluid ingestion during exercise.

In their study, Wyndham and Strydom [169] found that athletes who became dehydrated by more than 3% during a series of 32-km foot races had elevated postrace rectal temperatures. As also found by Adolph [5], there was a linear relationship between the athletes' levels of dehydration and their postrace rectal temperatures, at least for levels of dehydration greater than 3%. The authors concluded that: (*a*) the level of dehydration was the most important factor determining the rectal temperature during prolonged exercise so (*b*) the avoidance of dehydration would be the critical factor preventing heat injury during prolonged exercise [168, 169]. Interestingly, the authors did not speculate that dehydration might influence running performance. Their finding that the race winners had the highest rectal temperatures and were the most dehydrated [119], may have dissuaded them.

Although the basis for some of their conclusions has been challenged [119, 121, 125], there is no doubt that it was especially the study of Wyndham and Strydom [169] that stimulated the modern interest in the role of fluid replacement during exercise.

MODERN STUDIES OF FLUID LOSS AND FLUID INGESTION DURING EXERCISE

There are two experimental models that have been used to study the effects of fluid loss and fluid intake on the physiological responses during exercise.

As emphasized by Coyle et al. [35, 36], fluid loss (hypohydration) induced either by the administration of diuretics, or exposure to sauna, or fluid restriction *before* exercise, produces physiological effects that are more marked than those that result from the form of dehydration that develops voluntarily *during* exercise when the rate of fluid loss exceeds the rate of fluid ingestion. In particular, the reduction in plasma volume and in physical performance for a given level of dehydration is greater with hypohydration [22, 35, 107].

For this reason, the result of the hypohydration studies that are reviewed in detail elsewhere [147] are perhaps most relevant for activities in which subjects deliberately dehydrate themselves before exercise, usually to make a specific competitive weight. These studies will not be considered further in this review; we will focus principally on studies of exercise-induced dehydration.

Effect of Exercise-induced Dehydration on Physical Performance
At least six studies [5, 15, 49, 91, 136, 151] have evaluated the effects of progressive exercise-induced dehydration on physical performance. Most have compared the performance of a group of subjects, usually military personnel, who either ingested fluid or restrained from fluid ingestion during prolonged exercise of relatively low intensity (walking) in dry heat. The measure of physical performance was the number of subjects in each group able to complete the prescribed exercise task.

Although few of the studies were subject to rigorous statistical analysis, the trend in all was for fewer subjects to complete the exercise task when they did not ingest fluid. Furthermore, performance was least impaired in subjects who maintained fluid balance during exercise. Fluid ingestion reduced rectal temperatures and heart rates during exercise; this effect was greatest when the rate of fluid ingestion equalled the sweat rate. In general, sweat rates were not influenced by fluid ingestion and fell only when the fluid deficit exceeded 2.5 liters [91]. Fluid ingestion also prevented the development of postural hypotension on cessation of exercise [49].

Most researchers observed that fluid ingestion had more obvious effects on the psyche than on the soma. The description of Bean and Eichna [15] is typical for subjects who did not ingest fluid during exercise: "An important change which the chart does not show was the actual condition of the men, their low morale and lack of vigor, their glassy eyes, their apathetic, torpid appearance, their 'don't-give-a-damn-for-anything' attitude, their uncoordinated stumbling, shuffling gait. Some were incapable of sustained purposeful action and were not fit for work. All they wanted to do was rest and drink" (p. 155). Eichna et al. [49] reported that dehydrated subjects were "reduced to apathetic, listless, plodding men straining to finish the same task" that they completed "energetically and cheerfully" when fully hydrated. Similarly,

Strydom et al [151] reported that the fluid restriction caused their subjects to become morose, aggressive, and disobedient toward their superiors.

Since 1966, there have been relatively few studies that have looked specifically at the effects of fluid ingestion *alone* on athletic performance. Rather, the evaluation of *carbohydrate* ingestion has been emphasized [30, 36, 74, 75]. These studies generally show that carbohydrate ingestion enhances performance [30, 36] and the assumption is that this is due only to a metabolic effect. However, the addition of glucose to the ingested solution increases fluid absorption [66, 67]; hence, a part of the beneficial effect of carbohydrate ingestion during exercise could theoretically be due to an influence of the added carbohydrate on fluid balance.

Four modern studies have compared the exercise performance of subjects when they either ingested or did not ingest fluid during exercise. Maughan et al. [101] found that ingestion of either water or concentrated carbohydrate solutions did not increase endurance time at 70% $\dot{V}O_{2max}$, which exhausted subjects in 70–75 minutes. Endurance was prolonged, however, in subjects who ingested a dilute carbohydrate/ electrolyte solution.

In contrast, Barr et al. [14] showed that subjects who did not ingest fluid during prolonged exercise at 55% $\dot{V}O_{2max}$ terminated exercise approximately 90 min earlier than when they ingested fluid. Levels of dehydration at exhaustion were >6%. Montain and Coyle [108] also found that, when they did not ingest fluid, subjects were less likely to complete exercise in the heat at 65% $\dot{V}O_2max$.

Two studies have assessed the effects of fluid ingestion or infusion at higher exercise intensities. Deschamps et al. [43] reported that intravenous saline infusion did not enhance performance at 84% $\dot{V}O_{2max}$, which exhausted subjects in approximately 21 min. Walsh et al. [163], however, found that subjects were able to exercise significantly longer during a subsequent exercise bout at 90% $\dot{V}O_{2max}$ when they ingested fluid during a preceding 1-hr exercise bout at 70% $\dot{V}O_{2max}$ in the heat. This effect was not because of differences in any measured physiological variable including rectal temperature, and occurred despite a difference in fluid balance of only 1.1 kg between dehydrated and fluid-repleted subjects. Ratings of perceived exertion were significantly lower when fluid was ingested.

In summary, the balance of evidence indicates that the ingestion of water enhances performances during both very prolonged exercise of low intensity and during exercise of somewhat higher intensity but shorter duration. However, this effect may be somewhat less than that achieved when the fluid contains carbohydrate either alone [166] or with electrolytes [30, 101]. Possibly the most consistent finding is that fluid ingestion markedly reduces the perception of effort during exercise of both low [5] and high-intensity exercise [163]. It is also probable that exercise performance during high-intensity exercise is impaired at levels of dehydration that do not influence performance at lower exercise intensities [5].

Physiological Effects of Progressive Dehydration During Prolonged Exercise
The physiological effects of exercise-induced dehydration have been studied by comparing the physiological responses of athletes when they replace either none, some, or all of their fluid lost during prolonged exercise. More recent studies have infused fluid intravenously during exercise to reverse any dehydration-induced fall in plasma volume. These latter studies have attempted to differentiate the physiological effects caused by reduction in plasma volume from those caused by dehydration-induced changes in serum osmolality.

PLASMA VOLUME. Plasma volume falls at the initiation of exercise. This fall is influenced by the type and intensity of exercise, and by the posture adopted [35].

Thereafter, a progressive exercise-related fall in plasma volume is reduced in proportion to the amount of fluid ingested during exercise [14, 24, 100, 107, 108]. The change is least when most fluid is ingested [108] and can be prevented if the rate of fluid ingestion equals the rate of fluid loss [73].

There is some evidence that the ingestion of sodium-containing solutions during exercise may prevent the fall in plasma volume more effectively than the ingestion of pure water [23]; as discussed subsequently, water ingestion tends to reduce serum osmolality.

SERUM OSMOLALITY AND SERUM ELECTROLYTE CONCENTRATIONS. Serum osmolality rises if no fluid is ingested during prolonged exercise [24, 100, 101]. This rise is reduced by fluid ingestion [24, 100] and is least when the rate of fluid ingestion approximates the rate of fluid loss [108].

Changes in serum sodium concentrations parallel changes in serum osmolality because the serum sodium concentration is the major determinant of the serum osmolality. Hence, serum sodium concentrations rise with exercise-induced dehydration but are maintained when fluid is ingested [117, 120]. Interestingly, serum sodium concentrations and serum osmolality fall *only* when water is ingested during exercise [14, 23, 116]. This is a fundamental observation that invites explanation. No studies have yet reported that serum sodium concentrations fall in the absence of fluid ingestion during exercise; this would be unlikely as sweat is a hypotonic solution [32].

The rise in serum osmolality and serum sodium concentration correlates with the rise in esophageal temperature [108] and may be the stimulus for the reduction in sweating that develops at the higher levels of dehydration [91]. This suggests that an important goal of fluid ingestion during exercise may be to prevent changes in serum osmolality or serum sodium concentrations, as originally proposed by David Dill [46].

SWEAT RATE DURING EXERCISE. Some studies have shown that the sweat rate falls with increasing levels of dehydration [53, 71, 91, 149] whereas others have failed to show this effect [14, 24, 65, 73, 107, 108]. An early study found that sweat rate falls only above a certain level of dehydration [91].

Hypohydration studies indicate that sweat rate over the trunk but not the head may be selectively reduced by prior dehydration [25]. There may also be considerable individual variability in the effects of dehydration on sweat rates during exercise [149]; perhaps this explains the variable results reported in the literature. Hyperhydration prior to exercise increases sweat rate during subsequent exercise [110].

RECTAL OR ESOPHAGEAL TEMPERATURES DURING EXERCISE. The exercise-related rise in rectal temperature is attenuated by fluid ingestion during exercise [5, 14, 24, 33, 53, 65, 71, 73, 107, 108]. The rise is reduced in proportion to the amount of fluid ingested and is least when the rate of fluid ingestion approximates the sweat rate [71, 108]. Hence there is a linear relationship between the rise in esophageal temperature and the level of dehydration [107, 108] as also reported in some of the original field studies [5, 169].

Fluid ingestion reduces the rectal temperature response only after a minimum of 60–80 min of exercise [14, 73, 107, 108, 149, 150]. No effect of fluid ingestion on rectal temperature was found in a study of shorter duration but higher intensity [163], possibly because exercise terminated before 80 min.

The magnitude of this effect of fluid ingestion on the rise of rectal temperature is relatively small [122] so its real physiological relevance may be questioned. Most studies indicate that levels of dehydration of up to 5% (equivalent to a weight loss of 2–4 kg) usually increase rectal temperature by less than 1°C [14, 65, 73, 107, 108, 121]. Hyperhydration before exercise also decreases rectal temperature during subsequent exercise [111].

HEART RATE AND STROKE VOLUME. Heart rate is increased [5, 24, 71, 100, 149] and stroke volume reduced in proportion to the fluid deficit that develops during exercise [108]. Cardiac output and stroke volume do not fall when the rate of fluid ingestion is sufficient to prevent dehydration [73]. But heart rate is elevated even when dehydration is prevented by adequate fluid ingestion during exercise [73]; hence, dehydration is not the sole cause of the progressive increase in heart rate during prolonged exercise. Heart rate is also reduced by hyperhydration before exercise [110].

SKIN BLOOD FLOW. Fluid ingestion maintains higher rates of forearm blood flow during exercise [107, 108] and of forearm and calf blood flow at rest during prolonged heat exposure [82]. The reduction of forearm blood flow is proportional to the level of dehydration [108]. Hence, fluid ingestion during exercise may attenuate the development of hyperthermia by maintaining skin blood flow [107].

PERCEPTION OF EFFORT. The perception of effort during exercise is increased in proportion to the fluid deficit [108]. Even partial fluid replacement has a significant effect on the perception of effort during exercise of high intensity [163]. The major psychic effects of fluid restriction during prolonged exercise of low intensity and their rapid reversal with fluid ingestion, have been described.

HORMONAL CHANGES. Plasma concentrations or activities of the fluid and electrolyte-regulating hormones, specifically, atrial natriuretic peptide (ANP), antidiuretic hormone (ADH—also arginine vasopressin—AVP), aldosterone, and renin, increase during prolonged exercise [9, 17, 64, 162]. With the exception of ANP, these concentrations may remain elevated for up to 31 hr after exercise [9]. In general, ADH activities rise in response to increasing serum osmolality [159, 162], whereas plasma renin activity may follow changes in either plasma or extracellular fluid volumes.

There is also a paradoxical increase in the plasma activity of the diuretic and natriuretic hormone ANP during prolonged exercise when plasma volume is reduced [9, 162]. The diuretic effects of ANP are probably inhibited by the increased activity of the renin-angiotensin-aldosterone axis and the increased serum ADH concentrations [9, 161].

Fluid ingestion during exercise reduces the hormonal activities and concentrations during exercise; concentrations are further reduced when subjects hyperhydrate before exercise [17]. Of these, the rise in plasma ADH activity is most affected by either hyperhydration before or fluid ingestion during exercise; this effect may be relatively independent of the nature of the fluid ingested. In contrast, the increased activity of the renin-angiotensin-aldosterone axis is reduced more by the ingestion of sodium-containing solutions compared with pure water [17]. Thrasher et al. [159] reported essentially the same findings in dehydrated dogs; water ingestion reduced plasma ADH activity, whereas ingestion of an electrolyte solution with the same composition as the extracellular fluid volume reduced plasma renin activity.

As described, water ingestion, especially during exercise, causes serum osmolality either to remain the same or to fall; this would reduce ADH secretion. Why the ingestion of sodium-containing solutions specifically reduces plasma renin activity and aldosterone concentrations is not known. Possibly, the effect is because of the maintenance of higher plasma volumes when electrolyte-containing solutions are ingested [17, 23].

FLUID INGESTION AND RENAL FUNCTION. Renal function during prolonged exercise like marathon running is unaffected by levels of dehydration less than 4% [86–88] and is enhanced during recovery in those who retain fluid during exercise [85]. The classic studies also found that renal function was not influenced by levels of dehydration less than 7% [4]. Anuria has been reported in one runner who drank inadequately and lost 11% of her body weight during an 88-km ultramarathon [88].

Renal fluid and electrolyte excretion may be influenced by the nature of the fluid ingested during exercise, but this has been infrequently studied during exercise [14] or even at rest [20]. The renal response to the ingestion, during exercise, of fluids with different electrolyte contents will be influenced by a number of factors including the relative amount of sodium and water lost in sweat, the extent of the sodium movement from the interstitial space into the intestinal lumen [66, 67] and the relative rates of sodium and fluid absorption from the ingested solution. As yet, there are no studies that have addressed these issues, either singly or collectively.

GASTRIC EMPTYING AND INTESTINAL ABSORPTION. Dehydration impairs gastric emptying [113] and could theoretically limit fluid replacement during prolonged exercise. In contrast, intestinal absorption may increase when blood volume falls [148].

But gastric emptying should not limit fluid replacement during exercise as high rates of gastric emptying can always be achieved with the appropriate drinking patterns [127]. It is more probable that fluid absorption by the small bowel could limit fluid replacement especially when only plain water is ingested at high rates during prolonged exercise (see later).

INFLUENCE OF EXERCISE-RELATED FALL IN PLASMA VOLUME ON PHYSIOLOGICAL RESPONSES DURING EXERCISE. An important question is whether changes in serum osmolality or in plasma volume regulate the physiological responses to exercise-induced dehydration. The infusion of isotonic fluids that maintain plasma volume without altering serum osmolality can differentiate between these possibilities [62].

BODY TEMPERATURE, SKIN BLOOD FLOW AND SWEAT RATE. Fortney et al. [62] showed that the infusion of an isotonic saline solution reduced both the core temperature *and* total sweat output during exercise. The authors concluded that the maintenance of plasma volume increased skin blood flow thereby increasing convective heat losses. Hence, evaporative heat losses were reduced. In contrast, increased serum osmolality raises the temperature threshold at which skin blood flow increased and delayed the onset of sweating, thereby favoring heat retention [62, 63].

Montain and Coyle [107] infused a 6% dextran solution to increase plasma volume above the level maintained by fluid ingestion during exercise. Serum sodium concentrations and serum osmolality increased when subjects did not ingest fluid during exercise but were maintained at pre-exercise concentrations by saline infusion. Unlike the findings of

Fortney et al. [63], plasma volume expansion alone did not influence either the esophageal or rectal temperature response to exercise, or forearm skin blood flow. Nor did fluid infusion prevent the rise in the rating of perceived exertion as effectively as did fluid ingestion.

Thus, maintaining or increasing plasma volume by fluid ingestion does not explain the temperature-lowering effect of fluid ingestion during exercise. Rather, fluid ingestion may influence thermoregulation by preventing the rise in serum osmolality or serum sodium concentrations [107] with maintenance of forearm blood flow [128]. These findings support Dill's [46] proposal that the goal of fluid ingestion during exercise should be the maintenance of serum osmolality and serum sodium concentrations.

Cardiovascular Drift
Compared with the findings when no fluid was ingested, cardiac output and stroke volume were higher with intravenous infusion; but this effect was less than that achieved by full fluid replacement [107].

The authors concluded that the cardiovascular drift shown by an increase in heart rate and a fall in stroke volume and cardiac output during prolonged exercise is not solely caused by the fall in plasma volume. Thus, the beneficial physiological effects of fluid ingestion during exercise cannot be due solely to the maintenance of plasma volume and central cardiovascular function.

Hamilton et al. [73] have also shown that ingesting fluid at rates that prevent dehydration maintains cardiac output and stroke volume during prolonged exercise. Other components of cardiovascular drift, in particular the rise in heart rate and in oxygen consumption, were prevented only by the addition of a glucose infusion. They have proposed that especially the rise in oxygen consumption during prolonged exercise results from a catecholamine-mediated stimulation of metabolism that is prevented by glucose infusion.

OPTIMUM RATES OF FLUID INTAKE DURING EXERCISE

The evidence so far presented suggests that the principal aim of fluid ingestion during exercise is to prevent any rise in serum osmolality or serum sodium concentrations. A secondary goal is also to prevent any change in plasma volume. Few studies have considered the interacting influences of the rates of fluid loss and fluid ingestion, and the composition of the ingested solution on changes in these variables during exercise. Rather, it has been assumed that the optimum rate of fluid ingestion is always that which equals the rate of fluid loss. It is clear, however, that most subjects do not voluntarily replace all the fluid lost during exercise [5]. Therefore, it is appropriate first to discuss the factors that influence the rates of fluid loss and fluid ingestion during exercise as this may identify those exercising conditions when the development of voluntary dehydration is more likely. The possible effects of the nature of the ingested fluid on changes in serum osmolality and plasma volume under these conditions will also be briefly considered.

Rates of Fluid Loss During Exercise

The rate of sweat loss, which is the principal determinant of fluid loss from the body during exercise, is determined mainly by the metabolic rate [32, 39, 40, 69, 70, 125, 171]. At least in running, the metabolic rate is determined by the body mass and the running speed; in nonweight-bearing activities like cycling, the velocity of movement becomes the principal determinant of the metabolic rate. Barr and Costill [13] have predicted sweat rates for subjects of different masses running at different speeds. Figure 10.1, drawn from their data, shows the interaction of body mass and running speed on sweat rate and predicts, for example, that heavier athletes running quite slowly can have sweat rates equal to those of smaller runners running much faster.

FIGURE 10.1

Predicted sweat rates of athletes of different masses running at different speeds. Drawn from the data of Barr, S.I., and D.L. Costill. Water: can the endurance athlete get too much of a good thing? J. Am. Diet. Assoc. *89:1629–1632, 1989.*

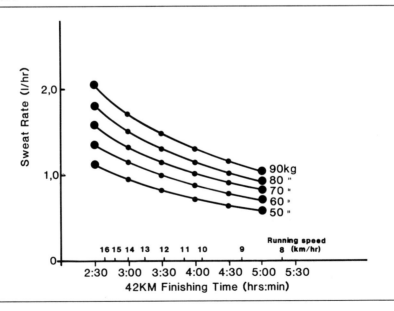

The prediction of this figure is that sweat rates will seldom be greater than 1.2 liters/hr in runners weighing less than 70 kg. Such high sweat rates are probable only in runners weighing 80 kg or more running faster than 12 km/hr. Heavier runners probably achieve these racing speeds only infrequently, at least for prolonged periods, for example, in marathon races.

The finding that sweat rates measured in runners during longer distance races are seldom greater than 1.2 liters/hr (for review, see [125]) confirms the general accuracy of these predictions. Higher sweat rates are usually recorded only when the environmental conditions are more severe (dry bulb temperature > 25°C) or when the activity is held indoors without the benefit of adequate convective cooling. For example, compared with sweat rates measured at the same metabolic rate in wind-still conditions indoors, sweat rates of cyclists are reduced by up to 38% during outdoor exercise [20].

Therefore, it seems probable that the reports of much higher sweat rates measured in the laboratory [10, 105] could possibly be explained, in part, by the absence of adequate convective cooling during exercise indoors.

Rates of Fluid Ingestion During Exercise
Table 10.1 lists the reported rates of fluid intake in both competitive and experimental studies both outdoors and in the laboratory, in runners, cyclists, and triathletes competing over a wide range of distances. Table 10.2 lists the absolute and relative exercise-induced weight changes in subjects competing in the same or similar events.

Table 10.1 shows that the rates of fluid intake during exercise vary considerably but are seldom more than about 500 ml/hr except in subjects cycling in the laboratory when forced to ingest fluid at higher rates. One conclusion might be that subjects voluntarily choose to drink about 500 ml/hr during exercise with little likelihood that rates > 1 liter/hr will be achieved except under laboratory conditions.

Because these rates of fluid ingestion are less than sweat rates, voluntary dehydration develops (Table 10.2), at least during those activities lasting less than about 6 hr. In longer events, especially those lasting many days, there is a tendency for body weight to increase during exercise.

A striking feature of Table 10.2, not previously noted, is the remarkable constancy of the weight loss (2–3 kg) experienced by athletes during prolonged exercise. This appears to be relatively independent of either the type or duration of the activity. It is as if total weight loss during exercise is a regulated variable.

Athletes develop symptoms of discomfort when they attempt to drink at rates equal to the higher sweat rates. Thus, both runners [33] and cyclists [106] develop symptoms of "fullness" when ingesting fluid at

TABLE 10.1
Reported Levels of Dehydration Developing in Athletes Competing in Running, Triathlon, and Cycling Races of Different Distances

Race Distance (km)	% Wt Loss	Kg Loss/Gain*	Reference
Running			
32	3.8	2.4	169
42	4.3	2.9	29
42	2.4	1.8	87
42	3.7	2.6	97
42	4.3	2.8	98
42	2.9	2.1	99
42	1.6–3.1	1.1–2.3	121
42	2.0	2.5	125
42	5.2	2.9	138
42	3.4 (male)†	2.5 (male)	140
	2.6 (female)	1.5 (female)	140
42	2.1	2.9	165
56	2.7	2.0	86
56	2.6–3.1	1.9–2.0	121
67	3.3 (male)†	2.4 (male)	139
	2.3 (female)	1.0 (female)	139
80	+0.3	+0.2	145
90	5.1	3.5	37
90	3.5	2.7	90
100–160	0.6	0.5	114
24-hr race (132–188 km)	3.6	2.3	61
24-hr race (121–242 km)	3.2	2.1	60
24-hr race (160–199 km)	3.6	2.7	123
960 km (5 days)	0.8	0.5	143
Triathlon			
52	4.0	2.9	105
52	1.7	1.2	134
110	3.3	2.3	158
113	2.8	2.1	134
160	4.5	3.2	160
174	3.2	2.2	61
226	4.1 (male)†	3.2 (male)	58
	2.4 (female)	1.4	58
226	3.6‡	2.8	59
226	3.7	2.8	134
Cycling race			
4800 km	+3.5	+2.8	96

*Weight gain during exercise.
†Note that weight loss is greater among males than females.
‡Most of weight loss in the triathlon occurred in the run section (1.6 kg vs. 0.7 kg in cycle section) despite the shorter duration of the run (04:34 vs. 06:08).

TABLE 10.2
Reported Rates of Fluid Intake of Athletes Competing in Running, Triathlon, and Cycling Races of Different Distances

Distance/Intensity/Duration (km) (% $\dot{V}O_2max$)* (hr:min)	Mean Rate of Fluid Intake (liters/hr)	Reference
Running		
25	0.05	140
32	0.15	169
42	0.40	29
42	0.41	97
42	0.19	98
42	0.38	99
42	0.45–0.49	121
42	0.48–0.59	121
42	0.60	125
42	0.12	138
42	0.15	140
56	0.49–0.62	121
56	0.40–0.46	121
67	0.40 (male)	139
	0.31 (female)	139
80	0.50	145
90	0.48	37
960	0.83	143
Running (Laboratory)		
70% $\dot{V}O_2max$ × 02:00	0.08–0.12	16
70% $\dot{V}O_2max$ × 04:00	0.21	41
71% $\dot{V}O_2max$ × 02:00	0.88	33
75% $\dot{V}O_2max$ × 02:00	0.60	65
76% $\dot{V}O_2max$ × 30 km	0.48	166
Triathlon		
52	0.6	105
Cycling (Competition)		
8 800 km	0.62	96
55% $\dot{V}O_2max$ × 06:00	1.2	14
60% $\dot{V}O_2max$ × 03:00	0.9	26
60% $\dot{V}O_2max$ × 03:00	1.1	144
70% $\dot{V}O_2max$ × 02:00	0.8–1.6	106
Rest		
00:40	1.5	48

*$\dot{V}O_2max$ = maximum oxygen consumption.

rates equal to or greater than 800 ml/hr. Runners were unable to sustain these high rates even for 2 hr [33] whereas cyclists reported increasing levels of discomfort when ingestion rates were greater than 800 ml/hr [106]. One-half of the cyclists ingesting 1200 ml/hr and all subjects ingesting 1600 ml/hr were "visibly uncomfortable." Interestingly, 25% of subjects developed diarrhea when ingesting 1.6 liters/hr [106] indicating that this rate of fluid ingestion exceeded the combined maximum rate of fluid absorption of both the small and large bowels.

Brouns et al. [18] showed that the rate of fluid ingestion of subjects encouraged to drink as much as possible during a simulated triathlon, was two to three times higher in the cycling leg (600–800 ml/hr) than in the running leg (100–300 ml/hr). This suggests that running reduces the desire to drink more than does cycling [19].

Hence, peak rates of fluid ingestion under ideal conditions are seldom greater than 800 ml/hr. Feelings of abdominal fullness seem to prevent higher rates of ingestion, especially during running.

Whereas this upper limit of voluntary fluid ingestion during exercise may be set by progressive gastric distension due to impaired gastric emptying [106], another possibility is that fluid ingested at such high rates may also accumulate at other sites, including the colon. The assumption that the small bowel has an unlimited capacity for both fluid and energy assimilation is currently under review [45]. Indeed, Buddington and Diamond [21] have suggested: ". . . the intestine never possesses an enormous excess absorptive capacity. Instead, just enough intestine and transporters are synthesized to absorb the expected nutrient loads so that biosynthetic energy is not wasted on unneeded tissue and molecules but ingested nutrients are not wasted either. The intestine exemplifies the motto, 'enough but not too much.' "

Their suggestion is that the maximum absorptive capacity of the small bowel at least for glucose is approximately twice the usual carbohydrate intake. If this holds also for fluid absorption, and if the usual fluid intake in humans is 180–200 ml/hr [56], then the maximum rates of small bowel fluid absorption might be approximately only 360–400 ml/hr. Interestingly, this value approximates the voluntary rates of fluid ingestion of most subjects during exercise (Table 10.2), but is well below both their average sweat rates [121] and the maximum rates of fluid ingestion of some athletes who develop fluid retention during prolonged exercise [85].

At present, the maximum rates of small bowel fluid and glucose absorption either at rest or during exercise are not known. There is sufficient information however, to suggest that these rates may be sufficiently low to limit optimum fluid and carbohydrate replacement during exercise.

Thus, a number of studies [74, 75, 109, 139, 141] have shown that less than about 40% of the carbohydrate ingested during exercise is oxidized by the muscles, possibly because intestinal glucose absorption is limiting. Peak rates of exogenous glucose oxidation by muscle are approximately 1 g/min regardless of the type of carbohydrate ingested [75]. This rate is equal to that given historically as the maximum rate of glucose absorption from the small bowel [1, 72]. As glucose absorption stimulates water absorption [65, 66], such low rates of glucose absorption might indicate that water absorption also occurs relatively slowly. Indeed,

Gisolfi et al. [66] have also calculated that only 37% of fluid infused into the duodenum and jejunum at rates of 900 ml/hr was absorbed; others have reported that the maximum rate of water absorption from an isotonic solution with a sodium concentration of 110 mmol/liter was only 800 ml/hr [42].

Similarly, studies in which fluid replacement either during [14] or after exercise [34] equalled fluid losses found that not all the ingested fluid could be accounted for by its appearance in the extracellular or intracellular fluid pools, suggesting that not all was rapidly absorbed [116]. Indeed, Costill and Sparks [34] suggested that: "a large fraction of the ingested water remained in the gastrointestinal tract or was shifted to the extravascular compartment."

In summary, the maximum rates of fluid absorption by the small bowel during exercise are not known but could be less than either the highest rates of fluid loss incurred by some athletes during more intensive exercise, or the highest rates of fluid ingestion of some less competitive runners especially during prolonged exercise [85]. Any unabsorbed fluid would accumulate in the large bowel where its presence might: (*a*) explain the symptoms of fullness experienced by some athletes ingesting large fluid volumes during prolonged exercise, and (*b*) lead to a potential "third space" effect that could be a factor in the etiology of the hyponatremia of exercise (see later).

Clearly, unless the maximum rates of fluid absorption by the small bowel are known, it is difficult to prescribe how much fluid should be ingested during exercise [116]. But, if intestinal absorptive capacity is regulated by demand and can increase when demand increases chronically [45], it follows that the chronic ingestion of large volumes of fluid either during or after exercise might increase intestinal absorptive capacity.

Influence of Changes in Serum Osmolality, Plasma Volume, and Other Factors on Drinking Behavior in Humans

In contrast to dogs [4, 159], the donkey (burro) [46], the monkey [11], and the Bedouin goat [27], only humans develop voluntary dehydration when given free access to fluid either during or after exercise in the heat; other mammals immediately replace all their fluid losses as soon as water is provided. The volume ingested by the dog appears to be regulated by receptors in the oropharynx [6, 159]. Drinking rapidly inhibits ADH release, probably in response to an oropharyngeal reflex [11].

Dill [46] proposed that humans develop voluntary dehydration during exercise because only they lose sodium chloride in sweat. As a result, serum osmolality rises less during exercise-induced dehydration in humans. But, as all mammals seemed to drink sufficiently to maintain a constant serum osmolality, Dill [46] postulated that the fluid intake of humans would always be inadequate to replace their sweat losses.

Nose et al. [130] have shown that the drinking behavior of dehydrated humans is regulated by changes in both serum osmolality and plasma volume. Hence, dipsogenic drive in dehydrated humans ceases when either osmolality *or* plasma volume is corrected by the ingestion of either plain water or a sodium-containing solution, respectively. Thus, the ingestion of plain water prematurely inhibits drinking by causing serum osmolality to return to isotonicity before either fluid or sodium losses are replaced; sodium chloride ingestion also terminates drinking prematurely by restoring plasma volume prematurely. But changes in osmolality and plasma volume during exercise-induced dehydration in humans are not independent of each other; the rising serum osmolality with dehydration acts to maintain plasma volume and to reduce the volume-dependent drive for fluid replacement [130]. The result is that whether or not they ingest plain water or sodium chloride solutions, dehydrated humans stop drinking before they are fully rehydrated.

In addition, water ingestion increases free water loss [130] whereas selective restoration of plasma volume with sodium-containing solutions inhibits secretion of sodium-retaining hormones [131], increasing osmotic diuresis.

Perhaps it is these complex interactions that also explain why humans are unable to prevent the development of voluntary dehydration during exercise. Others suggest that it is the rapid alleviation of the symptoms that initiate drinking including, among others, dryness of the mouth, which causes the premature cessation of drinking before full rehydration has occurred [84, 146]. Indeed, subjects can be classified as either "reluctant" or "avid" drinkers [153, 154] on the basis of the volume of fluid they ingest during exercise. Fluid ingestion during exercise is enhanced by drinking cold, sweet fluids [56, 84, 146]. Simultaneous food consumption also increases fluid consumption [5, 84].

There is a need to establish factors that will enhance fluid ingestion during exercise, thereby limiting the extent to which voluntary dehydration develops.

Role of Sodium Chloride Ingestion

The predictions of Adolph and Dill [7] that the fluid deficit that develops during exercise is corrected only when the sodium chloride deficit has been corrected so that "water cannot be held until the missing osmoles are made good" [92] has been confirmed by the detailed studies of Nose and colleagues [112, 129–131, 133]. The essential conclusion from these studies is that the sodium content of the extracellular space must regulate the extracellular fluid volume [112, 129]. As a result, the extracellular fluid volume must contract whenever a sodium deficiency develops. This explains why serum sodium concentrations remain constant (or increase slightly) during prolonged exercise when both sodium and water are lost, even if plain water in limited amounts is replaced [120].

There are two exceptions to this general rule that the extracellular fluid volume is regulated by its sodium chloride content so that serum sodium concentration will remain within a narrow range regardless of the degree of fluid or sodium deficit. The first is the condition of true sodium chloride deficiency [102–104]; the other is the hyponatremia of exercise [120]. These are discussed in subsequent sections. In both conditions, the volume of the extracellular space is increased out of proportion to its sodium chloride content.

Nose et al. [129] also found that, at any level of dehydration, the less sodium chloride lost in sweat, the greater the loss of fluid from the intracellular compartment. Thus, a reduction of sweat sodium losses with protection of the circulating volume is an important benefit of heat acclimatization and training.

It follows that an important benefit of ingesting sodium chloride during or after exercise might be better maintenance and more rapid restoration of the extracellular volume and possibly also the plasma volume [17, 23, 34, 116] although this is not always found [100, 137]. This effect would be enhanced by the addition of carbohydrate, which further increases the rate of fluid absorption from the solution ingested during exercise [67].

Figure 10.2 shows the rates of water, sodium, and carbohydrate absorption from different solutions ingested at rest. It shows that optimum fluid absorption occurs from isotonic carbohydrate/electrolyte solutions, whereas rates of absorption from water and electrolyte-containing solutions are not greatly different. Sodium absorption, however, is enhanced from electrolyte-containing solutions. This latter finding would explain why sodium-containing solutions are more likely to maintain plasma volume whereas the ingestion of water is more likely to influence plasma osmolality.

On the other hand, carbohydrate absorption is most rapid from concentrated (10%) carbohydrate solutions. But these solutions induce net water movement into the small bowel and could, therefore, be a factor contributing to the hyponatremia of exercise (see later).

APPLIED MEDICAL ASPECTS

"Salt-Deficiency" vs. "Water-Deficiency" Heat Exhaustion

An original classification of the heat illnesses distinguishes "salt-deficiency heat exhaustion" from "water-deficiency heat exhaustion" [28]. This distinction has persisted in the literature [83, 94]. Salt-deficiency heat exhaustion is considered to develop when fluid replace-

FIGURE 10.2

Rates of water, sodium, and carbohydrate absorption (secretion) from different solutions infused into the small bowel. Note that sodium and water absorption are greatest from the isotonic solution with modest sodium (25 mmol/liter) and carbohydrate (6%) content whereas carbohydrate absorption is greatest from the high (10%) carbohydrate solution; this solution causes net water secretion into the small bowel. Redrawn from data of Gisolfi, C.V., K.J. Spranger, R.W. Summers, H.P. Schedl, and T.L. Bleiler. Effects of cycle exercise on intestinal absorption in humans. J. Appl. Physiol. 71:2518–2527, 1991; and Gisolfi, C.V., R.W. Summers, H.P. Schedl, T.L. Bleiler, and R.A. Oppliger. Human intestinal water absorption: direct vs. indirect measurements. Am. J. Physiol. 258:G216–G222, 1990.

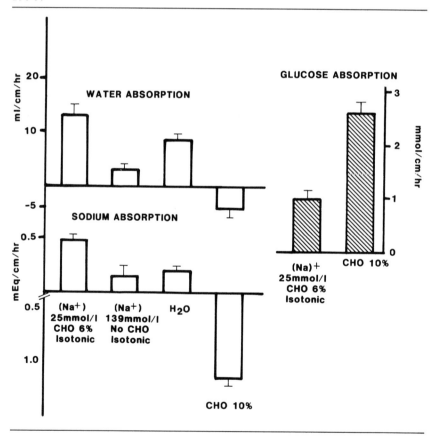

ment is adequate but replacement of salt is inadequate; water-deficiency heat exhaustion is believed to result from the converse. But if body sodium content regulates the extracellular fluid volume [112, 129–131], it is difficult to understand how there could be these distinct conditions. Nor do the accepted descriptions of the two conditions provide robust guidelines for their differentiation on either clinical or biochemical ground [83, 94].

The original distinction was made on the basis of an experimental model developed to induce salt deficiency in animals. In this model [38, 54, 81, 111], true sodium chloride deficiency was induced by injecting a 5% glucose solution into the peritoneal cavity of experimental animals; the solution that was withdrawn 4–5 hr later had a high sodium chloride content but a low protein content. The characteristics of this salt-deficiency syndrome were the following: hypotonic hyponatremia; a large fluid shift from the extracellular to the intracellular fluid compartments causing intracellular overhydration; and extracellular dehydration with a disproportionate reduction in plasma volume. The fall in plasma volume was greater than that developing in pure water loss and was associated with a large reduction in the total circulating protein content. Circulatory changes were more severe in salt-deficiency than in water-deficiency dehydration; animals with salt depletion were incapacitated whereas animals with pure water deficiency remained "vigorous and healthy" with no evidence of peripheral vascular collapse.

Elkinton et al. [54] concluded that the greater loss of circulating plasma protein content probably explained the larger fall in plasma volume and the more severe circulatory collapse with salt depletion than with water depletion. They concluded that "whenever there is any salt loss to the external environment or temporary segregation of salt *by pooling in the gut* (author's emphasis), peritoneum, or in the traumatized region, shock will be produced with greater ease than would otherwise be the case." It is understandable why these original researchers considered that subjects with more severe heat injury must be suffering from salt-deficiency heat exhaustion whereas those with less severe circulatory abnormalities had water deficiency alone.

It is extremely difficult, however, perhaps impossible, for healthy humans to develop salt deficiency regardless of the environment in which they live and the amount of exercise they perform [47, 56, 170]. Indeed, their inability to discover a single case of salt deficiency either in the literature or in their personal experience of 20 yr work in environmental physiology led Epstein and Sohar [56] to suggest that the mythical condition of "salt deficiency heat exhaustion" is another example of "christening by conjecture." "Such a syndrome" they conclude "has never been proven to exist."

Rather, sodium chloride deficiency has only ever been induced in healthy humans by combining a salt-free diet with daily exercise or sauna

FIGURE 10.3

Changes in body weight and body sodium content of subjects eating a sodium-free diet for 11 days (days 1–11) and during 5 days (days 11–16) of sodium repletion. Note that the rate of sodium loss is greater than the rate of weight loss between days 2 and 11. Hyponatremia developed during this period. Redrawn from McCance, R.A. The changes in plasma and cells during experimentally human salt deficiency. Biochemistry 31:1278–1284, 1937.

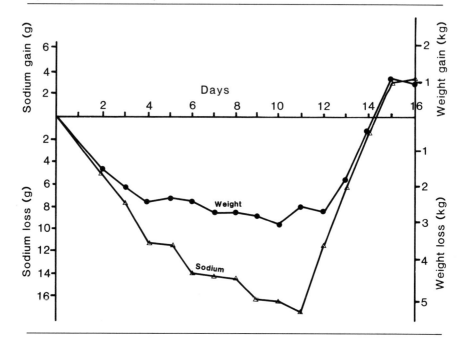

exposure to increase sodium chloride losses [102–104]. A cardinal feature of the syndrome was severe physical incapacitation that prevented any desire or attempt to exercise.

Figure 10.3 from McCance [102] depicts mean water and sodium balance in subjects from one of their studies. It shows that for the first 2 and the last 4 days of the experiment, water balance follows sodium balance, but from days 3–12, relative water conservation occurred despite a continuing sodium deficit. Hyponatremia developed during this period and became progressively more severe despite a contraction of the extracellular fluid volume by up to 38% [104].

These findings can be explained if the initial response to human salt deficiency is a contraction of the extracellular fluid volume with maintenance of a normal or elevated serum sodium concentration (days 0–2 on Fig. 10.2); thereafter there is relative conservation of the extracellular fluid volume despite increasing sodium deficit. During this period, hyponatremia develops. McCance [102] concluded: ". . . the human body comprised between (*a*) maintenance of its total osmotic pressure at the expense of anhydraemia, a reduction of blood volume, rise of haemoglobin, proteins and colloidal osmotic pressure in the serum, and (*b*) maintenance of its plasma and extracellular fluid volumes at the expense of a reduction in the concentrations of sodium and chloride in the serum, with a fall in its total osmotic pressure." The important point is that because the extracellular sodium content determines the extracellular fluid volume in health [112, 129, 130], any fall in serum sodium concentration can occur *only* if this interdependent relationship is lost so that the normal regulation of the extracellular fluid volume is disturbed.

The particular relevance of these studies is that they add important insights into the condition of the hyponatremia of exercise. This condition, which is reviewed in detail elsewhere [120], occurs typically in persons involved in very prolonged exercise during which they ingest large volumes of fluid, frequently containing 5–10% carbohydrate. Although it has been argued that large sodium chloride losses in sweat contribute to the pathogenesis of this condition [76–79], studies of runners with this condition have established that abnormal fluid retention, and not sodium deficiency, is the sine qua non for the development of the serious symptomatic form of this condition [85].

One proposal is that a third space effect similar to that produced in the experimental model of salt deficiency, may be operative. A large (± 2 liters) volume of unabsorbed fluid in the gut could, particularly if it has a high carbohydrate content, induce a sufficiently large sodium movement from the extracellular space into the unabsorbed fluid [66, 67, 139] to produce the changes found in experimental sodium chloride deficiency with hypotonic hyponatremia, intracellular overhydration, and a fall in plasma volume and in circulating protein content [120]. It is possible that sustained high rates of fluid intake (> 1 liter/hr), achieved uniquely only by some athletes during prolonged exercise [85] could exceed the fluid-absorbing capacity of the small bowel leading to this third space effect in the large bowel.

In summary, the hyponatremia of exercise appears to be due to the combination of at least three abnormalities: abnormal fluid retention, possibly on the basis of inappropriate ADH secretion; disturbed regulation of the extracellular fluid volume so that the normal relationship between its volume and sodium chloride content is lost, and possibly a third space effect with movement of sodium into unabsorbed fluid in the large bowel.

The sequence in which these abnormalities develops is not known. But the similarities between the hyponatremia of exercise and the experimental model of salt deficiency cannot be ignored [120]. This suggests that a third space effect may be crucial for the development of this condition.

Exercise-associated Collapse

After it had been found that rectal temperature rose as an apparently linear function of dehydration in marathon runners [169], it took only a small leap of faith to conclude that athletes who collapse after prolonged exercise must be suffering from a heat disorder caused by dehydration. As a result, it became fashionable to treat all athletes who collapsed during or after prolonged exercise with intravenous fluids [3, 51, 76–79, 93, 95, 132, 167].

But recent studies have shown that runners with this condition of exercise-associated collapse (EAC) [142] are not more likely to be hyperthermic than are control runners who do not collapse; indeed, a significant proportion may be hypothermic (Holtzhausen L.M., and Noakes, T.D. Unpublished observations). Nor is there any evidence that subjects with EAC are more dehydrated than are noncollapsed controls [118, 122]. In addition, intravenous fluid therapy retards rather than expedites the recovery of these subjects [55]; this form of therapy may also induce iatrogenic hyponatremia and hyperglycemia [122] and can be life-threatening in those with symptomatic hyponatremia due to fluid overload [85, 126].

On the basis of the evidence that: (*a*) the majority (> 85%) of subjects with EAC collapse after the cessation of exercise (Holtzhausen, L.M., and Noakes, T.D. Unpublished observations), and (*b*) that postural hypotension, often severe, is present in virtually all runners who complete ultramarathon races [80], we have proposed that postural hypotension probably caused by fluid displacement to the compliant veins of the lower limb, is the most likely cause of EAC [80, 118, 119]. This is not a novel proposal. For nearly 70 years it has been known that postural hypotension occurs frequently during exercise in the heat and is the principal abnormality in the condition incorrectly termed "heat exhaustion" [8, 49, 50, 155].

As the degree of postexercise postural hypotension is unrelated to the level of dehydration developed during exercise [80], it follows that intravenous fluid therapy is not the most rational form of therapy for EAC. Rather, therapy should aim to expedite return of blood from the peripheral pools in the lower limbs [19, 118]. This can be achieved by elevating the pelvis and legs; a form of therapy that has proven effective [68]. Failure to respond to this form of therapy may indicate the presence of dehydration.

Two additional points require emphasis. First, the most severe levels of exercise-induced dehydration yet reported [5] did not cause sudden collapse with circulatory failure, at least in the recumbent position. Rather, severely dehydrated subjects chose to lie down, possibly because they developed postural hypotension on standing. Hence, the development of postural hypotension could perhaps be the safety mechanism that prevents dehydrated subjects from continuing to exercise to levels of dehydration that would induce irreversible circulatory failure.

Second, Adolph [5] observed that blood biochemical markers were poor indicators of the level of dehydration, as also recently confirmed by us [80]. Adolph therefore proposed that the level of dehydration should be determined by conventional clinical parameters. In particular, intense thirst, a change in the timber of the voice, a dry mouth, and an inability to produce sputum indicated more severe dehydration.

In our experience, these are extremely uncommon findings in subjects whether or not they collapse after prolonged exercise. This observation is compatible with the finding that more severe levels of dehydration occur uncommonly in endurance athletes (Table 10.1).

SUMMARY

Current evidence indicates that adequate fluid ingestion during exercise enhances athletic performance, prevents a fall in plasma volume, stroke volume, cardiac output and skin blood flow, maintains serum sodium concentrations and serum osmolality, lowers rectal temperature and the perception of effort, and prevents a progressive rise in heart rate. Rates of sweating and urine flow are not influenced by fluid ingestion. The evidence suggests that the maintenance of serum osmolality and serum sodium concentrations at pre-exercise levels is the important determinant of these beneficial effects of fluid ingestion on cardiovascular function and thermoregulation. The provision of glucose in the ingested solution may be necessary to optimize performance; glucose ingestion that enhances fluid and sodium absorption in the small bowel may also prevent a progressive rise in oxygen consumption during exercise. Sweetened carbohydrate-containing drinks may also increase fluid intake during exercise, thereby minimizing voluntary dehydration.

Hence, the optimum solution for ingestion during exercise should provide carbohydrate, probably at rates of about 1 g/min and electrolytes in concentrations that, when drunk at the optimum rate, maintain serum osmolality and plasma volume at pre-exercise levels by replacing exactly the water and electrolyte losses from the extracellular space. At present, the composition of the fluid that will optimize electrolyte and fluid replacement of the extracellular space is not established. Neither are the optimum rates of fluid ingestion during exercise known. At low sweat rates (< 1 liter/hr), it is probable that all of the lost fluid can and should be replaced; rates of fluid ingestion needed to offset higher sweat rates may exceed the maximum intestinal absorptive capacity for water. Furthermore, high rates of fluid intake (> 1 liter/hr) are achieved with difficulty during exercise, especially when running, and are likely to lead to feelings of abdominal discomfort, possibly due to the accumulation of unabsorbed fluid in the small bowel or colon. Practicing to drink regularly during training might reduce the severity and frequency of these symptoms, possibly by increasing intestinal absorptive capacity.

Most athletes are "reluctant" drinkers during exercise and do not ingest fluid at rates equal to their rates of fluid loss; hence, they develop progressive (voluntary) dehydration during prolonged exercise. Surprisingly, the level of voluntary dehydration that develops during exercise is relatively independent of the duration or intensity of the activity. The factors that explain these phenomena remain elusive. Fluid consumption during exercise is enhanced by the ingestion of cold, sweet fluids. Simultaneous food consumption also stimulates fluid ingestion.

Despite the modest sodium losses in sweat, the serum sodium concentration remains relatively unchanged during exercise. This results from a regulated contraction of the extracellular volume, which develops in proportion to the sodium deficit. As its sodium content regulates the volume of the extracellular space, correction of any fluid loss incurred during exercise requires that electrolyte losses, especially sodium, also be corrected.

Failure of adequate contraction of the extracellular volume in response to sweat sodium losses is characteristic of the hyponatremia of exercise in which there is also abnormal fluid retention in subjects who sustain very high rates of fluid intake (> 1.3 liters/hr) for prolonged periods (> 6 hr). These subjects exhibit the extreme of "avid" drinking behavior during exercise.

It is frequently assumed that severe dehydration is the critical factor explaining the development of both exercise-induced heatstroke and the apparently related condition of EAC. Yet there is no evidence that dehydration plays an essential role in either condition. EAC, in particular, is not a heat disorder and appears to be caused by the rapid onset of postural hypotension with the cessation of exercise. Elevation of the lower limbs, rather than intravenous fluid therapy, is the initial treatment of choice.

Future research needs to establish (*a*) techniques that will increase the fluid intakes of "reluctant" drinkers during exercise so that the extent of the voluntary dehydration can be reduced or prevented; and (*b*) the nature of the ingested solution that will optimize maintenance of serum osmolality and plasma volume during exercise under different exercise conditions and in different individuals whose sweat sodium and water losses, and rates of intestinal absorption of electrolytes and water may differ substantially as a result of individual variability and levels of training. Indeed, the complex interrelationship between all of these diverse variables remains to be clarified.

ACKNOWLEDGMENTS

This work was supported by the Medical Research Council of South Africa, the Harry Crossley and Nellie Atkinson Staff Research Funds of the University of Cape Town, G.W. Leppin (Pty) Ltd, Wander A.G., Ltd., Bern, Switzerland and the South African Sugar Association. Ed Coyle, Ph.D. provided the author with unpublished manuscripts and other material in the preparation of this review.

REFERENCES

1. Abbott, W.O., W.G. Karr, P.M. Glenn, and R. Warren. Intubation studies of the human small intestine. XIV. The absorption of glucose from the duodenum. *Am. J. Med. Sci.* 200:532–536, 1940.
2. Abrahams, A. *The Disabilities and Injuries of Sport.* London: Elek Books Ltd, 1961.
3. Adner, M.M., J.J. Scarlet, J. Casey, W. Robison, and B.H. Jones. The Boston Marathon Medical Care Team: ten years of experience. *Phys. Sportsmed.* 16:99–106, 1988.
4. Adolph, E.F. Measurement of water drinking in dogs. *Am. J. Physiol.* 125:75–86, 1939.
5. Adolph, E.F. *Physiology of Man in the Desert.* New York: Interscience Publishers, 1947.
6. Adolph E.F. Thirst and its inhibition in the stomach. *Am. J. Physiol.* 161:374–384, 1950.
7. Adolph, E.F., and D.B. Dill. Observations on water metabolism in the desert. *Am. J. Physiol.* 123:369–378, 1938.
8. Adolph, E.F., and W.B. Fulton. The effects of exposure to high temperatures upon the circulation in man. *Am. J. Physiol.* 67:573–588, 1924.
9. Altenkirch, H.U., R. Gerzer, K.A. Kirsch, J. Weil, B. Heyduck, I. Schultes, and L. Rocker. Effect of prolonged physical exercise on fluid regulating hormones. *Eur. J. Appl. Physiol.* 61:209–213, 1990.
10. Armstrong, L.E., R.W. Hubbard, B.H. Jones, and J.T. Daniels. Preparing Alberto Salazar for the heat of the 1984 Olympic Games. *Phys. Sports Med.* 14:73–81, 1986.
11. Arnauld, E., and J. du Pont. Vasopressin release and firing of supraoptic neurosecretory neurones during drinking in the dehydrated monkey. *Pflugers Arch.* 394:195–201, 1982.
12. Bainbridge, F.A. (eds). A.V. Bock, and D.B. Dill, *The Physiology of Muscular Exercise,* 3rd edition. London: Longman, Green and Co., 1931.
13. Barr, S.I., and D.L. Costill. Water: can the endurance athlete get too much of a good thing? *J. Am. Diet. Assoc.* 89:1629–1632, 1989.
14. Barr, S.I., D.L. Costill, and W.J. Fink. Fluid replacement during prolonged exercise: effects of water, saline, or no fluid. *Med. Sci. Sports Exerc.* 23:811–817, 1991.
15. Bean, W.B., and L.W. Eichna. Performance in relation to environmental temperature. Reactions of normal young men to simulated desert environment. *Fed. Proc.* 2:144–158, 1943.
16. Bebb, J., J. Brewer, A. Patton, and C. Williams. Endurance running and the influence of diet on fluid intake. *J. Sports Sci.* 2:198–199, 1984.
17. Brandenberger, G., V. Candas, M. Follenius, and K.M. Kahn. The influence of the initial state of hydration on endocrine responses to exercise in the heat. *Eur. J. Appl. Physiol.* 58:674–679, 1989.
18. Brouns, F., E. Beckers, B. Knopfli, B. Villiger, and W. Saris. Rehydration during exercise: effect of electrolyte supplementation on selective blood parameters. *Med. Sci. Sports Exerc.* 23:S84, 1991.
19. Brouns, F., W.H.M. Saris, and N.J. Rehrer. Abdominal complaints and gastrointestinal function during long-lasting exercise. *Int. J. Sports Med.* 8:175–189, 1987.

20. Brown, S.L., and E.W. Banister. Thermoregulation during prolonged actual and laboratory-simulated bicycling. *Eur. J. Appl. Physiol.* 54:125–130, 1985.
21. Buddington, R.K., and J.M. Diamond. Ontogenetic development of intestinal nutrient transporters. *Annu. Rev. Physiol.* 51:601–619, 1989.
22. Caldwell, J.E., E.S.A. Ahonen, and U. Nousiainen. Differential effects of sauna-, diuretic-, and exercise-induced hypohydration. *J. Appl. Physiol.* 57:1018–1023, 1984.
23. Candas, V., J.P. Liebert, G. Brandenberger, J.C. Sagot, C. Amoros, and J.M. Kahn. Hydration during exercise. Effects on thermal and cardiovascular adjustments. *Eur. J. Appl. Physiol.* 55:113–122, 1986.
24. Candas, V., J-P. Libert, G. Brandenberger, J-C. Sagot, and J-M Kahn. Thermal and circulatory responses during prolonged exercise at different levels of hydration. *J. Physiol. (Paris)* 83:11–18, 1988.
25. Caputa, M., and M. Cabanac. Precedence of head homoeothermia over trunk homoeothermia in dehydrated men. *Eur. J. Appl. Physiol.* 57:611–615, 1988.
26. Carter, J.E., and C.V. Gisolfi. Fluid replacement during and after exercise in the heat. *Med. Sci. Sports Exerc.* 21:532–539, 1989.
27. Choshniak, I., C. Wittenberg, and D. Saham. Rehydrating Bedouin goats with saline: rumen and kidney function. *Physiol. Zool.* 60:373–378, 1987.
28. Climatic Physiological Committee. A classification of heat illness. *Br. Med. J.* 1:1533–1535, 1958.
29. Cohen, I., and A.L. Zimmerman. Changes in serum electrolyte levels during marathon running. *South Afr. Med. J.* 53:449–453, 1978.
30. Coggan, A.R., and E.F. Coyle. Carbohydrate ingestion during prolonged exercise: Effects on metabolism and performance. *Exerc. Sports Sci. Rev.* 19:1–40, 1991.
31. Costill, D.L. *A Scientific Approach to Distance Running.* Los Altos: Tafnews, 1979.
32. Costill, D.L. Sweating: its composition and effects on body fluids. *Ann. N.Y. Acad. Sci.* 301:160–174, 1977.
33. Costill, D.L., W.F. Kammer, and A. Fisher. Fluid ingestion during distance running. *Arch. Environ. Health* 21:520–525, 1970.
34. Costill, D.L., and K.E. Sparks. Rapid fluid replacement following thermal dehydration. *J. Appl. Physiol.* 34:299–303, 1973.
35. Coyle, E.F., and M. Hamilton. Fluid replacement during exercise: effects on physiological homeostasis and performance. In C.V. Gisolfi, and D.R. Lamb. (eds). *Perspectives in Exercise Science and Sports Medicine.* Vol. 3. *Fluid Homeostasis During Exercise.* Indianapolis: Benchmark Press, 1990; pp. 281–303.
36. Coyle, E.F., and S.J. Montain. Benefits of fluid replacement unit carbohydrate during exercise. *Med. Sci. Sports Exerc.* 24:S324–S330, 1992.
37. Dancaster, C.P., and S.J. Whereat. Fluid and electrolyte balance during the Comrades Marathon. *South Afr. Med. J.* 45:147–150, 1971.
38. Danowski, T.S., A.W. Winkler, and J.R. Elkinton. The treatment of shock due to salt depletion; comparison of the hemodynamic effects of isotonic saline, of hypertonic saline, and of isotonic glucose solutions. *J. Clin. Invest.* 25:130–138, 1946.
39. Davies, C.T.M. Influence of skin temperature on sweating and aerobic performance during severe work. *J. Appl. Physiol.* 47:770–777, 1979.
40. Davies, C.T.M., J.R. Brotherhood, and E. Zeidifard. Temperature regulation during severe exercise with some observations on effects of skin wetting. *J. Appl. Physiol.* 41:772–776, 1976.
41. Davies, C.T.M., and M.W. Thompson. Physiological responses to prolonged exercise in ultramarathon athletes. *J. Appl. Physiol.* 61:611–617, 1986.
42. Davis, G.R., C.A. Santa Ana, S.G. Morawski, and J.S. Fordtran. Development of a large solution associated with minimal water and electrolyte absorption or secretion. *Gastroenterology* 78:991–995, 1980.
43. Deschamps, A., R.D. Levy, M.G. Cosio, E.B. Marliss, and S. Magder. Effect of saline

infusion on body temperature and endurance during heavy exercise. *J. Appl. Physiol.* 66:2799–2804, 1989.

44. De Vries, H.A. *Physiology of Exercise.* London: Staples Press, 1967.
45. Diamond, J. Evolutionary design of intestinal nutrient absorption: enough but not too much. *NIPS* 6:92–96, 1991.
46. Dill, D.B. Physiological effects of hot climates and great heights. *Life, Heat, and Altitude.* Cambridge: Harvard University Press, 1938.
47. Dill, D.B., B.F. Jones, H.T. Edwards, and S.A. Oberg. Salt economy in extreme dry heat. *J. Biol. Chem.* 100:755–767, 1933.
48. Duchman, S.M., T.L. Bleiler, H.P. Schedl, R.W. Summers, and C.V. Gisolfi. Effects of gastric function on intestinal composition of oral rehydration solutions. *Med. Sci. Sports Exerc.* 22(Suppl):S89, 1990.
49. Eichna, L.W., W.B. Bean, W.F. Ashe, and N. Nelson. Performance in relation to environmental temperature. Reactions of normal young men to hot, humid (simulated jungle) environment. *Bull Johns Hopkins Hosp.* 76:25–58, 1945.
50. Eichna, L.W., S.M. Horvath, and W.B. Bean. Postexertional orthostatic hypotension. *Am. J. Med. Sci.* 213:641–654, 1947.
51. Eichner, E.R. Sacred cows and straw men. *Phys. Sportsmed.* 19:24, 1991.
52. Eggleton, M.G. *Muscular Exercise.* London: Kegan Paul, Trench, Truber, and Co., Ltd., 1936.
53. Ekblom, B., C.J. Greenleaf, J.E. Greenleaf, and L. Hermansen. Temperature regulation during exercise dehydration in man. *Acta. Physiol. Scand.* 79:475–483, 1970.
54. Elkinton, J.R., T.S. Danowski, and A.W. Winkler. Hemodynamic changes in salt depletion and in dehydration. *J. Clin. Invest.* 25:120–129, 1946.
55. Ellis, D., V. Verdile, M. Heller, D. Yealy, D. Deerwater, J. Irrgang, and P. Mazur-Ellis. The effectiveness of the addition of intravenous hydration to oral hydration in post-marathon patients. *Med. Sci. Sports Exerc.* 22(Suppl):S101, 1990.
56. Epstein, Y., and E. Sohar. Fluid balance in hot climates: sweating, water intake, and prevention of dehydration. *Publ. Health Rev.* 13:115–137, 1985.
57. Falls, H.B. *Exercise Physiology.* New York: Academic Press, 1968.
58. Farber, H., J. Arbetter, E. Schaefer, S. Hill, G. Dallal, R. Grimaldi, and N. Hill. Acute metabolic effects of an endurance triathlon. *Ann. Sports Med.* 3:131–138, 1987.
59. Farber, H.W., E.J. Schaefer, R. Franey, R. Grimaldi, and N.S. Hill. The endurance triathlon: metabolic changes after each event and during recovery. *Med. Sci. Sports Exerc.* 23:959–965, 1991.
60. Fellmann, N., M. Bedu, J. Giry, M. Pharmakis-Amadieu, M-J. Bezou, J-P. Barlet, and J. Coudert. Hormonal, fluid, and electrolyte changes during 72-h recovery from a 24-h endurance run. *Int. J. Sports Med.* 10:406–412, 1989.
61. Fellmann, N., M. Sagnol, M. Bedu, G. Falgairette, E. van Praagh, G. Gaillard, P. Jouanel, and J. Coudert. Enzymatic and hormonal responses following a 24 h endurance run and a 10 h triathlon race. *Eur. J. Appl. Physiol.* 57:545–553, 1988.
62. Fortney, S.M., N.B. Vroman, W.S. Beckett, S. Permutt, and N.D. LaFrance. Effect of exercise hemoconcentration and hyperosmolality on exercise responses. *J. Appl. Physiol.* 65:519–524, 1988.
63. Fortney, S.M., C.B. Wenger, J.R. Bove, and E.R. Nadel. Effect of hyperosmolality on control of blood flow and sweating. *J. Appl. Physiol.* 57:1688–1695, 1984.
64. Freund, B.J., J.R. Claybaugh, G.M. Hashiro, M. Buono, and S. Chrisney. Exaggerated ANF response to exercise in middle-aged vs. young runners. *J. Appl. Physiol.* 69:1607–1614, 1990.
65. Gisolfi, C.V., and J.R. Copping. Thermal effects of prolonged treadmill exercise in the heat. *Med. Sci. Sports* 6:108–113, 1974.
66. Gisolfi, C.V., K.J. Spranger, R.W. Summers, H.P. Schedl, and T.L. Bleiler. Effects of cycle exercise on intestinal absorption in humans. *J. Appl. Physiol.* 71:2518–2527, 1991.

67. Gisolfi, C.V., R.W. Summers, H.P. Schedl, T.L. Bleiler, and R.A. Oppliger. Human intestinal water absorption: direct vs. indirect measurements. *Am. J. Physiol.* 258:G216–G222, 1990.
68. Gough, K.J. Why marathon runners collapse. (Letter). *South Afr. Med. J.* 80:461, 1991.
69. Greenhaff, P.L. Cardiovascular fitness and thermoregulation during prolonged exercise in man. *Br. J. Sports Med.* 23:109–114, 1989.
70. Greenhaff, P.L., and P.J. Clough. Predictors of sweat loss in man during prolonged exercise. *Eur. J. Appl. Physiol.* 58:348–352, 1989.
71. Greenleaf, J.E., and B.L. Castle. Exercise temperature regulation in man during hypohydration and hyperhydration. *J. Appl. Physiol.* 30:847–853, 1971.
72. Guyton, A.C. *Textbook of Medical Physiology,* 2nd edition. Philadelphia, W.B. Saunders, 1961, p. 855.
73. Hamilton, M.C., J. Gonzalez-Alonso, S. Montain, and E.F. Coyle. Fluid replacement and glucose infusion during exercise prevent cardiovascular drift. *J. Appl. Physiol.* 71:871–877, 1991.
74. Hawley, J.A., S.C. Dennis, and T.D. Noakes. Oxidation of carbohydrate ingested during prolonged endurance exercise. *Sports Med.* 14:27–42, 1992.
75. Hawley, J.A., S.C. Dennis, A. Nowitz, F. Brouns, and T.D. Noakes. Exogenous carbohydrate oxidation from maltose and glucose ingested during prolonged exercise. *Eur. J. Appl. Physiol.* 64:523–527, 1992.
76. Hiller, W.D.B. Current and future research. *Report on the Ross Symposium on Medical Coverage of Endurance Athletic Events.* Ross Laboratories, Columbus, OH, 1987, pp. 114–115.
77. Hiller, W.D.B. Dehydration and hyponatremia during triathlons. *Med. Sci. Sports Exerc.* 21:S219–S221, 1989.
78. Hiller, W.D.B., M.L. O'Toole, E.E. Fortess, R.H. Laird, P.C. Imbert, and T.D. Sisk. Medical and physiological considerations in triathlons. *Am. J. Sports Med.* 15:164–167, 1987.
79. Hiller, W.D.B., M.L. O'Toole, and R.H. Laird. Hyponatremia and ultramarathons. (Letter). *JAMA* 256:213, 1986.
80. Holtzhausen, L-M., and T.D. Noakes. Postural hypotension after ultra marathon running is not related to levels of dehydration (Abstract). *Med. Sci. Sports Exerc.* 24:S44, 1992.
81. Hopper, J., J.R. Elkinton, and A.W. Winkler. Plasma volume of dogs in dehydration with and without salt loss. *J. Clin. Invest.* 23:111–117, 1944.
82. Horstman, D.H., and S.M. Horvath. Cardiovascular and temperature regulatory changes during progressive dehydration and euhydration. *J. Appl. Physiol.* 33:446–450, 1972.
83. Hubbard, R.W., and L.E. Armstrong. Hyperthermia: new thoughts on an old problem. *Phys. Sportsmed.* 17:97–113, 1989.
84. Hubbard, R.W., P.C. Szlyk, and L.E. Armstrong. Influence of thirst and fluid palatability on fluid ingestion during exercise. C.V. Gisolfi, and D.R. Lamb (eds). *Perspectives in Exercise Science and Sports Medicine.* Vol. 3. *Fluid Homeostasis During Exercise.* Indianapolis: Benchmark Press, 1990, pp. 39–85.
85. Irving, R.A., T.D. Noakes, R. Buck, R. van Zyl-Smit, E. Raine, J. Godlonton, and R.J. Norman. Evaluation of renal function and fluid homeostasis during recovery from exercise induced hyponatremia. *J. Appl. Physiol.* 70:342–348, 1991.
86. Irving, R.A., T.D. Noakes, S.C. Burger, K.H. Myburgh, D. Querido, and R. van Zyl-Smit. Plasma volume and renal function during and after ultramarathon running. *Med. Sci. Sports Exerc.* 22:581–587, 1990.
87. Irving, R.A., T.D. Noakes, G.A. Irving, and R. van Zyl-Smit. The immediate and delayed effects of marathon running on renal function. *J. Urol.* 136:1176–1180, 1986.
88. Irving, R.A., T.D. Noakes, R.I. Raine, and R. van Zyl-Smit. Transient oliguria with renal tubular dysfunction after a 90 km running race. *Med. Sci. Sports Exerc.* 22:756–761, 1990.

89. Karpovich, P.V. *Physiology of Muscular Activity*, 4th edition, London: W.B. Saunders, 1953.
90. Kelly, J.C., and J.D. Godlonton. The 1980 Comrades Marathon. *South Afr. Med. J.* 58:509–510, 1980.
91. Ladell, W.S.S. The effects of water and salt intake upon the performance of men working in hot and humid environments. *J. Physiol.* 127:11–46, 1955.
92. Ladell, W.S.S. Water and salt (sodium chloride) intakes. O. Edholm, and A. Bacharach (eds). *The Physiology of Human Survival*. New York: Academic Press, 1965; pp. 235–299.
93. Laird, R.H. Medical complications during the Ironman Triathlon World Championships 1981–1984 *Ann. Sports Med.* 3:113–116, 1987.
94. Leithead, C.S., and A.R. Lind. Heat stress and heat disorders. London: Cassell, 1964.
95. Lind, R.H. The Western States 100 mile run. *Report on the Ross Symposium on Medical Coverage of Endurance Athletic Events*. Ross Laboratories, Columbus, OH, 1987, pp. 22–34.
96. Lindeman, A.K. Nutrient intake of an ultraendurance cyclist. *Int. J. Sports Nutr.* 1:79–85, 1991.
97. Magazink, A., Y. Shapiro, D. Meytes, and I. Meytes. Enzyme blood levels and water balance during a marathon race. *J. Appl. Physiol.* 36:214–217, 1974.
98. Maron, M.B., S.M. Horvath, and J.E. Wilkerson. Acute blood biochemical alterations in response to marathon running. *Eur. J. Appl. Physiol.* 34:173–181, 1975.
99. Maughan, R.J. Thermoregulation in marathon competition at low ambient temperature. *Int. J. Sports Med.* 6:15–19, 1985.
100. Maughan, R.J., C.E. Fenn, M. Gleeson, and J.B. Leiper. Metabolic and circulatory responses to the ingestion of glucose polymer and glucose/electrolyte solutions during exercise in man. *Eur. J. Appl. Physiol.* 56:356–362, 1987.
101. Maughan, R.J., C.E. Fenn, and J.B. Leiper. Effects of fluid, electrolyte, and substrate ingestion on endurance capacity. *Eur. J. Appl. Physiol.* 58:481–486, 1989.
102. McCance, R.A. Experimental sodium chloride deficiency in man. *Proc. Roy. Soc. B.* 119:245–268, 1936.
103. McCance, R.A. The changes in the plasma and cells during experimentally human salt deficiency. *Biochemistry* 31:1278–1284, 1937.
104. McCance, R.A. The effect of salt deficiency in man on the volume of the extracellular fluids, and on the composition of sweat, saliva, gastric juice and cerebrospinal fluid. *J. Physiol.* 92:208–218, 1938.
105. Millard-Stafford, M., P.B. Sparling, L.B. Rosskopf, B.T. Hinson, and L.J. Dicarlo. Carbohydrate-electrolyte replacement during a simulated triathlon in the heat. *Med. Sci. Sports Exerc.* 22:621–628, 1990.
106. Mitchell, J.B., and K.W. Voss. The influence of volume on gastric emptying and fluid balance during prolonged exercise. *Med. Sci. Sports Exerc.* 23:314–319, 1991.
107. Montain, S.J., and E.F. Coyle. Fluid ingestion during exercise increases skin blood flow independent of increases in blood volume. *J. Appl. Physiol.* 73:903–910, 1992.
108. Montain, S.J., and E.F. Coyle. The influence of graded dehydration on hyperthermia and cardiovascular drift during exercise. *J. Appl. Physiol.* 73:1340–1350, 1992.
109. Moodley, D., T.D. Noakes, A.N. Bosch, J.A. Hawley, R. Schall, and S.C. Dennis. Oxidation of exogenous carbohydrate during prolonged exercise: the effects of the carbohydrate type and its concentration. *Eur. J. Appl. Physiol.* 64:328–334, 1992.
110. Moroff, S.V., and D.E. Bass. Effects of overhydration on man's physiological responses to work in the heat. *J. Appl. Physiol.* 20:267–270, 1965.
111. Nadal, J.W., S. Pedersen, and W.G. Maddock. A comparison between dehydration from salt loss and from water deprivation. *J. Clin. Invest.* 20:691, 1941.
112. Nadel, E.R., G.W. Mack, and H. Nose. Influence of fluid replacement beverages on body fluid homeostasis during exercise and recovery. C.V. Gisolfi, and D.R. Lamb (eds). *Perspectives in Exercise Science and Sports Medicine*. Vol. 3. *Fluid Homeostasis During Exercise*. Indianapolis: Benchmark Press, 1990; pp. 181–198.

113. Neufer, P.D., A.J. Young, and M.N. Sawka. Gastric emptying during exercise: Effects of heat stress and hypohydration. *Eur. J. Appl. Physiol.* 58:433–439, 1989.

114. Newmark, S.R., F.R. Toppo, and G. Adams. Fluid and electrolyte replacement in the ultramarathon runner. *Am. J. Sports Med.* 19:389–391, 1991.

115. Newton, A.F.H. Drinks and the marathon. *Athlet. Rev.* July:14–16, 1948.

116. Noakes, T.D. Hyponatremia during endurance running: a physiological and clinical interpretation. *Med. Sci. Sports Exerc.* 24:403–405, 1992.

117. Noakes, T.D. *Lore of Running.* Champaign, IL: Human Kinetic Publishers, 1991.

118. Noakes, T.D. Sacred cow revisited. *Physcn. Sportsmed.* 19:49, 1991.

119. Noakes, T.D. The collapsed endurance athlete—time to rethink our management? *Sports Training, Med. Rehab.* 2:171–191, 1991.

120. Noakes, T.D. The hyponatremia of exercise. *Int. J. Sports Nutr.* 2:205–228, 1992.

121. Noakes, T.D., B.A. Adams, C. Greeff, T. Lotz, and M. Nathan. The danger of an inadequate water intake during prolonged exercise. A novel concept revisited. *Eur. J. Appl. Physiol.* 57:210–219, 1988.

122. Noakes, T.D., N. Berlinski, E. Solomon, and L.M. Weight. Collapsed runners: Blood biochemical changes after IV fluid therapy. *Phys. Sportsmed.* 19:70–81, 1991.

123. Noakes, T.D., and J.W. Carter. Biochemical parameters in athletes before and after having run 160 kilometres. *South Afr. Med. J.* 50:1562–1566, 1976.

124. Noakes, T.D., E.V. Lambert, M.I. Lambert, P.S. McArthur, K.H. Myburgh, and A.J.S. Benade. Carbohydrate ingestion and muscle glycogen depletion during marathon and ultramarathon racing. *Eur. J. Appl. Physiol.* 57:482–489, 1988.

125. Noakes, T.D., K.H. Myburgh, J. du Plessis, L. Lang, M. Lambert, C. van der Riet, and R. Schall. Metabolic rate, not percent dehydration, predicts rectal temperature in marathon runners. *Med. Sci. Sports Exerc.* 23:443–449, 1991.

126. Noakes, T.D., R.J. Norman, R.H. Buck, J. Godlonton, K. Stevenson, and D. Pittaway. The incidence of hyponatremia during prolonged ultra-endurance exercise. *Med. Sci. Sports Exerc.* 22:165–170, 1990.

127. Noakes, T.D., N.J. Rehrer, and R.J. Maughan. The importance of volume in regulating gastric emptying. *Med. Sci. Sports Exerc.* 23:307–313, 1991.

128. Nose, H., G.W. Mack, X. Shi, K. Morimoto, and E.R. Nadel. Effect of saline infusion during exercise on thermal and circulatory regulations. *J. Appl. Physiol.* 69:609–616, 1990.

129. Nose, H., G.W. Mack, X. Shi, and E.R. Nadel. Shift in body fluid compartments after dehydration in humans. *J. Appl. Physiol.* 65:318–324, 1988.

130. Nose, H., G.W. Mack, X. Shi, and E.R. Nadel. Role of osmolality and plasma volume during rehydration in humans. *J. Appl. Physiol.* 65:325–331, 1988.

131. Nose, H., G.W. Mack, X. Shi, and E.R. Nadel. Involvement of sodium retention hormones during rehydration in humans. *J. Appl. Physiol.* 65:332–336, 1988.

132. Novak, D. Ironman Canada Triathlon Championships: Medical coverage of an ultradistance event. *Report on the Ross Symposium on Medical Coverage of Endurance Athletic Events.* Ross Laboratories, Columbus, OH, 1987, pp. 69–73.

133. Okuno, T., T. Yawata, H. Nose, and T. Morimoto. Difference in rehydration process due to salt concentration of drinking water in rats. *J. Appl. Physiol.* 64:2438–2443, 1988.

134. O'Toole, M.L. Prevention and treatment of electrolyte abnormalities. In: *Report on the Ross Symposium on Medical Coverage of Endurance Athletic Events.* Ross Laboratories, Columbus, OH, 1987, pp. 93–96.

135. Peters, J.H., J. Johnson, and J. Edmunson. *Modern Middle and Long Distance Running.* London: Nicholas Kaye, 1957.

136. Pitts, G.C., R.E. Johnson, and F.C. Consolazio. Work in the heat as affected by intake of water, salt and glucose. *Am. J. Physiol.* 142:253–259, 1944.

137. Powers, S.K., J. Lawler, S. Dodd, R. Tulley, G. Landry, and K. Wheeler. Fluid

replacement drinks during high intensity exercise: effects on minimizing exercise-induced disturbances in homeostasis. *Eur. J. Appl. Physiol.* 60:54–60, 1990.

138. Pugh, L.G.C.E., J.L. Corbett, and R.H. Johnson. Rectal temperatures, weight losses, and sweat rates in marathon running. *J. Appl. Physiol.* 23:347–352, 1967.

139. Rehrer, N.J. *Limits to Fluid Availability During Exercise.* Haarlem: B.V. Uitgeverij De Vrieseborch, 1990, pp. 1–239.

140. Rehrer, N.J., G.M.E. Janssen, F. Brouns, and W.H.M. Saris. Fluid intake and gastrointestinal problems in runners competing in a 25-km race and a marathon. *Int. J. Sports Med.* 10(Suppl 1):S22–S25, 1989.

141. Rehrer, N.J., A.J.M. Wagenmakers, E.J. Beckers, D. Halliday, J.B. Leiper, F. Brouns, R.J. Maughan, K. Westerterp, and W.H.M. Saris. Gastric emptying, absorption, and carbohydrate oxidation during prolonged exercise. *J. Appl. Physiol.* 72:468–475, 1992.

142. Roberts, W.O. Exercise-associated collapse in endurance events: A classification system. *Phys. Sportsmed.* 117:49–59, 1989.

143. Rontoyannis, G.P., T. Skoulis, and K.N. Pavlou. Energy balance in ultramarathon running. *Am. J. Clin. Nutr.* 49:976–979, 1989.

144. Ryan, A.J., T.L. Bleiler, J.E. Carter, and C.V. Gisolfi. Gastric emptying during prolonged cycling exercise in the heat. *Med. Sci. Sports Exerc.* 21:51–58, 1989.

145. Salvato, E.K., J.F. Nichols, and A.A. Sucec. Serum sodium and fluid balance during a fifty-mile ultraendurance race. *Int. J. Sports Med.* 11:320, 1990.

146. Sandick, B.L., D.B. Engell, and O. Maller. Perception of drinking water temperature and effects for humans after exercise. *Physiol. Behav.* 32:851–855, 1984.

147. Sawka, M.N., and K.B. Pandolf. Effects of body water loss on physiological function and exercise performance. C.V. Gisolfi, and D.R. Lamb (eds). *Perspectives in Exercise Science and Sports Medicine,* Vol 3. *Fluid Homeostasis During Exercise.* Indianapolis: Benchmark Press, 1990, pp. 1–30.

148. Sjovall, H., H. Abrahamsson, G. Westlander, R. Gillberg, S. Redfors, M. Jodal, and O. Lundgren. Intestinal fluid and electrolyte transport in man during reduced circulating blood volume. *Gut* 27:913–918, 1986.

149. Strydom, N.B., A.J.S. Benade, and A.J. van Rensburg. The state of hydration and the physiological responses of men during work in heat. *Aust. J. Sports Med.* 7:28–33, 1975.

150. Strydom, N.B., and L.D. Holdsworth. The effects of different levels of water deficit on physiological responses during heat stress. *Int. Z. angew. Physiol.* 26:95–102, 1968.

151. Strydom, N.B., C.H. Wyndham, C.H. van Graan, L.D. Holdsworth, and J.F. Morrison. The influence of water restriction on the performance of men during a prolonged march. *South Afr. Med. J.* 40:539–544, 1966.

152. Sullivan, J.E. *Marathon Running.* New York: American Sports Publishing Company, 1909.

153. Szlyk, P.C. I.V. Sils, R.P. Francesconi, and R.W. Hubbard. Patterns of human drinking: effects of exercise, water temperature, and food consumption. *Aviat. Space Environ. Med.* 61:43–48, 1990.

154. Szlyk, P.C. I.V. Sils, R.P. Francesconi, and R.W. Hubbard, and W.T. Matthew. Variability in intake and dehydration in young men during a simulated desert walk. *Aviat. Space Environ. Med.* 60:422–427, 1989.

155. Talbott, J.H., D.B. Dill, H.T. Edwards, E.H. Stumme, and W.V. Consolazio. The ill effects of heat upon workmen. *J. Indust. Hyg. Toxicol.* 19:258–274, 1937.

156. Talbott, J.H., H.T. Edwards, D.B. Dill, and L. Drastich. Physiological responses to high environmental temperature. *J. Trop. Med. Hyg.* 13:381–397, 1933.

157. Talbott, J.H., and J. Michelsen. Heat cramps. A clinical and chemical study. *J. Clin. Invest.* 12:533–549, 1933.

158. Thomas, B.D., and C.P. Motley. Myoglobinemia and endurance exercise: a study of

twenty-five participants in a triathlon competition. *Am. J. Sports Med.* 12:113–119, 1984.

159. Thrasher, T.N., J.F. Nistal-Herrera, L.C. Keil, and D.J. Ramsay. Satiety and inhibition of vasopressin secretion after drinking in dehydrated dogs. *Am. J. Physiol.* 240:E394–E401, 1981.

160. van Rensburg, J.P., A.J. Kielblock, and A. van der Linde. Physiologic and biochemical changes during a triathlon competition. *Int. J. Sports Med.* 7:30–35, 1986.

161. Vitali, E. DeP., F. Malacarne, M. Vedovato, R. Cavallini, B. Bagni, L. Nunzi, and P. Gilli. Atrial natriuretic peptide and urinary sodium balance during physical exercise. *Nephron* 57:60–63, 1991.

162. Wade, C.E., and B.J. Freund. Hormonal control of blood volume during and following exercise. C.V. Gisolfi, and D.R. Lamb. (eds). *Perspectives in Exercise Science and Sports Medicine.* Vol. 3. *Fluid homeostasis during exercise.* Indianapolis: Benchmark Press, 1990, pp. 207–241.

163. Walsh, R.M., and T.D. Noakes. Exercise tolerance is impaired at low levels of dehydration. (Abstract). *Med. Sci. Sports Exerc.* 24:543, 1992.

164. Webster, F.A.M. *The Science of Athletics.* London: Nicholas Kaye, 1948.

165. Whiting, P.H., R.J. Maughan, and J.D.B. Miller. Dehydration and serum biochemical changes in marathon runners. *Eur. J. Appl. Physiol.* 52:183–187, 1984.

166. Williams, C., M.G. Nute, L. Broadbank, and S. Vinall. Influence of fluid intake on endurance running performance. A comparison between water, glucose and fructose solutions. *Eur. J. Appl. Physiol.* 60:112–119, 1990.

167. Winslow, E.B.J. The Chicago Marathon. *Report on the Ross Symposium on Medical Coverage of Endurance Athletic Events.* Ross Laboratories, Columbus, OH, 1987, pp. 17–20.

168. Wyndham, C.H. Heat stroke and hyperthermia in marathon runners. *Ann. N.Y. Acad. Sci.* 301:128–138, 1977.

169. Wyndham, C.H., and N.B. Strydom. The danger of an inadequate water intake during marathon running. *South Afr. Med. J.* 43:893–896, 1969.

170. Wyndham, C.H., N.B. Strydom, A.J.S. Benade, and W.H. van der Walt. The effect on acclimatization of various water and salt replacement regimens. *South Afr. Med. J.* 47:1773–1779, 1973.

171. Wyndham, C.H., N.B. Strydom, A.J. van Rensburg, A.J.S. Benade, and A.J. Heyns. Relation between VO_2max and body temperature in hot humid air conditions. *J. Appl. Physiol.* 29:45–50, 1970.

11
Plasticity of Muscle Fiber and Motor Unit Types

TESSA GORDON, Ph.D.
MARY C. PATTULLO, Ph.D.

INTRODUCTION

More than 100 yr ago, characteristic differences were recognized in the structure and function of slow-tonic and fast-twitch muscles in lower vertebrates, and of slow- and fast-twitch mammalian muscles. Slow-twitch muscles were first distinguished from fast-twitch muscles by their red color, visibly slower contractile speed [152], and greater endurance for repeated contractions [33]. However, it is neither the purpose of this review to list in detail the myriad differences known to exist between slow- and fast-twitch muscles nor to enumerate the many conditions in response to which muscles demonstrate their remarkable plasticity. These are already well established, and equally well documented in both original papers and reviews [19, 25, 43, 83, 88, 158, 162, 165, 191]. Rather, it is our aim to present an overview of the multifactorial control of muscle phenotype with a particular emphasis on the role of neural activity. What do we now know about the extent to which muscle phenotype is under neural control and how much is controlled by other factors?

During the 1960s, two seminal series of experiments were carried out, in the laboratories of John Eccles in Australia and Elwood Henneman in North America, which provided the conceptual framework for the intensive study of the control of muscle phenotype. Buller et al. [16, 17] showed that differences in contractile speed of slow- and fast-twitch hindlimb muscles of the cat emerge during neonatal development and can be altered, even in adult life, by cross-reinnervation. This was the first demonstration of neural regulation of muscle phenotype and plasticity of muscle properties. The groundwork was laid for the experiments of Vrbova and her colleagues concerning the role of patterns of neural activity [146, 147, 191], and for the widespread study of muscle plasticity under both physiological and pathological conditions. Henneman and his colleagues [130] introduced their work on motor unit properties in the homogeneous cat soleus muscle with the statement that, "Although a muscle is no more than an assembly of motor units, the collective properties of the whole do not convey much information about its parts." (The motoneuron and the muscle fibers that it supplies had been termed the "motor unit" by Sherrington because the motor unit is the smallest functional unit of motor output of the central nervous system [167]. Henneman isolated single motor units and demonstrated that there was a wide range of contractile properties, consistent with histochemical studies of single muscle fibers that also showed considerable heterogeneity [44, 88, 89, 108, 130, 199]. A series of experiments, of which the motor unit studies were part, led to the formulation of Henneman's size principle, which related input and output properties of motoneurons, and stated that motor units are recruited into activity in order of their size [88, 89]. Identification of the heterogeneous muscle fiber and motor unit composition of muscle, and its significance for normal control of movement, has had enormous impact on our understanding of muscle plasticity and motor control [11]. This review is concerned with the issues of muscle plasticity only, although motor control will be alluded to where relevant.

Muscle fiber heterogeneity was first recognized by the histochemical demonstration of differences in the reaction intensities of myosin ATPases (mATPases) and oxidative and glycolytic enzymes in human and animal muscles [14, 39, 84]. Histochemical reactions for either mATPase [14, 84] or oxidative enzymes alone [39, 155], permitted at least three and as many as eight muscle fiber types to be discerned [155]. Histochemical procedures were modified to discriminate only three fiber types, and typing based on either ATPase alone (α, β, $\alpha\beta$, [84]; Type I, IIA, IIB [14]); or a combination of ATPase and metabolic enzymes (slow-oxidative [SO], fast-oxidative glycolytic [FOG], fast glycolytic [FG] [142]), has become routine practice [20, 70, 145]. In an effort to reconcile a continuous range of contractile properties with three different histochemical types, Henneman and Olson [89] used the slow units in the soleus muscle as the index of comparison to distinguish slow from fast. Burke et al. [21] developed an independent method, the "sag" test, to distinguish motor unit types without relying on twitch contraction times that are distributed along a continuum. This test identified differences in the force profile of unfused tetanic contractions of units; force increases throughout the contraction in slow units in contrast to a sag of peak force in fast units. In general terms, this sag criterion has been widely applied and, although not always applicable across muscles of different species, slow and fast motor units can normally be distinguished by their characteristic force profiles in unfused tetanic contractions [66, 188]. Furthermore, in motor units identified by glycogen depletion techniques, the physiological and histochemical types correspond reasonably well [21, 64, 188].

Susceptibility to fatigue was chosen as the criterion to subdivide fast units into fatigue resistant (FR) and fatigable (FF), to provide a physiological classification that corresponded with the histochemical division of type IIA (FOG) and IIB (FG) fibers [19, 20]. Whereas these classification systems are useful, it is important to recognize the continuous nature of the properties used in deriving them, and thus, realize that adherence to rigid systems may be inappropriate or misleading both in normal muscle and, even more, under conditions of plasticity. More recently, immunocytochemical analyses, using antibodies raised against slow and fast myosin heavy chains (MHCs), have complemented earlier classification systems and identified a fourth fiber type in rat muscle, type IIx, which is present in motor units physiologically classified as fast fatigue intermediate (FI), and histochemically as fast intermediate (F_{int}) [112, 188]. The multiple isoforms of contractile and regulatory proteins that have been identified can appear in many possible combinations [145], more consistent with a continuous range of muscle fibers rather than few discrete types.

Henneman and his colleagues [88, 199] argued that if each motor unit contained a random sample of heterogeneous muscle fibers with properties varying as widely as across the whole muscle, then all units would be similar because of the averaging effect of the distribution. However, as motor units demonstrate a wide range of properties, the variance of fiber properties within units must be less than between different units. This is consistent with neural determination of muscle properties, further supported by the low variance of metabolic enzyme activities observed within unit fibers when compared to nonunit fibers [108, 109, 124, 135, 136]. Nevertheless, variance within units was higher than expected if properties were regulated solely by the nerve [124]. Similarly, although the range of fiber size was generally smaller within a single unit than the range for the same fiber type throughout the muscle, it could still be as large as 5-fold [124, 187]. Furthermore, the size of any one type of muscle fiber was found to vary according to the region of the muscle in which it was located [149, 150, 187], suggesting that local influences contribute to determining fiber size.

These findings argue that, in normal muscle, the motoneuron cannot exert total control over fiber properties at the motor unit level. This review presents evidence from studies of reinnervation, and of conditions in which activity is controlled or reduced, to show that motor units retain heterogeneity that cannot be accounted for by the nerve. Muscle plasticity can be viewed as an adaptive phenomenon within a range that is controlled by muscle architecture and mechanical factors and/or intrinsic factors preset during development.

REINNERVATION: MUSCLE AND MOTOR UNIT PROPERTIES AND ORGANIZATION

Muscle Properties After Cross-reinnervation
In 1960, Buller et al. [17] discovered that the fast-twitch flexor digitorum longus (FDL) muscle contracted more slowly after cross-innervation with the soleus nerve, while the contractile speed of the slow-twitch soleus muscle increased after cross-innervation with the FDL nerve. The experimental paradigm was initially designed to examine whether synaptic rearrangement occurs after misdirection of nerves to antagonistic muscles, but the central plasticity was small as compared with the more obvious plasticity of the reinnervated muscles. This was an unanticipated finding of enormous importance suggesting that muscle phenotype was regulated by the motoneuron.

Several studies in the same decade confirmed these findings and provided physiological, morphological, and biochemical evidence for altered muscle phenotype after cross-reinnervation [25, 83, 191], thereby supporting the view that muscle phenotype was determined by neural input. However, closer examination of isometric and isotonic contractions, histochemical fiber types, and contractile and regulatory protein isoforms, in cross-reinnervated muscles, indicated that conversion of properties was incomplete with muscles often retaining some of their former characteristics [17, 18, 38, 152, 156, 175]. Either the muscle fibers did not fully transform their properties after cross-reinnervation or the new nerve supply was not homogeneously slow or fast [18, 153, 191]. These possibilities are best differentiated at the motor unit level.

Muscle Unit Properties in Reinnervated Muscles
Tetanic stimulation of single motor units to deplete the unit fibers of glycogen, followed by analysis of these fibers in glycogen-stained muscle cross-sections, was the ingenious method introduced by Edstrom and Kugelberg [44] to identify the fibers comprising single muscle units. Their data showed that muscle unit fibers were normally of the same histochemical type and that they were distributed in a mosaic pattern amid fibers of other muscle units. Later experiments showed that unit fibers in reinnervated muscles tended to be grouped together or "clumped" and that, after long-term reinnervation, the fibers were all of the same type [40, 61, 64, 109, 150, 187, 188]. This was true whether the reinnervating nerve was the original (self-reinnervation) or a foreign nerve (cross-reinnervation). As the regenerating nerve supplies muscle fibers that formerly belonged to different types of motor units, this is strong evidence that the nerve determines histochemical profile.

Muscle units in self- and cross-reinnervated cat and rat fast-twitch muscles obeyed the usual physiological criteria for classification [40, 54, 56, 66, 76, 77, 188]. Incomplete conversion of whole muscle twitch contractile speeds from fast to slow, and vice versa, was not caused by incomplete conversion of contractile speed of the constituent motor units because all parameters of contractile speed in slow and fast units were the same as in normal muscles [66]. Comparative analysis of whole muscle and motor unit contractile speeds in normal and reinnervated muscles showed that the rate of rise and fall of the whole muscle twitch contraction reflects the relative proportions of fast and slow motor units, respectively. Thus, findings that the rise time of the twitch contraction in cross-reinnervated fast-twitch muscles remained somewhat faster than that of normal slow-twitch muscles could be accounted for by the few remaining fast motor units that predominate in the rising phase of the contraction. Likewise, the slower than predicted twitch relaxation time persisting after cross-reinnervation of the soleus muscle could be accounted for by the remaining slow units that predominate in this contractile phase [66].

Thus, incomplete conversion of fast- and slow-twitch muscles following cross-reinnervation does not necessarily reflect incomplete control by the fast or slow nerve. There are, however, a number of lines of evidence suggesting that the nerve cannot fully transform muscle properties and that plasticity of reinnervated muscle fibers may be less than anticipated from the conclusions of Buller et al. [17].

Limited Muscle Fiber Plasticity
In reinnervation, the contractile speed of motor units is converted by the nerve but a more detailed examination of units and, in particular, of muscle fibers at the molecular level reveals that remnants of the previous phenotype remain. This is most obvious in the cross-reinnervated soleus that exhibits several examples of incomplete transformation. Soleus motor units retain their high endurance, with muscle fibers maintaining a high oxidative enzyme capacity despite reinnervation by nerves that formerly supplied muscles with large numbers of FF motor units [24, 41, 65]. Furthermore, motor units that are fast contracting do not always sag and are not necessarily composed of fibers with a type II histochemical profile: cat soleus muscle units that were cross-reinnervated by FDL nerves did not show the sag typical of the fast FDL units despite demonstrating the fast range of contractile speeds [41], and there were substantially more fast-contracting motor units in cross-reinnervated soleus in rat [65] and cat [53, 54, 77] than fast muscle fibers identified by pH sensitivity of the mATPase.

How then can conversion of muscle speed be reconciled with the lack of conversion of sag and endurance characteristics and muscle histochemical types? Expression of fast myosin and fast troponin isoforms in cross-reinnervated muscles can account for the increased contractile speed of cross-reinnervated slow muscle fibers [35, 64, 175]. However, muscle fibers that express fast myosin also continue to express slow myosin heavy and light chains [64]. The observed dissociation between physiological and histochemical types was, therefore, attributed to the presence of hybrid muscle fibers whose mixed fast and slow myosin composition was resolvable by immunohistochemistry but not by standard histochemistry [64, 65]. The incomplete transformation could not be accounted for by an insufficient time period as motor unit and muscle fiber properties were examined at least 5–18 months after reinnervation in the studies reported above. Thus, the retention of former slow properties in the soleus muscle following reinnervation by fast motor nerves argues that plasticity may be more limited than expected.

There are also examples of muscle fibers retaining remnants of their original phenotype in reinnervated fast-twitch muscles. Expression of MHCs varies considerably from one fiber to another within identified reinnervated muscle units, despite all fibers staining as the same histochemical type [61]. A significantly higher proportion of FI units consistently observed in reinnervated cat muscles [76, 77, 150] could be explained by remaining variations in fiber oxidative/glycolytic potential and endurance. Inclusion of fatigable and nonfatigable fibers in the same unit after reinnervation would result in a muscle unit displaying intermediate endurance characteristics. The range in muscle fiber size within reinnervated motor units was larger than normal, as if reinnervated fibers recovered their former size irrespective of the neural supply [187]. Indeed, the differences in size among SO, FOG, and FG fiber types were lost, with the size distributions becoming broader and overlapping extensively in both self- and cross-reinnervated muscles [77, 151, 187]. The increased variance in muscle fiber size within motor units, and the increased overlap of the size distributions of SO, FOG, and FG fibers are consistent with more similar tetanic forces in S, FR, and FF motor units after reinnervation [74, 76, 77].

It was also found that reinnervation restores regional distribution in the fast-twitch muscles, mouse tibialis anterior (TA) [138] and cat medial gastrocnemius (MG [150]), with more oxidative S and FR units in the deeper regions while FF units predominate in more superficial regions of the muscle. Because unit fibers were clumped in reinnervated muscles, the regionalization could not simply be attributed to the regenerating fibers finding their original muscle fibers. Rather, the tendency of fibers within different muscle regions to express their former phenotype suggests either an intrinsic regulation of phenotype or that local factors interact with neural supply in determining muscle phenotype. One possibility is that differential mechanical loading of muscle fibers in different regions may contribute to determining whether the fibers express one or another isoform of contractile protein, as well as regulating metabolic phenotype (see later). Another possibility is that restored regionalization of muscle fiber type after reinnervation reflects intrinsic properties of muscle fibers that originated in different clones of myoblasts during development, with deeper components derived from primary myoblasts and more superficial ones from secondary myoblasts (see Development of Muscle Phenotype).

Thus, although the motoneuron appears to respecify histochemical type and contractile speed by inducing gene expression for the appropriate contractile, regulatory, and metabolic enzymes in the muscle unit, the continued expression of the original phenotype in the same fibers argues that factors other than the nerve are also important in the regulation of muscle phenotype.

Rematching of Motoneuron and Muscle Unit Properties After Reinnervation: Functional Consequences and Mechanisms

Gordon and Stein [74] showed that the normal correlations between contractile force and speed in muscle units, and between muscle unit force and nerve size were lost during the early stages of self-reinnervation of cat MG muscle at which time muscle units are heterogeneous in their properties. Normal relationships returned as the nerves and muscles recovered from axotomy and denervation, respectively; this was during the same time-frame as the respecification of histochemical fiber type [74, 75]. Return of the size relationships was a general finding in reinnervated muscles whether the muscles were self- or cross-reinnervated [6, 7, 74–76, 114–116]. Further characterization of motoneuron properties after reinnervation showed that motoneuron properties recovered from axotomy to restore the normal relationships among input resistance, rheobase, and muscle unit force and contractile force [57].

Thus, with time, the formation of functional nerve-muscle connections restores the matching of nerve and muscle properties. Restored relationships among motoneuron size and excitability (the inverse of rheobase) and muscle unit size account for the orderly recruitment of motor units seen in self-reinnervated muscles [29, 184]. The apparent loss of recruitment order demonstrated in reinnervated from dorsal interosseus muscle, after injury and surgical repair of the ulnar nerve in human subjects, has been attributed to a random reinnervation of the muscle by ulnar motor nerves which formerly supplied several different hand muscles [184]. As a result, recruitment of motoneurons that formerly supplied one muscle, now results in contraction of several different muscles. Thus, misdirection of regenerating fibers may be associated with marked dysfunction, a problem that is particularly severe after cranial nerve injuries [71].

Rematching of reinnervated muscle unit force to motor nerve size was attributed to the respecification of the size of the muscle fibers, and their specific force, by the regenerated nerve [74, 77, 177]. The normal correlations between muscle unit contractile force and speed after reinnervation were similarly attributed to respecification of muscle properties by the motor nerve, in accordance with the prevalent ideas of muscle plasticity [191].

Later experiments determined the number of muscle fibers reinnervated by each motor nerve, or the innervation ratio (IR), by counting glycogen-depleted muscle fibers in isolated and characterized motor units [186, 187]. These showed that IR, and not muscle fiber size or specific force, is the major determinant of motor unit force in reinnervated muscles. Cross-sectional area (CSA) and specific force (SF) of the reinnervated unit fibers contributed little to the recovery of the normal range of unit force. A broader spectrum of fiber size within each reinnervated muscle unit, and more extensive overlap of fiber sizes between different units, reduced the impact of CSA as a factor contributing to the force range, while the range of SF values remained similar to normal.

Thus, IR, and not respecification of muscle properties, accounted for the restored range of unit force after reinnervation [177, 187]. IR, excitability, and conduction velocity of the motoneurons covaried with muscle unit force as in normal muscles and accounts for the rematching of nerve size with motor unit force. The smaller and most excitable motoneurons branch less extensively than the larger motoneurons, which require larger synaptic current to discharge as originally suggested by Henneman [88]. This is also apparent during reinnervation of partially denervated muscles by collateral sprouting from remaining healthy motoneurons [78, 150, 151]. All units in partially denervated muscles increased their force output by the same factor because the increase in numbers of muscle fibers per motoneuron was proportional to motoneuron size. Thus, the range in motor unit force remained the same, but mean force increased as sprouting compensated for reduced motor unit number. Unit size could increase 5- to 8-fold to compensate for reduced motor unit number [78, 151]. Whether the IR is restricted by a limited capacity of motoneurons to branch and innervate very large numbers of target muscles, or whether local factors in the partially denervated muscles limit collateral sprouting is still unclear.

Some of the rematching of nerve and muscle properties may also involve a retrograde influence on the motoneurons from the reinnervated muscle fibers. Reversal of axotomy-related changes may restore the original properties of the motoneurons, with the forming of functional target connections appearing to trigger the switch of gene expression from growth-related proteins to the original mature motoneuron phenotype, irrespective of the target muscle and even although muscle fibers may still be heterogeneous at this time [57, 72, 110]. On the other hand, some retrograde influence of the muscle fibers on motoneuron properties is suggested by findings of slower conduction velocity in former "fast" nerves after cross-reinnervation of soleus muscle [115]. After cross-reinnervation of soleus muscle, some MG motoneurons demonstrated electrophysiological characteristics more similar to soleus than MG motoneurons, which could not be accounted for by incomplete recovery from axotomy [53, 55]. Trophic interaction has been inferred as the mechanism for the observed matching of the motoneuron and muscle properties in cross-reinnervated soleus, and may be mediated by activity-dependent uptake or trophic substances from the muscle [32].

Muscle fiber and motor unit analysis of reinnervated muscles has shown that rematching of nerve and muscle properties is dynamic and involves plasticity of both nerve and muscle. Although the motoneuron respecifies histochemical type and contractile speed by inducing novel gene expression in reinnervated muscle fibers, evidence for continued expression of the original fiber phenotype argues that other factors are also important in the regulation of muscle phenotype. These factors will become more apparent during the consideration of muscle plasticity under conditions of imposed electrical stimulation (see Muscle Plasticity in Response to Chronic Electrical Stimulation), and conditions in which neuromuscular activity is reduced (see Muscle Plasticity in Models of Disuse).

Huxley suggested that the conversion of muscle properties by cross-reinnervation was mediated by the particular type of contraction that the muscle was subjected to by the novel innervation [17]. Another possibility suggested was that the neural influence was mediated by a trophic substance released from the new nerve. The latter suggestion has received little attention [46, 99], particularly since Salmons and Sreter [163] demonstrated that conversion of muscle properties by cross-reinnervation could be reversed by superimposing the original pattern of neuromuscular activity on the muscles by chronic electrical stimulation. On the other hand, the role of neuromuscular activity in controlling muscle phenotype has been extensively investigated.

MUSCLE PLASTICITY IN RESPONSE TO CHRONIC ELECTRICAL STIMULATION

Fast-to-Slow Muscle Conversion by Low-Frequency Stimulation

Vrbova [190] tenotomized cat and rabbit soleus as an experimental model to test Huxley's suggestion that the neural influence on muscle contractile speed was mediated by the pattern of neuromuscular activity. Tenotomy induced a significant increase in contractile speed, which could be reversed by stimulating soleus nerve continuously at low frequencies of 5–10 Hz, but not with intermittent stimulation at higher frequencies (40 Hz). Since the two patterns of stimulation resemble the discharge patterns of slow and fast motor units, respectively [33, 90], these findings supported the idea that the neural influence on contractile speed is mediated via neuromuscular activity.

Extension of these experiments to chronic stimulation of rabbit TA muscles with the "slow" activity pattern demonstrated dramatic conversion of fast muscle properties to slow without surgically altering the nerve supply [164]. As described for cross-reinnervation, fast-twitch muscle phenotype changes toward that of a slow-twitch muscle but the conversion is not always complete and may produce atypical hybrid fibers [99, 145–147]. In addition, there is considerable variation in the magnitude and time course of the induced changes under similar experimental conditions [147]. Nevertheless, the plasticity exhibited by chronically stimulated muscle has provided an excellent frame within which to determine the cellular basis for conversion of physiological properties and the control of gene expression in skeletal muscle [146, 147].

In most of these studies, bipolar electrodes are implanted close to the common peroneal nerve to stimulate the TA muscle continuously at 10 Hz for 8–24 hr daily over a 1- to 4-month period, using an external or internal stimulator [e.g., 15, 42, 45, 94, 102, 103, 163, 164]. Early increases in the time to peak twitch tension and relaxation rate are associated with rapid changes in Ca^{2+} sequestration, preceding the slower conversion of contractile and regulatory proteins from fast to slow isoforms [106, 144]. Increased endurance is associated with a rapid and marked increase in capillarization and oxidative capacity and decreased glycolytic enzyme activity [93, 144]. Reduced muscle fiber diameter is accompanied by a decline in muscle force [36, 103, 144]. This fast-to-slow fiber type transition is a "graded event" during which the number of type IIB fibers declines, type IID increases transiently, type IIA then increases, and finally, in most species but not in rats and mice, an increase in type I fibers is seen [147]. Transition between the different fiber types involves downregulation of mRNA for fast myosin isoforms and progressive upregulation of intermediate and eventually slow isoforms of both heavy and light chains [15, 105, 143]. Although changes in gene expression are induced within days of commencing stimulation, different rates of synthesis and degradation of the various myosin isoforms results in coexpression of different isoforms in the same fiber, particularly during the first month of stimulation [147, 183]. In chronically stimulated rat muscle, up to four different MHC isoforms have been found in a single muscle fiber [183]. Fast-to-slow transitions in troponin T isoforms occur over the same time course as for the contractile proteins, with a similar incidence of hybrid fibers [86]. The exchange of fast with slow isoforms of troponin C and I is less complete [87].

The rapid changes in Ca^{2+} sequestration, which account for the early changes in contractile speed, are caused by inactivation of the sarcoplasmic Ca-ATPase, which is later followed by a replacement of the fast with the slow isoform of Ca-ATPase, downregulation of calsequestrin and parvalbumin, and expression of phospholamban [42, 106, 113, 143, 168]. There is good temporal correlation between parvalbumin downregulation and slowing of the twitch relaxation in chronically stimulated muscles [106]. Transition from an anaerobic-glycolytic energy supply to a more aerobic-oxidative capacity, which correlates with increased muscle endurance, follows a similar time course with a rapid onset [144, 147]. There is a coordinated decline in the activity of glycolytic pathway enzymes and increased activity of enzymes involved in the citric acid cycle, the respiratory chain, and fatty acid oxidation; these have been correlated in some cases with corresponding changes in mRNA levels [147, 194, 195].

The nature of the coupling of electrical activity to altered gene expression is not yet understood although a rapid increase in internal Ca^{2+} concentration and/or reduced ATP relative to ADP and free inorganic phosphate have been identified as possible triggers [143, 147].

Pattern vs. Amount of Activity

In contrast to the many studies that have used low-frequency stimulation of fast-twitch muscles to investigate plasticity, the possibility of slow-to-fast conversions and a detailed analysis of stimulation patterns have been relatively neglected. This is mainly because of the technical difficulty of eliminating normal muscle activity to control the pattern and total amount of stimulus pulses.

Two different experimental approaches have been used since the pioneering work of Vrbova on tenotomized soleus [190]. First, Lomo and his colleagues denervated rat soleus muscle and independently varied the number and frequency of pulses imposed by chronic stimulation [79, 82, 119, 193]. Their results showed that denervated soleus developed force as rapidly as the fast-twitch EDL muscle after stimulation with high-frequency intermittent bursts of stimuli, and as slowly as normal soleus muscle after stimulation with a continuous low-frequency pattern. The increased contractile speed and associated induction of fast MHCs following intermittent high-frequency stimulation was attributed to the pattern of stimulation rather than any effects of denervation alone, as suggested by Al-Amood and Lewis [2], since denervation alone induces fast MHCs in only 40% of the muscle fibers as compared with 80% in the stimulated muscles [79]. In addition to stimulation frequency, the total number of pulses was found to be important for fast-to-slow but not slow-to-fast conversion. Increasing numbers of pulses at low frequencies led to further slowing of the denervated soleus, whereas increasing the pulse number in high-frequency strains had no additional effect in increasing contractile speed [193].

A second approach, taken by Kernell and his colleagues, was to reduce activity in the fast-twitch peroneous longus (PL) muscle of the cat by spinal cord hemisection and hindlimb deafferentation, and thereafter

control the frequency and total daily amount of stimulation independently [36, 45, 102, 103]. Under these conditions, it was shown that
fast-to-slow conversion was not frequency dependent, but rather depended on the total number of stimuli per day, in agreement with earlier
findings [94]. Irrespective of frequency (5–10 Hz or 20–40 Hz delivered
continuously, or in a 50% duty cycle of 1 sec on/1 sec off), chronically
stimulated PL muscles became slow contracting, fatigue resistant, and
exhibited tetanic force profiles typical of slow muscles within 4–8 weeks
[45]. When the duty cycle was reduced to 5% of the day, which
corresponds reasonably well with the daily amount of activity in FR units
in rat muscles [90], 10- or 100-Hz stimulation did not cause much slowing
but was effective in increasing the endurance of the muscle. When the
duty cycle was further reduced, to 0.5% of the day, to correspond more
closely with the low daily amount of activity typical of FF units, PL
muscles remained fast contracting but acquired intermediate fatigue
characteristics [102, 103]. Therefore, activation with total daily amounts
of activity of >30%, 5% and <0.5% of the day, corresponding roughly
with the daily activity of S, FR, and FF units, respectively, appeared to
convert the muscle contractile speed and endurance parameters toward
those of the predicted motor unit type. The normal order of recruitment
of unit types is S, FR, then FF, which determines their respective
amounts of daily activity. This, in turn, appears to be instrumental in
establishing and maintaining their contractile speed and endurance
properties. Findings that muscle force and fiber diameter also decreased
with progressively higher daily amounts of activity provided further
evidence for a coordinated rank-ordering of muscle force, speed, and
fatigability with recruitment order [88, 101].

Similarly, progressively increasing the total duration of low-frequency
stimulation of paralyzed TA muscles in spinal cord-injured human
subjects led to a progressive slowing of the muscle and an increase in
endurance [176]. Furthermore, the slowing of the muscles occurred with
type II to type I conversion [126], similar to the effects of low frequency
stimulation on paralyzed cat muscles [36]. Unlike the cat muscles,
however, the high-duration low-frequency stimulation was not associated with a decline in isometric force and decrease in muscle fiber
diameter. In the slower human muscles, the same frequency of
stimulation evokes more fused tetanic contractions. Muscle force increased under conditions in which brief strong contractions were
produced, by higher frequencies, during chronic stimulation of paralyzed cat [103] or denervated rat muscles [193]. These findings suggest
that pattern of stimulation is a contributing factor to determining muscle
force and fiber size. As Donselaar and colleagues [36] concluded, "The
higher rates of the fast patterns would produce stronger contractions
than those of the slow patterns, and a higher amount of 'force stress'
might favour the maintenance of factors of relevance for contractile

force.' Consideration of muscle building exercises [162, 165] and of disuse atrophy (see Muscle Plasticity in Models of Disuse) identifies muscle loading and length as important in determining contractile force.

Adaptive Range of Motor Unit Properties
In a recent study of chronically stimulated cat MG motor units, Gordon et al. [73] found that the mean contractile force, speed, and fatigability was significantly reduced, consistent with data on whole muscle. However, there remained almost as wide a range of contractile speed as normal, even when all muscle fibers expressed slow MHCs. This is contrary to the prediction that, if recruitment order determines motor unit properties and thereby mediates the effect of neural activity [101], synchronous activation of all motor units with the same amount and pattern of impulses should greatly diminish the range of unit properties. With prolonged periods of stimulation, this should result in a homogeneous population of units all exhibiting similar values of contractile force, speed, and endurance. In these experiments employing a "slow" pattern (20 Hz, 50% duty cycle), muscles became less forceful, slower, and more fatigue resistant. However, their muscle units were still heterogeneous in their properties, suggesting that neuromuscular activity modulates rather than determines muscle phenotype [73].

Normally, all muscle unit fibers "see" the same amount of activity from the common nerve and yet the range in fiber size is 3- to 5-fold [124, 187]. Chronic stimulation did not greatly reduce this range within single MG muscle units but did eliminate differences in size between units, thus dramatically reducing the range of fiber size across the muscle [73]. This reduced range of fiber size is consistent with several different studies of low-frequency stimulation [36, 144, 146, 147]. These data argue strongly that neuromuscular activity modulates, but does not determine muscle fiber size. Similarly, the remaining range in contractile speed and endurance of long-term stimulated motor units also supports the idea that neuromuscular activity modulates muscle phenotype within an adaptive range that is controlled by other factors. This adaptive range may arise from differences in mechanical loading within different regions of the muscle or it may be preset by the developmental origin of the muscle fibers ([5, 79]; see Adaptive Range of Muscle Properties).

It has been suggested that chronic stimulation may change muscle phenotype simply by selective degeneration of fast fibers, followed by satellite cell differentiation to produce the new slow phenotype [99]. This is supported by findings of a 20% reduction in muscle fiber number in chronically stimulated TA muscles, as this proportion corresponds with the proportion of type IIB fibers that do not have the oxidative capacity to adapt to increased neuromuscular activity [122]. The IIB fibers are rapidly depleted of glycogen and many undergo degeneration and are replaced [123]. Slow-to-fast transitions in chronically denervated muscles are similarly accounted for [3, 166] but this is not the case after short-term denervation [79, 82]. Replacement of muscle fibers could not account for change in phenotype of soleus muscles after stimulation because neonatal myosin isoforms were not found in the muscles [5, 79].

Adaptive Range of Muscle Properties
However, fast-twitch muscles of the rat are apparently resistant to transformation to slow phenotype by stimulation, be they denervated or normally innervated [5, 79, 82, 111]. This has been attributed to species differences, the thyroid status of the animal, different mechanical conditions, and/or a restricted adaptive range of muscle properties [79, 95, 104, 147, 193]. It was found that low-frequency stimulation of rat TA and EDL could produce fiber conversion from type IIA to type I if the rats were made hypothyroid, suggesting that normal levels of thyroid hormone in the rat prevent conversion by promoting fast over slow fiber types [104]. Thus, the thyroid status of the smaller mammals could account for the apparent resistance of fast-to-slow conversion of rat fast-twitch muscles, an explanation preferred by these authors to the proposal of Lomo and his colleagues [5, 79, 82, 193] that intrinsic properties of slow- and fast-twitch fibers set an adaptive range within which muscle properties can be modified but not fully converted by neuromuscular activity. However, the thyroid status of rats cannot account for the incomplete slow-to-fast conversion of soleus. Type I to IIA conversion never proceeded to IIB, and fibers continued to express slow MHCs as well as fast MHCs [79]. The fast MHC was later identified as IIx, which is found in FI motor units [5, 112]. The alternative explanation of a restricted adaptive range is based on the developmental origins of slow and fast muscle fibers, in primary and secondary generations, as described later (Development of Muscle Phenotype). Alternatively, tissue-specific differences may determine whether or not genes can be expressed [95]. However, Carraro et al. [23] have demonstrated slow MHCs in denervated fast laryngeal muscles after low-frequency stimulation. It is interesting that fast-to-slow transition is possible under conditions of architecture and mechanical loading different from those of the hindlimb. The phenotypic changes observed in several models of disuse also suggest that mechanical loading is an important factor underlying the wide range of fiber properties within muscles.

MUSCLE PLASTICITY IN MODELS OF DISUSE

The tendency of muscle to express fast phenotype and undergo atrophy in response to "disuse" has generally been attributed to reduced neuromuscular activity after the original observation of slow-to-fast fiber transitions resulting from spinal cord transection or tenotomy [16, 18]. However, the term disuse is more correctly defined as "altered neuronal discharge" [50] because activity is not always eliminated, or even greatly reduced, by such intervention [158]. In addition to any change in activity, paralysis by spinal cord transection results in altered muscle length and loss of weight-bearing function, as is also the case in several other models of disuse including limb immobilization, tenotomy, hind-limb suspension, and spaceflight. Despite the variation in the remaining muscle activity in these models, muscle contractions are generally unloaded suggesting that weight-bearing is an important factor influencing muscle phenotype. Physiological responses to the trauma associated with spinal cord injury, immobilization, and weightlessness may also contribute to the changes.

Sarah Tower [189] introduced the term "disuse atrophy" to describe the dramatic muscle wasting that occurred in paralyzed hindlimbs after spinal cord transection and bilateral deafferentation in the neonatal dog, and to distinguish it from the more rapid and severe denervation atrophy that follows direct injury to the motor nerve. The decline in muscle girth, weight and/or force, and fiber size, which follows muscle paralysis and/or loss of weight-bearing under conditions of spinal cord injury, immobilization, and limb or body suspension, have all been described as disuse atrophy. In human subjects, involvement of lower motoneurons at the injury site often reduces the number of motor units [200] and subsequent muscle wasting will then involve both disuse and denervation atrophy.

Spinal Cord Transection
Increased contractile speed associated with Type I to Type II fiber conversion, reduced endurance, and muscle strength are changes that commonly occur after spinal cord injury, particularly in physiological extensors. Spinal isolation [46, 80, 148], and spinal cord transection [28, 81, 92, 128, 132] or hemisection with or without deafferentation [45, 73], all produce some or all of these changes, irrespective of age. The extent of change varies considerably from study to study, and under different conditions, and does not necessarily correlate with the decline in neuromuscular activity. The slow-to-fast conversion is never complete. In general, postural weight-bearing muscles such as soleus muscle, are the most dramatically affected with respect to contractile speed, force, and muscle atrophy [28, 80, 81, 92, 141, 157, 160], but remain unaffected with respect to endurance [10, 28, 80, 92, 96]. The maintenance of high oxidative enzyme activities and fatigue resistance in paralyzed soleus even after complete elimination of neuromuscular activity is one of the most striking examples of resistance to change. This is reinforced by findings that type I to IIA conversions never proceeded to IIB in any species (cat [10, 28,96]; guinea pig [100]; human [81]). It

appears that glycolytic enzyme activity is more closely linked with neuromuscular activity, increasing in both slow- and fast-twitch muscles after spinal cord transection [10]. Paralyzed fast-twitch muscle becomes more fatigable [73, 141, 176], associated with a decrease in oxidative/glycolytic balance [97].

Qualitatively, the same changes are seen in hindlimb muscles after paralysis by blocking the sciatic nerve with tetrodotoxin (TTX) [172, 173, 179]. However, changes were smaller because of the shorter time course of study. Considerable atrophy also occurs after impulse blockade with maintained pressure [107].

It is interesting that in 1942 Solandt and Magladery [170] introduced their studies of muscle wasting after spinal cord injury with the following statement: "The wasting of paralyzed muscle has been recognized since antiquity. It received mention in the Bible. John Hunter, in his Croonian Lectures (in 1776) stated the fact as one generally familiar." Yet muscle wasting is not an invariant finding. Atrophy is extensive in slow-twitch muscles and in muscles that normally bear weight [28, 81, 100, 141, 157, 192], but is less (5–30%) in fast-twitch extensor muscles [73, 97, 98, 157, 192] and may be negligible in nonweight-bearing muscles, including the physiological flexors [148, 192]. Conclusions that there is a preferential Type II atrophy [100, 157] may be partially explained by the inclusion of converted fibers whose phenotype had changed to Type II but whose size remained small [98]. Similarly, reduced mean force in the FF unit population [73, 128, 132] could be explained by inclusion of less forceful FR units whose endurance had changed but strength remained unaffected. Consistent with this, the population distributions for Type II size, and FF force, were broader than normal but the range and distribution of properties of all fibers and motor units was the same as normal [73]. Where significant atrophy occurred, all muscle fiber and motor unit types were affected [128, 132, 192].

The direction of motor unit and fiber type conversion from S and Type I progressively to FF and Type IIB, respectively, is consistent with the scheme of Kernell [101] in which progressively less daily activity shifts properties from S → FR → FI → FF. Neuromuscular activity is generally reduced after paralysis, with summed EMG activity after spinal transection in cats and kittens reduced to less than 10% of normal [1]. This was the cause even when sufficient muscle activity could be induced to generate hindlimb locomotion and even weight-bearing [120]. To explain the incomplete conversion of Type I to Type II fibers after spinal transection or hemisection, it could be argued that the remaining neuromuscular activity is sufficient to maintain slow phenotype in some fibers. However, this argument cannot explain why many Type I fibers remain in soleus, gastrocnemius, and TA muscles that have been completely silenced by spinal isolation [80, 98, 148], nor why the mean and range of values of unit properties (force, speed, and endurance) in MG and TA muscles were strikingly normal [73, 148], nor why units could readily be classified into the four usual types using the normal criteria [73, 128, 132, 148].

The wide range of motor unit fatigability, histochemical phenotype, and metabolic enzyme activities demonstrated in several hindlimb muscles after substantial reduction or elimination of neuromuscular activity argues strongly that neither amount nor pattern of neuromuscular activity can account for the normal range of motor unit and fiber properties, or for the plasticity after paralysis. Indeed, slow-to-fast conversion and muscle atrophy can be remarkably similar under conditions in which the levels of activity vary substantially, with the converse also holding true: the extent of conversion and atrophy are notably different in different muscles despite very similar levels of EMG activity [157]. For these reasons, factors other than neuromuscular activity must be considered as determinants of muscle properties.

Because fiber conversion and atrophy are most pronounced in paralyzed muscles that normally bear weight and cross a single joint, loss of weight-bearing is likely to be an important contributing factor. In addition, effects associated with change in muscle length are well-recognized complications of muscle paralysis following higher or lower motoneuron disease. Whether the heterogeneity of muscle fibers and motor units can, therefore, be accounted for by differential mechanical loading or whether intrinsic, nerve-independent differences established during development are responsible is not known.

Limb Immobilization
After limb immobilization, muscles may also become faster and show partial Type I to Type II conversion in animals [12, 50, 52, 100, 121, 127, 198] and humans [85], but changes are smaller than after spinal transection. There is little or no change in fatigability even in fast-twitch muscles [127, 154, 197]. However, atrophic changes are particularly dramatic in slow-twitch muscles that act across a single joint [58, 117, 139, 170, 185, 198]. Muscle force, weight, and fiber size decline rapidly within the first 3 weeks of immobilization during which time there are dramatic alterations in protein synthesis and associated morphological changes [9, 137, 170]. Rate of protein synthesis falls within 6 hr of immobilization [13], with a later enhancement of the rate of protein degradation [68]. The greater atrophy of slow-twitch muscles may be partly caused by their more rapid protein turnover as compared to fast-twitch muscles [67].

Generally, there is an inverse relationship between muscle atrophy and the amount of stretch imposed on the immobilized muscle [58, 174]. In shortened immobilization, muscles adjust to the new length by segmental necrosis at the ends of the fibers, with a concomitant breakdown and subsequent reformation of myofibers with proper myofilament overlap and normal sarcomere length within the non-necrotic segment of the fiber [9]. In a shortened position, sarcomeres are removed in parallel as well as in series resulting in decreased muscle cross-sectional area and length [174, 180]. Removal of sarcomeres maintains the tight correlation between bone length and sarcomere number at any given joint angle ensuring optimal overlap between thick and thin filaments for maximal active force at the new joint position [180]. Adjustments in length also occur if the muscle is denervated although active shortening contractions in innervated muscles are associated with greater reductions in sarcomere number [69, 180]. Species differences in susceptibility of the same muscle to shortened immobilization can be explained by differences in the normal resting joint angles. For example, the normal resting ankle angle in the rabbit is 60–70° in comparison with 120° in a rat [12]. Consequently, when the ankle joint is fixed in plantar flexion, the soleus muscle of the rabbit undergoes relatively more shortening than in the rat or cat, and shows a correspondingly more extensive atrophy [139, 170].

Degenerative changes in the fibers may be sufficiently severe to disrupt neuromuscular connections resulting in partial denervation [48, 137]. This can account for the significant numbers of motor nerves that fail to elicit force in the shortened peroneus longus 3 weeks after immobilization [154].

Although Type I to Type II conversion and atrophy have been attributed to reduced activity, EMG analyses show that considerable neuromuscular activity persists after immobilization. Integrated EMG activity may be as low as 5–15% or as high as 50–80% of normal in immobilized soleus muscles [50, 58, 91, 139] and the pattern of discharge becomes more phasic presumably due to the unloading of the muscle spindles [50, 91]. In the flexor muscles EDL and TA, EMG activity was unchanged by immobilization [91, 140].

The procedures that are used to produce limb immobilization have several consequences. First, immobilized muscles can no longer bear weight. Under conditions of immobilization in which muscle length is reduced, unresisted muscle contractions are detrimental, causing significant muscle necrosis and associated loss in muscle bulk and strength (see earlier) similar to the effects of tenotomy [8, 129]. Necrosis that is associated with unresisted shortening contractions can be partly alleviated by reducing neuromuscular activity [129]. Not surprisingly, slow-twitch muscles, which usually contract against a load, are the most sensitive to chronic changes in length [117, 169]. Immobilization-induced Type I to Type II conversion has been attributed to a preferential Type I atrophy and replacement with Type II fibers that may arise through regeneration [12, 58, 85, 100, 174]. However, in the absence of any atrophic change, the opposite conversion, namely Type II to Type I, was found in fast-twitch rabbit TA muscles immobilized in a lengthened position [140]. This demonstrated that immobilization which resisted contractions of the elongated flexor muscles was sufficient to induce slow myosin genes. Thus, under conditions of immobilization, the expression of slow or fast myosin genes can be influenced differentially by resisting or unloading the contractions.

Second, methods of immobilization are generally traumatic themselves or associated with traumatic injury. Procedures such as plaster casting [12, 137], joint pinning [127, 171], or securing an external brace with pins through the bones [50, 58] are stressful. In human patients, casting is most often used to immobilize limbs during the repair of bone fracture or following tendon or ligament injury and repair [169]; both situations are painful and stressful. Physiological responses related to the pain and/or stress, including elevated levels of glucocorticoids, adrenal hypertrophy, and gastric ulcers, have been recorded in animal models and may promote atrophy [185]. Furthermore, glucocorticoid treatment of muscle can induce significant increases in contractile speed [63] it is conceivable that increased circulating glucocorticoids could contribute to the increased numbers of Type II fibers in immobilized muscle, particularly in light of the finding that the number of glucocorticoid receptors rises in immobilized muscles [37].

Reduced Load Bearing: Hindlimb Suspension and Spaceflight
Hindlimb suspension has been used as a model of reduced muscle activity and to simulate the weightlessness of spaceflight [133]. Contraction speed increases concurrent with Type I to Type II fiber conversion and considerable atrophy, particularly in unloaded soleus muscles [30, 51, 52, 133, 182, 185, 196]. Glycolytic enzyme activity increases in both fast and slow extensor muscle but soleus retains a high oxidative capacity in contrast to the fast extensor muscles that become more fatigable [159, 196].

Type I to Type II conversions may be due, at least in part, to preferential atrophy of Type I fibers: up to 80% of myofibrillar proteins are lost in the soleus muscle within 28 days of hindlimb suspension with relatively little effect on sarcoplasmic reticular proteins [185]. Relatively greater degradation of slow myosin [181] contributes to the Type I to Type II conversion in addition to de novo synthesis of fast myosin [185]. During suspension, EMG activity levels return to normal after a transient fall [4] and muscles are not prevented from length changes as in immobilization. Stress-induced changes, such as adrenal hypertrophy, which are attributable mainly to the handling involved in suspending the animals, are found to be transient [185]. Thus, atrophy and phenotypic change are more likely to be directly linked to unresisted contractions of the unloaded muscles.

Similar changes are observed after spaceflight with Type I to Type II fiber conversion apparent in hindlimb muscles of rats subjected to weightlessness aboard Cosmos biosatellite spaceflights [125] and American spacelabs [158]. Clearly, weight-bearing activity is normally an important determinant of slow phenotype and loss of this activity leads to expression of fast genes. Muscle atrophy during 7–12 days of spaceflight was comparable to atrophy in the hindlimb suspension model, particularly for the soleus muscles, although there was little evidence of preferential Type I atrophy within the shorter time course of the spaceflight study. In both cases, considerable degenerative changes were associated with active shortening of muscles that were not resisted by any load. Flexor muscles, which are slightly stretched during suspension and weightlessness, are relatively unaffected despite their high levels of EMG activity [4, 125].

Thus, unresisted shortening is detrimental, similar to the adverse effects of eccentric contractions, which are known to produce extensive muscle damage [49]. Apparently it is not simply reduced neural activity itself, but the contractions of muscles under abnormal mechanical conditions, which may lead to Type I to Type II conversion and disuse atrophy. When Huxley suggested that the pattern of activity may be important in determining muscle contractile properties, he suggested that it was the mechanical vibration of the postural muscles under load that maintained the slow contractile speed, in contrast to the forceful contractions produced at higher frequencies in fast muscles [17]. Data from chronic stimulation experiments and disuse models, which take into account the different loading conditions of muscle fibers, are consistent with this idea, suggesting that the pattern of muscle contraction is a very important factor in determining and maintaining mature muscle phenotype. Nevertheless, the partial retention of original phenotype noted under all of the conditions of plasticity described here has suggested that neuromuscular activity modulates muscle properties within an adaptive range set by intrinsic differences between early and later generations of developing muscle fibers.

DEVELOPMENT OF MUSCLE PHENOTYPE

It has long been recognized that developing muscles are initially slow contracting, and that fast and slow contractile speeds differentiate some time after the muscles become innervated [16, 17, 191]. These findings suggested that differentiation is nerve dependent. More recent studies of the early stages of myogenesis are consistent with a role for innervation. The first generation of muscle fibers, the primary myotubes, express slow MHCs and later generations of cells, the secondary myotubes, express neonatal MHC, the precursor of fast MHCs, and a fast Ca-ATPase when the muscle mass is invaded by motor nerves [26, 31, 34, 60, 134, 161]. In chick, a subgroup of primary myotubes express fast MHC and Ca-ATPase and become fast muscle fibers [60, 178]. Slow nerves are suggested to maintain slow phenotype by upregulating slow isoforms, which are otherwise suppressed [134].

Normally, secondary muscle fibers are generated along the walls of the primary myotubes under the basement membrane [60]. In muscles that lie close to the bone, such as the slow soleus muscle and the small fast ankle flexor muscles, generation of secondary myotubes leads to an intermingled pattern of fast and slow muscle fibers. In the more superficially placed muscles, secondary myotubes are generated primarily in the more superficial regions of the muscle that become predominantly fast regions [26]. Under neural control, the coexpression of slow MHCs with fast MHCs in secondary myotubes is progressively inhibited in the superficial portions of fast-twitch muscles, and may be amplified in the deeper regions to add to the slow muscle fiber population [26, 34, 60, 134].

However, several studies of aneural or paralyzed muscles in embryonic chicks [22, 59] and rats [27] have shown that the characteristic spatial distribution of slow and fast fibers in different muscle compartments, and the intermingling of slow and fast muscle fibers in the typical checkerboard or mosaic pattern can evolve in the absence of the nerve. Under conditions in which muscles were denervated or paralyzed by neural tube extirpation or injection of α-bungarotoxin or curare, the development of primary and secondary myotubes was found to proceed normally, resulting in the expression of slow and fast MHCs in the primary and secondary generations, respectively [27, 59]. However, substantial degeneration of myotubes then occurred, particularly the slow primary myotubes, with reduced generation of secondary myotubes possibly caused by the dependence of the formation of secondary myotubes on primary myotubes [59].

The normal generation of slow and fast fibers in aneural muscle in vivo [22, 27, 59] and in vitro [131] is consistent with intrinsic regulation of phenotype. Thereafter, the survival and maturation of muscle fibers is dependent on innervation and hormones, including thyroxin, which maintain and regulate the adult phenotype within the preset range. In addition, it is possible that the emergence of the unique architecture and function of each muscle during early myogenesis contributes to the expression of fast or slow phenotype in the developing fibers. The slow muscle fibers that are generated along the axis of the bone will be under different mechanical conditions to the second generation of fibers that develop on their walls, and will generally occupy the more superficial regions of most muscles.

CONCLUSION

Skeletal muscles have the capacity to change under many physiological, experimental, and pathological conditions but the diversity of muscle fiber and motor unit properties that is important for muscle function in motor control is retained. Elimination, reduction, or alteration of neuromuscular activity is insufficient to create a homogeneous population of motor units or muscle fibers. Thus, the nerve modulates the properties of the fibers it supplies within a limited or adaptive range, which is partly a function of the muscle's architecture and partly its developmental origin.

Diversity of muscle architecture is well recognized, but largely ignored when considering muscle plasticity. There is increasing evidence for the functional importance of regionalized specialization and structural organization within muscles [47, 62, 118]. The mechanical loading, length, and tension imposed upon different fibers within the same muscle vary according to the position, pinnation, and depth of the muscle. Even under conditions that change the innervation or control the level of neuromuscular activity of all units synchronously, each fiber is constrained by the muscle architecture.

It is clear that mechanical factors are of primary importance in determining and maintaining the diversity of muscle and motor unit properties as plasticity can often be attributed to changes in muscle length and/or loading, in addition to any changes in neuromuscular activity. The influence of length and loading factors will be particularly apparent after experimental manipulations or in clinical conditions that dramatically alter the muscle usage and, thus, the interactions between muscles. Finally, muscle function and plasticity under such conditions must be considered in the context of the whole organism, as factors such as hormonal status and blood flow also contribute to the dynamic nature of muscle, particularly if pain, discomfort, and/or stress are indicated.

ACKNOWLEDGMENTS

Our grateful thanks to the Medical Research Council and Muscular Dystrophy Association of Canada for their support of the work carried out in our laboratory, to the Alberta Heritage Foundation for Medical Research for personal support as an Alberta Heritage Scientist (T.G.) and the Canadian Network of Centers of Excellence for a postdoctoral fellowship (M.C.P.).

REFERENCES

1. Alaimo, M. A., J. L. Smith, R. Roy, and V. R. Edgerton. EMG activity of slow and fast ankle extensors following spinal cord transection. *J. Appl. Physiol.* 56:1608–1613, 1984.
2. Al-Amood, W. S., and D. M. Lewis. The role of frequency in the effects of long-term intermittent stimulation of denervated slow-twitch muscle in the rat. *J. Physiol. (London)* 392:377–395, 1987.
3. Al-Amood, W. S., D. M. Lewis, and H. Schmalbruch. Effect of chronic electrical

stimulation on contractile properties of long-term denervated rat skeletal muscle. *J. Physiol. (London)* 441:243–256, 1991.

4. Alford, E. K., R. R. Roy, J. A. Hodgson, and V. R. Edgerton. Electromyography of rat soleus, medial gastrocnemius, and tibialis anterior during hind-limb suspension. *Exp. Neurol.* 96:635–649, 1989.

5. Ausoni, S., L. Gorza, S. Schiaffino, K. Gundersen, and T. Lömo. Expression of myosin heavy chain isoforms in stimulated fast and slow rat muscles. *J. Neurosci.* 10:153–160, 1990.

6. Bagust, J., and D. M. Lewis. Isometric contractions of motor units in self-reinnervated fast and slow twitch muscles of the cat. *J. Physiol. (London)* 237:91–102, 1974.

7. Bagust, J., D. M. Lewis, and R. A. Westerman. Motor units in cross-reinnervated fast and slow twitch muscles of the cat. *J. Physiol. (London)* 313:223–235, 1981.

8. Baker, J. H. Segmental necrosis in tenotomized muscle fibres. *Muscle Nerve* 6:29–39, 1983.

9. Baker, J. H., and D. E. Matsumoto. Adaptation of skeletal muscle to immobilization in a shortened position. *Muscle Nerve* 11:231–244, 1988.

10. Baldwin, K. M., R. R. Roy, B. Sacks, C. Blanco, and V. R. Edgerton. Relative independence of metabolic enzymes and neuromuscular activity. *J. Appl. Physiol.* 56:1602–1607, 1984.

11. Binder, M. D., and L. M. Mendell (eds.), *The Segmental Motor System.* New York: Oxford University Press, 1990.

12. Booth, F. W., and J. R. Kelso. Effect of hind-limb immobilization on contractile and histochemical properties of skeletal muscle. *Pflügers Arch.* 342:231–238, 1973.

13. Booth, F. W., and M. J. Seider. Early change in skeletal muscle protein synthesis after limb immobilization of rats. *J. Appl. Physiol.* 47:974–977, 1979.

14. Brooke, M. H., and K. K. Kaiser. Three "myosin adenosine triphosphatase" systems: the nature of their pH lability and sulfhydryl dependence. *J. Histochem. Cytochem.* 18:670–672, 1970.

15. Brown, W. E., S. Salmons, and R. G. Whalen. The sequential replacement of myosin subunit isoforms during muscle type transformation induced by long term electrical stimulation. *J. Biol. Chem.* 258:14686–14692, 1983.

16. Buller, A. J., J. C. Eccles, and R. M. Eccles. Differentiation of fast and slow muscles in the cat hind limb. *J. Physiol. London* 150:399–416, 1960.

17. Buller, A. J., J. C. Eccles, and R. M. Eccles. Interactions between motoneurons and muscles in respect of the characteristic speeds of their responses. *J. Physiol.* 150:417–439, 1960.

18. Buller, A. J., and R. Pope. Plasticity in mammalian skeletal muscle. *Philos. Trans. Roy. Soc.,* B 278:295–305, 1977.

19. Burke, R. E. Motor units: anatomy, physiology, and functional organization. J. M. Brookhart and V. B. Mountcastle (eds). *Handbook of Physiology. The Nervous System. Motor Control.* Bethesda, MD: American Physiological Society, Vol. 2, Part 1, Section I, 1981, pp. 345–422.

20. Burke, R. E., and V. R. Edgerton. Motor unit properties and selective involvement in movement. *Exercise Sport Sci. Rev.* 3:31–81, 1975.

21. Burke, R. E., D. N. Levine, P. Tsairis, and F. E. Zajac. Physiological types and histochemical profiles in motor units of the cat gastrocnemius. *J. Physiol. (London).* 234:723–748, 1973.

22. Butler, J. E., E. Cosmos, and J. Brierly. Differentiation of muscle fibre types in aneurogenic brachial muscles of the chick embryo. *J. Exp. Zool.* 224:65–80, 1982.

23. Carraro, U., C. Catani, L. Saggin, et al. Isomyosin changes after functional electrostimulation of denervated sheep muscle. *Muscle Nerve* 11:1016–1028, 1988.

24. Chan M., V. R. Edgerton, G. E. Goslow, Jr., H. Kurata, S. Rasmussen, and S.A.

Spector. Histochemical and physiological properties of cat motor units after self- and cross-reinnervation. *J. Physiol. (London)* 332:343–361, 1982.

25. Close, R. Dynamic properties of mammalian skeletal muscles. *Physiol. Rev.* 32:129–197, 1972.

26. Condon, K., L. Silberstein, H. M. Blau, and W. J. Thompson. Development of muscle fiber types in the prenatal rat hindlimb. *Dev. Biol.* 138:256–274, 1990.

27. Condon, K., L. Silberstein, H. M. Blau, and W. J. Thompson. Differentiation of fiber types in aneural musculature of the prenatal rat hindlimb. *Dev. Biol.* 138:275–295, 1990.

28. Cope, T. C., S. C. Bodine, M. Fournier, and V. R. Edgerton. Soleus motor units in chronic spinal transected cats: physiological and morphological alterations. *J. Neurophysiol.* 55:1202–1220, 1986.

29. Cope, C., and B. D. Clark. Motor-unit recruitment in decerebrate cat: several unit properties are equally good predictors of order. *J. Neurophysiol.* 66:1127–1138, 1991.

30. Corley, K., N. Kowalchuk, and A. J. McComas. Contrasting effects of suspension on hind limb muscles in the hamster. *Exp. Neurol.* 85:30–40, 1984.

31. Crow, M. T., and F. E. Stockdale. Myosin expression and specialization among the earliest muscle fibers of the developing avian limb. *Dev. Biol.* 113:238–254, 1986.

32. Czeh G., R. Gallego, N. Kudo, and M. Kuno. Evidence for the maintenance of motoneurone properties by muscle activity. *J. Physiol. (London)* 281:239–252, 1978.

33. Denny-Brown, D. On the nature of postural reflexes. *Proc. Roy. Soc. (Biol).* 104:252–301, 1929.

34. Dhoot, G. K. Selective synthesis and degradation of slow skeletal myosin heavy chains in developing muscle fibers. *Muscle & Nerve* 9:155–164, 1986.

35. Dhoot, G. K., S. V. Perry, and G. Vrbova. Changes in the distribution of the components of the troponin complex in muscle fibers after cross-innervation. *Exp. Neurol.* 72:513–536, 1981.

36. Donselaar, Y., O. Eerbeek, D. Kernell, and B. A. Verhey. Fibre sizes and histochemical staining characteristics in normal and chronically stimulated fast muscle of cat. *J. Physiol. (London)* 382:237–254, 1987.

37. Dubois, D. C., and R. R. Almon. Disuse atrophy of skeletal muscle is associated with an increase in number of glucocortocoid receptors. *Endocrinology* 107:1649–1651, 1980.

38. Dubowitz, V. Cross-reinnervated mammalian skeletal muscle: histochemical, physiological, and biochemical observations. *J. Physiol. (London)* 193:481–496, 1967.

39. Dubowitz, V., and A. G. E. Pearse. Reciprocal relationship of phosphorylase and oxidative enzymes in skeletal muscle. *Nature* 185:701–702, 1960.

40. Dum, R. P., M. J. O'Donovan, J. Toop, and R. E. Burke. Cross-reinnervated motor units in cat muscle. I. Flexor digitorum longus muscle units reinnervated by soleus motoneurons. *J. Neurophysiol.* 54:818–836, 1985.

41. Dum, R. P., M. J. O'Donovan, J. Toop, P. Tsairis, M. J. Pinter, and R. E. Burke. Cross-reinnervated motor units in cat muscle. II. Soleus muscle reinnervated by flexor digitorum longus motoneurons. *J. Neurophysiol.* 54:837–851, 1985.

42. Dux, L., H. J. Green, and D. Pette. Chronic low-frequency stimulation of rabbit fast-twitch muscle induces partial inactivation of the sarcoplasmic reticulum Ca^{2+}-ATPase and changes in its tryptic cleavage. *Eur. J. Biochem.* 192:95–100, 1990.

43. Edstrom, L., and L. Grimby. Effect of exercise on the motor unit. *Muscle & Nerve* 9:104–126, 1986.

44. Edstrom, L., and E. Kugelberg. Histochemical composition, distribution of fibres and fatigability of single motor units. *J. Neurol. Neurosurg. Psychiat.* 31:424–433, 1968.

45. Eerbeek, O., D. Kernell, and B. A. Verhey. Effects of fast and slow patterns of tonic long-term stimulation on contractile properties of fast muscle in cat. *J. Physiol. (London)* 352:73–90, 1984.

46. Eldridge, L., W. F. H. M. Mommaerts, and D. Pette (eds). *Plasticity of Muscle.* Ability of

electrical silent nerves to specify fast and slow muscle characteristics. Berlin-New York: Walter de Gruyter, 1980, pp. 325–337.

47. English, A. W., and W. D. Letbetter. A histochemical analysis of identified compartments of cat lateral gastrocnemius muscle. *Anat. Rec.* 204:123–130, 1982.

48. Fahim, M. A., and N. Robbins. Remodelling of the neuromuscular junction after subtotal disuse. *Brain Res.* 383:353–356, 1986.

49. Faulkner J. A., D. A. Jones, and J. M. Round. Injury to skeletal muscles of mice by forced lengthening during contractions. *Q. J. Exp. Physiol.* 74:661–670, 1989.

50. Fischbach, G. D., and N. Robbins. Changes in contractile properties of disused soleus muscles. *J. Physiol.* 201:305–320, 1969.

51. Fitts, R. H., C. J. Brimmer, A. Heywood-Cooksey, and R. J. Timmerman. Single muscle fiber enzyme shifts with hindlimb suspension and immobilization. *Am. J. Physiol.* 256:C1082–C1091, 1989.

52. Fitts, R. H., J. M. Metzger, D. A. Riley, and B. R. Unsworth. Models of disuse: a comparison of hindlimb suspension and immobilization. *J. Appl. Physiol.* 60:1946–1953, 1986.

53. Foerhing, R. C., and J. B. Munson. Motoneuron and muscle-unit properties after long-term direct innervation of soleus muscle by medial gastrocnemius nerve in cat. *J. Neurophysiol.* 64:847–861, 1990.

54. Foerhing, R. C., G. W. Sypert, and J. B. Munson. Motor unit properties following cross-reinnervation of cat lateral gastrocnemius and soleus muscles with medial gastrocnemius nerve. I. Influence of motoneurons on muscle. *J. Neurophysiol.* 57:1210–1226, 1987.

55. Foerhing, R. C., G. W. Sypert, and J. B. Munson. Motor unit properties following cross-reinnervation of cat lateral gastrocnemius and soleus muscles with medial gastrocnemius nerve. II. Influence of muscle on motoneurons. *J. Neurophysiol.* 57:1227–1245, 1987.

56. Foerhing, R. C., G. W. Sypert, and J. B. Munson. Properties of self-reinnervated motor units of medial gastrocnemius of cat. I. Long-term reinnervation. *J. Neurophysiol.* 55:931–946, 1986.

57. Foerhing, R. C., G. W. Sypert, and J. B. Munson. Properties of self-reinnervated motor units of medial gastrocnemius of cat. II. Axotomized motoneurons and time course of recovery. *J. Neurophysiol.* 55:947–965, 1986.

58. Fournier, M., R. R. Roy, H. Perham, C. P. Simard, and V. R. Edgerton. Is limb immobilization a model of disuse? *Exp. Neurol.* 80:147–156, 1983.

59. Fredette, B. J., and L. T. Landmesser. A reevaluation of the role of innervation in primary and secondary myogenesis in developing chick muscle. *Dev. Biol.* 143:19–35, 1991.

60. Fredette, B. J., and L. T. Landmesser. Relationship of primary and secondary myogenesis to fiber type development in embryonic chick muscle. *Dev. Biol.* 143:1–18, 1991.

61. Fu, S., T. Gordon, D. J. Parry, and N. Tyreman. Immunohistochemical analysis of fiber types within physiological typed motor units of rat tibialis anterior muscle after long-term cross-reinnervation. *Soc. Neurosci.* 18:1557, 1992.

62. Gans, C., and A. S. Gaunt. Muscle architecture in relation to function. *J. Biomechanics* 24(Suppl 1):53–65, 1991.

63. Gardiner, P. G., D. S. Montanaro, and V. R. Edgerton. Effects of glucocortocoid treatment and food restriction on rat hindlimb muscles. *Pflügers Arch.* 385:147–153, 1980.

64. Gauthier, G. F., R. E. Burke, S. Lowey, and A. W. Hobbs. Myosin isozymes in normal and cross-reinnervated cat skeletal muscle fibers. *J. Cell. Biol.* 97:756–771, 1983.

65. Gillespie, M. J., T. Gordon, and P. R. Murphy. Motor units and histochemistry in rat lateral gastrocnemius and soleus muscles: evidence for dissociation of physiological and histochemical properties after reinnervation. *J. Neurophysiol.* 57:921–937, 1987.

66. Gillespie, M. J., T. Gordon, and P. R. Murphy. Reinnervation of the lateral gastrocnemius and soleus muscles in the rat by their common nerve. *J. Physiol. (London)* 372:485–500, 1986.
67. Goldberg, A. L. Protein synthesis in tonic and phasic skeletal muscles. *Nature* 216:1219–1220, 1967.
68. Goldspink, D. F. The influence of immobilization and stretch on protein turnover of rat skeletal muscle. *J. Physiol. (London)* 264:267–282, 1977.
69. Goldspink, G., C. Tabary, J. C. Tabary, C. Tardieu, and G. Tardieu. Effect of denervation on the adaptation of sarcomere number and muscle extensibility to the functional length of the muscle. *J. Physiol. (London)* 236:733–742, 1974.
70. Gollnick, P. D., and D. R. Hodgson. The identification of fiber types in skeletal muscle: a continual dilemma. *Exer. Sports Sci.* 14:81–104, 1986.
71. Gordon, T. Mechanisms for functional recovery of the larynx after surgical repair of injured nerves. *J. Voice* (in press).
72. Gordon, T. The dependence of peripheral nerves on their target organs. Burnstock, G., G. Vrbova, and R. R. O'Brien (eds). *Somatic and Autonomic Nerve-Muscle Interactions.* New York: Elsevier, 1983, pp. 289–325.
73. Gordon, T., M. C. Pattullo, and V. F. Rafuse. Motor unit heterogeneity with respect to speed and fatiguability in cat muscles after chronic stimulation or paralysis. Sargeant, A. J., and Kernell, D. (eds). *Problems of Neuromuscular Fatigue.* Springer-Verlag (in press).
74. Gordon, T., and R. B. Stein. Reorganization of motor-unit properties in reinnervated muscles of the cat. *J. Neurophysiol.* 48:1175–1190, 1982.
75. Gordon, T., and R. B. Stein. Time course and extent of recovery of reinnervated muscles of the cat. *J. Physiol. (London)* 323:307–323, 1982.
76. Gordon, T., R. B. Stein, and C. K. Thomas. Organization of motor units following cross-reinnervation of antagonistic muscles in the cat hind-limb. *J. Physiol. (London)* 374:443–456, 1986.
77. Gordon, T., C. K. Thomas, R. B. Stein, and S. Erdebil. Comparison of physiological and histochemical properties of motor units after cross-reinnervation of antagonistic muscles in the cat hindlimb. *J. Neurophysiol.* 60:365–378, 1988.
78. Gordon, T., J. Totosy de Zepetnek, V. Rafuse, and S. Erdebil. Motoneuronal branching and motor unit size after complete and partial nerve injuries. A. Wernig (ed). *Motoneuronal Plasticity.* Berlin: Springer Verlag, Ch. 22, 1991, pp. 207–216.
79. Gorza, L., K. Gundersen, T. Lömo, S. Schiaffino, and R. H. Westgaard. Slow-to-fast transformation of denervated soleus muscles by chronic high-frequency stimulation in the rat. *J. Physiol. (London)* 402:627–649, 1988.
80. Graham, S. C., R. R. Roy, C. Navarro, B. Jiang, D. Pierotti, S. Bodine-Fowler, and V. R. Edgerton. Enzyme and size profiles in chronically inactive cat soleus muscle fibers. *Muscle Nerve* 15:27–36, 1992.
81. Grimby, G., C. Broberg, I. Krotkiewska, and M. Krotkiewski. Muscle fiber composition in patients with traumatic cord lesion. *Scand. J. Rehab. Med.* 8:37–42, 1976.
82. Gundersen, K., E. Leberer, T. Lömo, D. Pette, and R. S. Staron. Fibre types, calcium-sequestering proteins and metabolic enzymes in denervated and chronically stimulated muscles of the rat. *J. Physiol. (London)* 398:177–189, 1988.
83. Guth, L. "Trophic" influences of nerve on muscle. *Physiol. Rev.* 48:645–687, 1968.
84. Guth, L., and F. J. Samaha. Procedure for the histochemical demonstration of actomyosin ATPase. *Exp. Neurol.* 28:365–367, 1970.
85. Haggmark, T., E. Eriksson, and E. Jansson. Muscle fiber type changes in human skeletal muscle after injuries and immobilization. *Orthopedics* 9:181–185, 1986.
86. Härtner, K.-T., B. J. Kirschbaum, and D. Pette. The multiplicity of troponin T isoforms. Normal rabbit muscles and effects of chronic stimulation. *Eur. J. Biochem.* 179:31–38, 1989.

87. Härtner, K.-T., and D. Pette. Effects of chronic low-frequency stimulation on troponin I and troponin C isoforms in rabbit fast-twitch muscle. *Eur. J. Biochem.* 188:261–267, 1990.

88. Henneman, E., and L. M. Mendell. Functional organization of the motoneurone pool and its inputs. V. B. Brooks and S. R. Geiger (eds). *Handbook of Physiology.* Section I. *The Nervous System.* Vol. 2. *Motor Control.* Part I. Bethesda, MD: American Physiological Society, 1981, pp. 423–508.

89. Henneman, E., and C. B. Olson. Relations between the structure and function in the design of skeletal muscles. *J. Neurophysiol.* 28:581–598, 1965.

90. Hennig, R., and T. Lomo. Firing patterns of motor units in normal rats. *Nature* 314:164–166, 1985.

91. Hnik, P., R. Vejsada, D. F. Goldspink, S. Kasicki, and I. Krekule. Quantitative evaluation of electromyogram activity in rat extensor and flexor muscles immobilized at different lengths. *Exp. Neurol.* 88:515–528, 1985.

92. Hoffmann, S. J., R. R. Roy, C. E. Bianco, and V. R. Edgerton. Enzyme profiles of single muscle fibers in the absence of normal neuromuscular activity. *J. Appl. Physiol.* 69:1150–1158, 1990.

93. Hudlicka, O. Development of microcirculation: capillary growth and adaptation. E. M. Renkin, C. C. Michel, and S. R. Geiger (eds). *Handbook of Physiology.* Section 2. *The Cardiovascular System.* Bethesda MD: American Physiological Society, 1984, pp. 165–216.

94. Hudlicka, O., K. R. Tyler, T. Srihari, A. Heilig, and D. Pette. The effect of different patterns of long-term stimulation on contractile properties and myosin light chains in rabbit fast muscles. *Pflügers Arch.* 393:164–170, 1982.

95. Izumo, S., B. Nadal-Ginard, and V. Mahdavi. All members of the MHC multigene family respond to thyroid hormone in a highly tissue-specific manner. *Science* 231:597–600, 1986.

96. Jiang, B., R. R. Roy, and V. R. Edgerton. Expression of a fast fiber enzyme profile in the cat soleus after spinalization. *Muscle Nerve* 13:1037–1049, 1990.

97. Jiang, B., R. R. Roy, and V. R. Edgerton. Enzymatic plasticity of medial gastrocnemius fibers in the adult chronic spinal cat. *Am. J. Physiol.* 259:C507–C514, 1990.

98. Jiang, B., R. R. Roy, C. Navarro, Q. Nguyen, D. Pierotti, and V. R. Edgerton. Enzymatic responses of cat medial gastrocnemius fibers to chronic inactivity. *J. Appl. Physiol.* 70:231–239, 1991.

99. Jolesz, F., and F. A. Sreter. Development, innervation and activity-pattern induced changes in skeletal muscle. *Ann. Rev. Physiol.* 43:531–552, 1981.

100. Karpati, G., and W. K. Engel. Correlative histochemical study of skeletal muscle after suprasegmental denervation, peripheral nerve section and skeletal fixation. *Neurology* 18:681–692, 1968.

101. Kernell, D. Organized variability in the neuromuscular system: a survey of task-related adaptations. *Arch. Ital. de Biol.,* 130:19–66, 1992.

102. Kernell, D., Y. Donselaar, and O. Eerbeek. Effects of physiological amounts of high- and low-rate chronic stimulation on fast-twitch muscle of the cat hindlimb. II. Endurance-related properties. *J. Neurophysiol.* 58:614–627, 1987.

103. Kernell, D., O. Eerbeek, B. A. Verhey, and Y. Donselaar. Effects of physiological amounts of high- and low-rate chronic stimulation on fast-twitch muscle of the cat hindlimb. I. Speed and force-related properties. *J. Neurophysiol.* 58:598–613, 1987.

104. Kirschbaum, B. J., H.-B. Kucher, A. Termin, A. M. Kelly, and D. Pette. Antagonistic effects of chronic low frequency stimulation and thyroid hormone on myosin expression in rat fast-twitch muscle. *J. Biol. Chem.* 265:13974–13980, 1990.

105. Kirschbaum, B. J., J.-A. Simoneau, A. Bär, P. J. R. Barton, M. E. Buckingham, and D. Pette. Chronic stimulation-induced changes of myosin light chains at the mRNA and protein levels in rat fast-twitch muscle. *Eur. J. Biochem.* 179:23–29, 1989.

106. Klug, G. A., E. Leberer, E. Leisner, J.-A. Simoneau, and D. Pette. Relationship between parvalbumin content and the speed of relaxation in chronically stimulated rabbit fast-twitch muscle. *Pflügers Arch.* 411:126–131, 1988.

107. Kowalchuk, N., and A. McComas. Effects of impulse blockade on the contractile properties of rat skeletal muscle. *J. Physiol.* 382:255–266, 1987.

108. Kugelberg, E., and B. Lindegren. Transmission and contraction fatigue of rat motor units in relation to succinate dehydrogenase activity of motor unit fibres. *J. Physiol. (London)* 288:285–300, 1979.

109. Kugelberg, E., L. Edstrom, and M. Abruzzese. Mapping of motor units in experimentally reinnervated rat muscle. *J. Neurol. Neurosurg. Psychiat.* 33:310–329, 1970.

110. Kuno, M., Y. Miyato, and E. J. Munoz-Martinez. Properties of fast and slow alpha-motoneurons following motor reinnervation. *J. Physiol. (London)* 242:273–288, 1974.

111. Kwong, W. H., and G. Vrbova. Effects of low-frequency electrical stimulation on fast and slow muscles of the rat. *Pflügers Arch.* 391:200–207, 1981.

112. Larsson, L., L. Edstrom, B. Lindergren, L. Gorza, and S. Schiaffino. MHC composition and enzyme-histochemical and physiological properties of a novel fast-twitch motor unit type. *Am. J. Physiol.* 261:C93–C101, 1991.

113. Leberer, E., U. Seedorf, and D. Pette. Neural control of gene expression in skeletal muscle Ca-sequestering proteins in developing and chronically stimulated rabbit skeletal muscles. *Biochem. J.* 239:295–300, 1986.

114. Lewis, D. M. Mammalian motor units. R. E. Davidoff (ed). *Handbook of the Spinal Cord.* New York: Dekker, 1984, pp. 269–314.

115. Lewis, D. M., J. Bagust, S. A. Webb, R. A. Westerman, and H. J. Finol. Axon conduction velocity modified by reinnervation of mammalian muscle. *Nature (London)* 270:745–746, 1977.

116. Lewis, D. M., A. Rowlerson, and S. Webb. Motor units and immunohistochemistry of cat soleus muscle after long periods of cross-reinnervation. *J. Physiol. (London)* 325:395–403, 1982.

117. Lieber, R. L., J. O. Friden, A. R. Hargens, L. A. Danzig, and D. H. Gershuni. Differential response of the dog quadriceps muscle to external skeletal fixation of the knee. *Muscle Nerve* 11:193–201, 1988.

118. Loeb, G. E., and F. J. R. Richmond. Architectural features of muscles with more than one action. *Proc. VIIth Eur. Soc. Biomech.* 245–247, 1992.

119. Lomo, T., R. H. Westgaard, and D. H. Dahl. Contractile properties of muscle: control by pattern of muscle activity in the rat. *Proc. Roy. Soc. B. (London)* 187:99–103, 1974.

120. Lovely, R. G., R. J. Gregor, R. R. Roy, and V. R. Edgerton. Effects of training on the recovery of full-weight-bearing stepping in the adult spinal cat. *Exp. Neurol.* 92:421–435, 1986.

121. Maier, A., J. L. Crockett, D. R. Simpson, C. W. Saubert IV, and V. R. Edgerton. Properties of immobilized guinea pig hindlimb muscles. *Am. J. Physiol.* 231:1520–1526, 1976.

122. Maier, A., B. Gambke, and D. Pette. Degeneration-regeneration as a mechanism contributing to the fast to slow conversion of chronically stimulated fast-twitch rabbit muscle. *Cell Tissue Res.* 244:635–643, 1986.

123. Maier, A., and D. Pette. The time course of glycogen depletion in single fibers of chronically stimulated rabbit fast twitch muscle. *Pflügers Arch.* 408:338–342, 1987.

124. Martin, T. P., S. C. Bodine-Fowler, R. R. Roy, E. Eldred, and V. R. Edgerton. Metabolic and fiber size properties of cat tibialis anterior motor units. *Am. J. Physiol.* 255:C43–C50, 1988.

125. Martin, T. P., V. R. Edgerton, and R. E. Grindeland. Influence of spaceflight on rat skeletal muscle. *J. Appl. Physiol.* 65:2318–2325, 1988.

126. Martin, T. P., R. B. Stein, P. H. Hoeppner, and D. C. Reid. Influence of electrical

stimulation on the morphological and metabolic properties of paralyzed muscle. *J. Appl. Physiol.* 72:1401–1406, 1992.

127. Mayer, R. F., R. E. Burke, J. Toop, J. A. Hodgson, K. Kanda, and B. Walmsley. The effect of long-term immobilization on the motor unit population of the cat medial gastrocnemius muscle. *Neuroscience* 6:725–739, 1981.

128. Mayer, R. F., R. E. Burke, J. Toop, B. Walmsley, and J. A. Hodgson. The effect of spinal cord transection on motor units in cat medial gastrocnemius muscles. *Muscle Nerve* 7:23–31, 1984.

129. McMinn, R. M. H., and G. Vrbova. Motoneurone activity as a cause of degeneration in the soleus muscle of the rabbit. *Q. J. Exp. Physiol.* 52:411–415, 1967.

130. McPhedran, A. M., R. B. Wuerker, and E. Henneman. Properties of motor units in a homogeneous red muscle (soleus) of the cat. *J. Neurophysiol.* 28:71–84, 1965.

131. Miller, J. B., and F. E. Stockdale. Developmental regulation of the multiple myogenic cell lineages of the avian embryo. *J. Cell. Biol.* 103:2197–2208, 1986.

132. Munson, J. B., R. C. Foerhing, S. A. Loften, J. E. Zengel, and G. W. Sypert. Plasticity of medial gastrocnemius motor units following cordotomy in the cat. *J. Neurophysiol.* 55:619–634, 1986.

133. Musacchia, X. J., J. M. Steffen, and D. R. Deavers. Rat hindlimb muscle responses to suspension hypokinesia/hypodynamia. *Aviat. Space Environ. Med.* 54:1015–1020, 1983.

134. Narusawa, M., R. B. Fitzsimons, S. Izumo, B. Nadal-Ginard, N. A. Rubinstein, and A. M. Kelly. Slow myosin in developing rat muscle. *J. Cell. Biol.* 104:447–459, 1987.

135. Nemeth, P., D. Pette, and G. Vrbova. Comparison of enzyme activities among single muscle fibres within defined motor units. *J. Physiol.* 311:489–495, 1981.

136. Nemeth, P.M., L. Solanki, D. A. Bordon, T. M. Hamm, R. M. Reinking, and D. G. Stuart. Uniformity of metabolic enzymes within individual motor units. *J. Neurosci.* 6:892–898, 1986.

137. Pachter, B. R., and A. Eberstein. Neuromuscular plasticity following limb immobilization. *J. Neurocytol.* 13:1013–1025, 1984.

138. Parry, D. J., and R. S. Wilkinson. The effect of reinnervation on the distribution of muscle fibre types in the tibialis anterior muscle of the mouse. *Can. J. Physiol. Pharmacol.* 68:595–602, 1990.

139. Pattullo, M. C. *The role of activity in the determination of skeletal muscle properties.* Ph.D. thesis, University of Aberdeen, Scotland, UK, 1989.

140. Pattullo, M. C., M. A. Cotter, N. E. Cameron, and J. A. Barry. Effects of lengthened immobilization of functional and histochemical properties of rabbit tibialis anterior muscle. *Exp. Physiol.* 77:433–442, 1992.

141. Peckham, P. H., J. T. Mortimer, and E. B. Marsolais. Alteration in the force and fatiguability of skeletal muscle in quadriplegic humans following exercise induced by chronic electrical stimulation. *Clin. Orthop.* 114:326–333, 1976.

142. Peter, J. B., R. J. Barnard, V. R. Edgerton, C. A. Gillespie, and K. E. Stempel. Metabolic profiles of three types of skeletal muscle in guinea pigs and rabbits. *Biochemistry* 11: 2627–2633, 1972.

143. Pette, D., and S. Düsterhöft. Altered gene expression in fast-twitch muscle induced by chronic low-frequency stimulation. *Am. J. Physiol.* 262:R333–R338, 1992.

144. Pette, D., W. Muller, E. Leisner, and G. Vrbova. Time dependent effects on contractile properties, fibre population, myosin light chains and enzymes of energy metabolism in intermittently and continuously stimulated fast twitch muscles of the rabbit. *Pflugers Arch.* 364:103–112, 1976.

145. Pette, D., and R. S. Staron. Cellular and molecular diversities of mammalian skeletal muscle fibers. *Rev. Physiol. Biochem. Pharmacol.* 116:1–76, 1990.

146. Pette, D., and G. Vrbova. Invited review: neural control of phenotypic expression in mammalian muscle fiber. *Muscle Nerve* 8:676–689, 1985.

147. Pette, D., and G. Vrbova. Adaptation of mammalian skeletal muscle to chronic electrical stimulation. *Rev. Physiol. Biochem. and Pharmacol.* 120:115–202, 1992.

148. Pierotti, D. J., R. R. Roy, S. C. Bodine-Fowler, J. A. Hodgson, and V. R. Edgerton. Mechanical and morphological properties of chronically inactive cat tibialis anterior motor units. *J. Physiol. (London)* 444:175–192, 1991.

149. Pullen, A. H. The distribution and relative sizes of three histochemical fibre types in the rat tibialis anterior muscle. *J. Anat.* 123:1–19, 1977.

150. Rafuse, V. Regulation of motor unit size after nerve injuries. Ph.D. Thesis, University of Alberta, Edmonton, Alberta, Canada, 1993.

151. Rafuse, V., T. Gordon, and R. Orozco. Proportional sprouting in partially denervated triceps surae muscles in the cat. *J. Neurophysiol.* 68:1261–1276, 1992.

152. Ranvier, L. Properties et structures differentes des muscles rouges et des muscles blanc chez les lapins et chez les raies. *C.R. Hebd. Seances Mem. Soc. Biol.* 77:1030–1034, 1873.

153. Robbins, N., G. Karpati, and W. K. Engel. Histochemical and contractile properties in the cross-reinnervated guinea pig soleus muscle. *Arch Neurol.* 20:218–329, 1969.

154. Robinson, G. A., R. M. Enoka, and D. G. Stuart. Immobilization-induced changes in motor unit force and fatigability in the cat. *Muscle Nerve* 14:563–573, 1991.

155. Romanul, F. C. A. Enzymes in muscle. I. Histochemical studies of enzymes in individual muscle fibres. *Arch. Neurol.* 11:355–368, 1964.

156. Romanul, F. C. A., and J. P. Van der Meulen. Slow and fast muscles after cross reinnervation. Enzymatic and physiological changes. *Arch. Neurol.* 17:387–402, 1967.

157. Roy, R. R., and L. Acosta, Jr. Fiber type and fiber size changes in selected thigh muscles six months after low thoracic spinal cord transection in adult cats: exercise effects. *Exp. Neurol.* 92:675–685, 1986.

158. Roy, R. R., K. M. Baldwin, and V. R. Edgerton. The plasticity of skeletal muscle: effects of neuromuscular activity. *Exer. Sports Sci. Rev.,* 19:269–312, 1992.

159. Roy, R. R., M. A. Bello, P. Bouissou, and V. R. Edgerton. Size and metabolic properties of fibers in rat fast-twitch muscles after hindlimb suspension. *J. Appl. Physiol.* 62:2348–2357, 1987.

160. Roy, H, R. D. Sacks, K. M. Baldwin, M. Short, and V. R. Edgerton. Interrelationships of contraction time, Vmax, and myosin ATPase after spinal transection. *J. Appl. Physiol.* 56:1594–1601, 1984.

161. Rubinstein, N. A., and A. M. Kelly. Development of muscle fiber specialisation in the rat hindlimb. *J. Cell Biol.* 90:128–144, 1981.

162. Salmons, S., and J. Henriksson. The adaptive response of skeletal muscle to increased use. *Muscle Nerve* 4:94–105, 1981.

163. Salmons S., and F. A. Sreter. Significance of impulse activity in the transformation of skeletal muscle type. *Nature* 263:30–34, 1976.

164. Salmons S., and G. Vrbova. The influence of activity on some contractile characteristics of mammalian fast and slow muscles. *J. Physiol.* 201:535–549, 1969.

165. Saltin, B., and P. D. Gollnick. Skeletal muscle adaptability: significance for metabolism and performance. L. D. Peachey (ed). *Handbook of Physiology. Skeletal Muscle. Specialization, Adaptation, and Disease.* Bethesda, MD: American Physiological Society, 1983, pp. 555–631.

166. Schmalbruch, H., W. S. Al-Amood, and D. M. Lewis. Morphology of long-term denervated rat soleus muscle and the effect of chronic electrical stimulation. *J. Physiol. (London)* 441:233–242, 1991.

167. Sherrington, C. The correlation of reflexes and the principle of the common final path. *Brit. Assoc. Rep.* 74:728–741, 1904.

168. Simoneau, J.-A., M. Kaufmann, K.-T Härtner, and D. Pette. Relations between chronic stimulation-induced changes in contractile properties and the Ca^{2+}-sequestering system of rat and rabbit fast-twitch muscles. *Pflügers Arch.* 414:629–633, 1989.

169. Sjostrom, M., A. Fugl-Meyer, and L. Wahlby. Achilles tendon injury: plantar flexion

strength and structure of soleus muscle after surgical repair. *Acta Chir. Scand.* 144:219–226, 1978.

170. Sjostrom, M., L. Wahlby, and A. Fugl-Meyer. Achilles tendon injury. III. Structure of rabbit soleus muscles after immobilization at different positions. *Acta Chir. Scand.* 145:509–521, 1979.

171. Solandt, D. Y., Partridge, R, and Hunter, J. The effect of skeletal fixation on skeletal muscle. *J. Neurophysiol.* 6:17–22, 1943.

172. Spector, S. A. Effects of elimination of activity on contractile and histochemical properties of rat soleus muscle. *J. Neurosci.* 5:2177–2188, 1985.

173. Spector, S. A. Trophic effects on the contractile and histochemical properties of rat soleus muscle. *J. Neurosci.* 5:2189–2196, 1985.

174. Spector, S. A., C. P. Simard, M. Fournier, E. Sternlicht, and V. R. Edgerton. Architectural alternations of rat hind-limb muscles immobilized at different lengths. *Exp. Neurol.* 76:94–110, 1982.

175. Sreter, F. A., A. R. Luff, and J. Gergely. Effect of cross-reinnervation on physiological parameters and on properties of myosin and sarcoplasmic reticulum of fast and slow muscles of the rabbit. *J. Gen. Physiol.* 66:811–821, 1976.

176. Stein, R. B., T. Gordon, J. Jefferson, A. Sharfenberger, J. Yang, J. E. Totosy de Zepetnek, and M. Belanger. Optimal stimulation of paralyzed muscle in spinal cord patients. *J. Appl. Physiol.* 72:1393–1400, 1992.

177. Stein, R. B., T. Gordon, and J. E. Totosy de Zepetnek. Mechanisms for respecifying muscle properties following reinnervation. L. Mendell and M. D. Binder (eds). *The Segmental Motor System.* London: Oxford University Press, 1990, pp. 278–288.

178. Stockdale, F. E., and J. B. Miller. The cellular basis of myosin heavy chain isoform expression during development of avian skeletal muscles. *Dev. Biol.* 123:1–9, 1987.

179. St-Pierre, D., and P. Gardiner. Effect of "disuse" on mammalian fast-twitch muscle: joint fixation compared to neurally applied tetrodotoxin. *Exp. Neurol.* 90:635–651, 1985.

180. Tabary, J. C., C. Tabary, C. Tardieu, G. Tardieu, and G. Goldspink. Physiological and structural changes in the cat's soleus muscle due to immobilization at different lengths by plaster casts. *J. Physiol.* 224:231–244, 1972.

181. Templeton, G., M. Padalino, J. Manton, T. Leconey, H. Halger, and M. Glasberg. The influence of rat suspension-hypokinesia on the gastrocnemius muscle. *Aviat. Space Environ. Med.* 55:381–386, 1984.

182. Templeton, G. H., H. L. Sweeney, B. F. Timson, M. Padalino, and G. A. Dudenhoeffer. Changes in fiber composition of soleus muscle during hindlimb suspension. *J. Appl. Physiol.* 65:1191–1195, 1988.

183. Termin, A., R. S. Staron, and D. Pette. Changes in myosin heavy chain isoforms during chronic low frequency stimulation of rat fast hindlimb muscles—a single fiber study. *Eur. J. Biochem.* 186:749–754, 1989b.

184. Thomas, C. K., R. B. Stein, T. Gordon, R. Lee, and G. Elleker. Patterns of reinnervation and motor unit recruitment in human hand muscles after complete ulnar and median nerve section and resuture. *J. Neurol. Neurosurg. Psychiatr.,* 50:259–268, 1987.

185. Thomason, D. B., and F. W. Booth. Atrophy of the soleus muscle by hindlimb unweighting. *J. Appl. Physiol.* 68:1–12, 1990.

186. Totosy de Zepetnek, J. E., T. Gordon, R. B. Stein, and H. V. Zung. Comparison of force and emg measures in normal and reinnervated tibialis anterior muscles of the rat. *Can. J. Physiol. Pharmacol.* 69:1774–1783, 1991.

187. Totosy de Zepetnek, J., H. V. Zung, S. Erdebil, and T. Gordon. Innervation ratio is an important determinant of force in normal and reinnervated rat tibialis anterior muscle. *J. Neurophysiol.* 67:1385–1403, 1992.

188. Totosy de Zepetnek, J. E., H. V. Zung, S. Erdebil, and T. Gordon. Motor unit

categorization based on contractile and histochemical properties: a glycogen depletion analysis of normal and reinnervated rat tibialis anterior muscle. *J. Neurophysiol.* 67:1404–1415, 1992.

189. Tower, S. S. Function and structure in the chronically isolated lumbo-sacral spinal cord of the dog. *J. Comp. Neurol.* 67:109–131, 1937.

190. Vrbova, G. The effect of motoneurone activity on the speed of contraction of striated muscle. *J. Physiol. (London)* 169:513–526, 1963.

191. Vrbova, G., T. Gordon, and R. Jones. *Nerve-Muscle Interaction.* London: Chapman & Hall, 1978.

192. West, S. P., R. R. Roy, and V. R. Edgerton. Fiber type and fiber size of cat ankle, knee, and hip extensors and flexors following low thoracic spinal cord transection at an early age. *Exp. Neurol.* 91:174–182, 1986.

193. Westgaard, R. H., and T. Lömo. Control of contractile properties within adaptive ranges by patterns of impulse activity in the rat. *J. Neurosci.* 8:4415–4426, 1988.

194. Williams, R. S., S. Salmons, E. A. Newsholme, R. E. Kaufman, and J. Mellor. Regulation of nuclear and mitochondrial gene expression by contractile activity in skeletal muscle. *J. Biol. Chem.* 261:376–380, 1986.

195. Williams, S. R., M. Garcia-Moll, J. Mellor, S. Salmons, and W. Harlan. Adaptation of skeletal muscle to increased contractile activity. Expression of nuclear genes encoding mitochondrial proteins. *J. Biol. Chem.* 262:2764–2767, 1987.

196. Winiarski, A. M., R. R. Roy, E. K. Alford, P. C. Chiang, and V. R. Edgerton. Mechanical properties of rat skeletal muscle after hind limb suspension. *Exp. Neurol.* 96:650–660, 1987.

197. Witzmann, F. A., D. H. Kim, and R. H. Fitts. Effect of hindlimb immobilization on the fatiguability of skeletal muscle. *J. Appl. Physiol.* 54:1242–1248, 1983.

198. Witzmann, F. A., D. H. Kim, and R. H. Fitts. Hindlimb immobilization: length-tension and contractile properties of skeletal muscle. *J. Appl. Physiol.* 53:335–345, 1982.

199. Wuerker, R. B., A. M. McPhedran, and E. Henneman. Properties of motor units in a heterogeneous pale muscle (m. gastrocnemius) of the cat. *J. Neurophysiol.* 28:85–99, 1965.

200. Yang, J. F, R. B. Stein, J. Jhamandas, and T. Gordon. Motor unit numbers and contractile properties after spinal cord injury. *Ann. Neurol.* 28:496–502, 1990.

12
Exercise and Weight Control

MARCIA L. STEFANICK, Ph.D.

INTRODUCTION

The first and second National Health and Nutrition Examination Surveys (NHANES-I and NHANES-II), conducted in the United States from 1971–1974 [67] and 1976–1980 [68], respectively, provided much of the overwhelming evidence of the adverse effects of obesity on health presented at the February 1985 National Institutes of Health (NIH) Consensus Development Conference on the Health Implications of Obesity [72]. The adverse effects of obesity, defined as excess body fat, include an excess of certain cancers and several of the major risk factors for coronary heart disease (CHD), including hypertension, hyper-cholesterolemia, and noninsulin-dependent diabetes mellitus, which has made it difficult to determine the direct relationship of obesity to CHD. Severe obesity, defined as being more than 30% above ideal body weight, was identified as an independent risk factor for CHD in the National Cholesterol Education Program (NCEP) Adult Treatment Guidelines, released by the National Heart, Lung and Blood Institute in 1987 [71], but even mild-to-moderate obesity was associated with a substantial elevation in risk of CHD, after controlling for other CHD risk factors, in over 100,000 middle-aged women followed for 8 yr in the Nurses' Health Study [64].

One of the confounding factors in the relationship of obesity to disease arises from differences in risk attributed to the regional distribution of excess body fat. Deposition of fat in the abdominal region is associated with a greater incidence of metabolic abnormalities and disease risk, including the incidence of CHD, than deposition in the gluteal and/or femoral region in both men and women, as determined by the ratio of waist girth to hip and/or thigh circumference, particularly with increasing obesity [56, 58, 59, 105].

Although a sedentary life-style is not listed among CHD risk factors in the 1987 NCEP guidelines, the Committee on Exercise and Cardiac Rehabilitation of the American Heart Association's Council on Clinical Cardiology recognized physical inactivity as a risk factor for coronary artery disease in a recent position statement and acknowledged that regular aerobic activity plays a role in both primary and secondary prevention of cardiovascular disease [29]. These conclusions followed critical evaluation [83] of several epidemiological and prospective studies, primarily of men, including the Harvard Alumni Study [79], the Multiple Risk Factor Intervention Trial (MRFIT [61]), and the Lipid Research Clinics (LRC) Mortality Follow-up Study [27], as well as a prospective study of fitness assessed by maximal treadmill exercise tests of 10,224 men and 3120 women [10]. Death caused by cancer was also related to inactivity [10, 79].

EXTENT OF THE PROBLEM

If obesity and inactivity affect the risk for heart disease and other chronic diseases independently, it is important to understand the prevalence of these life-style parameters.

Prevalence of Obesity

Data from NHANES-II revealed that 24.2% of men and 27.1% of women, aged 20–74 yr were overweight, defined as a body mass index (BMI—weight/height^2 as kg/m^2) $\geq$ the 85th percentile values of BMI distributions for men and women aged 20–29 yr, or BMI $\geq$ 27.8 kg/m^2 for men and BMI $\geq$ 27.3 kg/m^2 for women [57]. Men and women, 8% and 10.8%, respectively, were determined to be severely overweight, defined as BMI $\geq$ the 95th percentile of men and women aged 20–29 yr, or BMI $\geq$ 31.1 kg/m^2 for men and BMI $\geq$ 32.3 kg/m^2 for women. This totaled 34 million overweight adults, 12.5 million of whom were severely over-weight, in the United States alone. (Persons aged 20–29 yr are used as the reference group with the reasoning that no further increases in stature occur after this decade and most excess weight gain is associated with accumulation of adipose tissue.) It is likely that the prevalence of obesity, i.e., having excess body fat, is greater than the prevalence of overweight, since many individuals, particularly women, complete growth and accumulate considerable adipose tissue before age 20 yr.

Two major height and weight surveys were conducted in the Minneapolis-St. Paul metropolitan area; the first, in 1973–1974, in a sample of 1724 men and 1890 women, aged 25–59 yr, and the second in 1980–1981, in a sample of 913 men and 1024 women, aged 25–74 yr [41]. The prevalence of overweight, defined as BMI $\geq$ 27 kg/m^2 for men and BMI $\geq$ 26 kg/m^2 for women, increased significantly in men older than 40 yr whereas increases in younger men and women across all age ranges were not significant. Although prevalence of obesity did not change in women and younger men in this population, it is likely that most individuals who were overweight in the earlier survey remained overweight and may have gained further weight, thereby further increasing their risk for obesity-related disorders. The 10-yr incidence of major weight gain ($\geq$ 5 kg/m^2) by individuals in the U.S. population, as determined by the NHANES-I Epidemiologic Follow-up Study conducted in 1982–1984 [69], was twice as high in women as in men aged 25–74 yr, and major weight gain was highest in women aged 25–34 yr, compared with all sex-age groups [118]. Initial weight status predicted weight gain, and women aged 25–44 yr who were overweight initially, had the highest incidence (14.2%) of further gain.

Greater percentages of minority groups, especially minority women, are afflicted with obesity. Age-adjusted percentages of overweight and severely overweight Caucasian women (24.6% and 9.6%, respectively) were generally lower than corresponding percentages for African American (45.1% and 19.7%), Mexican (41.5% and 16.7%), Cuban (31.9% and 6.9%), and Puerto Rican (39.8% and 15.2%) women [57]. The differences among non-Caucasian ethnic groups is primarily because of the prevalence of severe overweight, as approximately 25% of each group met the criterion for overweight, but not for severely overweight; the corresponding percentile of overweight, but not severely overweight Caucasian women is 15%.

Prevalence of a Sedentary Life-style
Assessing physical activity in population-based surveys is a challenging task, as discussed in a recent document produced by the National Center for Health Statistics, during the developmental phase of the proposed 1988–1994 National Health and Nutrition Examination Survey (NHANES III [70]). Researchers have relied on a number of instruments, ranging from a few selected questions to detailed questionnaires, and occasionally, physical fitness measures. The response of 2319 men and 2067 women, all Caucasian, in the LRC North American Prevalence Study to two questions concerning performance of strenuous physical activity, revealed that 64.5% of men and 84% of women were inactive and only 29% of men and 12% of women did strenuous exercise or physical labor at least three times per week [35]. The remainder reported less regular exercise and younger males and females reported more activity than their older counterparts. In the Iowa Women's Health Study, a longitudinal cohort study of the relationship of body mass and fat distribution to cancer incidence, 47% of 40,980 women, aged 55–69 yr, reported a low activity level, 28% reported medium activity, and 25% reported high activity levels in response to two questions on frequency of moderate and vigorous leisure time physical activity [42].

Of 738 men and 878 women aged 25–74 yr surveyed in the Minnesota Heart Study, only 34% of men and 17% of women expended 2000 kcal or more per week in leisure time activity, as determined by the Minnesota Leisure Time Physical Activity (LTPA) questionnaire, which also showed that energy expenditure, especially heavy intensity activity, declined with age, especially in women [30]. A modified version of the LTPA questionnaire was used in the Framingham Offspring Study of

1598 men and 1762 women aged 20–69 yr, to reveal that only about 25% of men and 10% of women were expending more than 2000 kcal/week; as might be expected, LTPA showed substantial seasonal variation, being much greater in the summer than in winter [17]. In the northern California communities studied in the Stanford Five-City Project, the majority of 1006 men and 1120 women aged 20–74 yr reported some moderate activity in a physical activity recall interview covering the previous 7-day period; however, 75% of the men and 92% of the women reported no vigorous activity (6 METS), and virtually none of them practiced more than two vigorous activities regularly [91].

Epidemiological Relationships Between Weight Status and Activity Level
Because obesity and a sedentary life-style are highly prevalent in the U.S., the degree of overlap, interactions, and possible cause-and-effect nature of these two major health risks are of great interest to medical researchers and health promoters. What proportion of the millions of obese individuals are also inactive and what proportion of the millions of sedentary individuals are also obese? Unfortunately, it is difficult to tease apart the relationships between obesity and activity level in most epidemiological studies, largely because of the absence of adequate assessment of physical activity (including type, duration, and frequency) and of measures that provide information on body fat and lean body mass (such as skinfolds or hydrostatic weight data), or regional adiposity (such as the waist-to-hip ratio [WHR]). Interpretation of the data is further confounded by effects of dietary factors, which pose an equally challenging assessment task in free-living populations, particularly if ethnic foods are commonly consumed.

Unfortunately, even when measures of physical activity and obesity status have been made in the same individual, the overlap and relationship between these parameters are often not reported; but rather, the interaction of these parameters is presented only in relationship to a disease outcome [10, 61, 79]. LTPA, determined by a questionnaire patterned after the Minnesota LTPA questionnaire, was not associated with BMI (kg/m^2) in 1160 Caucasian men, 1150 Black men, 1300 Caucasian women or 1425 Black women in the Coronary Artery Risk Development in Young Adults (CARDIA) study, but activity was inversely associated with skinfold measures and the WHR in all groups, except Caucasian women [98]. Black women reported significantly less total, moderate, and intense activity and also had higher BMIs, individual and sum of skinfold thicknesses, and WHR than Caucasian women, whereas no such differences were seen between Black and Caucasian men [98]. Black women were also shown to be much less active and much more obese than Caucasian women in the smaller Pittsburgh Healthy Women Study sample of 48 Black and 490 Caucasian women, despite no difference in caloric intake between groups, as assessed by a 24-hour dietary recall [121].

In the Stanford Five-City Project, kcal expended per kg of total body weight per day, estimated from the 7-day physical activity recall, did not differ across BMI categories in women or men, nor was there any relationship between BMI and moderate or vigorous activity during the 7-day period prior to testing [91]. In contrast, greater high-intensity activity was associated with lower BMI in men and women in the Minnesota Heart Study, while BMI was not related to total kcal expended per day [30]. In the 40,980 women studied in the Iowa Women's Health Study, both BMI and WHR were negatively related to leisure time physical activity, as determined by two questions on frequency of moderate and vigorous activity [42]. A strong negative relationship between physical activity and BMI was also reported in the Nurses' Health Study in a sample of 141 women who completed a questionnaire similar to the Harvard Alumni Activity Survey [88]. These women also completed a food-frequency questionnaire, which showed that estimated energy intake was not related to BMI but was positively related to physical activity.

It is unclear whether disparities among studies arise from differences in activity assessment, population characteristics, or other factors; however, the observations collectively suggest that there are more overweight and/or obese individuals among sedentary study participants and/or more active individuals among the lean or less overweight participants. It is unclear how these samples compare to the general population; therefore, physical activity data collected in NHANES-III will be very valuable. Epidemiological data on physical activity and obesity across various age groups and in minority populations are also much needed.

It cannot be determined from cross-sectional observations whether activity causes leanness and/or inactivity causes obesity, or whether weight status influences activity level, or whether these associations are coincidental to genetic, behavioral, or other factors that predispose some individuals to a leaner body habitus and higher activity level and others to obesity and inactivity. Prospective studies might shed light on these questions and also provide information on the proportions of the population that respond one way or another to exercise, weight loss, or other behavioral changes, as well as the relationship of such changes to disease outcomes. It would be particularly valuable to know whether increasing the proportion of active individuals (and decreasing the proportion of inactive individuals) in the population would reduce the prevalence of obesity, and/or the incidence of chronic diseases associated with obesity, as well as those associated with a sedentary status. It could also be asked whether reducing the proportion of obese individuals, by whatever means, would bring about a more active population, and whether obese active individuals are clearly at lower risk for chronic disease than inactive obese people.

When weight changes were studied prospectively in 485 middle-aged women in the Pittsburgh Healthy Women Study, baseline activity level was associated with 3-yr weight change, with the greatest weight gains in those who had the lowest exercise levels at baseline; furthermore, a significant association was seen between decreases in exercise and increases in body weight across the 3 yr [122]. Weight changes in 571 men after 2 yr of participation in the Adelaide 1000 health and fitness program were significantly related to fitness changes, based on heart rate/workload relationships during a bicycle ergometer test; however, weight and fitness changes were not related in 430 women studied [94].

ROLE OF ACTIVITY LEVEL IN DETERMINING WEIGHT STATUS

The scope of the problem of obesity is vast and the influence of regular exercise on weight control is complex. It is frequently asked whether obesity is caused by overeating, inactivity, or a metabolic defect, but it is generally agreed that obesity occurs when energy intake chronically exceeds energy expenditure [96]. Kraemer et al. [52, 53] presented common methodological problems that lead to research inconsistencies in the answer to this question: (*a*) a lack of a precise and consistent conceptual definition of what is meant by obesity; (*b*) an inconsistent application of criteria to assess the quality of measures of obesity; (*c*) the frequent reporting of research results in terms of characteristics that are inferred from what was measured or observed, rather than what was actually measured or observed; (*d*) the fact that research designs are rarely based on an understanding of the normal developmental patterns of obesity in childhood and adolescence and the individual patterns of response to treatment; and (*e*) the fact that poor measurements frequently obscure individual differences in patterns, either developmental patterns or patterns of responses to treatments.

In the first volume of *Exercise and Sports Sciences Reviews* 20 yr ago, Oscai reviewed early studies of the role of exercise in weight control, with a primary focus on landmark studies of laboratory animals designed to shed further light on observations reported for humans [76]. Data were presented to dispel the concepts that the amount of exercise needed to change caloric balance is too great to be of practical use and that exercise is accompanied by a corresponding rise in appetite and food intake that impairs weight reduction. Exercise was reported to affect body composition favorably, by promoting loss of body fat and protecting against loss of lean mass. Oscai proposed that a decrease in physical activity may lead to the development of obesity, and that exercise may be effective in preventing weight gain and maintaining weight loss.

At least three major reviews on exercise and obesity or body composition appeared in the early 1980s. Epstein and Wing [28] reviewed the role of activity level in determining body weight and made several conclusions based on a meta-analysis of 13 studies of males, totaling 37 groups, 12 of which were no-treatment control groups, and three studies of women, totaling four groups, none of which were control groups. The analytic sample included studies that: (*a*) had at least five individuals per group; (*b*) provided pre- and postweights; (*c*) allowed calculation of energy expenditures by specifying exercise parameters; (*d*) excluded subjects who were not sedentary before the program; and (*e*) did not involve a planned diet. Duration of the study was not a factor. The authors concluded that overweight persons were more characterized by underexercising than by overeating; that exercise (without a planned diet) was associated with greater weight and fat loss than not exercising; that heavy persons lose more weight at the same exercise level than light persons, although the exercise effect was independent of initial weight; and that rate of weight loss was strongly related to number of exercise sessions per week or weekly caloric expenditure. Analysis of these studies suggested that people did not lose as much weight as might be expected from the amount of exercise reported and that exercise usually produced relatively slow weight loss, compared with dietary strategies.

Thompson et al. [106] concluded in their 1982 review of exercise and obesity that the roles of activity level and caloric intake in the development of obesity could not be determined, because of a failure to make a distinction between overweight subjects in *dynamic* and *static* phases of weight gain in observational studies and because of methodological problems in research studies, including: (*a*) failure to use body composition measures as dependent variables; (*b*) failure to report specifics regarding exercise tasks and participation rates; and (*c*) failure to divide subjects into homogeneous populations based on qualitative aspects of body fat type. The energy expenditure associated with the direct effect of exercise on metabolic rate was reported to depend on type, duration, and intensity of the activity, as was that associated with the indirect effect on metabolic rate subsequent to the activity. The wide variability reported across studies for this excess postexercise energy expenditure was considered to be caused by variability in exercise tasks and individual body composition, weight status, and fitness levels. Thompson et al. also concluded that exercise offsets the consistently reported reduction in basal metabolic rate (BMR) with caloric deprivation, but considered the effect of exercise on diet-induced thermogenesis to be unclear. In discussing intervention strategies, the authors emphasized that only minor body composition changes were found if the exercise program was of less than 3 months in duration.

Wilmore [119] reviewed relative weights of athletic men and women for a large number of sports and athletic groups and tabulated the results of 55 studies of body composition changes with physical training, which, in summary, showed moderate losses in total body weight, moderate-to-large losses in body fat, and small-to-moderate increases in lean body weight. The amplitude of these alterations varied directly with the frequency, intensity, and duration of the activity bout, as well as with the duration of the study. Wilmore also reviewed the literature on the effect of exercise on appetite, focusing on possible anorexigenic effects of exercise, following observations that male, but not female, rats showed appetite suppression with high-intensity work. The issue of possible sex differences in the exercise effect on appetite in humans could not be resolved with available studies, and the independent influences of initial body composition (which could underlie sex differences), exercise prescription, or diet composition were not discussed.

The past decade of research on exercise and weight control has generated studies in several major areas including: (*a*) fat metabolism and adaptations of muscle and fat tissue to exercise training, (*b*) multiple components of daily energy expenditure that may be affected by acute and chronic exercise; (*c*) body composition changes associated with exercise-induced weight loss; and (*d*) interactions between exercise and diet (both caloric intake and relative contributions from fat, carbohydrate, and protein) during weight loss.

Metabolism of Fat During and Subsequent to Exercise

What is the physiological rationale to support the notion that exercise could bring about loss of excess body fat and/or serve to maintain weight loss and/or prevent accumulation of excess adipose tissue over time? From the moment physical activity is initiated, fuel requirements of working muscle increase significantly from rest. The role of fat metabolism in exercise is of major interest, since fat is our most abundant energy reserve, with 1 lb of fat supplying enough energy to support about 30 miles of walking or running. This efficiency must be considered when one initiates the task of reducing fat weight by dieting or exercising. Fat weight loss may be slow, relative to weight loss strategies aimed at total weight, in which loss of water and stored carbohydrate or protein may occur quickly; on the other hand, it also takes longer to regain lost fat mass than it does to regain losses of lean body mass, although the time course of replacing lost muscle mass is unclear. Relevant issues addressed in this section include the use of fatty acids as a fuel source during and subsequent to an exercise bout, training-induced changes in adipose tissue, and the selective response of regional adipose tissue depots to exercise. The recent review of physical activity and lipid (and lipoprotein) metabolism lists further references [99].

FATTY ACIDS AS A FUEL SOURCE FOR AEROBIC EXERCISE. Fat utilization is under coordinated metabolic control and can only occur under aerobic conditions. To utilize lipids (fats) as fuel, muscles must take up, activate, and translocate free fatty acids (FFA) into mitochondria (to supply acetyl coenzyme A to the citric acid cycle). Oxidation of FFA is determined by the capacity of tissues to oxidize FFA and the availability of FFA. Sources of FFA include circulating FFA (which are released into the blood from adipose tissue, following hydrolysis of triglycerides by hormone-sensitive lipase); intramuscular triglycerides (which are hydrolyzed within muscle fibers); and circulating triglycerides (which are hydrolyzed on the surface of the muscle capillary endothelium by lipoprotein lipase [LPL]).

After an initial brief anaerobic phase followed by a phase of high glucose oxidation, fat is oxidized in progressively increasing amounts; consequently, lipids may cover up to 90% of the oxidative metabolism in prolonged exercise of moderate intensity (less than 50% of maximal oxygen intake, $\dot{V}o_2max$), as evidenced by a decrease in the respiratory exchange ratio (R-value). At high-intensity work (greater than 70% $\dot{V}o_2max$), fat is used in decreasing amounts and glycogen becomes the predominant energy source, as reflected by an increasing R-value. (Fat combustion corresponds to an R-value of 0.7; while glucose combustion has an R-value of 1.00. A typical resting R-value is 0.80–0.85.) Maximizing fatty acid consumption, therefore, involves exercising below the threshold at which glucose starts replacing fatty acid as fuel.

One of the adaptations that characterizes the trained state is an even greater reliance on FFA oxidation during submaximal exercise, as seen in a leg trained by bicycle exercise relative to the untrained leg of the same individual [37]. There is evidence that the proportion of energy derived from fatty acids steadily increases with increasing duration of a bout of exercise at a fixed work rate [123], suggesting that a single bout of long duration may be more beneficial in terms of fatty acid consumption than the same amount of exercise accumulated through several bouts of short duration [2].

It would be desirable to determine the optimal type, regimen, and intensity of exercise that would maximize oxidation of fatty acids for a sustained period, so that stored body fat is used as fuel during exercise in large enough quantities to bring about substantial fat loss. Shephard [97] and Andrews [2] each argued that an active life-style must be pursued systematically and that an exercise program must be sustained for months and years, rather than days and weeks, to bring about substantial fat weight loss. This is partially because many physiological adaptations that improve utilization of fat as fuel, discussed later, require a certain amount of time to become effective, but of greater significance is the fact that fat is a very efficient fuel, containing a high energy reserve per unit weight.

Even a lean athlete has tremendous energy reserves in stored fat. Because work done is a function of the total amount of weight that has to be carried, not the amount of lean or fat weight [95], this arrangement is clearly ideal; however, the consequence is that excess fat is depleted only slowly.

Investigations of the effect of gender on exercise substrate have yielded conflicting results, possibly because of differences in maximum oxygen consumption and training status (frequency and duration of training and weekly mileage) of subjects, and probably also because of differences in body composition. Several studies suggest that men and women who are equally trained derive similar fractions of energy from lipids. This was shown during treadmill running at 70% $\dot{V}O_2$max when $\dot{V}O_2$max values and muscle fiber composition were matched between the sexes [14]. No differences were seen in FFA increases or progressive (and significant) glycerol rises during a 15.5-km run at 65% $\dot{V}O_2$max between men and women matched for training status; however, women had significantly lower R-values than men and these differences appeared to result from less glycogen utilization by the women [102]. Nor were differences seen in FFA and glycerol increases during graded treadmill tests between similarly trained men and women, both of whom had significantly greater glycerol increases and lower FFA:glycerol ratios than men and women who were not endurance trained [32].

Capacity of Muscle Tissues to Oxidize Free Fatty Acids. Both cardiac and skeletal muscle are metabolically oxidative. Type I, "slow-twitch" (slow oxidative, SO) red, and Type IIa, "fast-twitch" (fast oxidative, FO) pink, skeletal muscle fibers have a greater oxidative capacity than Type IIb, "fast-twitch" (fast glycolytic, FG) white skeletal muscle fibers; therefore, the relative amount of SO and FO vs. FG muscle fiber contributes to an individual's ability to utilize fat metabolism. SO fibers are mainly activated during exercise of moderate intensity. Training has been shown to increase the proportion of SO and FO fibers, at the expense of the FG fibers [9], thereby increasing the oxidative capacity of the tissue. Training also leads to increases in mitochondrial number and size, particularly in the SO fibers, resulting in increased concentrations of enzymes for the citric acid cycle and electron transfer system [90], as well as for fatty acid oxidation [46]. The point at which muscles switch from fatty oxidation to anaerobic metabolism of glucose also increases with training, both absolutely and as a percentage of maximum capacity [2]. Increased endurance permits longer exercise bouts, which further promotes fat utilization.

Availability of Free Fatty Acids for Oxidation. Lipolysis and Mobilization from Adipose Tissue. The concentration of FFA in the blood is quite low at rest and relatively little fat is stored in muscle; therefore, lipids must be mobilized and transported to the working muscle. Between one-third and one-half of the fat that is oxidized during exercise comes from FFA liberated from adipose tissue by lipolysis. In human adipose tissue, which possesses stimulatory β-adrenoceptors and inhibitory α-adrenoceptors, norepinephrine and epinephrine are the principal lipolytic hormones; the only antilipolytic hormone of physiological importance is insulin. Acute exercise leads to increased sympathoadrenal activity and decreased insulin levels, thereby stimulating the activity of a hormone-sensitive lipase (HSL) in adipose tissue, which brings about hydrolysis of stored triglycerides, i.e., lipolysis. Liberated FFA are bound to plasma albumin and transported to active muscles in the blood. (HSL catalyzes the degradation of triacylglycerol to diacylglycerol and monoacylglycerol; whereas the hydrolysis of the third fatty acid is catalyzed by a specific monoacylglycerol lipase.) Glycerol formed by lipolysis cannot be reutilized in adipose tissue (because of low concentrations of the enzyme α-glycerokinase); therefore, the rate of lipolysis in adipose tissue can be estimated from plasma glycerol production.

Utilization of Intramuscular Lipid Stores. A small amount of fat is also stored as lipid droplets within the cytosol of muscle cells and/or between muscle fibers. An intracellular lipase is believed to mobilize FFA from these intramuscular triglyceride (TG) stores in response to exercise, depending on intensity [77]; thereby leading to a decreased muscle TG content. Intramuscular lipid stores were shown to be quantitatively larger in physically well-trained than untrained men at rest, but to be more reduced in the well-trained subjects following prolonged heavy exercise [63]. The reduction in quadriceps muscle TG concentrations after prolonged exercise were decreased even further in men after a strenuous 12-week program of endurance exercise training, relative to the untrained state [40]. This effect appears to be specific to the trained muscle as evidenced by the greater release of glycerol from the quadriceps muscle of a single leg trained by dynamic knee extensions, compared to the leg that served as the nontrained control [45]. Further evidence of the use of intramuscular TG during exercise appeared with the observation that lipid oxidation was decreased only 50% during exercise after complete inhibition of lipolysis by a nicotinic acid analogue, acipimox [117]. Increased hydrolysis of TG within the trained muscle could partially account for increased lipid utilization observed during exercise in trained vs. untrained muscle.

Utilization of Plasma Triglycerides. Dietary fatty acids are esterified and transported as TG in plasma chylomicrons and very low density lipoproteins (VLDL), which are metabolized into higher density lipoproteins through the action of LPL. LPL hydrolyzes circulating triglycerides, thereby reducing TG levels, so FFA can be taken up by muscle fibers, to be oxidized or re-esterified and stored within muscle tissue, or by adipocytes, to be re-esterified and stored in adipose tissue. (LPL is synthesized in cardiac and skeletal muscle cells, particularly in red [SO] fibers, as well as in adipocytes and cells of other tissues, then secreted and localized on the luminal surface of capillary endothelial cells.)

Following cross-sectional observations that endurance-trained men and women had higher skeletal muscle LPL activity than sedentary controls [75], a prolonged, exhaustive exercise bout (85-km 8-hour ski race) was shown to be followed by a 3-fold average increase in muscle LPL activity [63] and a 20-km run in the fasting state was shown to increase skeletal muscle LPL 2-fold [103]. Muscle LPL activity was also increased in men for at least 12 hr after days of heavy work during a 10-day march with heavy packs, and it decreased after days of rest [62]. Eight weeks of endurance training on cycle ergometers increased resting muscle LPL activity in sedentary, normal weight men [101] and the single-leg training model showed significant increases in skeletal muscle LPL activity of the quadriceps muscle of the leg trained by dynamic knee extensions vs. the untrained leg [45]. Endurance training also increased the activity of adipose tissue LPL, with a significant positive correlation between LPL changes and average weekly running mileage [73]. Cessation of exercise for 10 days in highly trained men significantly reduced postheparin plasma LPL activity [107]. Worth noting is that LPL activity of sprinters with nonendurance (power) training has been shown not to differ from sedentary controls [73].

Increased LPL activity in both skeletal muscle and adipose tissue following training would serve to decrease circulating plasma TG levels in trained individuals. It is well known that TG levels are generally much lower in trained individuals than sedentary controls [34]. Nonetheless, circulating TGs have not been shown to play a major role as a lipid source during exercise in the fasting state. TG levels were unchanged up to 4 hr after a marathon (42-km) run in trained male runners, in whom free glycerol levels were elevated five-fold immediately after the race, but TG levels were significantly reduced 18, 42, and 66 hr afterward [108]. In a study in which one leg was trained by dynamic knee extensions, a markedly higher arteriovenous VLDL-TG difference was seen in the trained thigh at rest, vs. the untrained leg, demonstrating greater VLDL-TG uptake in this leg; yet, a consistent degradation of VLDL-TG was not found during exercise with the trained thigh [45]. The quadriceps muscle of the trained leg showed significant increases with training in skeletal muscle LPL activity, relative to the untrained leg. The fact that VLDL-TG was taken up during the resting period, but not during the exercise bout, suggested to the authors that circulating TG may be more important in repleting intramuscular TG stores than in supplying a FFA source during exercise. High-fat diets were also shown to increase skeletal muscle LPL activity and TG concentration in quadriceps muscles of trained men [44]. Whether plasma TGs are utilized as a fuel source for exercise or as a means to replete intramuscular fat stores, the important implication here is that increased uptake of TGs by muscle precludes their being stored in adipose tissue.

In contrast to studies conducted on fasting individuals, a 45-minute bout of moderate intensity exercise enhanced the clearance of TGs in people with normal as well as elevated fasting TG levels after they ingested a fat-containing meal [74]. The clearance rate of exogenous fat increased 75% and fasting TG levels decreased 26% less than 24 hr after a marathon run by elite athletes, relative to before the race [89] and endurance training increased TG disappearance following intravenous administration of fat by 24% after 14 weeks and 49% after 32–48 weeks [109]. Therefore, in a postprandial state, the circulating TG pool represents a relatively rich source of lipid substrate for oxidation during exercise, particularly in trained individuals; however, this reduces the utilization of fatty acids liberated from adipose tissue. Consequently, a high-fat diet would reduce exercise-induced loss of fat weight.

Further Adaptations of Adipose Tissue to Exercise Training. Following the observation that suprailiac adipose cells of lean, highly trained runners had higher epinephrine-stimulated lipolysis (ESL) than sedentary controls [22], a similar enhanced lipolytic response was reported in suprailiac adipocytes of initially sedentary men and women who underwent a 20-week endurance training program, relative to individuals who remained sedentary throughout this period [19]. ESL of the 11 trained men responded better than that of 11 trained women and the males lost significant body fat, which was characterized by a decrease in mean fat cell size, with no decreases in cell number; whereas no such changes were seen in the women studied. Increased sensitivity of subcutaneous adipose tissue to the lipolytic action of catecholamines in trained vs. sedentary women was confirmed by others, who suggested that the differences were caused by functional differences in both the α_2-adrenergic and β-adrenergic pathways [16, 87].

Decreased fat cell size accompanied similar changes in body fat in 13 other men who underwent a similar 20-week training program [18]. Bjorntorp reported similar findings and provided evidence that hypertrophic (enlarged) fat cells may respond more favorably to an exercise intervention than hyperplastic adipose tissue, which is characterized by an increased number of adipocytes [9]. One's history of weight gain, which influences whether increased fat mass is characterized by increased fat cell size or increased fat cell number, may therefore play a role in the effectiveness of exercise for weight loss.

DIFFERENTIAL RESPONSES OF REGIONAL ADIPOSE TISSUE DEPOTS TO EXERCISE. The two largest fatty regions in humans are the subcutaneous and intra-abdominal (or "visceral") fat depots. The degree of obesity associated with excess subcutaneous fat has generally been studied by measuring skinfold thicknesses at specified body sites. It is well-recognized that women generally deposit subcutaneous fat at different sites than men do, such as the thighs, buttocks, and upper arms, vs. the abdominal region and torso in men. The subscapular-to-triceps skinfold ratio (STR) has been used to distinguish "peripheral" or "extremity" adiposity (low STR), often associated with a female-type "gynoid" pattern, from "central" or "truncal" obesity (high STR), generally associated with a male-type "android" pattern [111]. Waist and hip circumferences also provide relative information on excess storage of fat in the central area and the WHR has been used to distinguish "abdominal" (often linked to the android pattern) from "gluteal-femoral" (linked to the gynoid pattern) adiposity. WHR partially estimates intra-abdominal (visceral) depots, but also includes subcutaneous fat. In recent years, several noninvasive methods have been employed to distinguish intra-abdominal and subcutaneous depots, such as computed axial tomography (CAT) and magnetic resonance imaging (MRI) revealing, among other things, that men tend to have a greater ratio of intra-abdominal to subcutaneous abdominal fat than women [6].

There is mounting evidence that the regulation of intra-abdominal and subcutaneous fat depots differ, as does regulation among subcutaneous fat depots. Subcutaneous abdominal adipocytes have been shown to be four to five times more responsive to norepinephrine than gluteal fat cells [115]. Before a 1-week fast, lipolytic activity of femoral fat was 35% lower, while LPL activity was 20% higher, than in abdominal subcutaneous tissue; however, femoral lipolytic activity increased and LPL activity decreased to levels similar to abdominal fat during the fast [3]. Before fasting, femoral fat cells were 13% larger than abdominal cells; decreases in abdominal fat cell size during the fast increased this difference to 20%. Catecholamines have been shown to be more lipolytic in omental than in subcutaneous fat cells [26, 78] and omental fat is also less responsive to the antilipolytic effect of insulin than subcutaneous fat [11].

Arner et al. demonstrated that (bicycle) exercise mobilized fatty acid release from adipose tissue in the abdominal region more readily than in the gluteal area and these regional differences were more pronounced in women than men [4]. In addition to differential lipolytic responses, adipose tissue LPL activity has been shown to be higher in abdominal subcutaneous than gluteal adipose tissue in men, whereas the opposite was observed in women [5], for whom reproductive hormone status has been shown to relate to the activity of both femoral and subcutaneous abdominal adipose tissue LPL, and also the lipolytic responsiveness of these depots to catecholamines and insulin [85, 86].

Aerobic exercise training to bring about weight loss has been shown to result in greater mobilization of trunk fat than extremity fat in men, based on skinfolds [18]. An intensive 6-month endurance training program resulted in significant decrements, determined by CT, in intra-abdominal and abdominal subcutaneous fat depots in 13 young and 15 older men, although WHR improved only in the older men, who were shown to have two-fold greater intra-abdominal fat depot and about one-half the subcutaneous thigh fat of the younger men at baseline [93]. Greater loss of deep abdominal fat compared with midthigh adipose tissue was also seen by CT in obese premenopausal women after 14 months of training [21]. WHR was significantly reduced in moderately overweight men and premenopausal women, aged 25–49 yr, who exercised while adopting a low-fat diet, vs. controls, and these reductions were significantly greater in the men, relative to men who adopted the diet without exercise [126]. Changes in WHR over a 3-yr period were also significantly correlated with changes in activity in 108 women in the Healthy Women Study, and upper body fat distribution was associated with low exercise level [121].

Cross-sectional observations of 74 young and 200 older sedentary men and women and 59 young and 44 older endurance-trained men and women suggested that people who exercise regularly may accumulate less adipose tissue in upper, central body regions as they get older, than do their sedentary counterparts [50]. In support of this hypothesis, exercise training reduced skinfold thicknesses and waist and hip circumferences in 60- to 70-year-old women and men, who also lost fat weight, with no loss of lean weight after a 9- to 12-month exercise program; differences between sexes were not significant [51].

It has been suggested that women with a male distribution of fat may benefit more from exercise for weight reduction than do women who deposit fat in the more resistant gluteal and thigh areas, possibly due to preferential lipolysis of intra-abdominal fat with stimulation of the sympathetic nervous system during exercise [55]. It follows that obese men may benefit more from exercise training than women, in general. This may explain why individual changes in fatness over the course of a 20-week aerobic training correlated with the initial level of fat indices in 14 men, who reduced body fat and fat cell size, but not in 14 women [110]. It would be valuable to determine whether such sex differences would be seen if the sample included a majority of women with an android fat pattern. Further studies will be needed to determine the role of baseline regional fat distribution in the success of exercise-induced weight loss in men and women at various ages.

HEPATIC LIPID METABOLISM IN EXERCISE. Visceral fat cells have a unique position and relationship to the portal circulation, which means the liver is directly exposed to the lipolytic products of visceral adipocytes, whereas lipolysis in subcutaneous adipose tissue releases fatty acids into the systemic circulation. The significance of this has not been investigated. The liver is virtually the only organ of the body that produces ketone bodies, which generally occurs during periods of increased fatty acid oxidation. The concentration of plasma ketone bodies increases during prolonged exercise, presumably because of the abundant delivery of FFA to the liver, and continues to increase for several hours of the postexercise recovery period; however, this elevation is less pronounced in trained vs. untrained individuals, both during and after exercise [33].

Liver parenchymal cells synthesize a unique hepatic triglyceride lipase (HTGL), which can be studied following release from hepatic capillaries by heparin infusion. Postheparin HTGL activity correlated positively with intra-abdominal fat deposition, independent of total adiposity in obese women [20]. Postheparin HTGL activity was significantly reduced in 44 initially sedentary overweight men who were randomly assigned to a 1-yr exercise program with no dietary changes, vs. 41 controls; changes in HTGL activity were significantly related to changes in total and fat weight, which were also significant vs. control [100]. It is worth noting that 39 men assigned in the same study to weight loss by caloric restriction, with no change in diet composition or activity level, showed similar significant reductions in HTGL activity vs. controls. A 14-month training program also decreased postheparin HTGL activity in 13 obese premenopausal women; however, changes in HTGL activity were not related to total or abdominal fat loss in this sample [21].

Effects of Exercise on Daily Energy Expenditure
Recognizing that it is fat weight loss that should be the goal of a weight loss program, an expenditure (or deficit) of approximately 3000 calories above one's normal daily energy expenditure (or below one's normal caloric intake) is required for each pound of fat to be lost. If fat loss were to be achieved solely through the direct energy cost associated with increased physical exercise, a person must be committed to expending these calories over a reasonable period of time, with respect to his/her weight loss goal. The common argument that an inordinate quantity of activity is necessary to achieve weight loss seems to reflect a certain impatience on the part of the person who desires to lose the weight, since as little as one mile of walking a day (roughly 15–20 minutes of effort) would bring about more than 5 kg (11 lb) of fat weight loss over the course of a year, assuming one does not consume excess calories or expend less energy in the remaining 23.7 hr of the day. As previously suggested, it may be more cost-effective to engage in less frequent, longer duration exercise bouts, to utilize fatty acids maximally, and thereby promote fat weight loss. Mode and intensity of exercise are other important variables to consider with respect to the use of fat to meet any energy requirements.

The energy expenditure of physical activity includes the energy expended above the resting metabolic rate (RMR), i.e., that energy expenditure required to maintain normal physiological processes during rest in a postabsorptive state, the sleeping metabolic rate (SMR), and the thermic effect of food (TEF). The energy expenditure resulting from physical activity is highly variable and includes energy output associated with such muscular activities as fidgeting and shivering. In a sedentary individual, physical activity constitutes approximately 15% of total daily expenditure, whereas in individuals who engage in regular exercise, the contribution may increase to above 30% of daily energy output. Metabolic rate during exercise can increase up to 20 times above resting levels; therefore, it seems obvious that if a person were to engage in exercise regularly without increasing caloric intake appreciably, weight loss should occur. However, many individuals in clinical studies report that they have not increased food intake, but are not losing weight with exercise. Investigators interested in the etiology of obesity have focused attention on spontaneous activity, or fidgeting, thermoregulation, and other components of daily energy expenditure, in an attempt to resolve this apparent paradox.

POSTEXERCISE OXYGEN CONSUMPTION. One of these components is the postexercise metabolic rate, often referred to as the excess postexercise oxygen consumption (EPOC). Poehlman et al. [82] recently reviewed and tabulated studies that examined the effect of acute exercise on postexercise energy expenditure and concluded that prolonged submaximal exercise of moderate to high intensity along with meal ingestion during the postexercise period may result in elevation of metabolic rate for up to 24 hr after exercise, the magnitude and duration of which are related to both intensity and duration of the exercise bout. They predicted, however, that an exercise prescription which consists of exercise of low ($< 50\%$ $\dot{V}O_2$max) or moderate intensity (50–75% $\dot{V}O_2$max) would likely elevate the postexercise energy expenditure by only 9–30 kcal/bout, unless the bout was of long duration (80 minutes or longer), and would therefore probably not influence body weight significantly. The authors recognized, however, that there could be long-term implications of even such a small excess expenditure.

RESTING METABOLIC RATE. RMR constitutes about 60–75% of total daily energy expenditure in a sedentary human. RMR was shown to be higher in aerobically trained men, when expressed per kilogram of fat-free weight [81] and 3-day suspension of exercise training reduced RMR in nine trained women [38] and eight athletes of unspecified sex [11]; however, considerable controversy remains over the degree of the influence of exercise on RMR. Poehlman [81] recently outlined several methodological variations of investigators that contribute to the discrepant findings: timing of indirect calorimetry relative to last exercise bout; differences in intensity and duration of exercise training programs; mode of exercise (e.g., swimming vs. running); gender and other genetic differences of individuals studied; and changes in body composition. Insufficient sample size and statistical power to detect differences in RMR that vary by aerobic fitness and within subject variability because of preceding dietary practices were included among the reasons that cross-sectional studies do not provide a clear picture regarding the effects of the "trained state" on RMR [82].

Few training studies of adequate sample size and study duration appear in the literature of RMR. Frey-Hewitt et al. [31] found no change in RMR in 44 initially sedentary, overweight men assigned to a 1-yr weight loss program by exercise alone, with no changes in diet, compared with 41 controls; whereas a small, but significant reduction in RMR occurred in 36 men assigned to lose weight by moderate caloric restriction, with no changes in diet composition. The exercisers, who averaged 10 miles of running per week and showed significant fitness improvement, lost 4.1 kg of fat mass, with virtually no lean mass loss, while the dieters lost 5.5 kg of fat weight and 1.2 kg of lean weight, and controls did not change weight or body composition appreciably. Segal and collaborators conducted an elegant series of studies in which one of the three body-composition parameters was held constant by systematically matching lean and obese men with respect to total weight, lean weight, and fat weight [95]. These studies demonstrated that energy expenditure at rest is a function of lean body mass, which, when not controlled for in experiments, is frequently higher in obese individuals. Therefore, unless an exercise program brings about significant changes in lean body mass, RMR is not likely to be altered by training. Similarly, if a weight loss program does not reduce lean mass, there would be no reduction in RMR.

Prentice et al. [84] reported that almost all of 29 published studies on slimming, involving data from 515 subjects, showed a relatively modest suppression of RMR in response to energy restriction (dieting), ranging between 5% and 25%, with an average maximum change of about 15%. Among these studies, nine investigated the effect of exercise in preventing diet-induced reductions, six of which demonstrated protection of RMR, particularly those of van Dale [112, 114] and Mole [66], and their respective colleagues, and three of which did not show protection. There is some evidence that incorporation of any level of exercise may be of greater importance for women than men in preventing the decline in RMR during caloric restriction for weight loss [60]; however, the majority of RMR studies have included only men and this issue remains to be clarified.

THERMIC EFFECT OF FOOD. There are wide discrepancies in the literature regarding whether acute or chronic exercise affects postprandial thermogenesis. While several studies have not shown an enhancement of the thermic effect of food during exercise, a number of investigators have observed a potentiation of postprandial thermogenesis by exercise in lean, but not obese, subjects [95]. The effect of the sequence of a meal and exercise bout was also shown to differ between lean men and obese men; in lean men, the thermic effect was greater when the meal was eaten before exercise or when no exercise was performed, while in obese men, the thermic effect of food was significantly greater when the meal followed exercise, although it was blunted compared with lean subjects [95].

Effect of Exercise Training on Body Composition and Weight Status
The primary goal of a weight loss program should be to reduce fat weight, rather than total weight, particularly considering the value attributed to maintaining LBM. It has been shown repeatedly in volunteer-based studies that athletes and active individuals are leaner than sedentary, age-matched controls (who are often drawn from recruitment sources unrelated to those of the active subjects) [119]. Although it is often implied that participation in a sport is responsible for the differences in body composition between the active and inactive groups, the two groups are likely to differ with respect to many factors besides athletic and weight status. Randomized, controlled trials of the effects of increased physical activity level as the primary intervention provide the best way to answer questions about exercise effects on weight or body composition, provided the sample size is large enough to provide the statistical power to detect a difference between or among groups. The designs should specify mode, frequency, intensity, and duration of the exercise, all of which may profoundly alter the outcomes with respect to weight or body composition changes.

A recent meta-analysis by Ballor and Keesey [7] assessed the effects of type, duration, and frequency of exercise training on changes in body mass, fat mass, fat-free mass, and percent body fat both for adult males and females. Studies that contained at least five subjects per group and did not mix sexes were included in the analysis, if they also reported: pre- and postintervention body mass and percent body fat; adequate information to estimate exercise energy expenditure (except for weight training); type of exercise, with no mixing of exercise mode; and inclusion only of individuals who were sedentary at the outset. Studies that involved exercise sessions of longer than 60 minutes or programs of greater than 36 weeks were excluded, but the rationale for this was not presented. Studies involving subjects on weight reduction programs were also excluded. In the 53 studies that met these criteria (41 male, 12 female), of 500 published papers examined, weight loss after aerobic-type exercise training was shown to be modest in both sexes, but greater for males. All exercise was associated with reduction in fat mass; whereas an increase in fat-free mass was seen with cycling and weight training exercise in males, such that the actual fat mass loss was greater than total weight loss. No studies of weight training in females were included in the analysis. Energy expended during exercise and initial body fat levels or body mass accounted for most of the variance associated with changes in body composition; in females, weeks of training and duration of exercise per session were also significant predictors.

The role of resistance exercise in weight loss programs also intrigued Walberg [116] in a recent review, who reported preliminary evidence that suggests that weight-training may be more effective than aerobic exercise in preserving or increasing fat-free mass and RMR and has also been shown to reduce fat mass. Kreitzman also concluded that an exercise program of resistance training probably has much to offer individuals who are losing weight with a very low-calorie diet, and may be more valuable than aerobic training [54]. A recent survey of the literature showed that the use of weight training with low-calorie diets has not been thoroughly researched; although Donnelly et al. did not find additional retention of lean body mass in women who did weight training, it was acknowledged that further protocols should be explored [23].

SELECTED TRAINING STUDIES OF 12 WEEKS' DURATION OR LONGER. Few weight loss studies include exercise only arms (with no caloric restriction); on the other hand, the focus of most training studies (which generally attract relatively lean, active, and/or highly motivated volunteers) is often not weight loss, although body composition changes are generally significant in those assigned to exercise vs. control. Successful weight loss programs are often conducted in metabolic ward settings or situations in which weight and food intake are closely supervised. King and Tribble [49] recently reviewed and tabulated several weight loss studies involving exercise only arms and concluded that the programs which achieved the most weight loss either involved intensive training programs or were of relatively long duration. Fat weight loss is a slow, steady process that can be obscured by changes in lean weight if an exercise program causes initial increases in muscle mass and total weight is the only measure available; therefore, studies which focus on fat weight loss should be of at least 12 weeks' duration.

The Stanford Exercise Study [124] randomized 81 men, aged 30–55 yr, to either: (*a*) a 1-yr supervised jogging program (N = 48); or (*b*) 1 yr of no major change in activity level, i.e., "control" (N = 33), to determine the effects of exercise on high density lipoprotein (HDL) cholesterol. No instruction was given regarding diet. Initial BMI did not differ between groups and averaged about 25 kg/m^2, nor did percent body fat determined by hydrostatic weighing, averaging about 22%. Baseline fitness determined by maximal oxygen consumption during a maximal graded exercise treadmill test, averaged 34–35 ml/kg/min in both groups and 3-day food records revealed a baseline caloric intake of approximately 2500 kcal/day in both groups, with similar diet composition of about 40.5% of calories from fat, 16% from protein, 38% from carbohydrate, and 5% from alcohol. At 1 yr, maximal oxygen consumption increased nearly 10 ml/kg/min in exercisers vs. controls (P<0.0001), and worktime on the treadmill increased by nearly 4 minutes in exercisers vs. controls (P<0.0001). Despite no attempts on the part of investigators to bring about weight loss and no major differences detected in changes in caloric intake or percent of calories from any given food source between groups, the 48 exercising men lost significant weight relative to the 33 controls (2.5 kg; P<0.001), reducing percent body fat by 3.9% vs. control (P<0.0001).

Among exercisers, when men who reported active dieting were excluded from the analyses, miles run per week correlated significantly with change in body fat (Spearman's rho = −0.49; P<0.001), as well as with change in calories (r=0.45; P<0.005), which in turn correlated significantly with change in body fat (r=−0.57; P<0.0005). Furthermore, changes in HDL cholesterol were significantly related to all three of these parameters: miles/week (r=0.45; P<0.001); body fat changes (r=−0.47; P<0.001); and caloric changes (r=0.38; P<0.01), such that it was not possible to determine whether exercise or weight loss was responsible for HDL changes. Consequently, we designed two 1-yr, randomized controlled weight loss studies, to untangle the effects of weight loss from those of exercise on HDL cholesterol and other CHD risk factors.

The first Stanford Weight Control Project [125] randomized 155 moderately overweight men (20–50% above ideal body weight), aged 35–59 yr to 1-yr interventions of: (*a*) group instruction by a registered dietitian on moderate caloric restriction, without change in diet composition (N = 51); (*b*) supervised group walking or jogging sessions (N = 52); or (*c*) no change in caloric intake or activity. No significant baseline differences were seen among the three groups for total, lean or fat body mass assessed by hydrostatic weighing (approximately 94 kg, 68 kg, and 26 kg, respectively) or caloric intake determined by 7-day food records (about 2400 kcal/day), nor did groups differ with respect to initial fitness level of approximately 34.5 ml/kg/min for maximal oxygen consumption during a treadmill test. One-yr measurements were made after 6 weeks of weight stabilization in both groups. Exercisers did not reduce calories significantly vs. controls at 7 months or 1 yr, while caloric reduction was significant in dieters vs. controls at 7 months (about 335 kcal/day; P<0.01) and 1-yr (about 240 kcal/day; P<0.01), and was similarly reduced relative to exercisers at 7 months, while differences between dieters and exercisers at 1 yr were not significant. Maximal oxygen consumption was significantly improved in exercisers at 1 yr compared with dieters (4.1 ml/kg/min; P<0.001) and controls (6.5 ml/kg/min; P<0.001).

Seven months after baseline tests exercisers had lost 2.9 kg of fat weight vs. control (P<0.001), but only 0.3 kg of lean mass (n.s.) and by 1 yr, fat mass loss averaged 3.8 kg vs. control (P<0.001), with lean mass loss remaining insignificant. Although dieters lost 2.9 kg more fat weight than exercisers by 7 months (P<0.001), slight gains in fat by dieters and further fat loss by exercisers resulted in no significant differences between dieters and exercisers by 1 yr; furthermore, dieters lost significant lean mass vs. both exercisers (1.7 kg) and controls (2.0 kg). These data suggest that even 7 months is too short a period to see the long-term benefits of exercise vs. caloric restriction as a weight loss strategy. Furthermore, minimal intervention strategies were shown to be more effective in maintaining weight loss in men originally assigned to exercise over the course of a second year of follow-up than in men assigned to diet [47].

A 1-yr exercise training study conducted in the community of Sunnyvale California, the Stanford-Sunnyvale Health Improvement Program (SSHIP), randomly assigned 197 men and 160 women, aged 50–65 yr, to control or one of three exercise programs: high-intensity, group-based; high-intensity, home-based; and low-intensity home-based [48]. Adherence measures indicated that participants engaged in exercise at a level considerably above baseline, with no major differences between group (supervised) and home-based programs. Among the subjects randomized to the three exercise conditions, $\dot{V}O_2$max increased by approximately 5% and treadmill duration increased by 14% between baseline and 1 yr, yet there was no significant weight loss or body composition changes, assessed by hydrostatic weighing, despite the stated desire to lose weight on the part of many of the participants at entry. The previous Stanford studies did not include women. Possible differences between weight loss outcomes in the men in the previous Stanford clinical trials compared with those in this community study include lower exercise levels or greater dietary compensation, neither of which can be easily compared across studies, and age, which was slightly higher in the community sample. Arguing against age are results of a 9- to 12-month exercise training program in 60- to 70-year-old women and men, which resulted in weight loss averaging 1.6 kg and 3 kg of fat weight, respectively, with no loss of lean weight and no significant differences between sexes [51]; however, there were no controls in this study.

The role of appetite and diet compensation with exercise has interested researchers for years [76, 106, 119], but conclusive studies have not been conducted. In a recent 3-month uncontrolled training study of nine slightly obese men, seven obese women and 15 leaner women, neither men nor lean women altered caloric intake, while obese women significantly decreased energy intake; the men and obese women reduced body fat, whereas the leaner women did not [1]. It was argued that men, like male rats, become leaner during physical activity, due to a lack of energy-intake compensation, whereas women with similar body fat mass, like female rats, react with some compensation, causing a protection of their body fat. Such a conclusion does not seem to be supported by the data and only serves to confuse the issue as to whether true sex differences exist in the effectiveness of exercise for weight loss. Furthermore, the well-known greater adiposity of women vs. men is accompanied by differences in the regional distribution of the excess fat, which should be investigated before attributing sex differences to gender alone.

INFLUENCE OF DIET ON EXERCISE-INDUCED WEIGHT CHANGES. *Caloric Restriction, Without Change in Diet Composition.* It seems to be the general consensus among researchers in the area that the addition of exercise to a weight loss program involving caloric restriction results in much greater weight loss than caloric restriction alone [49, 116]. In a 12-week study of men, the addition of exercise to either a balanced caloric-deficit diet of 1000 kcal/day or a protein-sparing, ketogenic diet resulted in significantly greater weight loss and maintenance of weight loss over a 2-yr follow-up period during which participants resumed their normal diets [80]. Hill et al. also reported a significant main effect for exercise over a 12-week period of weight loss on either a constant 1200 kcal/day diet or diet alternating between 600 and 1800 kcal/day with and without exercise; exercisers had greater total weight loss and reduction of percent body fat, independent of diet type; furthermore, the drop out rate was lower in the exercise than in the no-exercise groups, suggesting valuable effects on adherence [39].

Saris and van Dale concluded that weight loss and especially fat loss is significantly promoted by exercise during a VLCD, of 400–800 kcal/day [92]. Investigators have used exercise to slow depletion of lean body mass during VLCD; however, the results are far from unequivocal. Donnelly et al. suggested that most studies had exercise programs of inadequate duration and suggested 90 days as the minimum duration necessary for adaptations to exercise [24].

Diet Composition. A role of diet composition in the etiology of obesity has been suggested by several investigators [96, 116]. Percent body fat, assessed by hydrostatic weighing, was significantly correlated with the intake of total, saturated, and monounsaturated fatty acids and negatively correlated with carbohydrates and plant protein, assessed by 7-day food records, in 155 sedentary overweight men, aged 30–59 yr [25]. In 107 men and in 109 women, aged 18–70 yr, who responded to advertisements for volunteers from the Indiana University Weight Loss Clinic, caloric intake expressed per kg lean body mass, assessed by hydrostatic weighing, was not related to adiposity; however, the percent of calories from fat and carbohydrate were significantly related to adiposity, as was caloric intake expressed per total body weight [65]. The macronutrient content of weight-reducing diets may also influence the effect of exercise on lean body mass [116].

The second Stanford Weight Control Project (SWCP-II; [126]) involved randomization of 132 moderately overweight men (BMI between 28 and 34 kg/m^2) and 132 moderately overweight women (BMI between 24 and 30 kg/m^2) to 1-yr interventions of (*a*) diet: group instruction by a registered dietitian on reduction of saturated fat and dietary cholesterol, with concomitant caloric restriction and a consistent message that women should not drop below 1200 kcal/day and men should not drop below 1500 kcal/day; or (*b*) diet plus exercise: identical diet instruction combined with supervised group walking or jogging sessions; or (*c*) control: no change in caloric intake or activity. Within each sex, the three study groups were well matched at baseline (combining the means of the three groups): for age (men, 40.3 ± 6.3 yr; women, 39.1 ± 6.4 yr); body composition by hydrostatic weighing (men, 70.7 kg lean mass, 27.7 kg fat mass; women, 48.1 kg lean mass, 26.9 kg fat mass); aerobic capacity during a maximal graded exercise treadmill test (men, 34.1 ± 4.9 ml/kg/min; women, 27.0 ± 4.2 ml/kg/min); total calories assessed by 7-day food records (men, about 2630 kcal/day; women, about 1945 kcal/day) and the intake of most nutrients.

One-yr measurements were completed on 40 of 45 men and 31 of 42 women randomized to the diet; on 39 of 43 men and 42 of 47 women assigned to the diet plus exercise; and on 40 of 44 men and 39 of 43 women randomized to control. Women assigned to diet only tended to drop out at a higher rate than any other sex/treatment assignment groups. Caloric reduction was significant in both men and women assigned to diet only or to diet plus exercise vs. control and did not differ between men or women assigned to diet only vs. diet plus exercise; furthermore, significant reductions in percent of calories from total fat and saturated fat vs. control, did not differ between diet only and diet plus exercise groups with the exception of a significantly greater reduction in percent of calories from total fat in men assigned to diet plus exercise versus diet only.

Figure 12.1 shows the fat weight changes from baseline to 1-yr for every individual who completed the trial and reveals the range of individual variability in response to the intervention programs. Both diet only and diet plus exercise women lost significant fat weight vs. controls (4.5 kg and 6.0 kg, respectively). Fat weight loss did not differ between women assigned to diet plus exercise vs. diet only, probably because of the higher drop-out rate for unsuccessful women assigned to diet only; similarly, significant decreases vs. control in percent body fat did not differ between exercising dieters (5.2%) and diet only women (3.5%). The WHR was significantly reduced in women assigned to diet plus exercise vs. control, but not vs. diet only; WHR reduction did not reach significance in diet-only women vs. control. Lean mass loss was negligible in women who lost weight by either diet only or diet plus exercise and also did not differ with the addition of exercise to the diet.

Both diet-only and diet plus exercise men lost significant fat weight vs. controls (5.5 kg and 9.0 kg, respectively), with loss of fat mass being significantly greater in men assigned to diet plus exercise vs. diet only. Percent body fat decreased 7.0% in men who exercised and dieted and 3.8% in men who dieted only (P<0.001). WHR was reduced in men assigned to either diet only or diet plus exercise vs. control, but significantly greater WHR reductions were seen in men assigned to diet plus exercise vs. diet only. Lean mass loss in men assigned to either diet

FIGURE 12.1

Fat weight change (kg) from baseline to 1-yr for each individual randomized in the second Stanford Weight Control Project (SWCP-II) to control, diet (hypocaloric low-fat/low cholesterol), or diet plus exercise (identical diet plus aerobic exercise). Numbers include 119 men (40 control; 40 diet only; 39 diet + exercise) and 112 women (39 control; 31 diet only; 42 diet + exercise) who were initially overweight and sedentary.

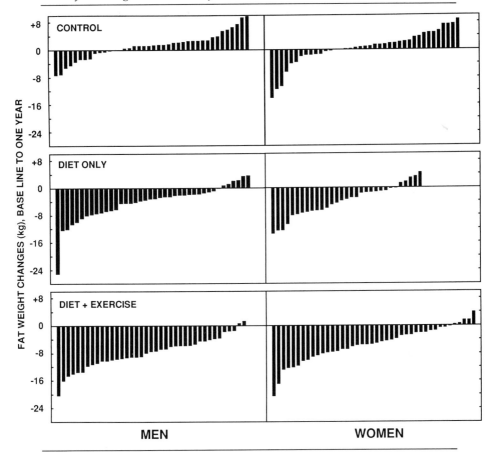

or diet plus exercise was significant vs. control and averaged 1.3 kg and 1.4 kg, respectively, with no difference between groups. When the weight and body composition changes of men in the second Stanford Weight Control Project (SWCP-II) are compared with those of SWCP-I, which was comprised of a similar sample of moderately overweight, sedentary men, albeit slightly younger, it would appear that weight loss achieved by a low-fat diet may result in greater fat weight loss than one characterized by caloric restriction only and that the combination of a hypocaloric low fat diet and routine aerobic exercise is a very effective strategy for long-term weight loss.

WEIGHT LOSS REGIMENS

Exercise was reported to be one of the few factors positively correlated with successful long-term body weight maintenance [12]. The Technology Assessment Conference on Methods for Voluntary Weight Loss and Control, convened by the NIH in March/April of 1992 [104], reported that participants who remain in weight loss programs in controlled settings usually lose about 10% of their weight; however, one- to two-thirds of the weight is regained within 1 yr of the end of the program and almost all is regained within 5 yr. Weight loss achieved by exercise programs alone was reported to be more limited than that by caloric restriction; however, exercise was described as an important adjunct to other strategies which could, if continued, diminish the tendency for rapid postprogram weight gain. Beneficial effects of exercise, independent of weight loss, were acknowledged.

The 1987 Behavioral Risk Factor Surveillance System (BRFSS), which compiled data from approximately 4500 adults through random-digit-dialed telephone interviews conducted through health departments in 32 states, plus the District of Columbia [13] revealed that the median prevalence of restricting calories to lose weight was 43.6% among men who reported being overweight and 63.9% among women who reported being overweight, while the median prevalence of increasing physical activity to lose weight was 24.3% for these men and 34.7% for these women. Only 20.2% of the men and 31.4% of the women reported using both weight-loss regimens. Data from 112,108 respondents to the 1985–1988 BRFSS from 21 states [8] revealed that overweight Caucasian and Black women reported a similar prevalence of simultaneously increasing physical activity and eating fewer calories (33% and 32%, respectively), despite a 1:2 ratio of overweight Caucasian to Black women at each age group examined, while both overweight Caucasian and Black men most frequently reported not trying to lose weight by any means (49% and 55%, respectively).

From 700 women recruited from a large health maintenance organization, 50 were randomly selected from each of the following self-chosen categories: relapsers (obese women who regained weight after successful weight reduction), maintainers (formerly obese, average weight), or always average weight, and data were obtained on 44 relapsers, 30 maintainers, and 34 controls, to reveal that few relapsers exercised (34%), whereas 90% of maintainers and 82% of controls exercised regularly [43].

Few exercise training studies have been conducted in minority populations. The potential value of prescribing exercise to treat the even greater problem of obesity in Black women and other minority women, who have higher WHRs than the majority of Caucasian women, as well as a greater incidence of hypertension and glucose intolerance, is unclear. The Zuni Diabetes Project, a community-based exercise and weight-control program, has demonstrated that regular exercise can produce significant weight loss in a community of Zuni [36], but similar programs are scarce.

The Council of Scientific Affairs of the American Medical Association stated that concern with weight control should begin sufficiently early in life to reduce the risk of developing obesity and that prevention is the treatment of choice [15]. The Council cited the three essential components of a weight control program as diet, exercise and behavior modification, emphasizing that gradual changes in eating habits and exercise levels were necessary for maintenance of weight loss.

SUMMARY AND CONCLUSIONS

Several important questions need to be answered to increase the likelihood that exercise will be accepted by the millions in the population who are obese. What is the minimum exercise "dose" (intensity, duration, frequency) and what is the optimal mode to bring about substantial fat weight loss, with minimal loss of lean mass? What is the best nutritional plan to optimize fat utilization during exercise, without impairing performance or loss of lean mass? Which diet and exercise programs maximally increase utilization of centrally deposited fat and how can hyperplastic obesity best be treated? Also of interest is the potential role of resistance exercise for weight loss, and the predictors of weight loss success. For instance, do individuals with gynoid obesity really differ from individuals with android obesity in their utilization and loss of body fat during exercise?

The potential advantages of exercise include: stimulation of fat as opposed to carbohydrate oxidation; increased energy use during the exercise itself and in the postexercise period; protection of lean body mass; possible reversal of the diet-induced suppression of BMR; and other health benefits. Among other parameters, the effectiveness of exercise on weight loss may be influenced by the type, intensity, frequency, and duration of exercise bouts and the duration of the training program, the nature of the excess fat stores, i.e., whether the person has obesity characterized by hyperplastic or hypertrophic adipose tissue or central (with large-intra-abdominal depot) or peripheral obesity, the composition and caloric content of the diet, and behavioral aspects that affect adherence to the program. With respect to this latter concern, even if a person has been very successful at weight loss in a metabolic ward or intensive program, he/she must eventually return to the outside world and figure out for himself/herself how to eat real food and/or maintain an activity level that promotes weight maintenance. Because diet and exercise habits are difficult to assess and to quantify in free-living populations, it continues to be difficult to evaluate the success of diet and/or exercise prescriptions for weight loss accurately and we continue to be plagued with questions regarding the effectiveness vs. efficacy of exercise as a means to control body weight. It would seem that the wide range of health benefits derived from regular exercise would justify emphasizing increased activity for inactive people, particularly for obese, sedentary individuals, whether or not ideal body weight or significant weight loss is achieved.

ACKNOWLEDGMENT

The National Institutes of Health, HL 24462 and HL 45733, are acknowledged as sources of support for our research in the area of exercise and weight control, some of which is described in this chapter. Sincere appreciation and gratitude is extended to my friend and colleague, Peter D. Wood, D.Sc., Ph.D., for carefully reviewing the manuscript, offering excellent suggestions for its revision, and providing collaborative support throughout the writing of this review.

REFERENCES

1. Anderson B., X. Xu, M. Rebuffe-Scrive, K. Terning, M. Krotkiewski, and P. Bjorntorp. The effects of exercise training on body composition and metabolism in men and women. *Int. J. Obesity* 15:75–81, 1991.
2. Andrews, J. F. Exercise for slimming. *Proc. Nutr. Soc.* 50:459–471, 1991.
3. Arner, P., P. Engfeldt, and H. Lithell. Site differences in the basal metabolism of subcutaneous fat in obese women. *J. Clin. Endocrinol. Metabol.* 53:948–952, 1981.
4. Arner, P., E. Kriegholm, P. Engfeldt, and J. Bolinder. Adrenergic regulation of lipolysis in situ at rest and during exercise. *J. Clin. Invest.* 85:893–898; 1990.
5. Arner, P., H. Lithell, H. Wahrenberg, and M. Bronnegard. Expression of lipoprotein lipase in different human subcutaneous adipose tissue regions. *J. Lipid Res.* 32:423–429, 1991.
6. Ashwell, M., T. J. Dole, and A. K. Dixon. Obesity: New insight into the anthropometric classification of fat distribution shown by computed tomography *Br. Med. J.* 290: 1692–1694, 1985.
7. Ballor, D. L., and R. E. Keesey. A meta-analysis of the factors affecting exercise-induced changes in body mass, fat mass and fat-free mass in males and females. *Int. J. Obesity* 15:717–726, 1991.
8. Bennett, E. M. Weight loss practices of overweight adults. *Am. J. Clin. Nutr.* 53:1519S–1521S, 1991.
9. Bjorntorp, P. Adipose tissue adaptation to exercise. C. Bouchard, R. J. Shephard, T. Stephens, J. R. Sutton, and B. D. McPherson (eds). *Exercise, Fitness and Health: A Consensus of Current Knowledge.* Champaign, IL: Human Kinetics: 1990, pp. 315–323.

10. Blair S. N., H. W. Kohl, R. S. Paffenbarger, D. G. Clark, K. H. Cooper, and L. W. Gibbons. Physical fitness and all-cause mortality: a prospective study of healthy men and women. *J.A.M.A.* 262:2395–2401, 1989.

11. Bolinder, J., L. Kager, J. Ostman, and P. Arner. Differences at the receptor and post-receptor levels between human omental and subcutaneous adipose tissue in the action of insulin on lipolysis. *Diabetes* 32:117–123; 1983.

12. Brownell, K. D., G. A. Marlat, E. Lichtenstein, and G. T. Wilson. Understanding and preventing relapse. *Am. J. Psychol.* 41:765–82, 1986.

13. Centers for Disease Control. Weight-loss regimens among overweight adults– behavioral risk factor surveillance system, 1987. *J.A.M.A.* 262:1163–167, 1989.

14. Costill, D. L., W. J. Fink, L. H. Getchell, L. J. Ivy, and F. A. Witzmann. Lipid metabolism in skeletal muscle of endurance-trained males and females. *J. Appl. Physiol.: Respir. Environ. Exerc. Physiol.* 47:787–791; 1979.

15. Council of Scientific Affairs. Treatment of obesity in adults. *J.A.M.A.* 260:257–2551, 1988.

16. Crampes, F., D. Riviere, M. Beauvill, M. Marceron, and M. Garrigues. Lipolytic response of adipocytes to epinephrine in sedentary and exercise-trained subjects: sex-related differences. *Eur. J. Appl. Physiol.* 59:249–255; 1989.

17. Dannenberg, A. L., J. B. Keller, P. W. F. Wilson, and W. P. Castelli. Leisure time physical activity in the Framingham Offspring Study: description, seasonal variation, and risk factor correlates. *Am. J. Epidemiol.* 129:76–88, 1989.

18. Despres, J. P., C. Bouchard, A. Tremblay, R. Savard, and M. Marcotte. Effects of aerobic training on fat distribution in male subjects. *Med. Sci. Sports Exerc.* 17:113–118; 1985.

19. Despres, J. P., C. Bouchard, A. Tremblay, R. Savard, and M. Marcotte. The effect of a 20-week endurance training program on adipose-tissue morphology and lipolysis in men and women. *Metabolism* 33:235–239, 1984.

20. Despres J. P., M. Ferland, S. Moorjani, et al. Role of hepatic-triglyceride lipase activity in the association between intra-abdominal fat and plasma HDL cholesterol in obese women. *Arteriosclerosis* 9:485–492, 1989.

21. Despres, J. P., M. C. Poulot, S. Moorjani, et al. Loss of abdominal fat and metabolic response to exercise training in obese women. *Am. J. Physiol.* 261 (*Endocrinol. Metab.* 24):E159–167; 1991.

22. Despres, J. P., R. Savard, A. Tremblay, and C. Bouchard. Adipocyte diameter and lipolytic activity in marathon runners: relationship with body fatness. *Eur. J. Appl. Physiol.* 51:223–230, 1983.

23. Donnelly, J. E., J. Jakicic, and S. Gunderson. Diet and body composition: effect of very low calorie diets and exercise. *Sports Med.* 12:237–249, 1991.

24. Donnelly, J. E., N. P. Pronk, D. J. Jacobsen, S. J. Pronk, and J. M. Jakicic. Effects of a very-low-calorie diet and physical-training regimens on body composition and resting metabolic rate in obese females. *Am. J. Clin. Nutr.* 54:56–61, 1991.

25. Dreon, D. M., B. Frey-Hewitt, N. Ellsworth, P. T. Williams, R. B. Terry, and P. D. Wood. Dietary fat: carbohydrate ratio and obesity in middle-aged men. *Am. J. Clin. Nutr.* 47:995–1000, 1988.

26. Efendic, S. Catecholamine and metabolism of human adipose tissue. III. Comparison between the regulation of lipolysis in omental and subcutaneous adipose tissue. *Acta Med. Scand.* 187:477–483, 1970.

27. Ekelund, L. G., W. L. Haskell, J. L. Johnson, F. S. Whaley, M. H. Criqui, and D. S. Sheps. Physical fitness as a predictor of cardiovascular mortality in asymptomatic North America men: the Lipid Research Clinics Mortality Follow-up Study. *N. Engl. J. Med.* 319:1379–1384, 1988.

28. Epstein, L. H., and R. R. Wing. Aerobic exercise and weight. *Addictive Behav.* 5:371–388, 1980.

29. Fletcher G. F., S. N. Blair, J. Blumenthal, et al. Statement on exercise: benefits and recommendations for physical activity programs for all Americans. *Circulation* 86:340–344, 1992.
30. Folsom, A. R., C. J. Caspersen, H. L. Taylor, et al. Leisure time physical activity and its relationship to coronary risk factors in a population-based sample: the Minnesota Heart Study. *Am. J. Epidemiol.* 121:570–579, 1985.
31. Frey-Hewitt, B., K. M. Vranizan, D. M. Dreon, and P. D. Wood. The effect of weight loss by dieting or exercise on resting metabolic rate in overweight men. *Int. J. Obesity* 14:327–334, 1990.
32. Friedmann, B., and W. I. Kindermann. Energy metabolism and regulatory hormones in women and men during endurance exercise. *Eur. J. Appl. Physiol.* 59:1–9, 1989.
33. Gorski, J., L. B. Oscai, and W. K. Palmer. Hepatic lipid metabolism in exercise and training. *Med. Sci. Sports Exer.* 22:213–221, 1990.
34. Haskell, W. L. The influence of exercise on the concentrations of triglyceride and cholesterol in human plasma. *Exer. Sports Sci. Rev.* 12:205–244, 1984.
35. Haskell, W. L., H. L. Taylor, P. D. Wood, H. Schrott, and G. Heiss. Strenuous physical activity, treadmill exercise test performance and plasma high-density lipoprotein cholesterol: the Lipid Research Clinics Program Prevalence Study. *Circulation* 62:IV–53–61, 1980.
36. Heath, G. W., R. H. Wilson, J. Smith, and B. E. Leonard. Community-based exercise and weight control: diabetes risk reduction and glycemic control in Zuni Indians. *Am. J. Clin. Nutr.* 53:1642S–6S, 1991.
37. Henriksson, J. Training induced adaptation of skeletal muscle and metabolism during submaximal exercise. *J. Physiol.* 270:661–675; 1977.
38. Herring, J. L., P. A. Mole, C. N. Meredith, and J. S. Stern. Effect of suspending exercise training on resting metabolic rate in women. *Med. Sci. Sports Exerc.* 24:59–64, 1992.
39. Hill, J. O., D. G. Schlundt, T. Sbrocco, et al. Evaluation of an alternating-calorie diet with and without exercise in the treatment of obesity. *Am. J. Clin. Nutr.* 50:248–254, 1989.
40. Hurley, B. F., P. M. Nemeth, W. H. Martin, J. M. Hagberg, G. P. Dalsky, and J. O. Holloszy. Muscle triglyceride utilization during exercise: effect of training. *J. Appl. Physiol.* 60:562–567, 1986.
41. Jeffery, R. W., A. R. Folsom, R. V. Luepker, et al. Prevalence of overweight and weight loss behavior in a metropolitan adult population: the Minnesota Heart Survey experience. *Am J. Public Health* 74:349–352, 1984.
42. Kaye, S. A., A. R. Folsom, R. J. Prineas, J. D. Potter, and S. M. Gapstur. The association of body fat distribution with lifestyle and reproductive factors in a population study of postmenopausal women. *Int. J. Obesity* 14:583–591, 1990.
43. Kayman, S., W. Bruvold, and J. S. Stern. Maintenance and relapse after weight loss in women: behavioral aspects. *Am. J. Clin. Nutr.* 52:800–807, 1990.
44. Kiens, B., B. Essen-Gastavsson, and H. Lithell. Lipoprotein lipase activity and intramuscular triglyceride stores after long-term high-fat and high-carbohydrate diets in physically trained men. *Clin. Physiol.* 7:1–9; 1987.
45. Kiens, B., and Lithell, H. Lipoprotein metabolism influenced by training-induced changes in human skeletal muscle. *J. Clin. Invest.* 83:558–564; 1989.
46. Kiens, B., and B. Saltin. Enhanced fat oxidation by exercising skeletal muscle after endurance training. *Clin. Physiol.* 5(Suppl 4):86a (Abstr.), 1985.
47. King, A. C., B. Frey-Hewitt, D. M. Dreon, and P. D. Wood. Diet vs. exercise in weight maintenance: the effects of minimal intervention strategies on long-term outcomes in men. *Arch. Intern. Med.* 149:2741–2746, 1989.
48. King, A. C., W. L. Haskell, C. B. Taylor, H. C. Kraemer, and R. F. DeBusk. Group- vs. home-based exercise training in healthy older men and women: a community-based clinical trial. *J.A.M.A.* 266:1535–1542, 1991.

49. King, A. C., and D. L. Tribble. The role of exercise in weight regulation in nonathletes. *Sports Med.* 11:331–349, 1991.
50. Kohrt, W. M., M. T. Malley, G. P. Dalsky, and J. O. Holloszy. Body composition of healthy sedentary and trained, young and older men and women. *Med. Sci. Sports Exer.* 24:832–837, 1991.
51. Kohrt, W. M., K. A. Obert, and J. O. Holloszy. Exercise training improves fat distribution patterns in 60- to 70-year-old men and women. *J. Gerontol.* 47:M99–M105, 1992.
52. Kraemer, H. C., R. I. Berkowitz, and L. D. Hammer. Methodological difficulties in studies of obesity. I. Measurement issues. *Ann. Behav. Med.* 12:112–118, 1990.
53. Kraemer, H. C., R. I. Berkowitz, and L. D. Hammer. Methodological difficulties in studies of obesity. II. Design and Analysis issues. *Ann. Behav. Med.* 12:119–124, 1990.
54. Kreitzman, S. N. Lean body mass, exercise and VLCD. *Int. J. Obesity* 13 (suppl. 2):17–25, 1989.
55. Krotkiewski, M., and P. Bjorntorp. Muscle tissue in obesity with different distribution of adipose tissue. Effects of physical training. *Int. J. Obesity* 10:331–341, 1986.
56. Krotkiewski, M., P. Bjorntorp, L. Sjostrom, and U. Smith. Impact of obesity on metabolism in men and women: importance of regional adipose tissue distribution. *J. Clin. Invest.* 72:1150–1162, 1983.
57. Kuczmarski, R. J. Prevalence of overweight and weight gain in the United States. *Am. J. Clin. Nutr.* 55:495S–502S, 1992.
58. Lapidus, L., C. Bengtsson, B. Larsson, K. Pennert, E. Rybo, and L. Sjostrom. Distribution of adipose tissue and risk of cardiovascular disease and death: 12-year follow-up of participants in the population study of women in Gothenburg, Sweden. *Br. Med. J.* 289:1257–1261, 1984.
59. Larsson, B., K. Svardsudd, L. Welin, L. Wilhelmsen, P. Bjorntorp, and G. Tibblin. Abdominal adipose tissue: distribution, obesity and risk of cardiovascular disease and death: 13-year follow-up of participants in the study of men born in 1913. *Br. Med. J.* 288:1401–1404, 1984.
60. Lennon, D., F. Nagle, F. Stratman, E. Shrago, and S. Dennis. Diet and exercise training effects on resting metabolic rate. *Int. J. Obesity* 9:39–47, 1985.
61. Leon, A. S., J. Connett, D. R. Jacobs, R. Rauramaa. Leisure-time physical activity levels and risk of coronary heart disease and death: the Multiple Risk Factor Intervention Trial. *J.A.M.A.* 258:2388–2395, 1987.
62. Lithell, H., M. Cedermark, J. Froberg, P. Tesch, and J. Karlsson. Increase of lipoprotein lipase activity in skeletal muscle during heavy exercise. Relation to epinephrine excretion. *Metabolism* 30:1130–1134; 1981.
63. Lithell, H., J. Orlander, R. Schele, B. Sjodin, and J. Karlsson. Changes of lipoprotein-lipase activity and lipid stores in human skeletal muscle with prolonged heavy exercise. *Acta Physiol. Scand.* 107:257–261, 1979.
64. Manson, J. E., G. A. Colditz, M. J. Stampfer, et al. A prospective study of obesity and risk of coronary heart disease in women. *N. Engl. J. Med.* 322:882–889, 1990.
65. Miller, W. C., A. K. Lindeman, J. Wallace, and M. Niederpruem. Diet composition, energy intake and exercise in relation to body fat in men and women. *Am. J. Clin. Nutr.* 52:426–430, 1990.
66. Mole, P. D., J. S. Stern, C. L. Schultz, E. M. Bernauer, and B. J. Holcomb. Exercise reverses depressed metabolic rate produced by severe caloric restriction. *Med. Sci. Sports Exercise* 21:29–33, 1989.
67. National Center for Health Statistics. Plan and operation of the Health and Nutrition Examination Survey, United States—1971–1973. *Vital and health statistics.* Series 1, No. 10. DHEW publication no. (HSM) 73–1310. Washington, D.C.: Government Printing Office, 1973.
68. National Center for Health Statistics. Plan and operation of the second National Health and Nutrition Examination Survey, United States—1976–1980. *Vital and health*

statistics. Series 1, No. 15. DHEW publication no. (PHS) 81–1317. Washington, D.C.: U.S. Government Printing Office, 1981.

69. National Center for Health Statistics (NCHS). Plan and Operation of the NHANES 1 Epidemiologic Follow-up Study, 1982–1984. *Vital and Health Statistics.* Series 1, No. 22. Washington, DC: Government Printing Office, 1987. U.S. Department of Health and Human Services publication (PHS) 87–1324.

70. National Center for Health Statistics. *Assessing physical fitness and physical activity in population-based surveys.* T. F. Drury, DHHS Pub. No. (PHS) 89–1253. Public Health Service. Washington, D.C.: U.S. Government Printing Office, 1989.

71. National Cholesterol Education Program. Highlights of the Report of the Expert Panel on Detection, Evaluation and Treatment of High Blood Cholesterol in Adults. Bethesda, MD: National Institutes of Health, 1987. (*DHHS publication* no. (NIH) 88–2926).

72. National Institutes of Health Consensus Development Panel. Health implications of obesity: National Institutes of Health consensus development conference statement. *Ann. Intern. Med.* 103:1073–1077, 1985.

73. Nikkila, E. A. Role of lipoprotein lipase in metabolic adaptation to exercise and training. J. Borensztajn (ed.). *Lipoprotein Lipase.* Chicago: Evener Publishers, Inc. 1987, pp. 187–199.

74. Nikkila, E. A., and A. Konttinen. Effect of physical activity on postprandial levels of fats in serum. *Lancet* I:1151–1154; 1962.

75. Nikkila, E. A., M. R. Taskinen, S. Rehunen, and M. Harkonen. Lipoprotein lipase activity in adipose tissue and skeletal muscle of runners: relation to serum lipoproteins. *Metabolism* 27:1661–1671; 1978.

76. Oscai, L. B. The role of exercise in weight control. *Exer. Sports Sci. Rev.* 1:103–123, 1973.

77. Oscai, L. B., and W. K. Palmer. Muscle lipolysis during exercise: an update. *Sports Med.* 6:23–28, 1988.

78. Ostman, J., P. Arner, P. Engfeldt, and L. Kager. Regional differences in the control of lipolysis in human adipose tissue. *Metabolism* 28:1198–1205, 1979.

79. Paffenbarger, R. S., R. T. Hyde, A. L. Wing, and C. C. Hsieh. Physical activity, all-cause mortality, and longevity of college alumni. *N. Engl. J. Med.* 314:605–613, 1986.

80. Pavlou, K. N., S. Krey, and W. P. Steffee. Exercise as an adjunct to weight loss and maintenance in moderately obese subjects. *Am. J. Clin. Nutr.* 49:1115–1123, 1989.

81. Poehlman, E. T. A review: exercise and its influence on resting energy metabolism in man. *Med. Sci. Sports Exercise* 21:515–525, 1989.

82. Poehlman, E. T., C. L. Melby, and M. I. Goran. The impact of exercise and diet restriction on daily energy expenditure. *Sports Med.* 11:78–101, 1991.

83. Powell, K. E., P. D. Thompson, C. J. Casperson, and J. S. Kendrick. Physical activity and the incidence of coronary heart disease. *Ann. Rev. Public Health* 8:253–287, 1987.

84. Prentice, A. M., F. R. Goldberg, S. A. Jebb, A. E. Black, P. R. Murgatroyd, and E. O. Diaz. Physiological responses to slimming. *Proc. Nutr. Soc.* 50:441–458, 1991.

85. Rebuffe-Scrive, M., L. Enk, N. Crona, et al. Fat cell metabolism in different regions in women: effect of menstrual cycle, pregnancy, and lactation. *J. Clin. Invest.* 75:1973–1976, 1985.

86. Rebuffe-Scrive, M., P. Lonnroth, P. Marin, et al. Regional adipose tissue metabolism in men and postmenopausal women. *Int. J. Obesity* 11:347–355, 1987.

87. Riviere, D., F. Crampes, M. Beauville, and M. Garrigues. Lipolytic response of fat cells to catecholamines in sedentary and exercise-trained women. *J. Appl. Physiol.* 66:330–335, 1989.

88. Romieu, I., W. C. Willett, M. J. Stampfer, et al. Energy intake and other determinants of relative weight. *Am. J. Clin. Nutr.* 47:406–412, 1988.

89. Sady, S. P., P. D. Thompson, E. M. Cullinane, M. A. Kantor, E. Domagala, and P. N. Herbert. Prolonged exercise augments plasma triglyceride clearance. *J.A.M.A.* 256:2552–2555, 1986.

90. Saltin, B., and P. D. Gollnick. Skeletal muscle adaptability: significance for metabolism and performance. L. D. Peachy, R. H. Adrian, and S. R. Geiger. (eds). *Handbook of Physiology*, Section 10, Chapt. 9, Baltimore: Williams & Wilkins, 1983.

91. Sallis, J. F., W. L. Haskell, P. D. Wood, S. P. Fortmann, T. Rogers, S. N. Blair, and R. S. Paffenbarger. Phsyical activity assessment methodology in the Five-City Project. *Am. J. Epidemiol.* 121:91–106, 1985.

92. Saris, W. H. M., and D. Van Dale. Effects of exercise during VLCD diet on metabolic rate, body composition and aerobic power: pooled data of four studies. *Int. J. Obesity* 13 (suppl. 2):169–170, 1989.

93. Schwartz, R. S., W. P. Shuman, V. Larson, et al. The effect of intensive endurance exercise training on body fat distribution in young and older men. *Metabolism* 40:545–551, 1991.

94. Sedgwick, A. W., D. W. Thomas, M. Davies, K. Baghurst, and I. Rouse. Cross-sectional and longitudinal relationships between physical fitness and risk factors for coronary heart disease in men and women: "The Adelaide 1000". *J. Clin. Epidemiol.* 42:189–200, 1989.

95. Segal, K. R., and F. X. Pi-Sunyer. Exercise and obesity. *Med. Clin. North Am.* 73:217–236, 1989.

96. Shah, M., and R. W. Jeffrey. Is obesity due to overeating and inactivity, or to a defective metabolic rate? A review. *Ann. Behav. Med.* 13:73–81, 1991.

97. Shephard, R. J. Nutritional benefits of exercise. *J. Sports Med.* 29:83–90, 1989.

98. Slattery, M. L., A. McDonald, D. E. Bild, et al. Associations of body fat and its distribution with dietary intake, physical activity, alcohol, and smoking in blacks and whites. *Am. J. Clin. Nutr.* 55:943–949, 1992.

99. Stefanick, M. L., and P. D. Wood. Physical activity, lipid and lipoprotein metabolism, and lipid transport. C. Bouchard, R. J. Shephard, and T. Stephens (eds). *Physical Activity, Fitness and Health 1992 Proceedings.* Champaign, IL: Human Kinetics Publishers, Inc. 1993, in press.

100. Stefanick, M. L., R. B. Terry, W. L. Haskell, and P. D. Wood. Relationships of changes in postheparin hepatic and lipoprotein lipase activity to HDL-cholesterol changes following weight loss achieved by dieting versus exercise. L. L. Gallo (ed). *Cardiovascular Disease: Molecular and Cellular Mechanisms, Prevention and Treatment.* New York: Plenum Press, 1987; pp. 61–68.

101. Svedenhag, J., H. Lithell, A. Juhlin-Dannfelt, and J. Henriksson. Increase in skeletal muscle lipoprotein lipase following endurance training in man. *Atherosclerosis* 49:203–207; 1983.

102. Tarnopolsky, L. J., J. D. MacDougall, S. A. Atkinson, L. J. Tarnopolsky, and J. R. Sutton. Gender differences in substrate for endurance exercise. *J. Appl. Physiol.* 68:302–308, 1990.

103. Taskinen, M. R., E. A. Nikkila, S. Rehunen, and A. Gordin. Effect of acute vigorous exercise on lipoprotein lipase activity of adipose tissue and skeletal muscle in physically active men. *Artery* 6:471–483, 1980.

104. Technology Assessment Conference Panel. Methods for voluntary weight loss and control: Technology Assessment Conference statement. *Ann. Intern. Med.* 116:942–949, 1992.

105. Terry, R. B., M. L. Stefanick, W. L. Haskell, and P. D. Wood. Contributions of regional adipose tissue depots to plasma lipoprotein concentrations in overweight men and women: possible protective effects of thigh fat. *Metabolism* 40:733–740, 1991.

106. Thompson, J. K., G. J. Jarvie, B. B. Lahey, and K. J. Cureton. Exercise and obesity: etiology, physiology, and intervention. *Psychol. Bull.* 91:55–79, 1982.

107. Thompson, P. D., E. Cullinane, R. Eshleman, S. P. Sady, and P. N. Herbert. The effects of calorie restriction or exercise cessation on the serum lipid and lipoprotein concentrations of endurance athletes. *Metabolism* 33:943–950, 1984.

108. Thompson, P. D., E. Cullinane, L. O. Henderson, and P. N. Herbert. Acute effects of prolonged exercise on serum lipids. *Metabolism* 29:662–665, 1980.

109. Thompson, P. D., E. Cullinane, S. P. Sady, et al. Modest changes in high density lipoprotein concentration and metabolism with prolonged exercise training. *Circulation* 78:25–34, 1988.

110. Tremblay, A., J. P. Despres, C. LeBlanc, and C. Bouchard. Sex dimorphism in fat loss in response to exercise-training. *J. Obes. Weight Regul.* 3:193–203, 1984.

111. Vague J. The degree of masculine differentiation of obesities: a factor determining predisposition to diabetes, atherosclerosis, gout, and uric calculous diseases. *Am. J. Clin. Nutr.* 4:20–34, 1956.

112. Van Dale, D., E. Beckers, P. F. M. Schoffelen, F. ten Hoor, and W. H. M. Saris. Changes in sleeping metabolic rate and glucose induced thermogenesis during a diet or a diet/exercise treatment. *Nutrit. Res.* 10:615–626, 1990.

113. Van Dale, D., and W. H. M. Saris. Repetitive weight loss and weight regain: effects on weight reduction, resting metabolic rate, and lipolytic activity before and after exercise and/or diet treatment. *Am. J. Clin. Nutr.* 49:409–416, 1989.

114. Van Dale, D., W. H. M. Saris, and F. ten Hoor. Weight maintenance and resting metabolic rate 18–40 months after a diet/exercise treatment. *Int. J. Obesity* 14:347–359, 1990.

115. Wahrenberg, H., J. Bolinder, and P. Arner. Adrenergic regulation of lipolysis in human fat cells during exercise. *Eur. J. Clin. Invest.* 21:534–541, 1991.

116. Walberg, J. L. Aerobic exercise and resistance weight-training during weight reduction: implications for obese persons and athletes. *Sports Med.* 47:343–346, 1989.

117. Walker, M., B. G. Cooper, C. Elliott, J. W. Reed, H. Orskov, and K. G. M. M. Alberti. Role of plasma non-esterified fatty acids during and after exercise. *Clin. Sci.* 81:319–325, 1991.

118. Williamson, D. F., H. S. Kahn, P. L. Remington, and R. F. Anda. The 10-year incidence of overweight and major weight gain in U.S. Adults. *Arch. Intern. Med.* 150:665–672, 1990.

119. Wilmore, J. H. Body composition in sport and exercise: directions for future research. *Med. Sci. Sports Exercise* 15:21–31, 1983.

120. Wing, R. R., L. H. Kuller, C. Bunker, et al. Obesity, obesity-related behaviors and coronary heart disease risk factors in black and white premenopausal women. *Int. J. Obesity* 13:511–519, 1989.

121. Wing, R. R., K. A. Matthews, L. H. Kuller, E. N. Meilahn, and P. Plantinga. Waist to hip ratio in middle-aged women: associations with behavioral and psychosocial factors and with changes in cardiovascular risk factors. *Arterioscler. Thromb.* 11:1250–1257, 1991.

122. Wing, R. R., K. A. Matthews, L. H. Kuller, E. N. Meilahn, and P. Plantinga. Weight gain at the time of menopause. *Arch. Intern. Med.* 151:97–102, 1991.

123. Wolfe, R. R. S. Klein, F. Carraro, and J. M. Weber. Role of triglyceride-fatty acid cycle in controlling fat metabolism in humans during and after exercise. *Am. J. Physiol.* 258 (*Endocrinol. Metabol.* 21):E382–E389, 1990.

124. Wood, P. D., W. L. Haskell, S. N. Blair, et al. Increased exercise level and plasma lipoprotein concentrations: a one-year, randomized, controlled study in sedentary, middle-aged men. *Metabolism* 32:31–39, 1983.

125. Wood, P.D., M. L. Stefanick, D. M. Dreon, et al. Changes in plasma lipids and lipoproteins in overweight men during weight loss through dieting as compared with exercise. *N. Engl. J. Med.* 319:1173–1179, 1988.

126. Wood, P.D., M. L. Stefanick, P. T. Williams, and W. L. Haskell. The effects on plasma lipoproteins of a prudent weight-reducing diet, with or without exercise, in overweight men and women. *N. Engl. J. Med.* 325:461–466, 1991.

13
Motor Cortex and Visuomotor Behavior

JOHN F. KALASKA, Ph.D.
TREVOR DREW, Ph.D.

As a result of his epochal studies of the motor deficits in neurological patients in the 1800s, John Hughlings Jackson proposed that the human motor system comprised a hierarchy of three levels [110]. Roughly speaking, the pons, medulla, and spinal cord were at the lowest level, the cerebral cortex around the central sulcus, including what is now called the primary motor cortex, formed part of the middle level, and a number of adjacent cerebral areas were at the highest level. Hughlings Jackson argued that the level at which movements were organized within this tripartite hierarchy varied in ascending sequence from the "most automatic," at the lowest level, to "least automatic " movements, at the highest level. These three levels did not form a rigid unidirectional hierarchy, however, and motor control depended on the interactions among the three levels.

The concept of automaticity of motor behavior goes beyond the dichotomy of "reflex" versus "voluntary" movements. A good example of the distinction is the use of the diaphragm and intercostal muscles during the highly automatic rhythmic motions of respiration generated by brainstem circuits, versus their use in speech, an act of low automaticity that is critically dependent on several cerebral cortical areas [110]. Least automatic movements encompass many nonstereotypical motor acts that are often guided by sensory information from the external world, and by motor strategies shaped by previous experience. They are the hallmark of the motor repertoire of higher mammals, especially primates, whose behavior has become progressively less stimulus-bound during phylogeny, and increasingly dependent on an intact cerebral cortex.

This perspective implies that the sequence of neuronal events controlling a movement is dependent on the nature and context of the movement. It also emphasizes that all descending supraspinal motor control is implemented through the intermediary of brainstem and spinal circuitry that has its own intrinsic ability to organize motor acts. These important points are often overlooked, especially in general textbooks and the clinical literature.

SCOPE

This essay examines the role of the primary motor cortex in motor control. In keeping with the Jacksonian perspective, the major premise of this article is that, although the motor cortex provides critical control signals for the performance of skilled or less automatic motor acts, the control of movement is best understood in terms of the interplay between supraspinal and spinal processes. This will be illustrated by considering two visually guided motor acts, reaching movements in primates and locomotor gait modifications in cats.

It may seem curious to review reaching in primates and locomotion in cats together. However, they are both examples of the use of the forelimbs in behaviors of differing degrees of automaticity. Stepping movements are a stereotypical rhythmic component of terrestrial locomotion in pedal animals. It is well documented that the isolated spinal cord of many vertebrates, including cats, is capable of generating the rhythmic automatism of the basic locomotor cycle [61]. Most neurophysiological studies of locomotion, therefore, have focused on its subcortical, especially spinal, mechanisms. In contrast, reaching is a quintessential example of a "voluntary" act. It often occurs during less stereotypical nonlocomotor behaviors, such as food gathering and manual exploration of the immediate environment. Neurophysiological studies of reaching and other less automatic acts have concentrated on the role of the cerebral cortex, especially the motor cortex.

A conceptual and experimental link between reaching and stepping is provided by precise visually guided gait modification during locomotion. While locomoting over the uneven ground of the normal environment, a cat must continually adjust its step cycle to compensate for observed irregularities in terrain and to step around or over obstacles. The motor cortex likely plays a key role in this gait modification [9, 36]. Moreover, reaching behavior may be an evolutionary elaboration of precise positioning of the forelimb during locomotion over irregular terrain that allowed for arboreal climbing [56]. Given that evolution is characterized by the adaptation of preexisting structures to new functions, it is probable, therefore, that reaching movements are mediated through much of the same neuronal circuitry as that used for precise gait control [56].

Furthermore, visually guided reaching and gait modifications are both multiarticular acts, and both require the transformation of visual input into a motor output. Many of the issues pertaining to these aspects of reaching and stepping movements have been discussed extensively in a number of reviews [23, 44, 49, 65, 67–69, 109, 121–124, 129]. It is worthwhile, however, to give a brief overview of some of the key concepts.

WHY STUDY MULTIARTICULAR ACTS?

Reductionism has a long and honorable history in science. The study of motor control is no exception. Research has often focused on the presumed elemental constituents of motor behavior, such as minimalist single-joint movements or reflex circuits. The assumption behind this reductionist approach is that all motor behavior can be explained by a limited number of universal organizing principles or strategies, such as reciprocal activation vs. cocontraction of antagonist muscles, or control or optimization of a variable, such as position, joint angles, muscle lengths, or energy expenditure. These universal features could be studied in simple movement tasks (to eliminate "superfluous" complexities), and then scaled up to more complex behaviors by a simple linear summation of the presumed individual "building blocks" of the behavior, such as single muscles or joints.

However, the validity of this approach has been challenged because multiarticular acts introduce fundamental motor control issues that cannot be addressed in reduced tasks (for excellent debates on this issue, see [60, 126]). For instance, the mechanical properties of a linked multiarticular chain, such as the arm, vary with its geometry, i.e., its posture [67, 68], and complex dynamic mechanical interactions occur among the limb segments during motion [49, 62, 65, 67, 68, 129]. These factors will have a profound influence on the muscle activity patterns required to produce a movement. A related complication of multiarticular acts is the need to coordinate the timing and strength of contraction of many muscles at many joints. Consequently, multiarticular acts cannot be executed by chaining together isolated closed-loop servo-control circuits for single joints and muscles [98, 101].

Moreover, the nervous system must select one of the theoretically infinite range of different sequences of joint motions and muscle activation patterns that can produce a particular movement or generate a desired output force. This is one manifestation of the so-called "degrees of freedom" problem in motor control [24, 65, 68]. Unlike the old joke about how you can't get there from here, there are usually *too many* ways to get there in motor control!

There is extensive evidence that the spinal cord is capable of resolving many of these mechanical complexities. Adult cats spinalized at the low thoracic level show a remarkable recovery of hindlimb motor function over a period of a month or so and are able to walk on a moving belt [20]. Nevertheless, the locomotor capacity of spinal cats is severely limited, and the movements lack the grace and coordination of normal locomotion. Locomotion is markedly improved if the cat is decerebrated just rostral to the thalamus, leaving intact the descending mesencephalic and brainstem projections to the spinal cord; such cats can support their own weight and demonstrate almost normal spontaneous locomotion and gait transitions (walk ↔ trot ↔ gallop) on a flat surface. Thus, subcortical circuits in cats are not merely passive relays for descending cortical motor signals; they possess sophisticated pattern-generating ability and may be responsible for much of the organization of stereotypical automatic multiarticular movements. Rather than having to reinvent solutions to the mechanics of multiarticular movements during less automatic behavior, cerebral motor centers could exploit this organizing capacity of midbrain and spinal systems by controlling movement through their intermediary.

Admittedly, the effects of spinal transection or decerebration in primates, especially in humans, are far more severe than in cats [40]. It is not yet clear whether this difference between cats and primates reflects a greater dependence of primate subcortical centers on a nonspecific descending facilitatory drive or a greater reliance on more specific descending control signals to initiate and to sustain motor behavior. Indeed, whether the primate spinal cord contains pattern-generating circuitry is still considered an open question, although both developmental and lesion studies suggest that some pattern-generating capacity probably exists [25, 31, 50, 93, 94]. Given the absence of evidence for fundamental physiological differences between local spinal circuitry in cats and monkeys, we will assume that spinal pattern-generating circuitry is retained in primates, but has lost much of the capacity to generate autonomous motor behavior, rendering them increasingly subservient to descending control signals from higher centers.

VISUOMOTOR COORDINATE TRANSFORMATIONS

The essential role of visual information in performing anticipatory locomotor gait adjustments is self-evident. Likewise, reaching movements are usually planned to position the hand at the spatial location of a visual target. The ability to perform these interactions with the environment is not completely innate. There is substantial evidence that this can be considered a motor skill that improves with early postnatal practice [63].

Pathways of Skilled Visuomotor Coordination
Several major pathways conveying visuospatial information ultimately converge on the motor cortex. Among these, the corticocortical pathway from the parietotemporal cortex to the prefrontal, premotor, and motor cortex appears to be particularly important [71, 109, 125]. The many potential roles for this pathway include: analyzing of the visual-flow input that arises during locomotion, defining the spatial location of potential movement targets, and transforming this visual information into appropriate motor responses [7, 125]. Lesions of both the primate

and feline parietal cortex do not impede the ability to move, *per se*, but do result in the visuomotor deficits encompassed under the term apraxia— the inability to make appropriate spatially directed motions in their proper context, such as misreaching [7, 43, 111, 125].

Lesions of the primary motor cortex in cats result in normal locomotion across a smooth surface, but major deficits in skilled locomotor tasks that require precise foot placement under visual guidance, such as walking along a curved surface or stepping on the rungs of a horizontal ladder [*see* 9]. As already noted, lesions of the motor cortex or pyramidal tract are far more devastating in primates than in cats, but monkeys eventually recover some use of the limbs. They can walk on all four limbs and climb [93], but the latter can be clumsy and slow [31, 64]. The least automatic movements are most severely compromised, particularly individual finger movements [64, 93]. Reaching movements can recover [64], but the graceful coordination of normal reaching is usually compromised; the movements are often initially reduced to crude swiping motions of the arm from the shoulder, with the elbow held in a fixed angle [31, 93]. Unfortunately, these observations have been largely anecdotal, and there has been no quantitative study of reaching skills after well-localized motor cortex lesions in monkeys. Nevertheless, these findings show that the capacity to perform reaching movements to visual targets is not entirely dependent on the motor cortex. An enduring question is the extent to which the residual ability to make reaching movements depends on other arm movement-related cerebral cortical areas [37, 71, 74, 85] vs. subcortical systems [3, 31, 89, 93, 94, 109].

Modeling Studies
A great deal of effort has been expended to deduce the planning processes by which the CNS generates the muscle activity patterns for discrete reaching movements to targets from a stationary starting position [23, 24, 44, 49, 62, 65, 67–69, 92, 109, 121–124, 129]. The central planning events are usually described in terms of a serial hierarchical "top-down" analysis of the control problem, progressing from more global attributes of the movement, such as behavioral objectives and general form, to increasingly more specific details concerning its execution [24, 65, 71, 82, 85]. A prominent approach is to view the planning of reaching movements as a problem of visuomotor coordinate transformations, beginning with a representation of the target location in external visual space and culminating in a representation of the movement in a multidimensional "space" of muscle activation patterns [24, 65, 68, 121–124]. Most of these models recognize three general levels of coordinate frameworks (Fig. 13.1), including representations of extrinsic kinematics, intrinsic kinematics, and dynamics (also often referred to as kinetics). Note that the terms kinematics and dynamics are used here simply to distinguish between spatiotemporal parameters that describe the form of a movement and

FIGURE 13.1

A general three-stage serial planning hierarchy for the control of arm reaching movements. Each arrow *represents a coordinate transformation. Candidate planned parameters are listed below each of the three general coordinate reference frames.*

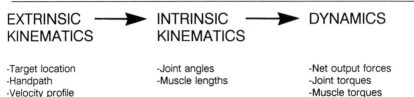

EXTRINSIC   →   INTRINSIC   →   DYNAMICS
KINEMATICS   KINEMATICS

-Target location	-Joint angles	-Net output forces
-Handpath	-Muscle lengths	-Joint torques
-Velocity profile		-Muscle torques
		-Muscle activation patterns

those related to causative forces and muscle activity, and so are amalgams of parameters that fall within statics, kinematics, and dynamics, as they are formally defined in Newtonian mechanics. We will use the terms kinematics-level and dynamics-level representations as convenient descriptors to distinguish between neuronal activity that covaries with the form of the movement and that which covaries with causal forces and muscle activity. However, this is not meant to imply that the central nervous system (CNS) plans a reaching movement by solving the Newtonian equations of motion to transform the handpath into joint motions (inverse kinematics), then to joint torques (inverse dynamics), before parcelling the net torques among the muscles acting across the joints [65] nor that it represents motor acts literally in terms of any of the parameters in Figure 13.1 [85].

Ample, albeit circumstantial, evidence supporting a hierarchical planning process comes from behavioral studies that have revealed a number of invariant properties of reaching movements, such as straight-line handpaths with bell-shaped velocity profiles [49, 65, 68, 69, 92], tightly coupled motions of the shoulder and elbow during reaching motions [124], and simple rules that define the relations between extrinsic kinematic parameters of the handpath of reaching and drawing motions and both intrinsic kinematic attributes, such as joint motions and limb segment angles [92, 121–124], and muscle activation patterns [44, 48, 60, 62, 86]. These stereotypical invariant patterns have been interpreted to reflect the natural coordinates and movement attributes by which the CNS represents the movement at different levels of the planning hierarchy, or to result from the transformations between coordinate representations [49, 65, 68, 92, 121–124].

However, there is still no consensus as to the nature of the putative reference frames and coordinate transformations underlying reaching movements, or where they arise in the CNS. For instance, whether or not the CNS explicitly plans the handpath of reaching movements remains controversial [24, 69, 92, 122, 124], A further important insight of these studies is that many movement attributes and invariants need not be explicitly planned by central processes. They may instead be products of peripheral musculoskeletal mechanics and the response of the combined spinal cord-musculoskeletal system to simpler central control signals. For example, the conversion from a putative kinematic representation of movement to dynamics and muscle activity is most problematic to solve by a top-down analytic approach [65, 68, 129]. However, controversial "equilibrium point" models have suggested that much of the apparent complexity of this stage in the planning process could be simplified if the CNS exploited the length-tension properties of muscles and controlled them like tunable springs [23, 44, 49, 67, 68]. These models propose that the causal dynamics and muscle activity are not explicitly computed, but arise implicitly through manipulation of the length-tension properties of muscles; for instance, by control of the stretch reflex recruitment threshold [23, 44] or by "virtual trajectory" signals that indicate the equilibrium position of the hand in space [49, 68]. According to these models, neural signals specifying muscle contractile activity originate in the spinal cord. As a result, the motor cortex need not be primarily concerned with the specific control of muscles, but with the extrinsic spatial attributes of movement, such as its direction or handpath [53, 54, 122, 123]. These models, therefore, would place the role of the motor cortex near the beginning of the putative planning hierarchy of Figure 13.1.

It is interesting to contrast these studies on the planning of reaching with the models used to explain the control of locomotion. As opposed to the top-down analytic structure of most of the models just described, locomotion is normally studied from a "bottom-up" perspective. Because the spinal cord of most vertebrates is capable of generating the complex muscle activation patterns that cause the basic locomotor movements, most effort has focused on such questions as how interacting populations of neurons can generate rhythmic patterns of activity, how peripheral input can modify this autonomous rhythmicity, and how different descending systems may enable and modify the basic locomotor rhythm. During visually guided gait modifications, motor cortex signals descend onto spinal systems that are already engaged in locomotor control. Thus, the motor cortex processes involved in producing gait modifications have been examined from the point of view of the changes in the amplitude and timing of muscle contractile activity needed to alter the movement, without consideration of any possible antecedent kinematic framework that might be required to plan such changes. This places the motor cortex nearer the end of the putative planning hierarchy than is suggested by some models for reaching movements. Nevertheless, the problem confronted by an animal in precise foot placement during locomotion is to control the path of limb motion so as to place the foot in a specific spatial location while avoiding obstacles along the path, just as in reaching movements. Although the goal of the movement is thus conceptually similar, a critical difference in the problems to be solved is that the descending signal from the cortex in this specific context does not initiate a movement from a stationary posture, but rather modifies an ongoing locomotor rhythm. In contrast, for discrete nonrhythmic fractionated movements, which occur with increasing frequency in primates, supraspinal and spinal circuits working in concert must initiate and generate de novo all the spinal activity subserving the motor act.

MOTOR CORTEX

The primary motor cortex corresponds approximately to the "agranular" cortex (lack of a well-defined cytoarchitectonic layer [45]) located in the pericruciate cortex in cats, and in the rostral bank of the central sulcus and the immediately anterior cortical surface in monkeys.

Corticospinal Tract

The motor cortex sends descending outputs to a number of subcortical motor structures, including the basal ganglia, red nucleus, pontine nuclei, and the pontine and medullary reticular formation. However, it is the corticospinal tract, which is unique to mammals, that affords the most direct cortical access to the spinal motor apparatus and has been the most intensely studied of all cortical motor systems. Although the cells of origin of the corticospinal tract are distributed over a large expanse of the precentral and postcentral cerebral cortex [37, 88], the primary motor cortex was thought for many years to be the major source of corticospinal axons [88]. Recently, however, it has become evident that the corticospinal output from arm-related areas outside of the primary motor cortex has been significantly underestimated [37], and may comprise the largest part of the tract. Therefore, the primary motor cortex is not, in the strictest sense, the "final common path" for the cerebral control of movement.

The spinal termination pattern of corticospinal tract neurons is different in the cat and monkey. In the cat, all corticospinal axons terminate in the spinal intermediate gray matter, and the minimal linkage to spinal motoneurons is disynaptic [8, 77, see 110 for review]. The corticospinal disynaptic pathway onto C5-C8 spinal motor neurons that innervate forelimb muscles is mediated not only via local segmental interneurons, but also through an identifiable class of propriospinal neurons located principally in cervical segments three and four (C3-C4 propriospinal interneurons), that project onto C5-C8 motor neurons, and receive collateral input from corticospinal axons that also innervate the cervical enlargement [70, 76–79, 119].

In contrast, along with the terminations on spinal interneurons, the primate's corticospinal tract also makes monosynaptic connections with spinal motoneurons of muscles acting around each of the major joints of the limb [89, 95, 110]. The cells of origin of this direct projection are found only in the primary motor cortex [88]. Electrophysiological [110] and anatomical [89] studies in nonhuman primates show that the monosynaptic projections are much stronger to digit motor neurons than they are to motor neurons controlling more proximal muscles. The major corticospinal control of proximal arm muscles in monkeys is, therefore, still primarily via spinal interneuronal relays. The direct monosynaptic pathway is larger in humans than in other primates and recent indirect evidence suggests that it may include significant mono-synaptic terminations on proximal arm motor neurons [29, 39]. The extent to which this monosynaptic pathway can be seen as augmenting the phylogenetically older polysynaptic pathway via spinal interneurons, or as supplanting it, is unknown.

Motor Cortex "Output" Map
Experiments designed to examine motor cortical functional topography have concentrated on two closely related issues, namely, how is the body represented upon the cortical surface, and what is the elemental output unit of the motor cortex?

Early electrical stimulation experiments by Fritsch and Hitzig, Ferrier, Sherrington and Woolsey gave rise to the now familiar concept of a somatotopic organization in which each part of the body is represented in a motor output map on the cortical surface [72, 96, 110]. Because of current spread, however, surface stimulation could not reveal the finer organization of the cortical projections. This problem was partially surmounted by the development of the technique of intracortical microstimulation (ICMS) [17], which permitted activation of a discrete, circumscribed volume of cortical tissue. The increased resolution of this method made it possible to examine the output map in more detail. Using this method, Asanuma and Sakata [17] showed that low-threshold currents of 10 μA or less frequently excited only a single spinal motoneuron pool. They proposed that the cortex was organized as a mosaic of vertical columns, each of which would preferentially control the activity of a single muscle [15].

One of the most detailed mapping studies using this technique was that of Kwan et al. [90], in which they identified the joint at which motions occurred in response to threshold ICMS in unanaesthetized monkeys. They reported that the motor map for the arm in rhesus monkeys was represented on the cortical surface in a series of nested, concentric rings. The digits and wrist were represented centrally and were surrounded by, respectively, areas activating the elbow and shoulder. The nested rings for each joint were not completely segre-gated; there was an extensive interdigitation of stimulation sites that evoked motions of the shoulder and elbow, and likewise, for the wrist and digits. The overlap between proximal (shoulder and elbow) vs. distal joints (wrist and digits) was much more modest. Other mapping studies in the fascicularis monkey [118] and squirrel monkey [32] and the baboon [128] also found extensive interdigitation of outputs to different muscles or joints, but a nested-ring configuration for arm segments was only reported in the fascicularis monkey.

Although the results of threshold ICMS studies suggested that the motor cortex output map was organized as a mosaic of multiple separate output zones for each muscle, separated by different combinations of output zones for other muscles, even low ICMS currents often facilitated more than one motoneuron pool in both cats [18] and monkeys [16]. This was more pronounced when slightly higher strengths of ICMS were used. In alert, unanaesthetized animals, stimuli at 20–35 μA frequently activated several muscles, including those acting at different joints [10, 11, 32, 72, 115, 116]. During movement, inhibitory effects also became evident [11, 28, 116]. This leads to a somewhat different perspective on the topographic organization of the motor cortex, whereby the cortical output zone activating any one particular muscle may occupy a broad patch of the motor cortex. At the same time, there is extensive overlap of output zones for different muscles, so that individual loci can activate several muscles acting around the same or different joints [32, 72, 96, 115]. Consequently, different parts of the arm portion of the map will contain different combinations of outputs to muscles acting across different joints.

However, even with ICMS, these results have to be interpreted with some caution because of the possibility that the apparent divergent multi-muscle output from single stimulus loci may be due, in part, to direct or transynaptic activation of several cortical output zones [96]. Moreover, it is important to appreciate that the responses observed in output mapping studies are the peripheral consequences of activation of a small part of the cortical map, as mediated via all intervening synaptic circuitry. In that sense, the motor cortex output map, as defined by ICMS, could be regarded as a property of the entire corticospinal system, and does not reside exclusively in the motor cortex.

Nevertheless, two further lines of compelling evidence indicate that small areas of cortex, and indeed, single corticospinal neurons, are likely to affect the contractile activity of several muscles in parallel. First, Fetz et al. [27, 45] used the technique of spike-triggered averaging to demonstrate that the discharge of some single motor cortex corticospinal neurons, which they called "corticomotoneurons," can simultaneously facilitate the activity of several muscles via divergent monosynaptic projections into different motoneuron pools [27, 45]. Similar results were reported by Lemon et al. for digit muscles [97]. The consensus from both groups is that individual corticomotoneurons can facilitate the activity of groups of synergistic muscles and may simultaneously disfacilitate, or inhibit, the motor neuron pools of antagonistic muscles

[28, 97]. Second, an anatomical and physiological basis for these findings has been provided by the elegant work of Shinoda and co-workers in both the cat and monkey [19, 52, 119, 120]. In one series of experiments, intraxonal injection of horseradish peroxidase (HRP) into corticospinal fibers in the monkey revealed axon terminal arborizations in several motor neuronal pools in one spinal segment [120; see also 95]. Further, individual corticospinal axons in the cat [119] and primate [19] not only branch profusely within any one segment, but also send collateral branches to neighboring segments. Thus, there is extensive divergence of the spinal projections of different cortical output clusters, and individual cortical neurons can influence the activity of several muscles. In addition, all of these experiments consider only the monosynaptic projections of corticospinal cells. It is probable that the functional divergence of corticospinal influences may be even more extensive than that already demonstrated when projections through interneuronal networks are considered.

Conversely, descending signals from different output clusters can interact by convergence onto spinal circuits and motoneuron pools. Furthermore, interactions among output clusters are not limited to the spinal level. Anatomical [75] and cross-correlation techniques [47, 91] have shown that functionally related output clusters throughout the motor cortex output map, such as clusters controlling the same joint or contiguous joints like the shoulder and elbow, can interact via a complex network of horizontal axonal connections within the motor cortex. Therefore, it might be best to think of the arm portion of the motor cortex map as a single integrated functional unit for the control of arm movement, and not as a patchwork of parallel independent output clusters controlling single muscles or joints.

Finally, a striking recent finding is that the functional relationship between a point on the motor cortex map and the peripheral musculature is flexible, within certain limits. For instance, the peripheral response to stimulation can vary from moment to moment during movement (see Segmental Interactions). Moreover, experimental interventions such as peripheral motor nerve transection [114], prolonged microstimulation of a single cortical locus [107], or iontophoretic application of bicuculline to the motor cortex [81] can induce a change in the set of muscles activated by microstimulation of a given point on the map. The alterations are too rapid to result from the formation of new synapses; they probably reflect rapid changes in the functional properties of corticospinal circuitry. Furthermore, stimulation of the somatosensory cortex and thalamus can induce long-term potentiation in motor cortical neurons [80, 113], allowing for changes of the input-output properties of the cortical output map. These important new findings suggest that the motor cortex output map, as defined by microstimulation, is not a static entity indelibly written onto the cortical surface. They further suggest a substantial potential for use-dependent modification of the functional organization of the motor cortex output map, which has important implications for the acquisition of motor skills, including the postnatal acquisition of accurate reaching.

RECORDING STUDIES IN MOTOR CORTEX DURING BEHAVIOR

Locomotion

During locomotion on a level treadmill, the discharge of many motor cortex neurons, including identified pyramidal tract neurons (PTNs), has been shown to be modulated at the rhythm of the locomotor cycle [9, 12, 38]. Most neurons showed a single peak of discharge, occurring at different times during the swing or stance phase of the contralateral limb in different cells. An ensemble average of motor cortical activity showed a clear maximum just before the onset of swing. This suggested that one role of the motor cortex during ordinary locomotion might be to regulate the timing of the transition between stance and swing [12].

While the role of the motor cortex may be facultative during ordinary treadmill locomotion, it is critical for walking over uneven terrain [9]. Recording studies have shown that motor cortex activity is selectively enhanced during visually guided gait modifications in cats, compared to walking on a flat surface. Morever, this activity may be closely correlated with specific details of the modification. For instance, Amos et al. [6] found that the discharge of six of 16 motor cortex neurons increased during locomotion on a circular ladder, compared to overground locomotion, which may have been related to the fine control of the distal musculature needed to place the forepaw accurately on the rungs of the ladder. This finding has been confirmed by Beloozerova and Sirota [22]. In addition, they recorded motor cortical discharge while cats stepped over a series of high barriers separated by varying distances. This required an increase in limb flexion to bring the foot over the barrier. Many motor cortex neurons showed a change in activity, the degree of which varied with the size of the interbarrier space within which the cat had to place its paw. This was interpreted as being related to the degree of foot-placement accuracy [22].

Recent experiments by Drew [34, 35] suggest that the alterations in corticofugal discharge could encode specific parts of the gait modification, rather than simply giving a generalized increased input to the spinal pattern generators (Fig. 13.2). In these experiments, cats stepped over obstacles of different shapes and sizes attached to a moving treadmill belt. Each obstacle required a different forelimb trajectory and muscle activity pattern to step over it [34]. Consequently, the gait modifications dissociated the activity patterns of muscles, which are often tightly coupled during ordinary treadmill locomotion (see, e.g., cleidobrachialis and brachialis in Fig. 13.2) A comparison of the timing of activity of recorded PTNs and muscles showed that the maximum alteration of cell activity occurred at different times in the modified step cycle for different cells, and that cell discharge was frequently better correlated with the activity of one (or a few) muscle(s) than with the others across the range of muscle activity patterns generated during gait modifications over all of the obstacles. For instance, the discharge of the cell in Figure 13.2 covaried better with the activity of the brachialis muscle than with either the cleidobrachialis or the extensor carpi radialis (Fig. 13.2C). This cell could be providing a signal for the increased activity in the brachialis and other flexors needed to bring the leg above the obstacle. A correlation with muscle activity during this initial stage of the gait modification was seen in 23 of 47 task-related PTNs. The discharge of a further 12 PTNs, which occurred later in the swing phase, covaried best with the activity of the wrist dorsiflexor muscles, implicating them in the control of the accurate placement of the foot.

Overall, the results from this study suggested that the motor cortex is supplying the detailed information about the altered step needed to modify the activity patterns of different groups of muscles at different times during the gait modification. It is assumed that this descending control is mediated via the interneuronal networks responsible for the generation of the basic locomotor rhythm.

Primates: Nonreaching Movements
To date, although no one has studied whether the same task-dependent difference occurs between more and less automatic limb movements in primates, some observations suggest that it does. For instance, many jaw movement-related motor cortex cells were very active when monkeys exerted small precise bite forces against a strain gauge, but were far less active when the animal chewed vigorously on a food pellet [66]. Similarly, wrist-related corticomotoneurons were often strongly active during accurate wrist movements but relatively inactive when the monkey made frustrated, brisk oscillatory motions of the wrist [27]. Finally, a number of corticomotoneurons were far more active during delicate precision-pinch movements of the thumb and index finger than during the more primitive power grip of the entire hand [102].

Therefore, many primate motor cortex cells can be preferentially recruited or show a selective enhancement of activity during precise skilled movements compared to brisk "ballistic" or more automatic behaviors, even though the output forces and muscle activity are often far greater in the latter situation. This important finding is all the more significant when one notes that the last two studies concern corticomotoneurons with monosynaptic access to spinal motoneurons. This

FIGURE 13.2

Discharge of a pyramidal tract neuron during voluntary gait modification. **A.** *Untreated data showing the activity of the PTN, along with electromyographic (EMG) activity from three flexor muscles and an extensor muscle during a step over an obstacle* (arrow). **B.** *Average activity of the neuron and muscles for a step over a round obstacle, together with the steps prior and subsequent to this* (thicker line). *The data have been normalized to the average step cycle duration during normal treadmill locomotion* (thinner line). **C.** *Raster displays and postevent histograms of the cell discharge compiled from steps over four different types of obstacles, each of which requires a different limb trajectory and thus pattern of muscle activity. The rasters are oriented to the onset of the indicated muscle* (vertical line). *The first series of* staggered, vertical ticks *indicates the time when muscle discharge ceases and therefore indicates the duration of the period of muscle activity during each step cycle. The rasters are rank-ordered according to the duration of each muscle burst. Note that the cell's discharge covaries better with the period of activity of* Br *than with either* ClB *or* ECR. *Threshold ICMS at the recording site caused elbow flexion.* CIB: *cleidobrachialis;* Br: *brachialis;* ECR: *extensor carpi radialis;* TRiL: *lateral head of triceps brachii;* CO: *contralateral to stimulation site.*

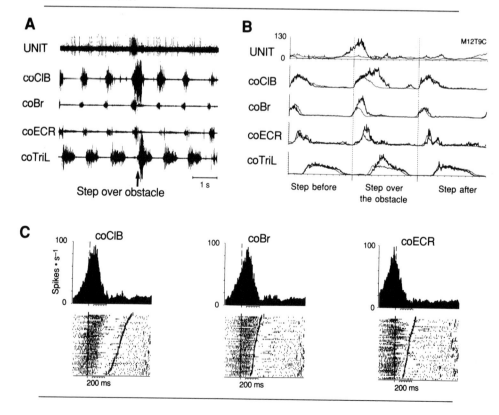

task-dependent property of primate motor cortex discharge may be more important than is currently appreciated, since relatively few studies have examined the behavior of the same motor cortex neurons during a range of behaviors of different degrees of automaticity.

On the contrary, most studies have tested cells under only a single task condition, usually requiring a significant degree of precise control. Typically, monkeys made movements of a single joint in two opposite directions, or exerted graded levels of isometric force. These "reductionist" tasks were designed to identify the movement parameters being signalled by motor cortex activity, and thus its position within the putative planning hierarchy for voluntary movement. Correlations were found among cell discharge and such experimental variables as movement direction, amplitude, velocity, and output force [1, 30, 41, 42, 73, 74, 127]. In particular, many motor cortex cells show some degree of covariation with the level of output force or torque (Fig. 13.3). The activity of populations of cells shows a better correlation with output torques and EMG activity than do individual cells [47, 73]. Thus, as is the case during visually guided stepping, motor cortex cells appear to signal detailed information about how to execute skilled precise movements, and so seem to function near the end of the presumed planning hierarchy.

However, not all motor cortex cells show a strong correlation with forces or muscles. Rather, this property may be most pronounced in corticospinal [42] and especially corticomotoneuronal cells [27], but less so in other cells, such as corticorubral [51] and corticostriatal [21] neurons. Indeed, it is a routine finding that many motor cortex cells show better correlations with aspects of movement other than forces or muscle activity, and the few experiments that have investigated this question have demonstrated that neuronal activity that reflects several different levels in the planning hierarchy may coexist in the motor cortex [1, 30, 53, 74, 82, 85, 127]. Therefore, it is possible that different subpopulations of motor cortex cells may preferentially encode quite different parameters of a movement.

Primates: Reaching Studies
Early studies using a limited range of reaching movements found that the activity of many cells appeared to correlate with the motions of specific joints during the movements [104, 105, 112]. Cells related to shoulder and elbow movement showed a tight temporal correlation during reach [104, 105], and cells related to proximal joints were active earlier in the reach movement than were cells related to more distal joints [105, 112]. This pattern of neuronal recruitment corresponds to the proximodistal sequence of joint motions and muscle activity during reach [105], and is probably analogous to the phase-specific activity of cat motor cortex cells observed during gait modification.

FIGURE 13.3

*Variation of the tonic activity rate of identified wrist-related PTNs as a function of the level of isometric torque exerted in the direction of wrist supination (**A**, 11 cells), and in pronation (**B**, 7 cells). Reproduced from Evarts, E.V., C. Fromm, J. Kroller, and V.A. Jennings. Motor cortex of finely graded forces. J. Neurophysiol. 49:1199–1215, 1983.*

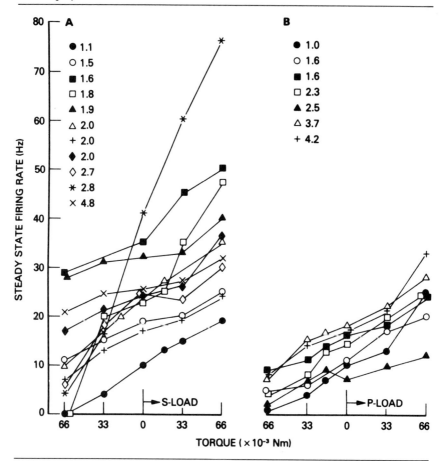

A more detailed series of experiments has been performed over the past decade using a wider range of reaching directions in 2D (planar) and 3D space [26, 53, 55, 58, 59, 82–85, 87, 117]. For the planar task, eight targets were uniformly dispersed in eight different directions in a circle around a common central starting position. For the 3D task, the eight targets were located at the corners of a cube and the start position was at the cube's center. Neuronal recordings were made of cells that were related to movements of the shoulder joint, whose 3 degrees of rotational freedom are critical for determining the initial direction of movement. A review of these results illustrates the difficulties that arise in studying the role of the motor cortex in the control of reaching [82, 83, 85].

The predominant task-related property of cell discharge was directional tuning (Fig. 13.4) [26, 58, 83, 85, 117]. Most shoulder-related cells showed a graded variation of response intensity as a function of

FIGURE 13.4

Activity of a motor cortex cell during eight directions of movement, displayed as rasters (left) *and as a polar plot* (right). *Each raster illustrates the activity during five repeated movements to one target, oriented to the onset of movement* (arrows). *The position of each raster corresponds to the direction of movement. The* heavier tick-marks *to the left and right of movement onset in each raster row represent the time of appearance of the target and the end of movement, respectively. Note the graded variation in the level of discharge with movement direction. This is emphasized in the polar plot, where the length of each axis is proportional to the mean discharge rate from the appearance of the target to the end of the trial. The* radius of the circle *represents the tonic rate of the cell while holding at the central starting position, waiting for a target to appear (i.e., to the* left of the first heavy tick *in the rasters). The calculated preferred movement direction of the cell was at 104°. Reproduced from Kalaska, J.F., D.A.D. Cohen, M.L. Hyde, and M. Prud'homme. A comparison of movement direction-related versus load direction-related activity in primate motor cortex, using a two-dimensional reaching task.* J. Neurosci. 9:2080–2102, 1989.

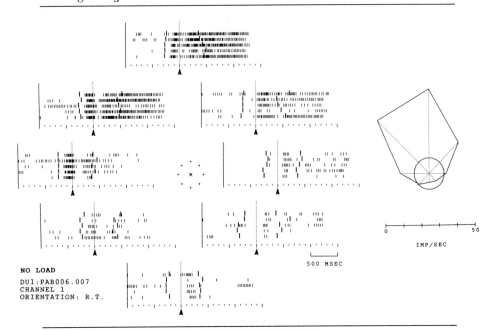

NO LOAD

DU1:PAB006.007
CHANNEL 1
ORIENTATION: R.T.

movement direction, centered on a preferred movement direction that was sufficiently broadly tuned and uniformly distributed about the preferred direction as to show a reasonably good but usually not exact fit to a cosine function. Different cells had different preferred directions, and all possible directions of movement away from the central start position were uniformly distributed in the cell sample in both tasks. The level of tonic activity of many motor cortex cells also covaried with the arm posture at the different target locations (Fig. 13.4) [55, 87].

Because of the broad and approximately symmetrical directional tuning of most motor cortex cells, a given rate of discharge of a single cell does not unambiguously signal the direction of movement, and many cells with widely different preferred directions would be active at different levels for any specific direction of movement. This suggested that an unambiguous signal about the direction of arm movement could only be ascertained at the level of the entire cell population [54, 59]. To test this hypothesis, the discharge of each cell was represented by a vector oriented along its preferred direction axis. The length of the vector for any given movement direction was scaled according to the mean change in discharge of the cell for that direction, recorded from the appearance of the target to the end of the movement. Two of the assumptions of this vector notation are that, whatever the actual information content of the activity of single cells, a change in activity of a cell was associated with (and possibly causal to) a displacement of the limb along a handpath corresponding to its preferred direction, and that the strength of each cell's directional influence was linearly proportional to its mean discharge rate. The population activity for any given movement could be represented by a cluster of vectors of different directions and lengths, and the net population signal could be estimated by a vectorial addition of the single-cell vector contributions. The result of this population analysis was a vector pointing approximately in the direction of movement (Fig. 13.5A). When the same vectorial analysis was done using the cell activity in 20-ms intervals, to capture its time-varying detail, and the 20-ms population vectors were linked head-to-tail, the resultant "neural trajectory" showed a reasonably good, but again not exact, correspondence to the displacement of the hand through space [59]. Since the neural trajectory led the actual movement by 160 ms, it cannot be generated only by reafferent input.

Therefore, the overall pattern of motor cortex population activity covaried with the spatial path and instantaneous tangential velocity of the hand during the reach to the target. This movement representation was encoded in distributed fashion across the neuronal population, and could not be extracted unambiguously from the discharge of single cells. This indicates that the motor command for any given movement is formed from the graded activation of many output clusters throughout the arm output map; different reach trajectories require different

FIGURE 13.5

Vector representation of the activity of a population of 262 motor cortex cells. **A.** *The movement-related change in activity during unloaded arm movements varied with movement direction. The position of each vector cluster corresponds to the direction of movement.* Heavy arrows: *net population vector sums.* **B.** *The change in activity induced by loads in different directions. The position of each cluster corresponds to the direction of external load. Reproduced from Kalaska, J.F., D.A.D. Cohen, M.L. Hyde, and M. Prud'homme. A comparison of movement direction-related versus load direction-related activity in primate motor cortex, using a two-dimensional reaching task.* J. Neurosci. 9:2080–2102, 1989.

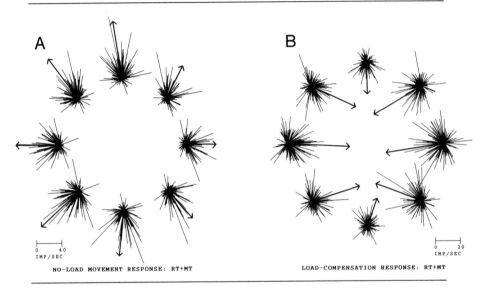

A

B

0   40
IMP/SEC

0   20
IMP/SEC

NO-LOAD MOVEMENT RESPONSE: RT+MT

LOAD-COMPENSATION RESPONSE: RT+MT

distributed patterns of activity. Therefore, all parts of the arm output map contribute a meaningful signal to the control of any reach movement, supporting the idea that it is a single functional unit for the control of multiarticular movement.

In what coordinate frame were the movements being represented? The covariation of the neural trajectory with the handpath would appear to support an extrinsic spatial coordinate system [53, 54, 59], such as target location or spatial vectors for hand displacement [23, 92, 122], as predicted by some modeling studies. However, the movement-related changes in cell activity did not explicitly signal the spatial location of the movement targets. When the monkeys made movements that all converged onto the central target from the eight outer target locations, cell activity continued to covary with movement direction in the same way as seen in the normal task [57]. Thus, the movement-related activity of each cell provided information about how to get to the target from the current arm position. Furthermore, the apparent correlation with extrinsic movement attributes could have arisen indirectly because of the stereotypical coupling between the handpath and joint motions during reaching movements [82, 83, 124]. Indeed, the neurons also discharged during isolated shoulder movements. The differences between the handpath and the neural trajectory may arise because cell activity covaries more closely with some intrinsic shoulder-centered movement attribute. To dissociate extrinsic and intrinsic variables, Caminiti et al. [26] trained monkeys to make reaching movements with parallel handpaths (the same direction in extrinsic space) from different starting points in space (different intrinsic joint angles and muscle activity). The preferred direction vectors of cells tended to rotate as a function of the shoulder joint angle at the different start positions [26], as if encoding movement in a shoulder-centered intrinsic coordinate framework, consistent with psychophysical studies [122]. However, along with the shifts in preferred direction, the level of movement-related activation of cells also varied with starting arm position. As a result, the population vectors continued to point in the direction of movement of the hand [26, 87].

These findings are only circumstantial evidence of an intrinsic representation, however. A more compelling test would be to have monkeys make reaching movements along the identical handpath but with different arm geometries, such as different degrees of shoulder abduction. If shoulder-related cell activity varies as a function of arm geometry, it will be difficult to argue that the motor cortical representation is extrinsic, at least at the single-cell level.

Although all of the reaching tasks described so far involved manipulation of kinematic movement parameters (target location, movement direction, start position), each of the movements also had a unique set of causal forces and muscle activity. To what degree could the movement-related activity of cells reflect a dynamics-level representation of movement, as was found in single-joint tasks? Indirect evidence on this question arises from the directional tuning of cells. If neurons were concerned only with extrinsic kinematic attributes of movement, such as direction, their tuning curves should be perfect cosines, reflecting the geometry of the target locations. However, because of the mechanics of multiarticular movements, the direction of hand displacement is often not colinear with the direction of forces required to produce those movements [62, 65, 123, 129]. As a result, cells that are signaling information about causal forces, or some combination of kinematic and dynamic information, would have tuning curves that deviate from a cosine. Whereas some motor cortex cells have tuning curves that are near-perfect cosines, many others have tuning curves that are narrower and somewhat skewed (Fig. 13.4) As with the differences between movement handpath and neural trajectories, the problem in interpreting the significance of this finding is to determine to what degree these deviations from cosine tuning correspond to the expected difference between the direction of hand movement and the direction of forces that produce that displacement. This requires a detailed knowledge of the biomechanics of the reaching movements.

To obtain a more direct answer to this question, motor cortex activity was studied in a task in which the kinematics and dynamics of the reach trajectories could be partially dissociated by applying different directions of external loads to the task handle in the planar movement task [83]. To compensate, the monkeys had to apply a continual force to the handle in the direction opposite to the applied load, to restore it over the target panel. The total force the monkey had to exert to produce a particular movement is the vector sum of the forces required to move the arm, plus that needed to compensate for the load, and so its direction and size would vary with load direction.

When motor cortex cells were studied in these conditions, cells continued to show activity that was tuned to movement direction under all task conditions [83] (Fig. 13.6*A*). However, many cells also showed strong response changes with the direction of external loads, the most pronounced effect being a variation in the level of tonic activity of the cells as the monkeys exerted continual compensatory forces against the handle (Fig. 13.6*A*) The load-related activity changes usually varied approximately as a cosine function of load direction centered on a load direction (the load axis) that was approximately opposite to each cell's preferred movement direction (Fig. 13.6*C*). Not every cell in the motor cortex was equally sensitive to the loads [83]. Rather, there was a broad continuum of sensitivity, from cells whose task-related activity was completely dominated by their load sensitivity (Fig. 13.6), to neurons that were strongly directional during movement but showed very little load-related response variation. As was the case for corticomotoneurons [27], the most load-sensitive cells also had tonic activity that varied with arm posture, while less load-sensitive cells tended to have a more phasic relation to movement.

Note that the directional tuning of the cell was relatively constant under the different load conditions (Fig. 13.6*A*), suggesting that the cell was *not* signaling either the direction of total output force or torque, or the direction of forces required to compensate for the loads. Correlations with both of the latter could be found in the pattern of population activity, however. A vector analysis of absolute cell activity revealed large load-related changes in the size and direction of the population signal [82, 83] (Fig. 13.7). A load opposite to the direction of movement resulted in an increased population vector length compared to the unloaded condition, while an assisting load caused a sharp reduction in length. Furthermore, loads perpendicular to the movement direction caused a deviation of the population vector signal away from the

FIGURE 13.6

A. *Variation of the response of the cell in Figure 13.4 as a function of external load direction. The activity during unloaded arm movements (Fig. 13.4) is represented by the central polar plot, and the responses during loaded arm movements are illustrated by the other eight polar plots. The position of each polar plot corresponds to the direction in which the load pulls the arm away from the central starting position. Note the large graded changes in overall activity, particularly tonic activity* (radius of the circles). Dashed line: *preferred movement direction;* dot-dashed line: *load axis.* **B.** *Cell activity varied approximately a cosine function of movement direction during unloaded arm movements, centered on the preferred direction.* **C.** *Cell activity varied approximately as a cosine function of load direction, centered on the load axis. Reproduced from Kalaska, J.F., D.A.D. Cohen, M.L. Hyde, and M. Prud'homme. A comparison of movement direction-related versus load direction-related activity in primate motor cortex, using a two-dimensional reaching task.* J. Neurosci. 9:2080–2102, 1989.

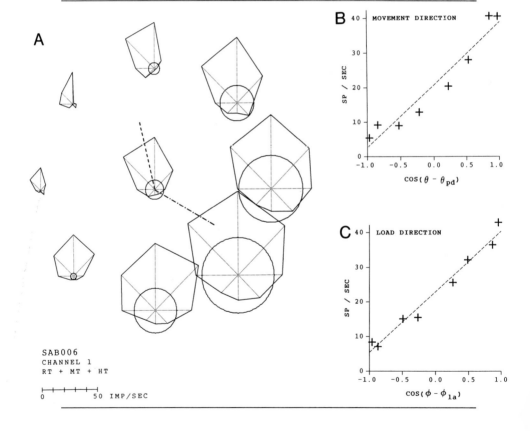

FIGURE 13.7

Vector representation of motor cortex cell activity during movements to the left (**A**) *and right* (**B**), *under all load conditions. Unlike Figure 13.5, this figure uses absolute response intensity, not changes in activity. The central vector clusters are population activity patterns during unloaded arm movements. The other clusters are the activity of the same neurons during loaded arm movements, and the position of each cluster corresponds to the direction of the applied load.* Heavy arrows: *net population vector sums.* **A** *reproduced from Kalaska, J.F. What parameters of reaching are encoded by discharges of cortical cells? D.R. Humphrey and H.-J. Freund (eds).* Motor Control Concepts and Issues. *Chichester: Wiley, 1991, pp. 307–330 and* **B** *from Kalaska, J.F., D.A.D. Cohen, M. Prud'homme, and M.L. Hyde. Parietal area 5 neuronal activity encodes movement kinematics, not movement dynamics.* Exp. Brain Res. *80:351–364, 1990.*

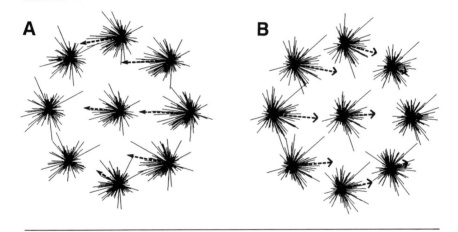

movement direction, so that the neural trajectory no longer corresponded well to the actual handpath. This deviation resulted mainly from load-induced alterations in the level of cell activity across the population, not from load-induced changes in single-cell preferred directions. The load-related *changes* in cell activity, compared to the unloaded condition, formed a population signal oriented approximately opposite to the applied load [83] (Fig. 13.5*B*). Once again, however, it is difficult to prove experimentally that these changes in population activity correspond exactly with the complex pattern of total output forces or changes in forces required to compensate for the loads.

If motor cortex activity covaries with the alterations in dynamics caused by external loads, to what degree could their movement-related activity transmit information about the dynamics of unloaded arm movements? Simplistically speaking, to produce a movement, the motor system must generate initial joint torque impulses to accelerate the limb toward the target, followed by transient torques in the opposite direction at about the time of peak velocity to halt the movement over the target, and then a second torque reversal to hold the new posture against gravity. The neural trajectory formed by the activity of a large population of cells sampled throughout the proximal-arm representation of the motor cortex does not appear to transmit information about these torque reversals [59]. This is not the case, however, for the most load-sensitive subpopulation of motor cortex cells [83] (Fig. 13.8). These cells have a characteristic temporal response profile during movements in their preferred direction, with a brief phasic burst before movement, a momentary pause during the movement and then a tonic response while the arm is held over the target (phasic-tonic cells) (Fig. 13.8*A*; see also Fig. 13.4). These cells often showed a reciprocal response pattern for movements in the opposite direction (Fig. 13.8*A*). A vectorial representation of the discharge of this group of cells at 20-ms intervals (Fig. 13.8*B*) shows the directional reversals expected for a representation of movement dynamics.

Nevertheless, these correlations with loads, forces, and torques are not proof that the motor cortex is trying to control force or any other Newtonian mechanical parameter, or that it is doing an inverse dynamics computation from joint motions to joint torques, or that the motor cortex knows anything at all about Newtonian mechanics [62, 82, 85]. They only show that an important component of reach-related activity in the motor cortex shows a better correlation with the causal forces of the movements than with its spatial form. Exactly what the cells are signaling is not clear.

Finally, the cell activity can be interpreted in terms of muscle activation patterns. The response profile of phasic-tonic cells is strikingly similar to the well-known triphasic electromyographic (EMG) pattern of muscles. Muscles tend to show the same broad directional tuning properties during movement, posture, and load compensation as do many motor cortex cells [82–84] (Fig. 13.9). This similarity suggests that at least some motor cortex cells could provide movement-related information in a code that is close to or readily transformable into muscle activation patterns. As already discussed, it is reasonable to expect that the discharge of a given corticospinal cell alters the contractile activity of several muscles (its muscle field) to different degrees [45, 54, 59, 117]. In this way, the directional tuning properties of a cortical cell could be transformed by spinal circuitry into a set of weighted muscle activations that would tend to deflect the limb in a direction corresponding to the cell's preferred direction [26, 53, 54, 59]. The shift in preferred direction with starting arm position [26] could reflect the change in arm displacement that would result from the activation of the cell's muscle field in different arm geometries. Since the discharge of many cells also covaries with dynamics parameters, the output signals of single cortical

FIGURE 13.8

A. *Raster representation of a phasic-tonic motor cortex cell during 10 movements in its preferred direction* (upper raster) *and in the opposite direction* (lower raster). Arrows *and* vertical dotted line: *onset of movement.* **B.** *Vector representation of the activity of a sample of 73 phasic-tonic cells at 20-ms intervals during movements to the right. Note that time advances downward in this figure.* GO: *mean and S.D. of time of appearance of the target.* Horizontal dotted line: *onset of movement.*

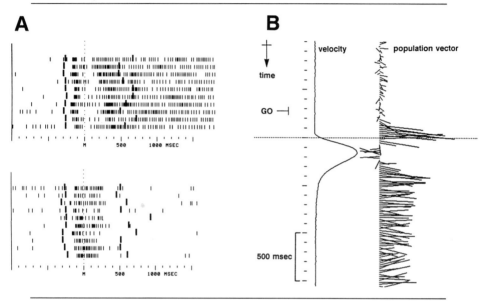

cells could also be transmitting information about the overall level of activity of the weighted combination of muscles during movements in different directions and during external load compensation.

An important unresolved question is whether the cells are specifically encoding a particular optimal weighted activation pattern of the muscles in their muscle field. If so, their discharge would be maximal whenever the EMG pattern required for a movement corresponds to their optimal activation pattern, and would be less for any other combination of muscle recruitment weightings. Conversely, each cell may be best correlated to the activity of only part of the overall field, but its activity is distributed to several motor pools, perhaps to facilitate the coordination of multimuscle activity at contiguous joints. It will be difficult to distinguish between these two alternatives, even for corticomotoneurons.

One final very important finding is that there may be a nonuniform anatomical distribution of response properties in the motor cortex.

FIGURE 13.9

A. *Activity of the latissimus dorsi muscle, represented as histograms of rectified EMG records from five movements to each of the targets, during unloaded arm movements.* **B.** *Variation of latissimus dorsi muscle activity as a function of external load direction. Same format as Figure 13.6. Kalaska, J.F., D.A.D. Cohen, M. Prud'homme, and M.L. Hyde. Parietal area 5 neuronal activity encodes movement kinematics, not movement dynamics.* Exp. Brain Res. 80:351–364, 1990.

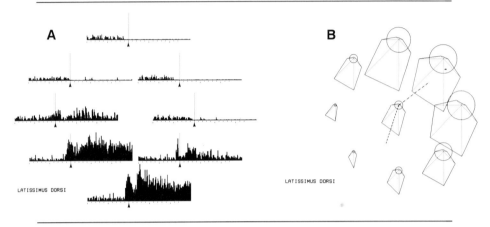

Preliminary evidence suggests that the most load-sensitive cells (especially phasic-tonic neurons) were in the cortex buried in the anterior bank of the central sulcus [83]. Cells in the anterior half of the motor cortex on the exposed surface of the cortex were less sensitive overall to loads. Furthermore, the most sensitive cells appeared to be in or near cortical layer 5, the origin of corticospinal and other descending output paths. Cells in more superficial layers were generally more phasic and less sensitive to loads, as if processing mainly kinematic information about the movement itself and may be less concerned with arm postures or the causal forces and muscle activity for movement. This suggests that different hierarchical levels of movement representation may coexist in the motor cortex and may be preferentially distributed among different anatomical subclasses of neurons in the motor cortex, as has also been observed in single-joint tasks [21, 27, 51, 74].

SEGMENTAL INTERACTIONS

To understand the role of the motor cortex, it is not sufficient to describe only the activity of motor cortical neurons. One also has to consider how this signal is further processed in the spinal cord. Although this aspect of motor control has received relatively little attention, two lines of research give some insight into the types of interactions that may occur between the motor cortex and the spinal cord.

Microstimulation During Locomotion
Microstimulation of the motor cortex during locomotion has been used to study how descending input interacts with the spinal pattern generators for locomotion. These studies have found that stimulation-evoked corticospinal volleys can cause transient changes in the amplitude of muscle activity, which may be either completely incorporated into the locomotor cycle without altering its overall rhythm or may override it, prematurely initiating a new step cycle.

An important finding is that the effect of stimulating a given point on the motor cortex map varies with the phase of the step cycle [11]. In Figure 13.10*A* it can be seen that a brief stimulus train during swing evoked a large, short-latency activation of the physiological flexor muscles (brachialis and extensor carpi radialis) but little or no response in the extensors (triceps and palmaris longus). The same stimulus applied at the same location during early stance, however, evoked the opposite pattern, short-latency activation of both extensors but little response in the flexors. Stimulation later in stance was less effective even though both extensor muscles were still active (Fig. 13.10*B* and *C*). Such effects are, in general, reduced or abolished by pyramidal tract section [10, 11].

It is unlikely that these phase-dependent variations are due to fluctuations in either the intensity of the descending volley or the level of depolarization of the spinal motor neurons [33]. Instead, they most likely reflect a differential mediation of the corticospinal volley at the spinal level, because of changes in the excitability of interposed interneurons which are either part of, or are influenced by, the spinal networks responsible for generating the locomotor rhythm.

Increasing the duration of the cortical stimulus can modify the pattern of muscle activity and ultimately the locomotor rhythm. Once again, the nature of the effect is determined by the phase of the step cycle, and thus, the functional status of spinal circuits. For example, stimulation in swing prolongs flexor muscle activity and retards the onset of extensor muscle activity (Fig. 13.11). In contrast, stimulation during stance may truncate the normal extensor muscle activity and initiate a new period of flexor muscle activity, effectively shortening the step cycle (see also [35] and [108]). Not all loci in the motor cortex map were equally capable of resetting the step cycle; such effects were much more prevalent from recording sites in which neurons change their activity during the gait modifications. This suggests that the alterations are not due to indiscriminate cortical stimulation, but are probably representative of a topographically organized functional system for movement control. Moreover,

FIGURE 13.10
Microstimulation of the motor cortex of an intact, unanaesthetized cat with short trains of stimuli (11 pulses at 300 Hz, 0.2-ms duration; 25 uA). **A.** *Effect of stimuli applied with the cat at rest or during different periods of the step cycle.* **B.** *and* **C.** *Quantitative analyses of the effects of such stimuli. The graphs show the variation of the integrated response to microstimulation as a function of the step cycle, plotted as a percentage of the maximum response evoked in each muscle. All data are synchronized to the onset of activity in the cleidobrachialis muscle. The* rectangles *above each graph indicate the time in the step cycle when the indicated muscle is active. For details of the methodology, see Drew [34].* Br: *brachialis;* TriL: *lateral head of triceps brachii;* ECR: *extensor carpi radialis;* PaL: *palmaris longus;* co: *contralateral to the stimulation site.*

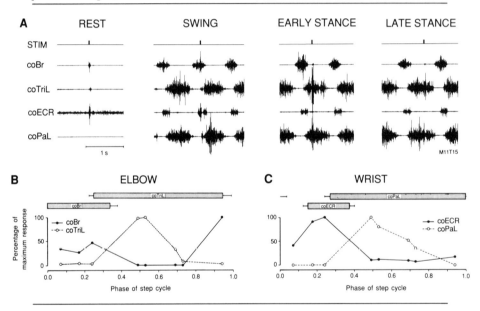

the step cycle modifications produced by stimulation of any one locus are only fragmentary components of the overall changes required to produce the graceful modified limb trajectories seen during normal behavior. Since the discharge of cells at each effective site similarly covaries with particular components of the overall gait change, the complete, coordinated multiarticular movement must result from the descending influence of many different neurons distributed across the forelimb output map, as is also the case for reaching movements.

C3-C4 Propriospinal System
The final expression of a motor cortical output is determined entirely (cat) or principally (primate) by the spinal interneuronal relays onto

FIGURE 13.11

Microstimulation in the same locus as Figure 13.10 with longer trains of stimuli (200 ms; other parameters the same). **B-E.** *Traces showing the effects of such stimuli at different times in the locomotor cycle with the time of stimulation expressed as a phase of the control step cycles. The data are all aligned on the onset of the activity in the brachialis, which was used to trigger the stimulator* (first dotted line). *The* second dotted line *indicates the time at which the next onset of brachialis would have been expected on the basis of the unperturbed, control step cycles* (rectangles in **A**). **F-H.** *Quantitative analysis of the effect of such stimuli on the duration of the step cycle, as well as the duration of the EMG burst in the brachialis and lateral head of triceps.* Horizontal dotted line *indicates the duration of these three parameters in the control step cycles.*

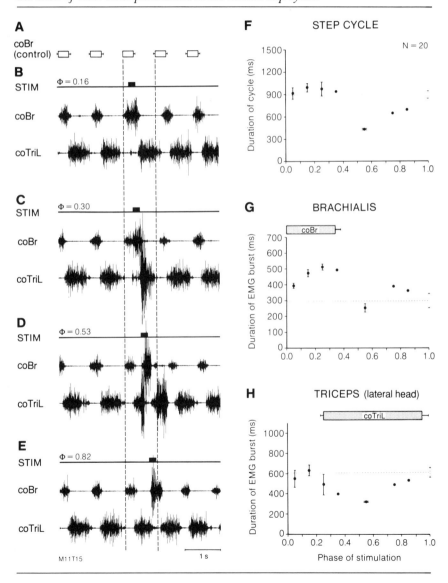

which the descending signals impinge. Much work needs to be done on the function of this interface during voluntary behavior, to forge a link between the wealth of data on spinal cord circuitry obtained mainly in acutely prepared cats and the equally large body of data on cortical function, mainly from primates.

Virtually every identified spinal reflex system receives descending inputs, and a number of models have been advanced to explain the control of movement via these circuits [70]. An early model, the "follow-up length servo" hypothesis (see [126]), suggested that higher brain structures controlled movement indirectly by excitation of δ-motor neurons, but has been discredited. The equilibrium-point hypothesis of Feldman [23, 44] is closely related, in that descending cortical activity shifts the stretch reflex threshold of motor neurons. Local spinal circuitry and peripheral input would then generate the neuronal activity that specifies the muscle activity patterns.

Other models have been based on data derived from electroanatomical circuit-tracing studies of identified interneurons in acute experiments. An example is the "flexor reflex afferent" (FRA) hypothesis [70,100]. This model states that the brain initiates movements indirectly by the selective activation of subsets of interneurons within the flexor reflex afferent system in the spinal cord. Once the movement begins, reafferent peripheral input into the same reflex system forms a positive feedback loop that helps sustain the movement until its completion, in cooperation with the influence of sustained descending inputs, particularly onto δ-motor neurons [100]. Again, this model suggests that cortical systems initiate movement by selective alterations of reflex gains within interneuronal networks, allying it conceptually with the length-servo and equilibrium-point models.

A further excellent example is the recent work of Lundberg, Alstermark, and their colleagues on the role of C3-C4 propriospinal interneurons in cats trained to make reaching movements to extract food from a horizontal tube at shoulder level [2, 3]. These neurons receive extensive convergent input from supraspinal structures including the motor cortex and from peripheral afferents, and project onto C5-T1 segmental motor neurons via axons that course in the ventrolateral fasciculus [76, 79]. Lesions of that fasciculus at C5 left intact the direct descending cortico- and rubrospinal projections into spinal segments C5-T1, and caused substantial ataxia in reaching but normal clasping movements of the wrist and digits to retrieve the food. Conversely, lesions of the dorsolateral fasciculus at C5, which interrupted the direct cortico- and rubrospinal input but left intact the propriospinal pathway, had only minor effects on the reaching movements but produced deficits in the distal grasping movements [3]. Use-dependent retrograde transsynaptic transport of HRP injected into the nerves of forelimb muscles showed that many C3-C4 interneurons are labeled when the cats perform reaching movements but very few when the cats walk on a flat surface [4, 5]. They concluded that C3-C4 propriospinal interneurons are critical for the elaboration of the descending cortical control signal for reaching movements and are preferentially activated during reaching. These same interneurons are also implicated in the on-line modification of reach trajectories in response to changes in target location [2].

Some questions still remain about this hypothesis, however. For instance, to what degree are the same circuits used in nonreaching behaviors, such as during visually guided gait modifications and even during normal locomotion? Whereas the HRP studies [4, 5] suggested that the C3-C4 system is selectively activated during reaching, recordings of these same interneurons showed them to be rhythmically active during fictive locomotion [14]. Although the applicability of the fictive preparation to normal locomotion has been challenged [5], the failure to label these interneurons during normal locomotion may indicate only that the level of activity in these neurons is too low during locomotion over a flat surface to be detected by activity-dependent retrograde HRP transport. Moreover, to what degree is the enhanced activation of C3-C4 propriospinal interneurons causally related to the reaching movements themselves, or to the concomitant postural adjustments and stabilization of the shoulder girdle? The latter role is suggested by the fact that C3-C4 propriospinal interneurons are labeled on both sides of the spinal cord during reaching movements with one forelimb [4, 5].

Finally, the C3-C4 propriospinal system is only one of many spinal interneuronal networks that can contribute to the control of reaching. C5-T1 segmental interneurons undoubtedly also play a major role [5, 77, 79]. Many of the corticospinal axons terminating on C3-C4 interneurons also project to the cervical enlargement, and so coactivate interneurons in both spinal regions [52, 76, 119]. Indeed, during both reaching and locomotion, the majority of HRP-labeled neurons were in segments C5-T1, outnumbering C3-C4 interneurons by an order of magnitude [5]. The circuits involved in controlling both types of movements are undoubtedly both segmental and propriospinal and probably involve many elements in common.

Unfortunately, predictions of the C3-C4 and FRA hypotheses have not yet been tested by recording studies in behaving animals, so the nature of their role in the spinal implementation of cortical motor signals remains largely inferential. Moreover, these models may be inappropriately constrained by arbitrarily subdividing the spinal interneuronal network into isolated "reflex" circuits [98, 99, 101]. It might be more appropriate to regard the interneuronal networks as a more integrated distributed system designed to cope with the complex mechanics of the limb, to facilitate the organization of multiarticular motor acts [98, 99, 101]. Determining how these interneuronal networks transform inputs from descending systems and integrate them with the function of local pattern-generating circuitry represents a formidable experimental and conceptual challenge.

SYNTHESIS AND CONCLUSION

We have considered the role of the motor cortex in visuomotor control using data from two different behaviors, primate reaching movements and cat locomotor gait modifications. In each situation, motor cortex activity is correlated to different aspects of the movement. The activity of individual pyramidal tract neurons during locomotor gait modifications and unidentified neurons during reaching covaries with the temporal phasing, sequencing, and direction of motion of different limb segments, and even with the activation patterns of specific muscles. Many neurons, however, are emitting signals that are not obviously correlated with output forces, nor are they replicas of single-muscle activity. This supports the Jacksonian hypothesis that the motor cortex lies neither at the highest level of motor control (abstract global planning) nor at the end point (spinal motor neurons and muscles) but rather occupies a middle level, bridging the gap between the two. Expressed in terms of the hierarchical planning model (Fig. 13.1), the motor cortex appears to play a critical role in the transformation from kinematics-level representations of movement to a dynamics-level representation. The corticospinal output is then distributed onto spinal interneuronal networks and, in primates, directly onto the motor neuron pools of several muscles, and thus also contributes to the determination of muscle activity patterns.

However, despite a great deal of effort, it is still not possible to define the role of the motor cortex more precisely, nor is there a definitive conclusion about the information content of the control signal(s) generated by the motor cortex. Some of the reasons for this failure are methodological. In many studies, the "task-related" discharge of unidentified neurons or pyramidal tract cells was correlated with arbitrarily chosen parameters of the movements, without consideration of the biomechanics of the movement or of the possible relation of the neurons to the muscles producing the movement. At least in the case of corticomotoneurons, one can define their target muscle fields and then make a detailed analysis of their response correlations with increased confidence. For most cells, however, this is not possible because they are at least two synapses removed from any measurable peripheral event. The complex biomechanics of multiarticular behavior compounds the problem of attempting to identify the peripheral correlates. An equally important reason, however, may be the tendency to treat cells in the motor cortex as a homogeneous population that encode movement in a similar fashion. Evidence is growing that cells in different layers and with different projection patterns may play different roles in the visuomotor transformation process. Therefore, the primary motor cortex may not be a functionally homogeneous structure with only one role. The answer to the question "what is the motor cortex doing?" may depend, to a large degree, on the neuron one asks! At the very least, one should not equate motor cortex function with corticospinal neuron activity.

Similarly,we still do not know what the fundamental unit of representation is within the motor cortex motor map. The consensus of most recent studies is that each small part of the motor map influences the contractile activity of a set of muscles. Yet the distribution of output clusters is complex and its organizational basis remains elusive [32, 72, 96, 128]. If there is a single overriding organizing principle that is mapped systematically across the motor cortex, its basis may be more functional [32, 72, 85], such as the direction of movement or forces, or combinations of muscle activity, than it is anatomical, such as single muscles or joints. For instance, the topographic organization of the motor cortex map has features that could contribute to the coordination of multiarticular behavior. The extensive interdigitation of output clusters to shoulder and elbow muscles, but relative segregation of proximal-arm and distal-arm representations [90] is consistent with the tight coupling of shoulder and elbow joint motions and their dissociation from wrist motions during reaching [124]. A local aggregate of output clusters directed to different muscle sets at different joints may be maximally activated during a particular reaching movement, while cluster aggregates at different locations on the map would be preferentially activated during different reach trajectories [72, 91, 103]. The activity of output clusters throughout the motor cortex map would, in turn, be coordinated by the network of intracortical horizontal connections [75]. Of course, this analysis may be relevant only for the corticospinal output system. Other motor cortex output systems (corticorubral, corticostriatal, corticocortical, etc.) may have other functions and organizing principles. If any one conclusion can be drawn from this discussion, it is that there undoubtedly exist important features of the functional organization of the motor cortex that will only be revealed and understood during multiarticular behavior; while reductionist single-joint studies have made important contributions to our understanding of motor cortex function, there is a limit to what they can tell us.

Finally, it is doubtful that one will ever fully understand the role of the motor cortex in visuomotor control by studying it in isolation. For instance, further investigations should be made into the degree of task-specificity of motor cortex activity, and the relative contribution of the motor cortex to more or less automatic behaviors. Furthermore, the graceful execution of even nonstereotyped or less automatic voluntary acts can best be understood in terms of the interaction between cortical, subcortical, and spinal systems. Descending signals address the appropriate parts of the spinal pattern-generating circuitry and associated interneuronal networks, exploiting their power to resolve many of the complexities inherent in the organization and execution of multiarticular movement. The fact that the motor cortex exerts its major effects through interneuronal networks is often overlooked in primates where the emphasis is frequently placed on the monosynaptic connections with the distal musculature. The nature of the interaction between descending and spinal networks remains one of the most fundamental challenges to an understanding of the role of the motor cortex in the control of movement.

ACKNOWLEDGEMENTS

The preparation of this article was supported by the Medical Research Council of Canada and les Fonds de Recherche en Santé de Québec.

REFERENCES

1. Alexander, G.E., and M.D. Crutcher. Preparation for movement: Neural representations of intended direction in three motor areas of the monkey. *J. Neurophysiol.* 64:133–150, 1990.
2. Alstermark, B., T. Gorska, A. Lundberg, and L.-G. Pettersson. Integration in descending motor pathways controlling the forelimb in the cat. 16. Visually guided switching of target-reaching. *Exp. Brain Res.* 80:1–11, 1990.
3. Alstermark, B., A. Lundberg, U. Norrsell, and E. Sybirska. Integration in descending motor pathways controlling the forelimb in the cat. 9. Differential behavioural defects after spinal cord lesions interrupting defined pathways from higher centres to motoneurones. *Exp. Brain. Res.* 42:299–318, 1981.
4. Alstermark, B., and H. Kümmel. Transneuronal transport of wheat germ agglutinin conjugated horseradish peroxidase into last order spinal interneurones projecting to acromio- and spinodeltoideus motoneurones in the cat. 1. Location of labelled interneurones and influence of synaptic activity on the transneuronal transport. *Exp. Brain Res.* 80:83–95, 1990.
5. Alstermark, B., and H. Kümmel. Transneuronal transport of wheat germ agglutinin conjugated horseradish peroxidase into last order spinal interneurones projecting to acromio- and spinodeltoideus motoneurones in the cat. 2. Differential labelling of interneurones depending on movement type. *Exp. Brain Res.* 80:96–103, 1990.
6. Amos, A., D.M. Armstrong, and D.E. Marple-Horvat. Changes in the discharge patterns of motor cortical neurones associated with volitional changes in stepping in the cat. *Neurosci. Lett.* 109:107–112, 1990.
7. Andersen, R.A. Inferior parietal lobe function in spatial perception and visuomotor integration. F. Plum (ed.). *Handbook of Physiology, Section I, The Nervous System*, Vol. 5. Baltimore: Williams & Wilkins, 1987, pp. 483–518.
8. Armand, J., G. Holstege, and H.G.J.M. Kuypers. Differential corticospinal projections in the cat. An autoradiographic tracing study. *Brain. Res.* 343:351–355, 1985.
9. Armstrong, D.M. Supraspinal contributions to the initiation and control of locomotion in the cat. *Prog. Neurobiol.* 26:273–361, 1986.
10. Armstrong, D.M., and T. Drew. Electromyographic responses evoked in muscles of the forelimb by intracortical stimulation in the cat. *J. Physiol.* 367:309–326, 1985.

11. Armstrong, D.M., and T. Drew. Forelimb electromyographic responses to motor cortex stimulation during locomotion in the cat. *J. Physiol.* 367:327–351, 1985.
12. Armstrong, D.M., and T. Drew. Locomotor-related neuronal discharges in cat motor cortex compared with peripheral receptive fields and evoked movements. *J. Physiol.* 346:497–517, 1984.
13. Armstrong, D.M., and T. Drew. Topographical localisation in the motor cortex of the cat for somatic afferent responses and evoked movements. *J. Physiol.* 350:33–54, 1984.
14. Arshavsky, Y.I., G.N. Orlovsky, G.A. Pavlova, and L.B. Popova. Activity of C3–C4 propriospinal neurons during fictitious forelimb locomotion in the cat. *Brain. Res.* 363:354–357, 1986.
15. Asanuma, H. Recent developments in the study of the columnar arrangement of neurons within the motor cortex. *Physiol. Rev.* 55:143–156, 1975.
16. Asanuma, H., and I. Rosen. Topographical organisation of cortical efferent zones projecting to distal forelimb muscles in the monkey. *Exp. Brain. Res.* 14:243–256, 1972.
17. Asanuma, H., and H. Sakata. Functional organisation of a cortical efferent system examined with focal depth stimulation in cats. *J. Neurophysiol.* 30:35–54, 1967.
18. Asanuma, H., S.D. Stoney, and C. Abzug. Relationship between afferent input and motor outflow in cat motosensory cortex. *J. Neurophysiol.* 31:670–681, 1968.
19. Asanuma, H., P. Zarzecki, E. Jankowska, T. Hongo, and S. Marcus. Projection of individual pyramidal tract neurons to lumbar motor nuclei of the monkey. *Exp. Brain. Res.* 34:73–89, 1979.
20. Barbeau, H., and S. Rossignol. Recovery of locomotion after chronic spinalization in the adult cat. *Brain. Res.* 412:84–95, 1987.
21. Bauswein, E., C. Fromm, and A. Preuss. Corticostriatal cells in comparison with pyramidal tract neurons: Contrasting properties in the behaving monkey. *Brain Res.* 493:198–203, 1989.
22. Beloozerova, I.N., and M.G. Sirota. Role of motor cortex in control of locomotion. V.S. Gurfinkel, M.E. Ioffe, J. Massion, and J.P. Roll (eds.). *Stance and Motion: Facts and Concepts.* New York: Plenum Press, 1988, pp. 163–176.
23. Berkinblit, M.B., A.G. Feldman, and O.I. Fukson. Adaptability of innate motor patterns and motor control mechanisms. *Behav. Brain Sci.* 9:585–638, 1986.
24. Bernstein, N. *The Co-ordination and Regulation of Movements.* Oxford: Pergamon Press, 1967.
25. Bussel, B., A. Roby-Brami, P. Azouvi, A. Biraben, A. Yakovleff, and J.P. Held. Myoclonus in a patient with spinal cord transection. Possible involvement of the spinal stepping generator. *Brain* 111:1235–1245, 1988.
26. Caminiti, R., P.B. Johnson, and A. Urbano. Making arm movements within different parts of space: Dynamic aspects in the primate motor cortex. *J. Neurosci.* 10:2039–2058, 1990.
27. Cheney, P.D., and E.E. Fetz. Functional classes of primate corticomotoneuronal cells and their relation to active force. *J. Neurophysiol.* 44:773–791, 1980.
28. Cheney, P.D., E.E. Fetz, and S.S. Palmer. Patterns of facilitation and suppression of antagonistic forelimb muscles from motor cortex sites in the awake monkey. *J. Neurophysiol.* 53:805–820, 1985.
29. Colebatch, J.G., J.C. Rothwell, B.L. Day, P.D. Thompson, and C.D. Marsden. Cortical outflow to proximal arm muscles in man. *Brain* 113:1843–1856, 1990.
30. Crutcher, M.D., and G.E. Alexander. Movement-related neuronal activity selectively coding either direction or muscle pattern in three motor areas of the monkey. *J. Neurophysiol.* 64:151–163, 1990.
31. Denny-Brown, D., N. Yanagisawa, and E.J. Kirk. The localization of hemispheric mechanisms of visually directed reaching and grasping. K.J. Zulch, O. Creutzfeldt, and E.C. Galbraith (eds). *Cerebral Localization.* New York: Springer-Verlag, 1975, pp. 63–75.

32. Donoghue, J.P., S. Leibovic, and J.N. Sanes. Organization of the forelimb area in squirrel monkey motor cortex: representation of digit, wrist and elbow muscles. *Exp. Brain Res.* 89:1–19, 1992.

33. Drew, T. Functional organization within the medullary reticular formation of the intact unanaesthetized cat. III. Microstimulation during locomotion. *J. Neurophysiol.* 66:919–938, 1991.

34. Drew, T. Motor cortical cell discharge during voluntary gait modification. *Brain Res.* 457:181–187, 1988.

35. Drew, T. The role of the motor cortex in the control of gait modification in the cat. M. Shimamura, S. Grillner, and V.R. Edgerton (eds.). *Neurobiological Basis of Human Locomotion.* Tokyo: Japan Scientific Societies Press, 1991, pp. 201–212.

36. Drew, T. Visuomotor coordination in locomotion. *Current Opinion in Neurobiology* 1:652–657, 1991.

37. Dum, R.P., and P.L. Strick. The origin of corticospinal projections from the premotor areas in the frontal lobe. *J. Neurosci.* 11:667–689, 1991.

38. Durelli, L., E.M. Schmidt, J.S. McIntosh, and M.J. Bak. Single unit chronic recordings from the sensorimotor cortex of unrestrained cats during locomotion. *Exp. Neurol.* 62:580–594, 1978.

39. Edgley, S.A., J.A. Eyre, R.N. Lemon, and S. Miller. Excitation of the corticospinal tract by electromagnetic and electrical stimulation of the scalp in the macaque monkey. *J. Physiol.* 425:301–320, 1990.

40. Eidelberg, E., J.G. Walden, and L.H. Nguyen. Locomotor control in macaque monkeys. *Brain. Res.* 104:647–663, 1981.

41. Evarts, E.V. Relationship of pyramidal tract activity to force exerted during voluntary movement. *J. Neurophysiol.* 31:14–27, 1968.

42. Evarts, E.V., C. Fromm, J. Kröller, and V.A. Jennings. Motor cortex control of finely graded forces. *J. Neurophysiol.* 49:1199–1215, 1983.

43. Fabre, M., and P. Buser. Effects of suprasylvian lesions on visually guided performances in cats. *Exp. Brain Res.* 41:81–88, 1981.

44. Feldman, A.G., S.V. Adamovich, D.J. Ostry, and J.R. Flanagan. The origin of electromyograms—explanations based on the equilibrium point hypothesis. J.M. Winters and S.L. Y. Woo (eds.). *Multiple Muscle Systems: Biomechanics and Movement Organization.* New York: Springer-Verlag, 1990, pp. 195–213.

45. Fetz, E.E., and P.D. Cheney. Postspike facilitation of forelimb muscle activity by primate corticomotoneuronal cells. *J. Neurophysiol.* 44:751–772, 1980.

46. Fetz, E.E., P.D. Cheney, K. Mewes, and S. Palmer. Control of forelimb muscle activity by populations of corticomotoneuronal and rubromotoneuronal cells. J.H.J. Allum and M. Hulliger (eds.). Afferent Control of Posture and Locomotion. *Prog Brain Res* 80:437–449, 1989.

47. Fetz, E., K. Toyama, and W. Smith. Synaptic interactions between cortical neurons. A. Peters (ed.). *Cerebral Cortex*, Vol. 9. New York: Plenum Press, 1991, pp. 1–47.

48. Flanders, M. Temporal patterns of muscle activation for arm movements in three-dimensional space. *J. Neurosci.* 11:2680–2693, 1991.

49. Flash, T. The organization of human arm trajectory control. J.M. Winters and S.Y.-L. Woo (eds.). *Multiple Muscle Systems. Biomechanics and Movement Organization.* New York, Springer-Verlag, 1990, pp. 282–301.

50. Forssberg, H. Ontogeny of human locomotor control: I. Infant stepping, supported locomotion and transition to independent locomotion. *Exp. Brain. Res.* 57:480–493, 1985.

51. Fromm, C. Contrasting properties of pyramidal tract neurons located in the precentral and postcentral areas and of corticorubral neurons in the behaving monkey. *Adv. Neurol.* 39:329–345, 1983.

52. Futami T., Y. Shinoda, and J. Yokota. Spinal axon collaterals of corticospinal neurons identified by intracellular injection of horseradish peroxidase. *Brain. Res.* 164:279–284, 1979.

53. Georgopoulos, A.P. Higher order motor control. *Annu. Rev. Neurosci.* 14:361–377, 1991.
54. Georgopoulos, A.P. Neural integration of movement: Role of motor cortex in reaching. *FASEB J.* 2:2849–2857, 1988.
55. Georgopoulos, A.P., R. Caminiti, and J.F. Kalaska. Static spatial effects in motor cortex and area 5: quantitative relations in a two-dimensional space. *Exp. Brain. Res.* 54:446–454, 1984.
56. Georgopoulos, A.P., and S. Grillner. Visuomotor coordination in reaching and locomotion. *Science* 245:1209–1210, 1989.
57. Georgopoulos, A.P., J.F. Kalaska, and R. Caminiti. Relations between two-dimensional arm movements and single-cell discharge in motor cortex and area 5: movement direction versus movement end point. *Exp. Brain Res. Suppl. 10,* Berlin: Springer-Verlag, 1985, pp. 175–183.
58. Georgopoulos, A.P., J.F. Kalaska, R. Caminiti, and J.T. Massey. On the relations between the direction of two-dimensional arm movements and cell discharge in primary motor cortex. *J. Neurosci.* 2:1527–1537, 1982.
59. Georgopoulos, A.P., R.E. Kettner, and A.B. Schwartz. Primate motor cortex and free arm movements to visual targets in three-dimensional space. II. Coding of the direction of arm movement by a neuronal population. *J. Neurosci.* 8:2928–2937, 1988.
60. Gottlieb, G.L., D.M. Corcos, and G.C. Agarwal. Strategies for the control of voluntary movements with one mechanical degree of freedom. *Behav. Brain Sci.* 12:189–250, 1989.
61. Grillner, S. Control of locomotion in bipeds, tetrapods and fish. V.B. Brooks (ed.). *Handbook of Physiology,* Vol II, Part 2. Bethesda, MD: American Physiological Society, 1981, pp. 1179–1236.
62. Hasan, Z. Biomechanics and the study of multijoint movements. D.R. Humphrey and H.-J. Freund (eds.). *Motor Control: Concepts and Issues.* Chichester: Wiley, 1991, pp. 75–84.
63. Held, R., and J.A. Bauer. Development of sensorially-guided reaching in infant monkeys. *Brain Res.* 71:265–271, 1974.
64. Hepp-Reymond, M.C., and M. Wiesendanger. Unilateral pyramidectomy in monkeys: Effect on force and speed of a conditioned precision grip. *Brain. Res.* 36:117–131, 1972.
65. Hildreth, E.C., and J.M. Hollerbach. Artificial intelligence: Computational approach to vision and motor control. F. Plum (ed.). *Handbook of Physiology, Section I, The Nervous System,* vol. 5. Baltimore: Williams & Wilkins, 1987, pp. 605–642.
66. Hoffman, D.S., and E.S. Luschei. Responses of monkey precentral cortical cells during a controlled jaw bite task. *J. Neurophysiol.* 44:333–348, 1980.
67. Hogan, N. Mechanical impedance of single- and multi-articular systems. J.M. Winters and S.L.-Y. Woo (eds.). *Multiple Muscle Systems: Biomechanics and Movement Organization.* New York: Springer-Verlag, 1990, pp. 149–164.
68. Hogan, N., E. Bizzi, F.A. Mussa-Ivaldi, and T. Flash. Controlling multi-joint motor behavior. *Exercise Sport Sci. Rev.* 15:153–190, 1987.
69. Hollerbach, J.M., and C.G. Atkeson. Deducing planning variables from experimental arm trajectories: Pitfalls and possibilities. *Biol. Cybern.* 56:279–292, 1987.
70. Hultborn, H., and M. Illert. How is motor behaviour reflected in the organization of spinal systems? D.R. Humphrey and H.-J. Freund (eds.). *Motor Control: Concepts and Issues.* Chichester: Wiley, 1991, pp. 49–73.
71. Humphrey, D.R. On the cortical control of visually directed reaching: contributions by nonprecentral areas. R.E. Talbott and D.R. Humphrey (eds.). *Posture and Movement.* New York: Raven Press, 1979, pp. 51–112.
72. Humphrey, D.R. Representation of movements and muscles within the primate precentral motor cortex: Historical and current perspectives. *Fed. Proc.* 45:2687–2699, 1986.

73. Humphrey, D.R., E.M. Schmidt, and W.D. Thompson. Predicting measures of motor performance from multiple cortical spike trains. *Science* 170:758–761, 1970.

74. Humphrey, D.R., and J. Tanji. Parameters of motor control encoded by neuronal populations in different arm-hand regions of the motor cortex. D.R. Humphrey and H.-J. Freund (eds.). *Motor Control: Concepts and Issues.* Chichester, Wiley, 1991, pp. 413–443.

75. Huntley, G.W., and E.G. Jones. Relationship of intrinsic connections to forelimb movement representations in monkey motor cortex: A correlative anatomical and physiological study. *J. Neurophysiol.* 66:390–413, 1991.

76. Illert, M., A. Lundberg, Y. Padel, and R. Tanaka. Integration in descending motor pathways controlling the forelimb in the cat. 5. Properties of and monosynaptic excitory convergence on C3-C4 propriospinal neurones. *Exp. Brain. Res.* 33:101–130, 1978.

77. Illert, M., A. Lundberg, and R. Tanaka. Integration in descending motor pathways controlling the forelimb in the cat. 1. Pyramidal effects on motoneurons. *Exp. Brain. Res.* 26:509–519, 1976.

78. Illert, M., A. Lundberg, and R. Tanaka. Integration in descending motor pathways controlling the forelimb in the cat. 2. Convergence on neurones mediating disynaptic cortico-motoneuronal excitation. *Exp. Brain. Res.* 26:521–540, 1976.

79. Illert, M., A. Lundberg, and R. Tanaka. Integration in descending motor pathways controlling the forelimb in the cat. 3. Convergence on propriospinal neurones transmitting disynaptic excitation from the corticospinal tract and other descending tracts. *Exp. Brain. Res.* 29:323–346, 1977.

80. Iriki A., C. Pavlides, A. Keller, and H. Asanuma. Long-term potentiation of thalamic input to the motor cortex induced by coactivation of thalamocortical afferents. *J. Neurophysiol.* 65:1435–1441, 1991.

81. Jacobs, K.M., and J.P. Donoghue. Reshaping the cortical motor map by unmasking latent intracortical connections. *Science* 251:944–947, 1991.

82. Kalaska, J.F. What parameters of reaching are encoded by discharges of cortical cells? D.R. Humphrey and H.-J. Freund (eds.). *Motor Control: Concepts and Issues.* Chichester: Wiley, 1991, pp. 307–330.

83. Kalaska, J.F., D.A.D. Cohen, M.L. Hyde, and M. Prud'homme. A comparison of movement direction-related versus load direction-related activity in primate motor cortex, using a two-dimensional reaching task. *J. Neurosci.* 9:2080–2102, 1989.

84. Kalaska, J.F., D.A.D. Cohen, M. Prud'homme, and M.L. Hyde. Parietal area 5 neuronal activity encodes movement kinematics, not movement dynamics. *Exp. Brain Res.* 80:351–364, 1990.

85. Kalaska, J.F., and D.J. Crammond. Cerebral cortical mechanisms of reaching movements. *Science* 255:1517–1523, 1992.

86. Karst, G.M., and Z. Hasan. Initiation rules for planar, two-joint arm movements: Agonist selection for movements throughout the work space. *J. Neurophysiol.* 66:1579–1593, 1991.

87. Kettner, R.E., A.B. Schwartz, and A.P. Georgopoulos. Primate motor cortex and free arm movements to visual targets in three-dimensional space. III. Positional gradients and population coding of movement direction from various movement origins. *J. Neurosci.* 8:2938–2947, 1988.

88. Kuypers, H.G.J.M. Anatomy of the descending pathways. V. Brooks (ed.). *Handbook of Neurophysiology,* Vol II, Part 1. Bethesda, MD: American Physiological Society, 1981, pp. 597–666.

89. Kuypers, H.G.J.M., and J. Brinkman. Precentral projections to different parts of the spinal intermediate zone in the rhesus monkey. *Brain. Res.* 24:29–48, 1970.

90. Kwan, H.C., W.A. MacKay, J.T. Murphy, and Y.C. Wong. Spatial organization of precentral cortex in awake primates. II. Motor outputs. *J. Neurophysiol.* 41:1120–1131, 1978.

91. Kwan, H.C., J.T. Murphy, and Y.C. Wong. Interaction between neurons in precentral cortical zones controlling different joints. *Brain. Res.* 400:259–269, 1987.

92. Lacquaniti, F. Central representations of human limb movement as revealed by studies of drawing and handwriting. *Trends Neurosci.* 12:287–291, 1989.

93. Lawrence, D.G., and H.G.J.M. Kuypers. The functional organization of the motor system in the monkey. I. The effects of bilateral pyramidal lesions. *Brain.* 91:1–14, 1968.

94. Lawrence, D.G., and H.G.J.M. Kuypers. The functional organization of the motor system in the monkey. II. The effects of lesions of the descending brain-stem pathways. *Brain.* 91:15–36, 1968.

95. Lawrence, D.G., R. Porter, and S.J. Redman. Corticomotoneuronal synapses in the monkey: Light microscopic localization upon motoneurons of intrinsic muscles of the hand. *J. Comp. Neurol.* 232:499–510, 1985.

96. Lemon, R. The output map of the primate motor cortex. *Trends Neurosci.* 11:501–506, 1988.

97. Lemon, R.N., R.B. Muir, and G.W.H. Mantel. The effects upon the activity of hand and forearm muscles of intracortical stimulation in the vicinity of corticomotor neurones in the conscious monkey. *Exp. Brain. Res.* 66:621–637, 1987.

98. Loeb, G.E. Hard lessons in motor control from the mammalian spinal cord. *Trends Neurosci.* 10:108–113, 1987.

99. Loeb, G.E., and W.S. Levine. Linking musculoskeletal mechanics to sensorimotor neurophysiology. J.M. Winters and S.L.-Y. Woo (eds.). *Multiple Muscle Systems: Biomechanics and Movement Organization.* New York: Springer-Verlag, 1990, pp. 165–181.

100. Lundberg, A., K. Malmgren, and E.D. Schomberg. Reflex pathways from group II muscle afferents. 3. Secondary spindle afferents and the FRA: a new hypothesis. *Exp. Brain. Res.* 65:294–306, 1987.

101. McCrea, D.A. Spinal cord circuitry and motor reflexes. *Exercise Sport Sci. Rev.* 14:105–141, 1986.

102. Muir, R.B., and R.N. Lemon. Corticospinal neurons with a special role in precision grip. *Brain. Res.* 261:312–316, 1983.

103. Murphy, J.T., H.C. Kwan, W.A. MacKay and Y.C. Wong. Spatial organization of precentral cortex in awake primates. III. Input-output coupling. *J. Neurophysiol.* 41:1132–1139, 1978.

104. Murphy, J.T., H.C. Kwan, W.A. MacKay and Y.C. Wong. Precentral unit activity correlated with angular components of a compound arm movement. *Brain. Res.* 246:141–145, 1982.

105. Murphy, J.T., Y.C. Wong, and H.C. Kwan. Sequential activation of neurons in primate motor cortex during unrestrained forelimb movement. *J. Neurophysiol.* 53:435–445, 1985.

106. Nieoullon, A., and L. Rispal-Padel. Somatotopic localization in cat motor cortex. *Brain Res.* 105:405–422, 1976.

107. Nudo, R.J., W.M. Jenkins, and M.M. Merzenich. Repetitive microstimulation alters the cortical representation of movements in adult rats. *Somatosens. Motor Res.* 7:463–483, 1990.

108. Orlovsky, G.N. The effect of different descending systems on flexor and extensor activity during locomotion. *Brain Res.* 40:359–371, 1972.

109. Paillard, J. Basic neurophysiological structures of eye-hand coordination. C. Bard, M. Fleury, and L. Hay (eds.). *Development of Eye-Hand Coordination Across the Life Span.* Columbia: University of South Carolina Press, 1990, pp. 26–74.

110. Phillips, C.G., and R. Porter. *Corticospinal neurones. Their role in Movement.* London, New York, and San Francisco: Academic Press, 1977.

111. Poizner, H., L. Mack, M. Verfaellie, L. Gonzalez Rothi, and K.M. Heilman. Three-dimensional computergraphic analysis of apraxia. *Brain* 113:85–101, 1990.

112. Porter, R., and M.McD. Lewis. Relationship of neuronal discharges in the precentral gyrus of monkeys to the performance of arm movements. *Brain. Res.* 98:21–36, 1975.

113. Sakamoto, T., L.L. Porter, and H. Asanuma. Long-lasting potentiation of synaptic potentials in the motor cortex produced by stimulation of the sensory cortex in the cat: A basis of motor learning. *Brain. Res.* 413:360–364, 1987.

114. Sanes, J.N., S. Suner, and J.P. Donoghue. Dynamic organization of primary motor cortex output to target muscles in adult rats. I. Long-term patterns of reorganization following motor or mixed peripheral nerve lesions. *Exp. Brain Res.* 79:479–491, 1990.

115. Sato, K.C., and J. Tanji. Digit-muscle responses evoked from multiple intracortical foci in monkey precentral motor cortex. *J. Neurophysiol.* 62:959–970, 1989.

116. Schmidt, E.M., and J.S. McIntosh. Microstimulation mapping of precentral cortex during trained movements. *J. Neurophysiol.* 64:1668–1682, 1990.

117. Schwartz, A.B., R.E. Kettner, and A.P. Georgopoulos. Primate motor cortex and free arm movements to visual targets in three-dimensional space: I. Relations between single cell discharge and direction of movement. *J. Neurosci.* 8:2913–2927, 1988.

118. Sessle, B.J., and M. Wiesendanger. Structural and functional definition of the motor cortex in the monkey (Macaca Fascicularis). *J. Physiol.* 323:245–265, 1982.

119. Shinoda, Y., T. Yamaguchi, and T. Futami. Multiple axon collaterals of single corticospinal axons in the cat spinal cord. *J. Neurophysiol.* 55:425–448, 1986.

120. Shinoda, Y., J.I. Yakota and T. Futami. Divergent projection of individual corticospinal axons to motoneurons of multiple muscles in the monkey. *Neurosci. Lett.* 23:7–12, 1981.

121. Soechting, J.F., and M. Flanders. Arm movements in three-dimensional space: Computation, theory and observation. *Exercise Sport Sci. Rev.* 19:389–417, 1991.

122. Soechting, J.F., and M. Flanders. Deducing central algorithms of arm movement control from kinematics. D.R. Humphrey and H.-J. Freund (eds.). *Motor control: Concepts and Issues.* Chichester, Wiley, 1991, pp. 293–306.

123. Soechting, J.F., and M. Flanders. Moving in three-dimensional space: Frames of reference, vectors, and coordinate sytems. *Annu. Rev. Neurosci.* 15:167–191, 1992.

124. Soechting, J.F., and C.A. Terzuolo. Sensorimotor transformations underlying the organization of arm movements in three-dimensional space. *Can. J. Physiol. Pharmacol.* 66:502–507, 1988.

125. Stein, J.F. Representation of egocentric space in the posterior parietal cortex. *Quart. J. Exp. Physiol.* 74:583–606, 1989.

126. Stein, R.B. What muscle variable(s) does the nervous system control in limb movements? *Behav. Brain Sci.* 5:535–577, 1982.

127. Thach, W.T. Correlation of neural discharge with pattern and force of muscular activity, joint position and direction of intended next movement in motor cortex and cerebellum. *J. Neurophysiol.* 41:654–676, 1978.

128. Waters, R.S., D.D. Samulack, R.W. Dykes, and P.A. McKinley. Topographic organization of baboon primary motor cortex: Face, hand, forelimb, and shoulder representation. *Somatosens. Motor Res.* 7:485–514, 1990.

129. Zajac, F.E., and M.E. Gordon. Determining muscles' force and action in multi-articular movement. *Exercise Sport Sci. Rev.* 17:187–230, 1989.

Index